Foodborne Parasites in the Food Supply Web: Occurrence and Control

Related titles

Tracing pathogens in the food chain
ISBN 978-1-84569-496-8

Foodborne pathogens: hazards, risk analysis and control
ISBN 978-1- 84569-362-6

Woodhead Publishing Series in Food Science, Technology and Nutrition: Number 288

Foodborne Parasites in the Food Supply Web

Occurrence and Control

Edited by

Alvin A. Gajadhar

ELSEVIER

AMSTERDAM • BOSTON • CAMBRIDGE • HEIDELBERG
LONDON • NEW YORK • OXFORD • PARIS • SAN DIEGO
SAN FRANCISCO • SINGAPORE • SYDNEY • TOKYO
Woodhead Publishing is an imprint of Elsevier

WP WOODHEAD PUBLISHING

Woodhead Publishing is an imprint of Elsevier
80 High Street, Sawston, Cambridge, CB22 3HJ, UK
225 Wyman Street, Waltham, MA 02451, USA
Langford Lane, Kidlington, OX5 1GB, UK

British Library Cataloguing-in-Publication Data
A catalogue record for this book is available from the British Library.

Library of Congress Control Number: 2015931795

ISBN 978-1-78242-332-4 (print)
ISBN 978-1-78242-350-8 (online)

For information on all Woodhead Publishing publications visit our website at http://store.elsevier.com/

Typeset by Spi Global
www.spi-global.com
Printed and bound in the United Kingdom

Contents

List of contributors

B. Al-Adhami Canadian Food Inspection Agency, Saskatoon, SK, Canada

L. Alban Danish Agriculture and Food Council, Copenhagen, Denmark

S. Bach Pacific Agri-Food Research Centre, Summerland, BC, Canada

S. Bidaisee St. George's University, Grenada, West Indies

P. Boireau ANSES, Animal Health Laboratory, OIE Collaborating Centre Foodborne Zoonotic Parasites, Maisons-Alfort, France

J. Conlan Food Standards Australia New Zealand, Barton, ACT, Australia

L. Cuttell Safe Food Production Queensland, Spring Hill, QLD, Australia

P. Delaquis Pacific Agri-Food Research Centre, Summerland, BC, Canada

B.R. Dixon Health Canada, Ottawa, ON, Canada

H.L. Enemark Technical University of Denmark, Frederiksberg, Denmark

A.A. Gajadhar Canadian Food Inspection Agency, Saskatoon, SK, Canada

H.R. Gamble National Research Council, Washington, DC, USA

S. Geerts Institute of Tropical Medicine, Antwerp, Belgium

M.V. Johansen University of Copenhagen, Frederiksberg, Denmark

S.R.M. Jones Pacific Biological Station, Nanaimo, BC, Canada

A. Lal Australian National University, Canberra, ACT, Australia

L.F. Lalonde Canadian Food Inspection Agency, Saskatoon, SK, Canada

V. Lobanov Canadian Food Inspection Agency, Saskatoon, SK, Canada

C.N.L. Macpherson St. George's University, Grenada, West Indies

L. Mingyuan Jilin University, Institute of Zoonosis, OIE Collaborating Centre Foodborne Zoonotic Parasites, Changchun, PR China

L.R. Polley University of Saskatchewan, Saskatoon, SK, Canada

E. Pozio Istituto Superiore di Sanità, Rome, Italy

M. Sato Niigata University, Niigata, Japan

M.O. Sato Universidade Federal do Tocantins, Palmas, Brazil

W.B. Scandrett Canadian Food Inspection Agency, Saskatoon, SK, Canada

B.B. Singh Guru Angad Dev Veterinary and Animal Science University, Ludhiana, India

R.C.A. Thompson Murdoch University, Murdoch, WA, Australia

R.J. Traub The University of Melbourne, Parkville, VIC, Australia

I. Vallée ANSES, Animal Health Laboratory, OIE Collaborating Centre Foodborne Zoonotic Parasites, Maisons-Alfort, France

J. Waikagul Mahidol University, Bangkok, Thailand

X. Wang Jilin University, Institute of Zoonosis, OIE Collaborating Centre Foodborne Zoonotic Parasites, Changchun, PR China

Woodhead Publishing Series in Food Science, Technology and Nutrition

1 **Chilled foods: A comprehensive guide**
Edited by C. Dennis and M. Stringer
2 **Yoghurt: Science and technology**
A. Y. Tamime and R. K. Robinson
3 **Food processing technology: Principles and practice**
P. J. Fellows
4 **Bender's dictionary of nutrition and food technology Sixth edition**
D. A. Bender
5 **Determination of veterinary residues in food**
Edited by N. T. Crosby
6 **Food contaminants: Sources and surveillance**
Edited by C. Creaser and R. Purchase
7 **Nitrates and nitrites in food and water**
Edited by M. J. Hill
8 **Pesticide chemistry and bioscience: The food-environment challenge**
Edited by G. T. Brooks and T. Roberts
9 **Pesticides: Developments, impacts and controls**
Edited by G. A. Best and A. D. Ruthven
10 **Dietary fibre: Chemical and biological aspects**
Edited by D. A. T. Southgate, K. W. Waldron, I. T. Johnson and G. R. Fenwick
11 **Vitamins and minerals in health and nutrition**
M. Tolonen
12 **Technology of biscuits, crackers and cookies Second edition**
D. Manley
13 **Instrumentation and sensors for the food industry**
Edited by E. Kress-Rogers
14 **Food and cancer prevention: Chemical and biological aspects**
Edited by K. W. Waldron, I. T. Johnson and G. R. Fenwick
15 **Food colloids: Proteins, lipids and polysaccharides**
Edited by E. Dickinson and B. Bergenstahl
16 **Food emulsions and foams**
Edited by E. Dickinson
17 **Maillard reactions in chemistry, food and health**
Edited by T. P. Labuza, V. Monnier, J. Baynes and J. O'Brien
18 **The Maillard reaction in foods and medicine**
Edited by J. O'Brien, H. E. Nursten, M. J. Crabbe and J. M. Ames
19 **Encapsulation and controlled release**
Edited by D. R. Karsa and R. A. Stephenson

20 **Flavours and fragrances**
Edited by A. D. Swift
21 **Feta and related cheeses**
Edited by A. Y. Tamime and R. K. Robinson
22 **Biochemistry of milk products**
Edited by A. T. Andrews and J. R. Varley
23 **Physical properties of foods and food processing systems**
M. J. Lewis
24 **Food irradiation: A reference guide**
V. M. Wilkinson and G. Gould
25 **Kent's technology of cereals: An introduction for students of food science and agriculture Fourth edition**
N. L. Kent and A. D. Evers
26 **Biosensors for food analysis**
Edited by A. O. Scott
27 **Separation processes in the food and biotechnology industries: Principles and applications**
Edited by A. S. Grandison and M. J. Lewis
28 **Handbook of indices of food quality and authenticity**
R. S. Singhal, P. K. Kulkarni and D. V. Rege
29 **Principles and practices for the safe processing of foods**
D. A. Shapton and N. F. Shapton
30 **Biscuit, cookie and cracker manufacturing manuals Volume 1: Ingredients**
D. Manley
31 **Biscuit, cookie and cracker manufacturing manuals Volume 2: Biscuit doughs**
D. Manley
32 **Biscuit, cookie and cracker manufacturing manuals Volume 3: Biscuit dough piece forming**
D. Manley
33 **Biscuit, cookie and cracker manufacturing manuals Volume 4: Baking and cooling of biscuits**
D. Manley
34 **Biscuit, cookie and cracker manufacturing manuals Volume 5: Secondary processing in biscuit manufacturing**
D. Manley
35 **Biscuit, cookie and cracker manufacturing manuals Volume 6: Biscuit packaging and storage**
D. Manley
36 **Practical dehydration Second edition**
M. Greensmith
37 **Lawrie's meat science Sixth edition**
R. A. Lawrie
38 **Yoghurt: Science and technology Second edition**
A. Y. Tamime and R. K. Robinson
39 **New ingredients in food processing: Biochemistry and agriculture**
G. Linden and D. Lorient
40 **Benders' dictionary of nutrition and food technology Seventh edition**
D. A. Bender and A. E. Bender
41 **Technology of biscuits, crackers and cookies Third edition**
D. Manley

42 **Food processing technology: Principles and practice Second edition**
P. J. Fellows
43 **Managing frozen foods**
Edited by C. J. Kennedy
44 **Handbook of hydrocolloids**
Edited by G. O. Phillips and P. A. Williams
45 **Food labelling**
Edited by J. R. Blanchfield
46 **Cereal biotechnology**
Edited by P. C. Morris and J. H. Bryce
47 **Food intolerance and the food industry**
Edited by T. Dean
48 **The stability and shelf-life of food**
Edited by D. Kilcast and P. Subramaniam
49 **Functional foods: Concept to product**
Edited by G. R. Gibson and C. M. Williams
50 **Chilled foods: A comprehensive guide Second edition**
Edited by M. Stringer and C. Dennis
51 **HACCP in the meat industry**
Edited by M. Brown
52 **Biscuit, cracker and cookie recipes for the food industry**
D. Manley
53 **Cereals processing technology**
Edited by G. Owens
54 **Baking problems solved**
S. P. Cauvain and L. S. Young
55 **Thermal technologies in food processing**
Edited by P. Richardson
56 **Frying: Improving quality**
Edited by J. B. Rossell
57 **Food chemical safety Volume 1: Contaminants**
Edited by D. Watson
58 **Making the most of HACCP: Learning from others' experience**
Edited by T. Mayes and S. Mortimore
59 **Food process modelling**
Edited by L. M. M. Tijskens, M. L. A. T. M. Hertog and B. M. Nicolaï
60 **EU food law: A practical guide**
Edited by K. Goodburn
61 **Extrusion cooking: Technologies and applications**
Edited by R. Guy
62 **Auditing in the food industry: From safety and quality to environmental and other audits**
Edited by M. Dillon and C. Griffith
63 **Handbook of herbs and spices Volume 1**
Edited by K. V. Peter
64 **Food product development: Maximising success**
M. Earle, R. Earle and A. Anderson
65 **Instrumentation and sensors for the food industry Second edition**
Edited by E. Kress-Rogers and C. J. B. Brimelow
66 **Food chemical safety Volume 2: Additives**
Edited by D. Watson

67 **Fruit and vegetable biotechnology**
Edited by V. Valpuesta
68 **Foodborne pathogens: Hazards, risk analysis and control**
Edited by C. de W. Blackburn and P. J. McClure
69 **Meat refrigeration**
S. J. James and C. James
70 **Lockhart and Wiseman's crop husbandry Eighth edition**
H. J. S. Finch, A. M. Samuel and G. P. F. Lane
71 **Safety and quality issues in fish processing**
Edited by H. A. Bremner
72 **Minimal processing technologies in the food industries**
Edited by T. Ohlsson and N. Bengtsson
73 **Fruit and vegetable processing: Improving quality**
Edited by W. Jongen
74 **The nutrition handbook for food processors**
Edited by C. J. K. Henry and C. Chapman
75 **Colour in food: Improving quality**
Edited by D. MacDougall
76 **Meat processing: Improving quality**
Edited by J. P. Kerry, J. F. Kerry and D. A. Ledward
77 **Microbiological risk assessment in food processing**
Edited by M. Brown and M. Stringer
78 **Performance functional foods**
Edited by D. Watson
79 **Functional dairy products Volume 1**
Edited by T. Mattila-Sandholm and M. Saarela
80 **Taints and off-flavours in foods**
Edited by B. Baigrie
81 **Yeasts in food**
Edited by T. Boekhout and V. Robert
82 **Phytochemical functional foods**
Edited by I. T. Johnson and G. Williamson
83 **Novel food packaging techniques**
Edited by R. Ahvenainen
84 **Detecting pathogens in food**
Edited by T. A. McMeekin
85 **Natural antimicrobials for the minimal processing of foods**
Edited by S. Roller
86 **Texture in food Volume 1: Semi-solid foods**
Edited by B. M. McKenna
87 **Dairy processing: Improving quality**
Edited by G. Smit
88 **Hygiene in food processing: Principles and practice**
Edited by H. L. M. Lelieveld, M. A. Mostert, B. White and J. Holah
89 **Rapid and on-line instrumentation for food quality assurance**
Edited by I. Tothill
90 **Sausage manufacture: Principles and practice**
E. Essien

91 **Environmentally-friendly food processing**
Edited by B. Mattsson and U. Sonesson
92 **Bread making: Improving quality**
Edited by S. P. Cauvain
93 **Food preservation techniques**
Edited by P. Zeuthen and L. Bøgh-Sørensen
94 **Food authenticity and traceability**
Edited by M. Lees
95 **Analytical methods for food additives**
R. Wood, L. Foster, A. Damant and P. Key
96 **Handbook of herbs and spices Volume 2**
Edited by K. V. Peter
97 **Texture in food Volume 2: Solid foods**
Edited by D. Kilcast
98 **Proteins in food processing**
Edited by R. Yada
99 **Detecting foreign bodies in food**
Edited by M. Edwards
100 **Understanding and measuring the shelf-life of food**
Edited by R. Steele
101 **Poultry meat processing and quality**
Edited by G. Mead
102 **Functional foods, ageing and degenerative disease**
Edited by C. Remacle and B. Reusens
103 **Mycotoxins in food: Detection and control**
Edited by N. Magan and M. Olsen
104 **Improving the thermal processing of foods**
Edited by P. Richardson
105 **Pesticide, veterinary and other residues in food**
Edited by D. Watson
106 **Starch in food: Structure, functions and applications**
Edited by A.-C. Eliasson
107 **Functional foods, cardiovascular disease and diabetes**
Edited by A. Arnoldi
108 **Brewing: Science and practice**
D. E. Briggs, P. A. Brookes, R. Stevens and C. A. Boulton
109 **Using cereal science and technology for the benefit of consumers: Proceedings of the 12PthP International ICC Cereal and Bread Congress, 24 – 26PthP May, 2004, Harrogate, UK**
Edited by S. P. Cauvain, L. S. Young and S. Salmon
110 **Improving the safety of fresh meat**
Edited by J. Sofos
111 **Understanding pathogen behaviour: Virulence, stress response and resistance**
Edited by M. Griffiths
112 **The microwave processing of foods**
Edited by H. Schubert and M. Regier
113 **Food safety control in the poultry industry**
Edited by G. Mead

114 **Improving the safety of fresh fruit and vegetables**
Edited by W. Jongen
115 **Food, diet and obesity**
Edited by D. Mela
116 **Handbook of hygiene control in the food industry**
Edited by H. L. M. Lelieveld, M. A. Mostert and J. Holah
117 **Detecting allergens in food**
Edited by S. Koppelman and S. Hefle
118 **Improving the fat content of foods**
Edited by C. Williams and J. Buttriss
119 **Improving traceability in food processing and distribution**
Edited by I. Smith and A. Furness
120 **Flavour in food**
Edited by A. Voilley and P. Etievant
121 **The Chorleywood bread process**
S. P. Cauvain and L. S. Young
122 **Food spoilage microorganisms**
Edited by C. de W. Blackburn
123 **Emerging foodborne pathogens**
Edited by Y. Motarjemi and M. Adams
124 **Benders' dictionary of nutrition and food technology Eighth edition**
D. A. Bender
125 **Optimising sweet taste in foods**
Edited by W. J. Spillane
126 **Brewing: New technologies**
Edited by C. Bamforth
127 **Handbook of herbs and spices Volume 3**
Edited by K. V. Peter
128 **Lawrie's meat science Seventh edition**
R. A. Lawrie in collaboration with D. A. Ledward
129 **Modifying lipids for use in food**
Edited by F. Gunstone
130 **Meat products handbook: Practical science and technology**
G. Feiner
131 **Food consumption and disease risk: Consumer–pathogen interactions**
Edited by M. Potter
132 **Acrylamide and other hazardous compounds in heat-treated foods**
Edited by K. Skog and J. Alexander
133 **Managing allergens in food**
Edited by C. Mills, H. Wichers and K. Hoffman-Sommergruber
134 **Microbiological analysis of red meat, poultry and eggs**
Edited by G. Mead
135 **Maximising the value of marine by-products**
Edited by F. Shahidi
136 **Chemical migration and food contact materials**
Edited by K. Barnes, R. Sinclair and D. Watson
137 **Understanding consumers of food products**
Edited by L. Frewer and H. van Trijp

138 **Reducing salt in foods: Practical strategies**
Edited by D. Kilcast and F. Angus
139 **Modelling microorganisms in food**
Edited by S. Brul, S. Van Gerwen and M. Zwietering
140 **Tamime and Robinson's Yoghurt: Science and technology Third edition**
A. Y. Tamime and R. K. Robinson
141 **Handbook of waste management and co-product recovery in food processing Volume 1**
Edited by K. W. Waldron
142 **Improving the flavour of cheese**
Edited by B. Weimer
143 **Novel food ingredients for weight control**
Edited by C. J. K. Henry
144 **Consumer-led food product development**
Edited by H. MacFie
145 **Functional dairy products Volume 2**
Edited by M. Saarela
146 **Modifying flavour in food**
Edited by A. J. Taylor and J. Hort
147 **Cheese problems solved**
Edited by P. L. H. McSweeney
148 **Handbook of organic food safety and quality**
Edited by J. Cooper, C. Leifert and U. Niggli
149 **Understanding and controlling the microstructure of complex foods**
Edited by D. J. McClements
150 **Novel enzyme technology for food applications**
Edited by R. Rastall
151 **Food preservation by pulsed electric fields: From research to application**
Edited by H. L. M. Lelieveld and S. W. H. de Haan
152 **Technology of functional cereal products**
Edited by B. R. Hamaker
153 **Case studies in food product development**
Edited by M. Earle and R. Earle
154 **Delivery and controlled release of bioactives in foods and nutraceuticals**
Edited by N. Garti
155 **Fruit and vegetable flavour: Recent advances and future prospects**
Edited by B. Brückner and S. G. Wyllie
156 **Food fortification and supplementation: Technological, safety and regulatory aspects**
Edited by P. Berry Ottaway
157 **Improving the health-promoting properties of fruit and vegetable products**
Edited by F. A. Tomás-Barberán and M. I. Gil
158 **Improving seafood products for the consumer**
Edited by T. Børresen
159 **In-pack processed foods: Improving quality**
Edited by P. Richardson
160 **Handbook of water and energy management in food processing**
Edited by J. Klemeš, R.. Smith and J.-K. Kim
161 **Environmentally compatible food packaging**
Edited by E. Chiellini

162 **Improving farmed fish quality and safety**
Edited by Ø. Lie
163 **Carbohydrate-active enzymes**
Edited by K.-H. Park
164 **Chilled foods: A comprehensive guide Third edition**
Edited by M. Brown
165 **Food for the ageing population**
Edited by M. M. Raats, C. P. G. M. de Groot and W. A Van Staveren
166 **Improving the sensory and nutritional quality of fresh meat**
Edited by J. P. Kerry and D. A. Ledward
167 **Shellfish safety and quality**
Edited by S. E. Shumway and G. E. Rodrick
168 **Functional and speciality beverage technology**
Edited by P. Paquin
169 **Functional foods: Principles and technology**
M. Guo
170 **Endocrine-disrupting chemicals in food**
Edited by I. Shaw
171 **Meals in science and practice: Interdisciplinary research and business applications**
Edited by H. L. Meiselman
172 **Food constituents and oral health: Current status and future prospects**
Edited by M. Wilson
173 **Handbook of hydrocolloids Second edition**
Edited by G. O. Phillips and P. A. Williams
174 **Food processing technology: Principles and practice Third edition**
P. J. Fellows
175 **Science and technology of enrobed and filled chocolate, confectionery and bakery products**
Edited by G. Talbot
176 **Foodborne pathogens: Hazards, risk analysis and control Second edition**
Edited by C. de W. Blackburn and P. J. McClure
177 **Designing functional foods: Measuring and controlling food structure breakdown and absorption**
Edited by D. J. McClements and E. A. Decker
178 **New technologies in aquaculture: Improving production efficiency, quality and environmental management**
Edited by G. Burnell and G. Allan
179 **More baking problems solved**
S. P. Cauvain and L. S. Young
180 **Soft drink and fruit juice problems solved**
P. Ashurst and R. Hargitt
181 **Biofilms in the food and beverage industries**
Edited by P. M. Fratamico, B. A. Annous and N. W. Gunther
182 **Dairy-derived ingredients: Food and neutraceutical uses**
Edited by M. Corredig
183 **Handbook of waste management and co-product recovery in food processing Volume 2**
Edited by K. W. Waldron
184 **Innovations in food labelling**
Edited by J. Albert

185 **Delivering performance in food supply chains**
Edited by C. Mena and G. Stevens
186 **Chemical deterioration and physical instability of food and beverages**
Edited by L. H. Skibsted, J. Risbo and M. L. Andersen
187 **Managing wine quality Volume 1: Viticulture and wine quality**
Edited by A. G. Reynolds
188 **Improving the safety and quality of milk Volume 1: Milk production and processing**
Edited by M. Griffiths
189 **Improving the safety and quality of milk Volume 2: Improving quality in milk products**
Edited by M. Griffiths
190 **Cereal grains: Assessing and managing quality**
Edited by C. Wrigley and I. Batey
191 **Sensory analysis for food and beverage quality control: A practical guide**
Edited by D. Kilcast
192 **Managing wine quality Volume 2: Oenology and wine quality**
Edited by A. G. Reynolds
193 **Winemaking problems solved**
Edited by C. E. Butzke
194 **Environmental assessment and management in the food industry**
Edited by U. Sonesson, J. Berlin and F. Ziegler
195 **Consumer-driven innovation in food and personal care products**
Edited by S. R. Jaeger and H. MacFie
196 **Tracing pathogens in the food chain**
Edited by S. Brul, P. M. Fratamico and T. A. McMeekin
197 **Case studies in novel food processing technologies: Innovations in processing, packaging, and predictive modelling**
Edited by C. J. Doona, K. Kustin and F. E. Feeherry
198 **Freeze-drying of pharmaceutical and food products**
T.-C. Hua, B.-L. Liu and H. Zhang
199 **Oxidation in foods and beverages and antioxidant applications Volume 1: Understanding mechanisms of oxidation and antioxidant activity**
Edited by E. A. Decker, R. J. Elias and D. J. McClements
200 **Oxidation in foods and beverages and antioxidant applications Volume 2: Management in different industry sectors**
Edited by E. A. Decker, R. J. Elias and D. J. McClements
201 **Protective cultures, antimicrobial metabolites and bacteriophages for food and beverage biopreservation** *Edited by C. Lacroix*
202 **Separation, extraction and concentration processes in the food, beverage and nutraceutical industries**
Edited by S. S. H. Rizvi
203 **Determining mycotoxins and mycotoxigenic fungi in food and feed**
Edited by S. De Saeger
204 **Developing children's food products**
Edited by D. Kilcast and F. Angus
205 **Functional foods: Concept to product Second edition**
Edited by M. Saarela
206 **Postharvest biology and technology of tropical and subtropical fruits Volume 1: Fundamental issues**
Edited by E. M. Yahia

207 **Postharvest biology and technology of tropical and subtropical fruits Volume 2: Açai to citrus**
Edited by E. M. Yahia
208 **Postharvest biology and technology of tropical and subtropical fruits Volume 3: Cocona to mango**
Edited by E. M. Yahia
209 **Postharvest biology and technology of tropical and subtropical fruits Volume 4: Mangosteen to white sapote**
Edited by E. M. Yahia
210 **Food and beverage stability and shelf life**
Edited by D. Kilcast and P. Subramaniam
211 **Processed Meats: Improving safety, nutrition and quality**
Edited by J. P. Kerry and J. F. Kerry
212 **Food chain integrity: A holistic approach to food traceability, safety, quality and authenticity**
Edited by J. Hoorfar, K. Jordan, F. Butler and R. Prugger
213 **Improving the safety and quality of eggs and egg products Volume 1**
Edited by Y. Nys, M. Bain and F. Van Immerseel
214 **Improving the safety and quality of eggs and egg products Volume 2**
Edited by F. Van Immerseel, Y. Nys and M. Bain
215 **Animal feed contamination: Effects on livestock and food safety**
Edited by J. Fink-Gremmels
216 **Hygienic design of food factories**
Edited by J. Holah and H. L. M. Lelieveld
217 **Manley's technology of biscuits, crackers and cookies Fourth edition**
Edited by D. Manley
218 **Nanotechnology in the food, beverage and nutraceutical industries**
Edited by Q. Huang
219 **Rice quality: A guide to rice properties and analysis**
K. R. Bhattacharya
220 **Advances in meat, poultry and seafood packaging**
Edited by J. P. Kerry
221 **Reducing saturated fats in foods**
Edited by G. Talbot
222 **Handbook of food proteins**
Edited by G. O. Phillips and P. A. Williams
223 **Lifetime nutritional influences on cognition, behaviour and psychiatric illness**
Edited by D. Benton
224 **Food machinery for the production of cereal foods, snack foods and confectionery**
L.-M. Cheng
225 **Alcoholic beverages: Sensory evaluation and consumer research**
Edited by J. Piggott
226 **Extrusion problems solved: Food, pet food and feed**
M. N. Riaz and G. J. Rokey
227 **Handbook of herbs and spices Second edition Volume 1**
Edited by K. V. Peter
228 **Handbook of herbs and spices Second edition Volume 2**
Edited by K. V. Peter
229 **Breadmaking: Improving quality Second edition**
Edited by S. P. Cauvain

230 **Emerging food packaging technologies: Principles and practice**
Edited by K. L. Yam and D. S. Lee
231 **Infectious disease in aquaculture: Prevention and control**
Edited by B. Austin
232 **Diet, immunity and inflammation**
Edited by P. C. Calder and P. Yaqoob
233 **Natural food additives, ingredients and flavourings**
Edited by D. Baines and R. Seal
234 **Microbial decontamination in the food industry: Novel methods and applications**
Edited by A. Demirci and M.O. Ngadi
235 **Chemical contaminants and residues in foods**
Edited by D. Schrenk
236 **Robotics and automation in the food industry: Current and future technologies**
Edited by D. G. Caldwell
237 **Fibre-rich and wholegrain foods: Improving quality** *Edited by J. A. Delcour and K. Poutanen*
238 **Computer vision technology in the food and beverage industries**
Edited by D.-W. Sun
239 **Encapsulation technologies and delivery systems for food ingredients and nutraceuticals**
Edited by N. Garti and D. J. McClements
240 **Case studies in food safety and authenticity**
Edited by J. Hoorfar
241 **Heat treatment for insect control: Developments and applications**
D. Hammond
242 **Advances in aquaculture hatchery technology**
Edited by G. Allan and G. Burnell
243 **Open innovation in the food and beverage industry**
Edited by M. Garcia Martinez
244 **Trends in packaging of food, beverages and other fast-moving consumer goods (FMCG)**
Edited by N. Farmer
245 **New analytical approaches for verifying the origin of food**
Edited by P. Brereton
246 **Microbial production of food ingredients, enzymes and nutraceuticals**
Edited by B. McNeil, D. Archer, I. Giavasis and L. Harvey
247 **Persistent organic pollutants and toxic metals in foods**
Edited by M. Rose and A. Fernandes
248 **Cereal grains for the food and beverage industries**
E. Arendt and E. Zannini
249 **Viruses in food and water: Risks, surveillance and control**
Edited by N. Cook
250 **Improving the safety and quality of nuts**
Edited by L. J. Harris
251 **Metabolomics in food and nutrition**
Edited by B. C. Weimer and C. Slupsky
252 **Food enrichment with omega-3 fatty acids**
Edited by C. Jacobsen, N. S. Nielsen, A. F. Horn and A.-D. M. Sørensen
253 **Instrumental assessment of food sensory quality: A practical guide**
Edited by D. Kilcast

254 **Food microstructures: Microscopy, measurement and modelling**
Edited by V. J. Morris and K. Groves
255 **Handbook of food powders: Processes and properties**
Edited by B. R. Bhandari, N. Bansal, M. Zhang and P. Schuck
256 **Functional ingredients from algae for foods and nutraceuticals**
Edited by H. Domínguez
257 **Satiation, satiety and the control of food intake: Theory and practice**
Edited by J. E. Blundell and F. Bellisle
258 **Hygiene in food processing: Principles and practice Second edition**
Edited by H. L. M. Lelieveld, J. Holah and D. Napper
259 **Advances in microbial food safety Volume 1**
Edited by J. Sofos
260 **Global safety of fresh produce: A handbook of best practice, innovative commercial solutions and case studies**
Edited by J. Hoorfar
261 **Human milk biochemistry and infant formula manufacturing technology**
Edited by M. Guo
262 **High throughput screening for food safety assessment: Biosensor technologies, hyperspectral imaging and practical applications**
Edited by A. K. Bhunia, M. S. Kim and C. R. Taitt
263 **Foods, nutrients and food ingredients with authorised EU health claims: Volume 1**
Edited by M. J. Sadler
264 **Handbook of food allergen detection and control**
Edited by S. Flanagan
265 **Advances in fermented foods and beverages: Improving quality, technologies and health benefits**
Edited by W. Holzapfel
266 **Metabolomics as a tool in nutrition research**
Edited by J.-L. Sébédio and L. Brennan
267 **Dietary supplements: Safety, efficacy and quality**
Edited by K. Berginc and S. Kreft
268 **Grapevine breeding programs for the wine industry**
Edited by A. G. Reynolds
269 **Handbook of antimicrobials for food safety and quality**
Edited by T. M. Taylor
270 **Managing and preventing obesity: Behavioural factors and dietary interventions**
Edited by T. P. Gill
271 **Electron beam pasteurization and complementary food processing technologies**
Edited by S. D. Pillai and S. Shayanfar
272 **Advances in food and beverage labelling: Information and regulations**
Edited by P. Berryman
273 **Flavour development, analysis and perception in food and beverages**
Edited by J. K. Parker, S. Elmore and L. Methven
274 **Rapid sensory profiling techniques and related methods: Applications in new product development and consumer research,**
Edited by J. Delarue, J. B. Lawlor and M. Rogeaux
275 **Advances in microbial food safety: Volume 2**
Edited by J. Sofos

276 **Handbook of antioxidants for food preservation**
Edited by F. Shahidi
277 **Lockhart and Wiseman's crop husbandry including grassland: Ninth edition**
H. J. S. Finch, A. M. Samuel and G. P. F. Lane
278 **Global legislation for food contact materials**
Edited by J. S. Baughan
279 **Colour additives for food and beverages**
Edited by M. Scotter
280 **A complete course in canning and related processes 14th Edition: Volume 1**
Revised by S. Featherstone
281 **A complete course in canning and related processes 14th Edition: Volume 2**
Revised by S. Featherstone
282 **A complete course in canning and related processes 14th Edition: Volume 3**
Revised by S. Featherstone
283 **Modifying food texture: Volume 1: Novel ingredients and processing techniques**
Edited by J. Chen and A. Rosenthal
284 **Modifying food texture: Volume 2: Sensory analysis, consumer requirements and preferences**
Edited by J. Chen and A. Rosenthal
285 **Modeling food processing operations**
Edited by Serafim Bakalis, Kai Knoerzer and Peter J. Fryer
286 **Foods, Nutrients and Food Ingredients With Authorised EU Health Claims Volume 2**
Edited by Michele Sadler
287 **Feed and Feeding Practices in Aquaculture**
Edited by D. Allen Davis
288 **Foodborne Parasites in the Food Supply Web: Occurrence and Control**
Edited by Alvin Gajadhar
289 **Brewing microbiology: design and technology applications for spoilage management, sensory quality and waste valorisation**
Edited by Annie Hill

Part One

Perspectives

Introduction to foodborne parasites

1

A.A. Gajadhar
Canadian Food Inspection Agency, Saskatoon, SK, Canada

1.1 Introduction

A safe food supply is essential to the survival of humankind. As people have multiplied and technology has advanced, the food supply has evolved from a base of local consumer production to large-scale integrated production and distribution practices. Consumers, particularly those in urban regions, are largely unaware of the origin and processing of their food. Similarly, most producers are unaware of the variety of potential public health hazards that are transmissible by food. Both consumers and producers rely on government regulations and oversight for guidance and protection. Although information regarding foodborne hazards is widely available from many sources, especially regarding hazards such as bacteria and chemical residues, there is limited information on foodborne parasites. This is becoming an urgent matter as the food supply web is now global and expertise in parasitology in developed countries has waned. This complacency has been driven primarily by improved hygiene standards and the increasingly effective control of zoonotic parasites in food animals in those regions. This chapter introduces the diversity and unique characteristics of foodborne parasites, the food vehicles by which they are transmitted, and their significance to consumers. A ranking of these foodborne parasites by various socioeconomic factors and information relevant to their control are presented.

The world's population currently exceeds 7 billion consumers living in regions where foodborne parasites are endemic or where there is risk of infection from imported food. Yet, relatively little is known about parasites, and their identity and characteristics are often confused with those of bacteria and viruses. Parasites are eukaryotic organisms that are classified within diverse taxa ranging from single-cell protozoa to complex hermaphroditic helminths. Foodborne parasites that are prevalent globally or regionally include the flagellated protozoon Giardia, the coccidian protozoa *Cryptosporidium* and *Toxoplasma*, the roundworms (nematodes) *Trichinella* and *Anisakis*, the tapeworms (cestodes) *Taenia* and *Echinococcus*, and the flukes (trematodes) *Opisthorchis*, *Clonorchis*, and *Fasciola*. The diversity of their structural and life-cycle characteristics that are employed in astounding strategies for survival, transmission, host adaptation, and replication makes parasites difficult to control but also fascinating to study.

Foodborne Parasites in the Food Supply Web. http://dx.doi.org/10.1016/B978-1-78242-332-4.00001-1

1.2 Parasites transmitted by food

Human parasitic infections originate from many sources and are acquired by various modes of transmission. Oral transmission via food and water represents the most common route of infection. Because food is produced globally in a wide range of microenvironments, and because it originates from a variety of aquatic or terrestrial animals and plants, there is a diverse range of strategies for parasite survival, replication, and transmission. A list of various food products and examples of the parasites they transmit is provided in Table 1.1. Although many waterborne parasites such as *Giardia* and *Entamoeba* have simple, direct life cycles, foodborne parasites often have life cycles that involve multiple stages and various host species that exploit both the exogenous and endogenous environments and food habits of consumers. Generally, meatborne parasites replicate and attain infectivity in protective structures such as cysts within muscle, established during the animal's development (Table 1.1). Examples include *Toxoplasma gondii*, *Sarcocystis hominis*, and *Trichinella spiralis*. Other parasites such as *Giardia* and *Cryptosporidium* can infect consumers by contaminating surfaces of ready-to-eat fruits and vegetables.

Most foodborne parasites in food animals or the external environment have stages that are capable of survival in a variety of conditions for long periods of time. For example, coccidian protozoa are protected immunologically as they develop within host cells and are located in sites to facilitate replication and exit from the host or to allow for long-term survival in the host. *Trichinella* spp. larvae also develop within the

Table 1.1 Food groups and products that can serve as transmission vehicles for parasites capable of infecting consumers

Food		Parasites	
Major food groups	**Food source**	**Species/family**	**Transmission stage**
Animals: aquatic	Amphibians (frogs)	*Alaria americana*	Metacercaria
		Spirometra spp.	Plerocercoid
	Crustaceans (crab, shrimp, etc.)	Anisakidae	Larva (L3)
		Paragonimus spp.	Metacercaria
	Freshwater fish	*Alaria Americana*	Metacercaria
		Clonorchis sinensis	Metacercaria
		Diphyllobothriidae	Plerocercoid
		Heterophyidae	Metacercaria
		Metrochis spp.	Metacercaria
		Opisthorchis spp.	Metacercaria
	Marine fish	Anisakidae	Larva (L3)
		Diphyllobothriidae	Plerocercoid
		Heterophyidae (brackish water)	Metacercaria
	Shellfish	*Cryptosporidium* spp.	Oocyst
		Giardia duodenalis	Cyst
		Toxoplasma gondii	Oocyst

Table 1.1 Continued

Food		Parasites	
Major food groups	**Food source**	**Species/family**	**Transmission stage**
Animals: terrestrial	Beef	*Sarcocystis hominis*	Tissue cyst
		Taenia saginata	Cysticercus
		Toxoplasma gondii	Tissue cyst
	Dairy products	*Toxoplasma gondii*	Tachyzoite
		Cryptosporidium spp.	Oocyst
	Game meat	*Alaria americanum*	Metacercaria
		Toxoplasma gondii	Tissue cyst
		Trichinella spp.	Larva (L1)
	Horse	*Toxoplasma gondii*	Tissue cyst
		Trichinella spp.	Larva (L1)
	Pork	*Paragonimus* spp.	Metacercaria
		Sarcocystis suihominis	Tissue cyst
		Taenia solium	Cysticercus
		Toxoplasma gondii	Tissue cyst
		Trichinella spp.	Larva (L1)
	Reptiles	*Alaria Americana*	Metacercaria
		Spirometra spp.	Plerocercoid
		Trichinella spp.	Larva (L1)
	Small ruminants	*Toxoplasma gondii*	Tissue cyst
	Snake	*Spirometra* spp.	Plerocercoid
Animals: birds	Chicken	*Toxoplasma gondii*	Tissue cyst
	Water fowl (geese, ducks)	*Toxoplasma gondii*	Tissue cyst
Plants: aquatic	Fresh produce	*Fasciola* spp.	Metacercaria
		Fasciolopsis buski	Metacercaria
Plants: terrestrial	Fresh produce (berries, leafy greens, etc.)	*Ascaris* spp.	Egg
		Balantidium coli	Cyst
		Cryptosporidium spp.	Oocyst
		Cyclospora cayetanensis	Oocyst
		Echinococcus granulosus	Egg
		Echinococcus multilocularis	Egg
		Entamoeba histolytica	Cyst
		Giardia duodenalis	Cyst
		Taenia solium	Egg
		Toxocara spp.	Egg
		Toxoplasma gondii	Oocyst
		Trichuris trichiura	Egg
	Fruit juice	*Cryptosporidium* spp.	Oocyst
		Trypanosoma cruzi	Trypomastigote

protective environment afforded by host cells, and most species remain encapsulated as such until consumed by a new host. Many species of cestodes and trematodes are also protected in enclosures such as cysts and eggs in their respective hosts, environments, or food products as they await transmission to consumers. Exogenous stages of many species of parasites can resist a wide range of chemicals and survive for long periods of time under various environmental conditions such as mild heat and extreme cold, drought, and seasonality (Gajadhar and Allen, 2004). Therefore, strategies and measures traditionally used for controlling other foodborne pathogens are often ineffective for parasites. The unique characteristics of their life cycles, and the epidemiology of parasites must be considered when designing control programs and implementing intervention measures for farms or contaminated food products.

1.3 Foods that transmit parasites

The expanding culinary preferences for fresh, slightly cooked, and ready-to-eat food and the increasing demands for meat in developing countries are increasing the risks posed by foodborne parasites. To promote and enhance the natural flavors of food, meat producers are advocating the use of cooking temperatures that would achieve a lower level of cooking thoroughness. This practice inherently increases the risk of survival of parasites such as *Trichinella* spp. and *Taenia solium* in pork, and *T. gondii* in chicken and lamb.

The numbers of tourists venturing to exotic locations are increasing exponentially and so are their insatiable appetite to indulge in local traditions involving food and drink. Not infrequently, such food and beverages harbor parasites to which native residents are relatively immune, but which pose risks of serious illness for nonresidents (Motarjemi and Adams, 2006). Tourists naive to exotic pathogens can become severely ill before or long after returning home. As many areas of the developing world encounter unprecedented increases in economic and social growth, there are increasing demands for meals with higher levels of protein and for fresh meats, fruits, and vegetables. This is in addition to the ongoing demands for these products from developed countries with affluence, but often a limited agricultural land base and climate that prohibits continuous, large-scale domestic production. Globalization of the food supply and animal transit have been the response. Although guidelines for controlled production and traceability have been proposed for food animals, meat, and plant products to assure the origin and quality of food-reaching consumers, widespread implementation has not occurred in most countries. Very few countries monitor food products for parasites, and when it is done, the number of samples tested is minimal and provides little or no added security for consumers.

1.4 Public health and economy

Foodborne parasites are important for public health reasons and/or trade. Recently, an expert committee from the Food and Agricultural Organization/World Health

Organization (FAO/WHO) ranked the importance of foodborne parasites by socioeconomic and trade impact (Figures 1.1 and 1.2). The entire human population is at risk of becoming infected with foodborne parasites. Particularly for some of the ubiquitous zoonotic protozoan parasites, it is quite likely that all adults have previously been infected once or repeatedly, although the vast majority have never been aware of it because of the lack of pathognomonic symptoms or misdiagnosis. The outcomes of parasitic infection in humans vary widely depending on factors such as the species, strain, or genotype of the parasite, dose, and life stage of parasite, condition of the host, infection site, and incubation period. Infection with *T. gondii*, for example, may

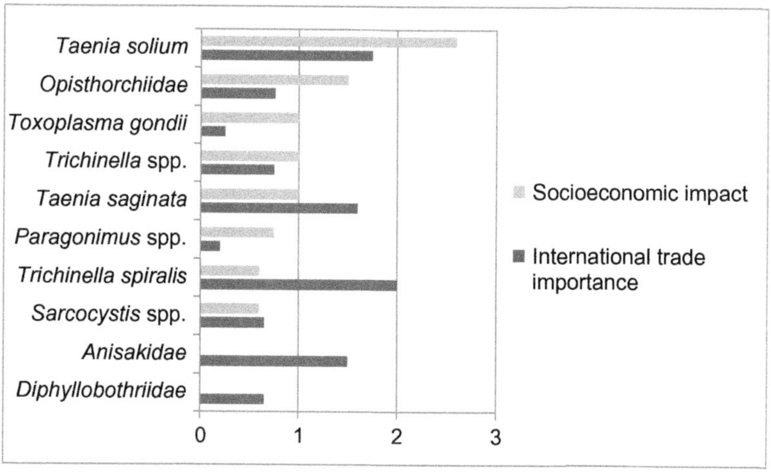

Figure 1.1 FAO/WHO ranking of terrestrial and aquatic meatborne zoonotic parasites by importance for socioeconomic impact and international trade. Parasites include those that are common globally or regionally.

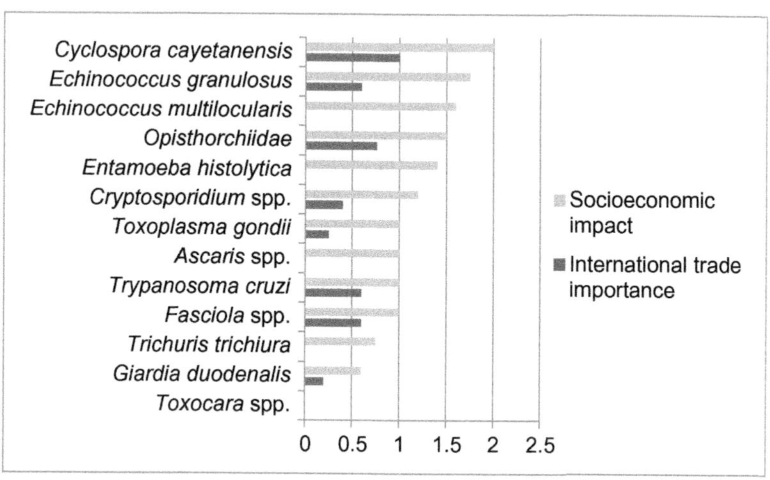

Figure 1.2 FAO/WHO ranking of terrestrial and aquatic plantborne parasites that are common globally or regionally.

be influenced by any of these factors. Disease form, virulence, and tissue predilection differ by genotype and whether transmission occurs via tachyzoites, cysts with bradyzoites, or oocysts with sporozoites of the infecting organisms. Additionally, a single *T. gondii* oocyst containing eight sporozoites and contaminating fruits or vegetables is capable of establishing infection and causing disease, whereas infected meat usually contains numerous cysts each of which contains thousands of infectious bradyzoites. Depending on these factors and the immune competence of the infected person, clinical illness may be mild to severe, and manifested within days to weeks, or it may appear as long-term developmental and neurological pathology including loss of organ function, deformation, or fetal loss. Parasitic infections are known to persist for the life of the host, and the availability and effectiveness of treatments vary according to the species and stage of parasite and site of infection.

Foodborne parasitic infection that is solely gastrointestinal usually results in short-term diarrhea and related illness; in an otherwise healthy individual, this is followed by apparent complete recovery. Such infections, including cryptosporidiosis, cyclosporosis, and giardiosis, are more readily recognized and diagnosed in episodes of outbreaks, but not as isolated individual cases. Tissue infections caused by foodborne parasites, however, tend to be more insidious, protracted, and pathogenic. Examples of such diseases attributed to infected food include gastric ulceration from anasakids in fish, myalgia from *Trichinella* in pork and horsemeat, neurocysticercosis from *T. solium* in pork, hydatidosis from *Echinococcus* on produce, cholangiocarcinoma from *Clonorchis sinensis* and *Opisthorchis viverrini* in fish, and bile duct obstruction from *Fasciola* on aquatic plants. Further examples and details are provided in Table 1.1.

1.5 Challenges and future trends

There is much misconception about parasites, their occurrence, the risk they pose to public health, and their control. Although much is known about the life cycle and epidemiology of common foodborne parasites such as *Cryptosporidium* and *Giardia*, limited information is available or readily assessable to stakeholders. Generally, the food industry, regulators, public health workers, and consumers have little knowledge of foodborne parasites, their nature, and the potential for their occurrence in the food chain. As the distribution and occurrence of these parasites expand globally, accurate and up-to-date information is required by a wide range of stakeholders, from producers, risk assessors, regulators, and food scientists to consumers and anyone with an interest in foodborne parasitology. Newly established resources for further information and updates in this area include the journal *Food and Waterborne Parasitology* and the International Association of Food and Waterborne Parasitology.

The food supply chain has evolved into an intricate system fueled by technological advances enabling enormous efficiencies and opportunities, as well as creating unforeseen challenges. Modern forms of production, transportation, and trade practices have played a large role in this evolution of the global food supply web and in providing consumers with an unprecedented variety of choices. Foodborne parasites, which previously did not have a significant presence or were even ignored in some regions of the world, are now among the emerging challenges facing society. Nevertheless, notification of foodborne parasitic diseases to public health authorities is not compulsory, but recently such acquired diseases have been recognized as neglected diseases (FAO/WHO, 2014). Education, research, and surveillance are urgently needed to assist risk assessors, regulators, food scientists, and other stakeholders in addressing the challenges related to emerging foodborne parasites. The provision of science-based guidelines and technical and financial support is essential to ensure improvements across the global food supply web for the control of foodborne parasites.

References

Food and Agriculture Organization of the United Nations/World Health Organization (FAO/WHO), 2014. Multicriteria-Based Ranking for Risk Management of Foodborne Parasites. Microbiological Risk Assessment Series No. 23, Rome, Italy, 302 pp.

Gajadhar, A.A., Allen, J.R., 2004. Factors contributing to the public health and economic importance of waterborne zoonotic parasites. Vet. Parasitol. 126, 3–14.

Hunter, P.R., Hughes, S., Woodhouse, S., Raj, N., Syed, Q., Chalmers, R.M., Verlander, N.Q., Goodacre, J., 2004. Health sequelae of human cryptosporidiosis in immunocompetent patients. Clin. Infect. Dis. 39, 504–510.

Motarjemi, Y., Adams, M. (Eds.), 2006. Emerging Foodborne Pathogens, second ed. Woodhead Publishing, Cambridge.

Trends in food production practices relative to foodborne parasites

2

H.R. Gamble
National Research Council, Washington, DC, USA

2.1 Introduction

Foodborne parasites can be transmitted to humans through ingestion of infective stages on, or in, food. Foodborne sources include meat, fish, shellfish, vegetables, and fruits. Human exposure to parasites can be prevented by interventions or mitigations at various stages of the production-to-consumption continuum. Interventions during the production phase will generally be targeted to avoid exposure to, or contamination with, infective parasite stages. Postharvest methods will generally target detection (testing), removal (e.g., washing), or inactivation (by further processing) of infective parasite stages.

The efficacy of these interventions or mitigations is determined by the pathways in which parasites are transmitted during production and the effectiveness of postharvest processes. This chapter addresses general aspects of production practices that reduce or eliminate the risk of exposure to infective parasitic stages. Postharvest decisions about risk mitigation should consider steps taken during food production to reduce or eliminate parasite risk. The *Codex Alimentarius General Principles of Food Hygiene* (Codex Alimentarius, 2003) states the following:

> *The potential effects of primary production activities on the safety and suitability of food should be considered at all times. In particular, this includes identifying any specific points in such activities where a high probability of contamination may exist and taking specific measures to minimize that probability. The HACCP-based approach may assist in the taking of such measures....*
>
> *Producers should as far as practicable implement measures to:*
>
> - *control contamination from air, soil, water, feedstuffs, fertilizers (including natural fertilizers), pesticides, veterinary drugs, or any other agent used in primary production;*
> - *control plant and animal health so that it does not pose a threat to human health through food consumption, or adversely affect the suitability of the product; and*
> - *protect food sources from fecal and other contamination.*
>
> *In particular, care should be taken to manage wastes, and store harmful substances appropriately. On-farm programmes which achieve specific food safety goals are becoming an important part of primary production and should be encouraged.*

Although the *Codex Alimentarius* does not provide specific guidance for most commodities with respect to parasites, many of the general production principles included in this general code contribute to the prevention of exposure to or contamination with foodborne parasites.

Foodborne Parasites in the Food Supply Web. http://dx.doi.org/10.1016/B978-1-78242-332-4.00002-3

2.2 Parasite transmission pathways in food production

Transmission pathways relevant to food production include contamination of food or water with infective parasite stages or direct infection of food animals by tissue-dwelling parasite stages.

2.2.1 *Controlled versus noncontrolled food production*

For the purposes of discussion, it is necessary to distinguish production that is under some form of controlled management from food that is harvested from the environment without any control over production stages. Examples of noncontrolled production include wild-caught fish and other seafood, game meats (wild/feral animals), or fruits and vegetables that grow wild. Parasite risk from food in these categories cannot generally be controlled preharvest, and therefore risk assessment, testing, and postharvest mitigations must be used to protect human health.

For food that is produced under controlled conditions, specific steps may be taken to reduce the risk of exposure to parasites. The steps necessary for control can be derived from assessing the risk through a hazard analysis critical control point (HACCP) process. Some general concepts for reducing risk of exposure to parasites during food production will be addressed here.

2.2.2 *Classes of parasites*

Parasites that pose a risk to human health include protozoa, trematodes, cestodes, and nematodes. Among these classes of parasites, some are specific to a certain commodity, such as *Taenia saginata* tapeworm larvae in cattle, whereas others are found as contaminants on a variety of products such as *Cryptosporidium* and *Giardia* on fruits and vegetables or even more broadly, posing a threat from both produce and livestock (e.g., *Toxoplasma*).

2.2.3 *Parasites important in food production*

Because an integrated approach to food safety must begin with the prevention of exposure during production, it is important to understand the potential hazards that occur where food is being produced. Hazards will vary by commodity, region, production system, etc., and it is important to understand what the risks are to manage them during production.

The Food and Agricultural Organization (FAO) and World Health Organization (WHO) have jointly published an assessment of the importance of various parasites in food production (FAO/WHO, 2014). Based on the expert consultation and global public health data, the FAO/WHO report lists 24 parasites that are of primary importance in food production. These include eight protozoa, four trematodes, five cestodes, and seven nematodes. The report further lists 18 general commodity groups including land animals, aquatic animals, dairy products, plants, and others. Among the 24 parasites listed, 13 pose a human health risk through ingestion of contaminated land plants (fruits and vegetables), 5 pose a risk from ingestion of meat from infected livestock, 3 pose a risk from ingestion of fresh/brackish water fish and shellfish, 2 pose a risk from ingestion of marine fish, game meats, and juice/milk, and 1 poses a risk from the ingestion of amphibians/reptiles (*Spirometra*) and aquatic plants (*Fasciola*). Information on important parasite genera affecting livestock, produce, and fish are discussed in Chapter 1.

2.2.4 General principles

Basic principles apply to food production as related to reducing or preventing exposure to parasites. These basic principles are related to the potential sources of introduction of parasite stages which include primarily feed, water, soil, manure/fecal material, and animal tissue (Table 2.1). Some infective parasite stages are extremely resistant to desiccation and heat, and this must be considered when developing plans to avoid risk. Common sources of parasites can be categorized as follows:

2.2.4.1 Water

Water supplies can contain parasite oocysts, eggs, or other stages that are shed in the feces of animals or humans. These environmentally resistant stages may remain viable for extended periods of time; water supplies can become more heavily contaminated from soil runoff following heavy rains or when animals defecate in or near water sources. The risk of parasite contamination should be taken into consideration when a water supply is selected for the irrigation of land crops or as a source for use in animal production. When risk exists, steps should be taken to mitigate that risk (e.g., sampling/testing, treatment, etc.).

Several important groups of foodborne parasites, including trematodes, cestodes, and nematodes, complete all or part of their life cycles in an aquatic environment. Stages that are infective to humans occur in fish, shellfish, or aquatic plants (see Chapter 1 and elsewhere). For fish, shellfish, and aquatic plants harvested from the

Table 2.1 Major sources of risk for parasite infection/contamination among broad commodity groups

Livestock and poultry	Drinking water Feed (source and storage) Rodents in or around production facilities Wildlife in or around production facilities Contamination of soil with animal or human feces
Fresh fruits and vegetables	Water for irrigation Water from overflow/flooding of rivers/lakes Manure applied to fields prior to or during production Contamination of soil with animal or human feces
Fish and shellfish	Water used in production Water runoff from land areas Feed (source and storage)

wild, there will always be risk for contamination with these parasites, although the risk may vary regionally based on the global distribution of the parasite species.

2.2.4.2 Soil

Like water, when parasites' stages are shed into the environment via animal or human feces, they may disperse into soil. Animals that graze or eat off the ground may ingest infective parasite stages. These stages could be further carried into barns, on shoes or boots, or be dispersed onto fields via wind, runoff, etc. and may remain viable for long periods of time. Soil may serve to protect parasite stages from desiccation and damage due to radiation, thus increasing chances for dispersal and subsequent contamination of water, animal feed or the animal environment.

2.2.4.3 Fertilizer/manure

Manure can harbor infectious stages of parasites that are shed in human or animal feces. The source of manure should be assessed for risk and appropriate treatments applied to manure prior to use as fertilizer.

2.2.4.4 Animal feed

Animal feed that includes meat products should be treated in such a way that any pathogens that might be contained in the meat are inactivated. Likewise, feed may be contaminated from environmental sources (e.g., rodents or other animals that defecate in feed) or by contamination with organic material. Feed must be stored in such a way that contamination does not occur.

2.2.4.5 Animals/biotic risks

Wild animals may harbor tissue stages which, if ingested by another animal, pose a risk for parasite infection. Notable examples are *Trichinella* in rodents and small mammals and *Toxoplasma* in mice. Isolating livestock from wild animals and rodents is important in preventing transmission of parasitic, as well as other diseases, to food animals.

2.3 Illustrations of food production systems for parasite control

2.3.1 Preventing parasites in pork production systems

The principal foodborne parasitic hazards found in pork include *Toxoplasma gondii* (a protozoan coccidium), *Taenia solium* (a tapeworm), and *Trichinella spiralis* (a nematode). Pigs become infected with *T. gondii* by ingestion of oocysts (in, for example, water, feed, or soil) or by ingestion of animal tissue containing cysts. *T. gondii* oocysts are only shed by felids, and domestic and feral cats are the most common source of contamination. Pigs become infected with *T. solium* by the ingestion of eggs in the environment (in, for example, water, feed, or soil). *T. solium* eggs are only passed by human tapeworm carriers, so fecal contamination from infected persons is the only source of exposure. Pigs become infected with *T. spiralis* by ingestion of animal tissue harboring infective larvae. *T. spiralis* and other species of the genus *Trichinella* can only be passed to a new host by ingestion of skeletal muscle containing infective larvae. Sources of infection include exposure of pigs to wildlife and rodents, deliberate feeding of uncooked meat waste, and cannibalism of infected pig carcasses.

Understanding the risks for exposure to infectious parasite stages is important for implementing effective preventative measures for foodborne parasites. Potential sources of infection for the three parasites important to pork production include water, feed, soil/organic material contaminated with oocysts or eggs, feed contaminated with infected animal tissue, and exposure to and ingestion of tissue from rodents, pigs, or wildlife carcasses.

Modern pork production systems address the risks of exposure to these three parasites through biosecurity measures. Only systems that utilize controlled housing can be relied on to prevent preharvest exposure to one or more of these parasites. Management practices that dramatically reduce the potential risk for exposure to parasites include components of building construction including physical barriers, external and internal rodent control systems, good feed manufacturing practices, feed storage requirements, water quality requirements, personnel hygiene requirements, building and equipment wash-down, and animal movement. Examples of pork industry production standards that address biosecurity can be found in the Danish Product Standard (2014) (http://www.pigresearchcentre.dk/~/media/Files/DANISH/DANISH%20produktstandard/Produkt_Standard_UK.ashx), the US Pork Quality Assurance Program (http://porkcdn.s3.amazonaws.com/sites/all/files/documents/PQAPlus/V2.0/TrainingAdults/PQAPlusEducationHandbookVersion2.0.pdf), and the OIE Terrestrial Animal Health Code, Chapter 8.15 (http://www.oie.int/index.php?id=169&L=0&htmfile=chapitre_trichinella_spp.htm).

2.3.1.1 A biosecure pork production system

Building construction

Buildings' housing pigs are constructed to exclude animals and birds, and the area around buildings is maintained to reduce the presence of animals and animal harborage (Figure 2.1). Stepwise exclusion is accomplished by creating barriers external to the buildings, such as open spaces which contain no animal harborage and keeping these areas free of vegetation. Often, gravel is used to line the perimeter of buildings; this enhances other efforts to control rodents. Buildings are constructed and maintained so there are no openings that could be accessed by animals or birds. General guidance is that an opening of ¼ in. in diameter can be accessed by a rat (Tobin and Fall, 2004). Pipe entries, door perimeters, roof joints, and other potential access points are inspected and repaired as necessary to ensure the integrity of the building.

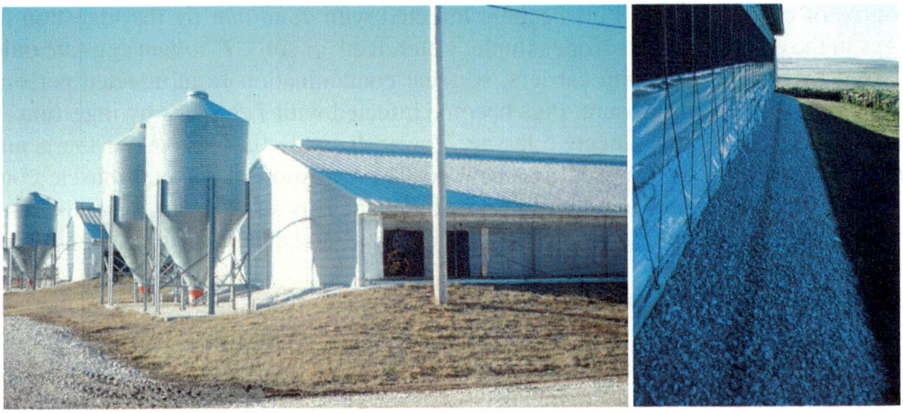

Figure 2.1 A typical confinement pork management system that is constructed to provide a biosecure environment for pigs. Areas around barns are kept clear of harborage for rodents, and a barrier is established along the perimeter. Feed is stored securely with no spills.

Rodent control systems

Building construction alone cannot eliminate access of rodents to pork production facilities. Steps in rodent control include open perimeters, as previously described, as well as exterior and interior bait stations. Generally these stations are installed and maintained by professional pest control operators, who can recognize signs of rodent infestation. Bait stations are regularly inspected and the perimeters of buildings are also inspected for the signs of rodent, especially rat, activity.

Exclusion of domestic and feral cats

Based on the transmission of *T. gondii*, cats pose a special risk to all farms, including the pork and poultry industries. Almost all cats that are outdoors for all or part of their lives are exposed to *T. gondii* and, for several weeks following exposure, shed environmentally resistant oocysts (up to millions per day). Oocysts are dispersed in the environment; pigs raised outdoors may have infection prevalence rates of 50% or higher (Gamble et al., 1999). Even in confinement barns, oocysts can be transported inside on shoes; therefore, boot changes are essential for reducing risk of exposure of pigs to this parasite. Excluding cats from the local production environment is a basic principle for reducing the risk of exposure to foodborne parasites.

Water

To prevent the introduction of infective parasite stages in water, it is important to determine that the source of water is not subject to contamination. Water may also be periodically tested and if necessary treated prior to providing it to animals. In the case of *Toxoplasma*, oocysts shed by cats can enter a watershed in runoff and can persist for months or years. Similarly, water that may have been contaminated with human feces can contain eggs of *T. solium*.

Feed manufacturing and storage

To reduce the risk of feed as a source of parasites, feed produced either on-site or off-site, should meet the requirements of good manufacturing practices (GMPs) and other quality assurance standards recognized by the feed industry. Ingredients do not include any meat and bone meal. Prior to and during the manufacturing process, feed and feed ingredients are stored to prevent contamination with fecal material or animal tissue. Adherence to GMPs or other quality assurance standards is normally documented in a feed mill quality assurance affidavit. The principles of GMP for feed are described in the International Feed Industry Federation, FAO Feed manual (FAO, IFIF, 2010; http://www.ifif.org/uploadImage/2012/1/17/0a9131729326f9a2a111ae84024a851f1326840707.pdf), and other relevant sources, such as the American Feed Industry Association (https://www.afia.org/Afia/Home.aspx).

Feed storage is also important, as contamination with parasites can occur on the farm, and feed is an attraction to rodents, feral cats, and wildlife. To protect feed from contamination with feces and rodent carcasses, feed is stored in elevated bins that do not afford points of entry to mice and other rodents. Rodent control, especially baiting, is maintained in feed storage areas. Feed spills, including those occurring during delivery, are promptly cleaned up to avoid attracting rodents.

Personnel hygiene

Worker (and visitor) hygiene is critical to prevent exposure to parasites. Workers can be a direct source of parasite stages, in the case of human tapeworm carriers, or can mechanically introduce parasite stages into the swine environment, by transporting oocysts, for example, into barns on boots. Due to these risks, producers restrict entry into biosecure pork production facilities. Workers who enter barns should wear coveralls or completely change clothes prior to entering barns. Likewise, barn-only boots are generally worn inside, and care is taken to isolate footwear that is used inside and outside. In the best facilities, workers shower prior to entry, although this is more critical for the control of pathogens other than parasites. Similar hygiene measures are applied to anyone who works in or around the production site, including feed truck drivers, transport drivers, and others.

Facility cleaning

Modern pork production facilities follow an animal flow pattern of all-in/all-out, in which animals move as a group; this means no new animals are entered into the population during the grow-out phase. Between grow-out cycles, a thorough wash-down is done in production facilities using very hot water. This assures that organic material that may have entered or accumulated in the facility during the production cycle is removed. Also, any residual feed that could attract rodents is also removed.

2.3.1.2 Changes resulting from good pork production practices

The impact of good management in the pork industry is most obvious in the decline of *Trichinella* in domestic pork in countries where modern or industrialized pork production is practiced. Historically, pigs were fed raw garbage and, in many cases,

Trichinella cycled from pig to pig by feeding infected pork meat. Likewise, when pigs were raised outdoors, they were exposed to rodents and other wild mammals which served as sources of infection. Over time, the feeding of raw garbage, or any garbage, has been banned in many countries, and pork production has moved into a very controlled environment including increasing levels of biosecurity. As the pork industry has progressed in this way, *Trichinella* has disappeared as a common zoonotic infection (Gamble et al., 2007).

Toxoplasma is another example of how good management can greatly reduce the risk of parasite infection in pigs. The prevalence of infection in pigs is dramatically different in outdoor pigs as compared to pigs raised in confinement (Gamble et al., 1999). Outdoor husbandry can result in a prevalence of 50% or more in a pig herd, whereas in confinement systems *Toxoplasma* infection is rare (Dubey, 2009). Nevertheless, risks for exposure to *Toxoplasma* remain in confinement systems, and additional provisions for biosecurity are necessary (Hill et al., 2009). For example, improvements in boot hygiene have been shown to reduce exposure of pigs raised in confinement.

Although *T. solium* infection is rare in pigs raised under good management conditions, it persists in regions where the parasite can cycle between humans and pigs (Garcia et al., 2003). When humans and pigs live in close proximity and sanitation is poor, eggs shed by human carriers can contaminate the pigs' environment and result in pigs infected with cysticerci. Humans then acquire the tapeworm by ingesting cysticerci in insufficiently cooked pork. The implementation of sanitation systems, targeted treatment of tapeworm carriers, and education can break this cycle in rural areas where infection rates may be high (Sarti et al., 1997).

2.3.1.3 Other considerations in pork production practices

Organic production and food safety

Specific guidelines govern organic production in some countries. For example, the US Department of Agriculture National Organic Program (7 CFR PART 205) states, "The producer of an organic livestock operation must establish and maintain year-round livestock living conditions which accommodate the health and natural behavior of animals, including: (1) Year-round access for all animals to the outdoors…" Under these conditions, it is virtually impossible to isolate animals from exposure to parasites such as *Toxoplasma* if there have been domestic or feral cats in the pig environment. Consumers should be aware of the additional risks posed by outdoor husbandry of livestock and take appropriate precautions in food handling and preparation to avoid exposure to parasites and other pathogens.

Animal welfare and food safety

Animal welfare is an important issue for livestock producers both from an ethical and economic perspective, as stress and disease affect productivity. Likewise, the welfare of food animals is an ethical concern for consumers. It does not follow, however, that welfare requires free access to an outdoor environment as is required for organic production. Outdoor exposure in the case of parasites increases, sometimes dramatically, the risk of exposure to infection. There have been many examples of "free-range" or backyard-raised pork implicated in human trichinellosis. Likewise, the risk for pigs to acquire *Toxoplasma* infection can be manyfold higher when pigs are raised outdoors. As with organic production, consumers should be aware of the additional risks posed by outdoor husbandry of livestock and take similar precautions in food handling and preparation.

2.3.2 Prevention of parasite contamination in vegetable and fruit production

Contamination of produce (vegetables and fruit crops grown close to or in contact with soil) can occur from a variety of sources. The major parasites that pose a risk for produce are described in the FAO/WHO report (FAO/WHO, 2014) and include protozoa (infective stages are cysts and oocysts), as well as cestode and nematode eggs on land plants and trematodes (metacercariae) on aquatic plants. For produce, as with other food production systems, understanding possible contamination risk is important prior to initiating production. The major sources for the contamination of produce include water, soil, and manure that have been contaminated with infected feces from animals or humans (Agri-Food and Veterinary Authority of Singapore, 2005).

2.3.2.1 Water

Water may be used for a variety of reasons in crop production, but irrigation is of primary importance in most systems. Irrigation water must be assessed for possible risk of parasite contamination. For example, surface waters from rivers and lakes often contain fecal material shed by land animals, and these are sources of parasite stages. Likewise, human fecal contamination could introduce parasites into irrigation water. Thus, irrigation-holding ponds, for example, should not be in proximity to portable lavatories, where ground seepage can cause contamination. In general, ground water (well water) is a safer source of water for irrigation as compared to surface water. However, well water can be contaminated by runoff from heavy rains or flooding or any event in which animal or human fecal material could enter the system.

Water should be tested frequently for all forms of microbial contamination: coliform bacteria and parasite stages. Surface water is particularly susceptible to contamination after a significant rainfall. Where risk occurs, filtration is one method commonly used to reduce microbial contamination. Application methods can also reduce contamination of produce by minimizing the amount of water that directly contacts edible portions of the plant. Thus, methods of furrow or underground irrigation are preferred when parasites may be a risk.

2.3.2.2 Manure

The source of manure used to fertilize fields where produce is grown should be evaluated for potential risks of harboring zoonotic parasites and should be treated appropriately to mitigate those risks. Likewise, the location and method of manure storage should take into account possible risks of contamination from animals. This is particularly important if manure will come into contact with edible potions of produce during the growing or harvesting process. Specific guidelines for good management govern the intervals required from manure application to harvest, and these intervals are longer when manure has not been composted (USDA, National Organic Standards, 2011). Human waste should never be used for fertilization of produce.

2.3.2.3 Animal exclusion

Steps should be taken to exclude domestic and wild animals from fields where produce is grown. Various approaches are taken including fencing or other physical barriers. Rodent control programs, as described for pork production, also may be used. When possible, netting should be used as an additional barrier to protect produce from contamination with fecal material from mammals and birds.

2.3.2.4 Worker hygiene

Field workers may also spread parasite stages during harvest or postharvest production. Workers should have adequate toilet facilities with a proper sewage disposal system, as well as access to hand-washing stations with hot water and drying options. Workers should have specific guidelines for hand washing and other protocols associated with hygiene when working with produce.

2.3.2.5 Equipment hygiene

Equipment and containers used in fields should be cleaned and sanitized prior to use. Equipment should be stored in such a way as to avoid possible contamination with fecal material from animals.

2.3.2.6 Postharvest contamination

Postharvest processing (e.g., washing) is an important intervention for decontamination of the surfaces of fresh fruits and vegetables; however, water used for washing may also pose a risk for additional contamination. Although it is not the subject of this chapter, facility and worker hygiene as well as water quality all can play a role in contamination with parasites, and any program to reduce or eliminate risks should consider primary production as well as postharvest risk assessment and mitigations. The various control components for foodborne parasites in the food production chain are discussed in Chapter 16.

2.4 Conclusion and future trends

In developed countries, major advances have been made in farming systems with respect to food safety in general and parasites in particular. However, the sanitary level of farming varies greatly by country and economic situation. Even in developed countries, not all farmers and producers can afford to follow the highest levels of sanitation for food production. Understanding the economic and public health value of following practices that support food safety and having the resources available to support this implementation of good production practices are critical to continuous improvement in both developed and developing countries.

A cornerstone for advancing safe food production is education of the producer regarding the specific risks for parasite contamination. Sources of information available to farmers and producers may include government personnel, academic (extension) personnel, or commodity/producer organizations. Numerous documents exist on the Web, many of which describe best practices for the production of individual commodities. A good example is the very detailed Pork Quality Assurance Program (National Pork Board, 2014), which has been used by the US pork industry for many years. Understanding how good production practices ensure safe food and add value to the product provides the incentive for farmers and producers to implement best practices.

Once risks are understood, the next step to preventing exposure of food animals to, or contamination of produce with, parasites, is risk assessment and a specific risk-mitigation plan following an HACCP process. As described for pork production, there are specific risk factors for the three parasites discussed. Modern pork production systems effectively mitigate these risks through controls that are in place at each stage of food production. Likewise, for field crops, there are specific risks for contamination with infective parasite stages, and adherence to good production practices will largely mitigate these risks.

It is essential that there are standards by which food can be produced in a safe manner. There are many sources of national and international guidances on safe food production, and some of these have been referenced in this chapter. Some of this guidance is regulatory in nature, and some guidance serves to regulate trade. As these guidelines and regulatory documents are developed and revised, food producers should pay attention to the best scientific information that reduces risks for parasites in food.

Finally, the safety of our food, especially food that is produced in developed countries, is a direct result of scientific research and the application of that research to food production. Safe practices in food production systems have been developed and implemented in an incremental process, over time, with clear results in reducing human illness. Developing countries still face significant challenges in food safety. As these economies grow, more emphasis is placed on quality and safety of food, and good production systems will become increasingly important.

The global demand for food will continue to grow. There cannot be complacency in our efforts to improve the technology that we use in food production. Increased productivity must go hand in hand with increased safety, and that will result from continued research to support food production systems.

References

Agri-Food and Veterinary Authority of Singapore, 2005. Good Agricultural Practice for Vegetable Farming. http://caff.org/wp-content/uploads/2012/06/Codes-of-GAP-from-Department-of-Agriculture.pdf.

Codex Alimentarius, 2003. General Principles of Food Hygiene, CAC-RCP 1-1969. http://www.codexalimentarius.org/standards/list-of-standards/en/?no_cache=1?provide=standards&orderField=ccshort&sort=asc&num1=.

Danish Pig Research Center, 2014. Danish Product Standard. http://www.pigresearchcentre.dk/~/media/Files/DANISH/DANISH%20produktstandard/Produkt_Standard_UK.ashx.

Dubey, J.P., 2009. Toxoplasmosis of Animals and Humans, second ed. CRC Press, Boca Raton, FL, USA, 313 pp.

FAO, IFIF, 2010. Good practices for the feed industry—implementing the Codex Alimentarius Code of practice on good animal feeding. FAO Animal Production and Health Manual No. 9. FAO and IFIF, Rome.

FAO/WHO, 2014. Multicriteria-based ranking for risk management of food-borne parasites. Microbiological Risk Assessment Series No. 23. FAO/WHO, Rome, 302 pp.

Gamble, H.R., Brady, R.C., Dubey, J.P., 1999. Prevalence of *Toxoplasma gondii* infection in domestic pigs in the New England states. Vet. Parasitol. 82, 129–136.

Gamble, H.R., Boireau, P., Noeckler, K., Kapel, C.M.O., 2007. Prevention of *Trichinella* infection in the domestic pig. In: Dupouy-Camet, J., Murrell, K.D. (Eds.), FAO/WHO/OIE Guidelines for the Surveillance, Management, Prevention and Control of Trichinellosis. FAO/WHO/OIE, Rome, pp. 101–110.

Garcia, H.H., Gilman, R.H., Gonzalez, A.E., Verastegui, M., Rodrigues, S., Gavidia, C., Tsang, V.C.W., Falcon, N., Lescano, A.G., Moulton, L.H., Bernal, T., Tovar, M., The Cysticercosis Working Group in Peru, 2003. Hyperendemic human and porcine *Taenia solium* infection in Peru. Am. J. Trop. Med. Hyg. 68, 268–275.

Hill, D.E., Haley, C., Wagner, B., Gamble, H.R., Dubey, J.P., 2009. Seroprevalence of and risk factors for *Toxoplasma gondii* in the U.S. swine herd using sera collected during the National Animal Health Monitoring Survey (Swine 2006). Zoonosis Public Health 57, 53–59.

National Pork Board, 2014. Pork Quality Assurance Program. http://porkcdn.s3.amazonaws.com/sites/all/files/documents/PQAPlus/V2.0/TrainingAdults/PQAPlusEducationHandbookVersion2.0.pdf.

Sarti, E., Flisser, A., Schantz, P.M., Gleizer, M., Loya, M., Plancarte, A., Avila, G., Allan, J., Craig, P., Bronfman, M., Wijeyaratne, P., 1997. Development and evaluation of a health education intervention against *Taenia solium* in a rural community in Mexico. Am. J. Trop. Med. Hyg. 56, 127–132.

Tobin, M.E., Fall, M.W., 2004. Pest Control: Rodents. USDA National Wildlife Research Center, Staff Publications, Paper 67.

U.S. Code of Federal Regulations, Title 7: Agriculture, Part 205—National Organic Program, Subpart C—Organic Production and Handling Requirements, Washington, DC.

USDA, 2011. National Organic Program, Guidance on Compost and Vermicompost in Organic Crop Production. http://www.ams.usda.gov/AMSv1.0/getfile?dDocName=STELPRDC5090756.

Foodborne parasites and climate change: Possible impacts and challenges

3

L.R. Polley
University of Saskatchewan, Saskatoon, SK, Canada

3.1 Introduction

A look around the world reveals many patterns for the occurrence and importance of foodborne parasites. Whether the foods consumed come from a vertically integrated, globalized supply system, from a farmers' market, from a single local producer, from a small garden, from or a hunting trip or favorite fishing spot, the determinants of these patterns are similar. They include the foods and parasites involved, the structure and function of the food supply system "from farm to fork," the likelihood of foods being infected or contaminated by parasites transmissible to people, and the risk of these infected animals or contaminated animal tissues or plants being consumed by people. Also important are the overall health and well-being of the people at risk and of animal sources of the parasites, the vitality of public health programs, and cultural practices, which can have several points of contact with a food supply system. Despite many advances in our understanding of these parasites, they remain an important health burden in many parts of the world (Torgerson et al., 2014).

The current episode of climate change has many components, but most often listed are warming temperatures, rising and warming oceans, shifts in precipitation patterns, and an increase in the frequency and severity of extreme climate and weather events. These are continuing to evolve, with shifts in their spatial and temporal distributions and force. Climate change envelops our world, affecting land, freshwater, oceans, flora, and fauna, including people, together with the links within and between these components of our planet's biosphere (IPCC, 2014a). The persistence and transmission of foodborne parasites among animal and human hosts depend on many of these links, and the parasites, hosts, and links all have vulnerabilities to the new climate, which can affect parasite occurrence and significance in two ways: directly and indirectly (Mas-Coma et al., 2008). In many situations, these effects of climate change might result in quantitative or temporal shifts in preexisting parasite transmission patterns, but sometimes these shifts, perhaps coupled with other changes in the local ecosystem, are such that a tipping point is reached, and transmission and many other features of the host–parasite system are radically altered (e.g., Kutz et al., 2005).

The new climate also has the potential to affect many aspects of the structure and function of ecosystems, generating a range of consequences for human and animal health, many of which will likely not be recognized or quantified until they have major

Foodborne Parasites in the Food Supply Web. http://dx.doi.org/10.1016/B978-1-78242-332-4.00003-5

effects on people and/or animals. Looking at all foodborne pathogen groups, it is clear that the links between the pathogens and the new climate are very complex, as are the steps required to develop and implement plans for surveillance, prevention, management of infection and disease in people, and the prediction of future possibilities (Tirado et al., 2010). It is interesting that a search of the 2014 report from Working Group II of Intergovernmental Panel on Climate Change (IPCC) found no mention of foodborne parasites under food security and food production systems (Chapter 7), or under human health (Chapter 11) (IPCC, 2014a). This is perhaps because the infections and the diseases they cause in people are considered to be of limited significance relative to all the other impacts of climate change. Similarly, literature searches using "climate change" and the complete or abbreviated genus names of the parasites on the FAO/WHO 2014 list of priority foodborne parasites (FAO/WHO, 2014) result in few publications for many of the parasites (Web of Science, 1900–2014, accessed March 1, 2014): anisakids—8; *Ascaris lumbricoides*—1; *Toxocara canis*—5; *Trichinella* in pigs—3; *Trichinella* in wildlife—9; *Trichuris trichiura*—5; *Diphyllobothrium*—3; *Echinococcus granulosus*—4; *Echinococcus multilocularis*—11; *Spirometra*—0; *Taenia saginata*—0; *Taenia solium*—0; *T. solium* cysticercosis—0; *Fasciola hepatica*—34; Heterophyids—1; *Opisthorchis*—3; *Paragonimus*—5; *Balantidium coli*—1; *Cryptosporidium*—46 (many of these include *Giardia* and/or waterborne transmission); *Cyclospora cayetanensis*—5; *Entamoeba histolytica*—5; *Giardia*—30 (many of these include *Cryptosporidium* and/or waterborne transmission); *Toxoplasma gondii*—30; and *Trypanosoma cruzi*—11. Also noteworthy is that many of these publications make reference only to climate change as a possible driver for shifts in the ecology of the parasites, without empirical data.

The direct effects of climate change result from exposure of parasites to the climate while in the environment or in ectothermic hosts. For example, shifts in environmental temperatures, and/or in the amount and spatial and temporal distributions of precipitation, can alter development and mortality rates of parasite life-cycle stages thus exposed, local to global spatial distributions of parasites, and contacts between hosts and parasites (van Dijk et al., 2010). These direct effects of climate change can also be important in the ecology of ectothermic hosts, whether those consumed by people (e.g., fish, crustaceans, bivalves) or those essential for the development of immature stages of parasites (e.g., snails for trematodes). The spatial distributions, health, reproduction, development and mortality rates, and sustainability of these ectothermic hosts are all linked in some way to climate. Some ectotherms, however, can exhibit adaptive behavior which, within limits, protects them from unfavorable changes in their local environment. For example, warm temperatures induce some terrestrial gastropods to move to cooler areas of their habitats (Rollo, 1991). Also, local spatial distributions of aquatic ectothermic hosts (e.g., snails) often follow shifts in the distribution of surface water, in some cases resulting from climate change. These shifts can, therefore, alter the footprints of parasite transmission, and of parasite infection and disease in people and in animals (Mas-Coma et al., 2009).

The indirect effects of climate change on the parasites are mediated through the hosts, including ectotherms and their shared ecosystems (Figure 3.1). For example, changes in the overall health and well-being of the animal and/or human hosts might

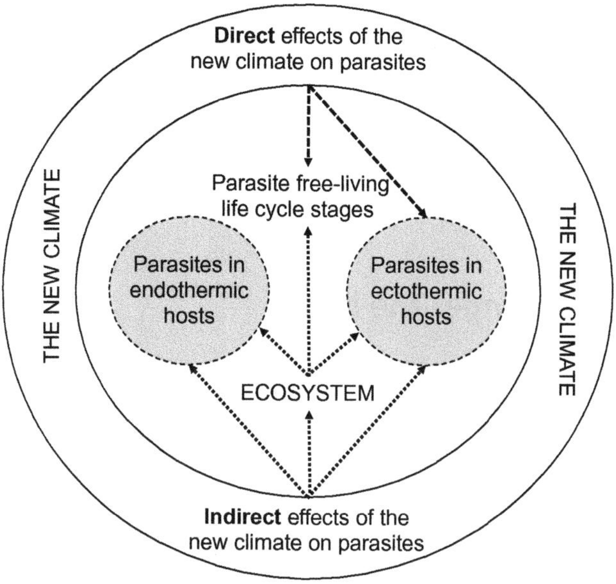

Figure 3.1 Possible linkages between climate change, hosts, parasites, and ecosystems.

result from, and/or lead to, shifts in the prevalence and abundance of foodborne parasites in these hosts, and thereby in the availability of life-cycle stages capable of infecting other animals and people, or of contaminating foods. As well as these possible host-centered effects of the changing climate, others are ecosystem-centered and could have a major influence, both positive and negative, on the occurrence of foodborne parasites and their significance for human and animal health. Examples include the availability of hosts—definitive, intermediate, and paratenic—required for the completion of life cycles and/or important as reservoirs of infection, an environment that will sustain hosts and parasites, freedom from pathogens that can adversely affect the hosts and from biotic factors that can adversely affect the parasites (Thieltges et al., 2008), and freedom from other stressors. In some instances, reduction or removal of some of these ecosystem-based supports can be used to reduce the occurrence of parasites in or on foods of animal and plant origin (e.g., draining habitats used by the snail intermediate hosts of *F. hepatica*).

After introductions to climate change, foodborne parasites, and food supply systems, and using specific examples where available, this chapter explores the possible impacts of the shifting climate on each phase of supply systems for foods of animal and plant origin, bearing in mind variations in the scale and complexity of the systems—from hunter-gatherers to multinational food businesses. Parasite infection in animal tissues is differentiated from parasite contamination of plants and animals, as are direct and indirect effects of the new climate on the parasites. Finally, some general priorities for climate change and this important group of parasites are discussed, together with some of the possibilities for future developments in their occurrence and management in a changing world. Because of the scarcity of empirical data on the linkages between climate change and foodborne parasites, many of the possible outcomes presented include elements of conjecture, but what is known now about the new climate and the parasites can form a useful basis for peering into the future.

This chapter is not intended to be a catalog of all the published observations on climate change and foodborne parasites. Its goal instead is to offer a landscape illustrating the nature and extent of this globally important focus in animal and human health and to provide a context for understanding its past, present, and future.

3.2 Climate change: The basics

The current episode of global climate change includes warming temperatures; shifts in the amounts, types, and spatial and temporal distributions of precipitation; shifts in hydrology; shifts in the timing of the seasons; melting glaciers and icecaps; reduced snow cover; warming oceans and rising sea levels; and increased frequency and severity of extreme climate and weather events (IPCC, 2014a). These changes vary with time and place, and it is often difficult to predict with any accuracy what, when, where, how much, and with what results. They can, however, be linked to at least some of the heatwaves (e.g., western Europe, 2003; Australia 2014), frigid winters (e.g., North America, 2013–2014), floods (Sudan and Somalia, 2013), droughts (e.g., northeastern Brazil and southern China, 2013), and storms and coastal inundations (e.g., typhoon Haiyan, Philippines, 2013) (see World Meteorological Organization, 2014). However, attributing these events to the new climate can be difficult (see IPCC, 2014a; World Meteorological Organization, 2014). Nevertheless, individually and in various combinations, components of climate change could affect the ecology of foodborne parasites, most importantly the risk of transmission to people. Also often difficult to predict is the degree to which the results of shifts in the climate will trend "positive," "negative," or "neutral" for the occurrence of foodborne parasites, and how the trend for a particular location might change with time (see Paull and Johnson, 2014).

As the new climate has come to affect ever more aspects of life on earth, people around the world are developing strategies for adaptation and mitigation (IPCC, 2014a,b). The former seeks to alter systems and behaviors to take advantage of the positive features of climate change and to minimize its negative effects, and the latter to reduce or neutralize the drivers of the change. Where needed, these strategies can be applied to supply systems for foods of animal and plant origin, especially the production phase (Morgan and Wall, 2009). The degree of development and adoption of mitigation and adaptation strategies depends on the severity of local shifts in the climate, and on many political, economic, and sociological factors and therefore tend to vary with place and time. Over the long term, domestic animal and wildlife hosts, plants, and the foodborne parasites might also take advantage of opportunities to adopt adaptation strategies to help them survive, and sometimes thrive, in the midst of the new climate.

For the parasites there is empirical evidence for some of the direct effects of climate change, particularly on the free-living life-cycle stages of helminths (e.g. *Ascaris* spp., *Echinococcus* spp.) and enteric protozoans (e.g., *Cryptosporidium* spp. and *Giardia* spp.). The indirect effects are less well understood, however, primarily because of the complexity of the mechanisms generating the effects, of the methods needed to detect and measure them, and of the inevitable variations with parasite and host species, local ecosystems, foods involved, and the precise structure and functioning of the affected food supply system. Despite these limitations, it is possible to identify, or to hypothesize, some of the impacts that the new climate might have on the risks of foodborne parasite transmission to people.

3.3 Food supply systems: The basics

Regardless of the location around the world, and the scale (from local to global), foods pass through some or all of the various phases of a food supply system (farm to fork): production, harvest, inspection, storage, processing, distribution, retailing, and in-home practices, particularly storage and preparation (Vermeulen et al., 2012; Chapters 2 and 14). Components of many of these phases are susceptible to the effects of climate change, and the characteristics of each phase vary with food, location, economic well-being, infrastructure, and cultural practices. To infect people, parasites must survive a wide range of environmental conditions in the supply system, as well as any measures taken to neutralize them or remove them from the system (Figure 3.2).

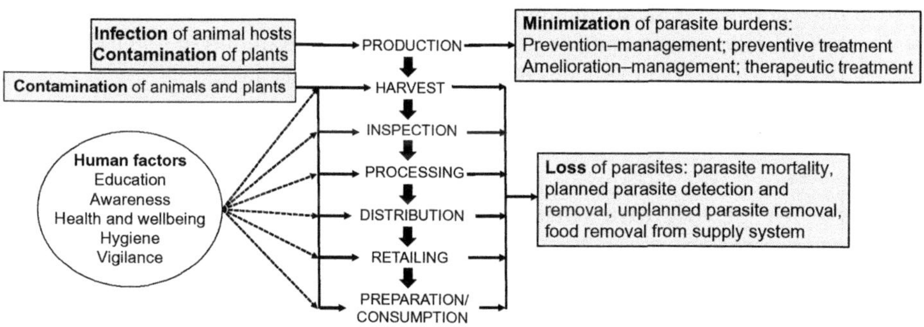

Figure 3.2 Parasites and the phases of food supply systems.

A particular concern, primarily in regions of the world with emerging economies, are parasites in or on foods originating from wildlife or from wild plants (see Chapter 4). Some of these parasites (and other pathogens) might not yet have been identified, nor have their life cycles elucidated, or their potential impacts on human health known, or their sensitivities to climate change understood. Some of these wildlife, and probably to a lesser extent plants, are exported and consumed as "exotic" foods in other, often more affluent parts of the world. Estimates indicate that the scale of consumption of these wildlife where harvested, and elsewhere, is very significant (Karesh and Cook, 2005; Lindsey et al., 2013), although accurate data are difficult to find. Globally, this bushmeat trade is also a significant threat to wildlife conservation.

An additional risk linked to climate change that might affect the ability of food supply systems to deliver safe foods is relaxation by government and other agencies of system monitoring to detect and manage foodborne parasites and to minimize the possibility of human infection. The extent and effectiveness of this monitoring varies around the world (Chapter 17), and relaxation can result from a number of factors including reduced human and financial resources, problems with the infrastructure supporting the monitoring, climatic events disrupting the food supply system, and the overall health and well-being of those responsible for inspection.

3.4 Foodborne parasites: The basics

Globally, foodborne parasites include many helminths and protozoa. Multiple species have been identified (Chapters 6–10), but a recent report from an FAO/WHO Expert Committee identified 24 as high global priorities (Tables 3.1 and 3.2; FAO/WHO, 2014). These and other foodborne parasites can be usefully grouped into those that are present in the tissues of infected animals consumed by people and those that contaminate foods of animal and plant origin prior to consumption by people.

Foodborne parasites that infect animals include the larval stages of a variety of nematodes (e.g., *Trichinella* spp.), cestodes (e.g., *T. saginata*), and tissue cysts of the protozoan *T. gondii* (Table 3.1). Animals acquire these parasites only prior to harvest (slaughter), most often by the ingestion of infective stages (e.g., larvae of *Trichinella* spp. in muscle tissue of many mammals, eggs of *T. saginata* in human feces, oocysts of *T. gondii* in felid feces), and less commonly by skin penetration (e.g., larvae of the trematodes *Opisthorchis* in fish and *Paragonimus* in crustaceans).

Table 3.1 Parasites infecting foods: parasite life-cycle stages infective for people and sources of these stages

Parasite	Parasite group	Parasite life-cycle stage infective for people	Source(s) of infection for people
Taenia saginata	Cestode	Cysticercus	Cattle
Taenia solium	Cestode	Cysticercus	Pigs
Sarcocystis spp.	Protozoan	Sarcocyst	Cattle, pigs
Toxoplasma	Protozoan	Tissue cyst	Various mammals (pigs, sheep, wildlife); chickens
Trichinella spp.	Nematode	Larva	Various mammals (pigs, wildlife, horses); crocodiles
Anisakids	Nematode	Larva	Marine fish
Diphyllobothridae	Cestode	Plerocercoid	Marine and freshwater fish
Spirometra spp.	Cestode	Procercoid or plerocercoid	Freshwater crustaceans and fish; various mammals, reptiles, and amphibians
Opisthorchidae	Trematode	Metacercaria	Freshwater fish
Heterophyidae	Trematode	Metacercaria	Brackish and freshwater fish
Paragonimus spp.	Trematode	Metacercaria	Freshwater crustaceans; pigs

Table 3.2 Parasites contaminating foods: parasite life-cycle stages infective for people and sources of these stages

Parasite	Parasite group	Parasite life-cycle stage contaminating foods	Source(s) of life-cycle stage contaminating foods
Ascaris lumbricoides	Nematode	Egg	Human feces
Trichuris trichiura	Nematode	Egg	Human feces
Cyclospora cayetanensis	Protozoan	Oocyst	Human feces
Entamoeba histolytica	Protozoan	Cyst	Human feces
Cryptosporidium spp.	Protozoan	Oocyst	Human and various animal feces
Giardia spp.	Protozoan	Cyst	Human and various animal feces
Toxocara spp.	Nematode	Egg	Canid feces
Echinococcus granulosus	Cestode	Egg	Canid feces
Echinococcus multilocularis	Cestode	Egg	Canid (and felid) feces
Toxoplasma gondii	Protozoan	Oocyst	Felid feces
Ascaris suum	Nematode	Egg	Pig feces
Balantidium coli	Protozoan	Cyst	Pig feces
Fasciola hepatica	Trematode	Metacercaria	Snails (acquire parasite from feces of various mammals)

Foodborne parasites that contaminate plant and animal products consumed by people include the eggs of a variety of nematodes (e.g., *A. lumbricoides*) and cestodes (e.g., *E. granulosus*), together with oocysts (e.g., *Cryptosporidium*, *Cyclospora*, *T. gondii*) and cysts (e.g., *Giardia* spp.) of a variety of protozoans (Table 3.2). The eggs, oocysts, and cysts come ultimately from the feces of infected hosts, human and/or animal. Other life-cycle stages are occasionally involved in contamination, for example, infective larvae of the nematode *Angiostrongylus* spp., free or in gastropod and other intermediate and paratenic hosts and consumed with salads and other plants (Wang et al., 2008), and infective stages of the protozoan *T. cruzi* in fruit juices containing the parasite's hemipteran vectors and/or their feces contaminating the fruit used for juice production (Alarcón de Noya et al., 2010).

Parasite contamination of plants consumed by people can occur during any phase of the food supply system, including production, whereas contamination of foods of animal origin, other than some invertebrates (e.g., bivalves), can occur only during harvest and subsequently. For some foodborne parasites (e.g., *F. hepatica* metacercariae on aquatic plants) contamination of plants is essential for parasite transmission, for others it is incidental (e.g., *Cyclospora* oocysts on raspberries). Contamination of both animal and plant products poses a particular risk where the food is consumed, especially shortly after harvest, without inspection or measures to remove or neutralize the parasites.

Several features of the biology of foodborne parasites are important determinants of their vulnerabilities to the various components of climate change, of their responses, and of the consequences for people consuming the affected foods. For example, depending on the species, during completion of their life cycles, many foodborne parasites pass through a range of external environments, as well as one or more hosts, in some species including ectotherms, thereby exposing them to both the direct and indirect effects of climate change (Table 3.3).

Parasites infecting animals require a period of development in the host to become infective for people (days, weeks, or months, depending primarily on the parasite species). Similarly, parasites of many of the species contaminating foods require a period of development in the environment (generally days to weeks, depending on parasite species and temperature and moisture) to become infective (e.g., oocysts of *Toxoplasma*; eggs of *A. lumbricoides*), but some contaminating parasites are infective when they are excreted by the definitive hosts (e.g., oocysts of *Cryptosporidium* and cysts of *Giardia*; eggs of *Taenia* and *Echinococcus*). Additionally, for many of the contaminating parasites there are many sources of human infection other than contaminated foods, including the feces of people, and/or domestic animals and/or wildlife.

3.5 Climate change, food supply systems, and foodborne parasites: From producer to consumer

Within any food supply system there are four factors that can have major effects on the parasite's significance for human health. One, education and awareness of people involved in all phases of the system regarding the potential risks linked to foodborne parasites, both with and without the complications of climate change, and how these risks can be minimized. Two, the effectiveness of public health programs, particularly those related to food safety. Three, the health and well-being of the animal and human hosts, particularly in terms of nutrition, resistance and immunity, and concurrent disease; healthy hosts are usually less susceptible to parasitic infection and disease, and healthy people are likely more interested in learning about the parasites and more vigilant in protecting foods from parasitic infection and contamination, and in avoiding potentially infected and contaminated foods; as a result, healthy hosts, both human and animal, are less likely to become sources of parasites for others. Four, the availability and use of clean, pathogen-free water during all phases of the food supply system, from production to consumption (see Kirby et al., 2003); clean water is particularly important for fruits and vegetables, other foods of plant origin, and foods that are eaten without cooking, or without pickling, salting, drying, or other methods of preservation, the effects of which on the viability of infecting or contaminating parasites are uncertain.

Each component of climate change also has the potential to impact the various phases of a food supply system (Table 3.4). Some of these impacts will be seen commonly, some occasionally, and others rarely, and their occurrence and extent will vary

Table 3.3 **Foodborne parasites with life-cycle stages in the environment and/or in ectothermic hosts, and source(s) of human infection**

Parasite	Life-cycle stages in the environment	Life-cycle stages in ectothermic hosts	Source(s) of human infection
Nematodes			
Anisakids	+	+	Marine mammals > marine fish and squid
Ascaris lumbricoides	+		People > environment[a]
Ascaris spp.	+		Pigs > environment
Toxocara spp.	+		Canids > environment
Trichinella spiralis			Muscle tissue of various mammals > muscle tissue of various mammals
Trichinella spp.			Muscle tissue of various mammals and crocodiles > muscle tissue of various mammals and crocodiles
Trichuris trichiura	+		People > environment
Cestodes			
Diphyllobothridae	+	+	Piscivorous mammals and birds > copepods > freshwater/marine fish
Echinococcus granulosus	+		Canids > environment
Echinococcus multilocularis	+		Canids/felids > environment
Spirometra spp.	+	+	Mammals > copepods > freshwater crustaceans and fish and various mammals, reptiles and amphibians[b]
Taenia saginata/T. solium	+		People > muscle tissue of cattle/pigs
Taenia solium cysticercosis in people	+		Pig tissues > people > environment
Trematodes			
Fasciola spp.	+	+	Various mammals > snails > freshwater plants
Heterophyidae	+	+	Piscivorous mammals > snails > fresh/brackish water fish
Opisthorchidae	+	+	Piscivorous mammals > snails > freshwater fish
Paragonimus spp.	+	+	Piscivorous mammals > snails > freshwater crustaceans
Protozoa			
Balantidium coli	+		Pigs/people > environment
Cryptosporidium spp.	+		People/animals/birds > environment
Cyclospora cayetanensis	+		People > environment
Entamoeba histolytica	+		People > environment
Giardia spp.	+		People/animals/birds > environment
Sarcocystis spp.	+		Various carnivores > cattle/pig tissues
Toxoplasma gondii	+		Felids > environment[a] > animal tissues
Trypanosoma cruzi	+	+	Arthropod vectors/fruit juices

Notes: Sources underlined transmit infection directly to people. Sources preceding these are required for life-cycle completion but are not involved in this direct transmission.

[a] Environment includes water as a possible source of infection.

[b] People are the second intermediate, not definitive hosts.

Table 3.4 Potential linkages between the major components of climate change and food supply systems

Phase of food supply system	Climate change feature							
	Warming air temperatures	Shifts in precipitation patterns	Shifts in hydrology	Shifts in timing of seasons	Reduced snow cover	Melting glaciers and icecaps	Warming oceans and rising sea levels	Increased incidence and severity of extreme climatic events
Production	●	●	●	●	●	●	●	●
Harvest	●	●	●	●	●	●	●	●
Inspection	●	●	●	●	●	●	●	●
Storage	●	●	●	●	●	●	●	●
Processing	●	●	●	●	●	●	●	●
Distribution	●	●	●	●	●	●	●	●
Retailing	●	●	●	●	●	●	●	●
In-home practices	●	●	●	●	●	●	●	●

The frequency and significance of these linkages vary with parasite, place, and time.

with the climatic component(s) involved, the parasites, the type of food, the location, and the structure and resilience of the affected food supply system (Table 3.5).

3.6 Examples of linkages between foodborne parasites and climate change

Although the new climate seems to have a role in changes in the distribution and occurrence of some foodborne parasites, these shifts could also be influenced by many other structural and functional features of the ecosystems they share with the hosts. These components include increasing urbanization, changes in land use, and movements of hosts and parasites, either actively into new areas that support the life cycles of both or passively and sometimes inadvertently as a result of human intervention. In many cases it is proving difficult to determine which of the various drivers, including climate change, are involved in a particular situation, and their precise roles in the shifts in parasite ecology, and in the occurrence of human infection and disease. Another complicating factor is that in any location at any time, different climatic factors can have opposing effects on the parasites and hosts. For example, warming temperatures might speed development of a parasite's free-living stages, while concurrent drought might increase their mortality rates.

Table 3.5 Potentially climate-sensitive factors affecting animal and plant production and food supply systems

	Potential to affect key requirements for an animal production system	Potential to affect key requirements for a plant production system	Potential to affect key requirements for a food supply system
Food quality, quantity, and supply	●		
Soil quality and fertility		●	
Water quality, quantity, and supply reliability	●	●	●
Energy availability and supply reliability	●	●	●
Other infrastructure	●	●	●
Overall animal management	●		
Animal reproduction	●		
Seed quality, quantity, and supply reliability		●	
Overall animal and plant health status	●	●	
Food supply system integrity			●
Compliance with internal and external regulations	●	●	●
Production and supply system economics	●	●	●
Structure and function of production ecosystem host fauna: definitive, intermediate and paratenic, other animals, invasive species, and pests	●	●	
Structure and function of production ecosystem flora, invasive species, and pests	●	●	
Structure and function of production ecosystem parasite fauna, including invasive species	●	●	
Worker health and well-being	●	●	●
Worker education and awareness	●	●	●
Worker vigilance	●	●	●
Worker and system hygiene	●	●	●
Anticipated and unanticipated external and internal challenges to system structure and function	●	●	●

Among regions of the world hardest hit already by climate change is the North American Arctic (Davidson et al., 2011; Jenkins et al., 2013; Kutz et al., 2005). Here the effects of the new climate on foodborne parasites are potentially important because local residents, following traditional cultural practices, consume many wildlife species, sometimes with the risk of human infections.

3.6.1 Echinococcus canadensis *and* Echinococcus multilocularis—*Source: Contaminated foods*

Empirical data for *Echinococcus* spp. demonstrating the possible linkages between the new climate and the occurrence of foodborne infection of people is more or less limited to the effects of various climatic factors on the development and mortality rates of the eggs in the feces of carnivore definitive hosts. There are, however, many other factors that could have a role in determining occurrence, transmission patterns, and health significance of these parasites. For example, Jenkins et al. (2011, 2013), considering *E. canadensis*—a species currently maintained in wildlife in many parts of Canada—mentioned climate-linked changes in the geographic distribution and abundance of cervid intermediate hosts as perhaps shifting the footprint and abundance of the parasite in carnivore definitive hosts, which are sources of human infections. Also listed was the possibility that heavy rains might wash the eggs of *Echinococcus* into sources of water consumed or otherwise used by people. For *E. multilocularis* in North America, Jenkins et al. (2011, 2013) listed climate-induced shifts in the geographic distribution and abundance of definitive and intermediate hosts as possible influences on the occurrence and transmission of the parasite, and on its potential to infect people. Similar drivers were identified by Atkinson et al. (2013) for *Echinococcus* species. Also, for *E. multilocularis*, it is possible that the various genotypes recently described in Canada (Gesy et al., 2014) might have different ecological characteristics and vary in their susceptibility to climate change and in their effects on human and animal hosts. A similar approach might prove useful for other foodborne parasites with multiple genotypes (e.g., *Cryptosporidium*, *Giardia*, and *Toxoplasma*).

3.6.2 Trichinella *spp.—Source: Infected foods*

As with several other foodborne parasites, much of the discussion of the possible effects of climate change on *Trichinella* spp. has focused on the parasite in northern North America. For example, Rausch et al. (2007) suggested that changes in the extent and duration of sea ice in this region could impact the feeding behavior, diet, and parasite fauna of pagophilic (ice-dependent) marine mammals, especially walrus, seal, and polar bear, which are important sources of food for northern peoples. These changes might affect transmission patterns of *T. nativa* and *Trichinella* T6, the northern species of *Trichinella*, which could become more prevalent and more abundant in wildlife consumed by people, with possibly an increased risk of human disease. Also migration routes of marine and terrestrial mammals might change in response to the new climate, which could lead to shifts in the food webs essential for *Trichinella* transmission (Jenkins et al., 2013).

3.6.3 Toxoplasma gondii—*Source: Infected and contaminated foods*

Climate change could affect the occurrence and significance of this parasite in both terrestrial and marine ecosystems. In the first, changes in the distribution and abundance of the felid definitive hosts and in food webs, both key elements of transmission for *T. gondii* and potentially sensitive to climate change, could lead to shifts in environmental contamination with oocysts, in the occurrence and significance of the tissue stages of the parasite in animals consumed by people, and in the parasite's significance in people. In marine systems, increases in precipitation on land can lead to increased runoff of *T. gondii* oocysts into rivers and oceans, with altered risk of infection in marine mammals and invertebrates (Miller et al., 2008; Van Bressem et al., 2009) as a result of ingestion of either the oocysts or of invertebrates, particularly bivalves, that accumulate oocysts through filter-feeding. Consumption by people of either the infected mammals or the contaminated invertebrates risks *T. gondii* infection and disease. In the North American Arctic, where *T. gondii* occurs despite the absence of felids, a recent hydrological modeling study suggested that the spring snowmelt in inland areas where felids are present might result in oocysts being carried downstream, with contamination of estuarine areas sufficient to infect mammals and invertebrates feeding there (Simon et al., 2013). Additionally, ocean warming linked to climate change could affect the development and survival of *T. gondii* oocysts. In marine and presumably terrestrial systems, shifts in climate could also result in increased animal mortalities leading to increased transmission by scavenging (see Burek et al., 2008).

3.6.4 Fasciola hepatica—*Source: Contaminated foods*

In common with other trematodes, the life cycle of *F. hepatica* has many points of sensitivity to a changing climate, most notably the essential ectothermic snail intermediate hosts, the fluke's free-living life-cycle stages in the environment, and the developing stages in the snails. The links between climate and fluke transmission are much studied, and in the 1950s led to the development of a forecasting system for *F. hepatica* infection and disease in livestock in the United Kingdom (Ollerenshaw and Rowlands, 1959). Subsequently, additional approaches have been developed for fluke forecasting and applied in several areas of the world where *F. hepatica* is a significant threat to animal and/or human health (see Fox et al., 2011). While very few data are available for *F. hepatica*, within minimum and maximum limits and assuming adequate moisture, warming temperatures were thought to increase development rates of the immature stages of trematodes in snails (Paull and Johnson, 2011) as well as increasing the production and release of cercariae (Poulin, 2006). These effects appear not to be consistent among trematodes, however, leaving uncertain the links between climate and these components of fluke transmission (Morley and Lewis, 2013).

Climate can also affect the ecology of the snails which, in turn, can influence *F. hepatica* transmission and its occurrence and significance (Rapsch et al., 2008). A key feature of this ecology is the ability of the snails to colonize new environments, and thus facilitate the spread of *F. hepatica* into new areas (Mas-Coma et al., 2009).

Hydrological changes resulting from climate change—specifically the creation of temporary or permanent habitats supportive of the snails—could facilitate this colonization. *F. hepatica* is also able to infect a wide range of domestic animal and wildlife definitive hosts, which can serve as reservoirs of the parasite. Any effects of climate change on the availability of these hosts might, therefore, enhance or inhibit the fluke's geographic spread and maintenance in traditional and in newly occupied areas.

Fasciolosis (fascioliasis) is considered an emerging and reemerging disease of livestock and people in several areas of the world, an evolving status likely to be the result of many factors, including climate change. A recent study in the United Kingdom combining Ollerenshaw's forecasting method with climate records for 1970–2000 and climate projections for 2020–2070 indicated a steady increase in the risk of livestock infection over these periods, although this change did not affect all areas equally (Fox et al., 2011). These findings provide some support for potential linkages between climate change and the occurrence of fasciolosis in livestock in the United Kingdom.

3.7 Direct effects of climate change during production

Climate change can directly affect both survival and development rates, and thus abundance, of any parasite life-cycle stages that are free-living or in ectothermic hosts in either terrestrial or aquatic environments. Examples of these stages include eggs and developing larvae of nematodes (e.g., anisakids), eggs and aquatic life-cycle stages of trematodes (e.g., eggs, miracidia, and cercariae of *Opisthorchis*), cestodes (e.g., eggs of *Taenia* and eggs and coracidia of *Diphyllobothrium*), and protozoa (e.g., cysts of *Giardia* and oocysts of *Toxoplasma*). Particularly important are shifts in temperature and in patterns of precipitation. In general, given adequate moisture, and within limits, warmer temperatures accelerate parasite development in the environment and in ectothermic hosts, but too warm or too cool temperatures can slow development and/or increase parasite mortality, and increase host mortality, especially if there is insufficient moisture. This linkage between parasites, hosts, and the environment is complicated, however, by species differences in both the ideal conditions for the parasites in the environment and in ectothermic hosts, and in the nature and magnitude of the parasite's response to minor and major changes in climate. In terrestrial ecosystems, excessive precipitation (e.g., severe rain storms, large-scale melts of snow and ice, and floods) can lead to contamination of drinking water supplies with the infective stages of foodborne parasites (e.g., oocysts of *Cryptosporidium* and *Toxoplasma* and cysts of *Giardia*) and to potentially parasite-contaminated overflows from sewage treatment plants (Patz et al., 2008).

Ocean warming as a result of climate change, sometimes in combination with other drivers, can affect the distribution, abundance, species richness, and ecology of many of the organisms—both hosts and parasites—living in the oceans (Kaschner et al., 2011; Marcogliese, 2008; Sadorus et al., 2014). Of particular concern for foodborne parasites are the various vertebrates and invertebrates consumed by people. Some of these foods, for example, fish, marine mammals, and crustaceans can be infected; and others, for example, filter-feeding bivalves, can be contaminated with the life-cycle stages of parasites infective for people.

Short-term, long-term, or permanent shifts in ocean boundaries, whether natural (perhaps linked to climate change) or managed, also risk introduction of aquatic host and parasite species into new areas. Rising sea levels, caused in part by increased water flow from the land, can lead to erosion and inundation of coastal areas, with disruption of local ecosystems, natural or managed, from which fish, crustaceans, and bivalves are harvested for food. These changes in ocean boundaries, even when temporary, together with the ocean-warming characteristic of climate change, might also result in altered development and mortality rates and abundance of the parasites' life-cycle stages in the water and in ectothermic hosts, and of the aquatic hosts, and thereby could affect the risk of infection in the fish and other seafood consumed by people.

3.8 Indirect effects of climate change during production

Climate change could shift the local to global spatial distributions, abundance, and transmission of foodborne parasites indirectly through effects on the animal hosts, including the ectotherms, on people at risk of infection, and on other constituents of the ecosystem essential for the sustainability of these hosts and parasites. Possible results of these shifts include altered contacts between hosts and parasites causing transient or permanent interruptions, increases, or decreases in parasite transmission, with subsequent changes in the risk of animal and human infection. Also important are the ways in which the new climate might alter the overall health and well-being of the human and animal hosts, making them more or less susceptible to infection with these parasites and to other diseases. Among the triggers for these changes in health status are shifts in several factors linked to the local ecosystem, especially the level of nutrition, the availability of clean water, immune competence, concurrent disease, shelter, and social structure, including access to appropriate medical and veterinary care. Also, for some foodborne parasites, if climate change affects the timing and characteristics of seasons, there could be disruption of synchronies linking parasite infective stages with susceptible animal hosts, the several host species required by some foodborne parasites for life-cycle completion, and those linking increased host needs for nutrients with food availability, especially during reproduction and rearing of young.

There are many ways in which climate change might indirectly affect ecosystem structure and function. Most important are shifts in ecosystem services, especially the production of foods essential to animals and/or people, the availability and quality of water, and the ability to adapt to the new climate and other stressors while sustaining sufficient productivity. Key threats to these services are climate-driven changes in the structure of the flora and fauna, especially shifts in the relative abundance of native species and the establishment of invasive species that could curtail or even obliterate native animals and plants, including those harvested for animal and human food. These reorderings of the flora and fauna might also lead to changes in the animal species involved in food webs, many of which are important in the transmission of some foodborne parasites.

One of the key features of animal, fruit, and vegetable production around the world is the use of animal and sometimes human feces as fertilizer applied by or for the producer. Additionally, defecation by farm workers and other people in areas shared with animals or with fruits or vegetables can lead to infection of the animals or contamination of the fruits and vegetables. These animal and human feces sometimes contain the infective stages of zoonotic parasites that can eventually infect or contaminate foods consumed by people (e.g., *Cryptosporidium*, *Giardia*, *T. saginata*). Some food producers are particularly dependent on these natural fertilizers and also often discourage or prohibit the use of many drugs for parasite control in their animals. Despite measures taken to neutralize parasite life-cycle stages in manure, it is possible that in some circumstances this type of food production might result in a greater risk of human infection with foodborne parasites, in part because in some situations animals and perhaps people might be more likely to serve as reservoirs of infection.

The various elements of climate change might also lead to alterations in food production systems such that the parasite–food contacts are increased or reduced. Additionally, if the new climate becomes hostile, the stress generated in food producers and others working in food supply systems might lead to less vigilance in minimizing the risk of infection in animals and contamination of plants destined for consumption by people.

3.9 Climate change and harvest

There are many similarities between the direct effects of climate change on the free-living life-cycle stages of parasites contaminating foods and of those infecting foods of animal origin. As mentioned previously, however, there are more opportunities throughout the food system for climate change to impact contaminating parasites, perhaps most importantly by shifting parasite prevalence and abundance in both animals and people. These shifts could affect the risk of contamination of the foods during harvest, and of water in contact with the foods or with any of the equipment and tools used during the harvest, or that is consumed by the harvesters. Climate change could also disrupt sanitary facilities and other infrastructure, increasing the risk of fecal contamination of the foods and their surroundings during harvest. Another potentially important risk at harvest, and also at inspection, is cross-contamination of parasites among carcasses and animal products, and among fruits, vegetables, and other foods of plant origin. These problems might become more common if climate change or other stressors are adversely affecting the harvesters.

3.10 Climate change and food inspection

In many parts of the world, efforts are made during harvest to visually detect foodborne parasite species (e.g., cysticerci of *T. saginata* and *T. solium*, larvae of anisakids) in the tissues of their animal hosts and to neutralize them by treating the carcass so that the parasites are killed, or to remove all or part of the affected animal from the food supply. Some helminths (e.g., larvae of *Trichinella* and *Angiostrongylus*) and most protozoans (e.g., cysts of *Giardia* and tissue cysts of *Toxoplasma*) infecting or contaminating foods can be detected and identified only by the use of laboratory procedures, in the past microscopy and more recently immunological and molecular approaches. Routine use of these procedures is, however, beyond the current resources of many food-producing regions.

Climate change might indirectly affect the inspection process if it generates an increased risk of parasite infection in the inspectors or others involved in the process, or of contamination of the immediate surroundings or of any water used. The new climate might have other indirect effects on food inspection. For example, as for the production and harvest phases, it could result in compromised nutrition, inadequate shelter, and disease, which might reduce the ability of those involved in the inspections to maintain the required level of vigilance and in some cases might result in the reduction or termination of inspection efforts. Stress linked to climate might also result in lower levels of hygiene during the inspection process. These problems at the point of inspection could also spread within food safety systems, particularly if climate change adversely affected communication and integrity within the systems. A possible consequence could be the onward movement of foods in which infecting or contaminating parasites had not been detected and, therefore, of which consumers were not aware. Individually and together, these failures in food inspection can result in increased risks of human infection and disease.

3.11 Climate change and food storage

The storage of food might be required at any postproduction phase of food supply systems, and methods and duration vary considerably. For meat, other animal products, and fruits and vegetables, other than those consumed very soon after harvest or preserved in some way, cooling or freezing are required for storage, the latter particularly for meat and meat products. Freezing of foods can be an effective method to inactivate many, but not all, foodborne parasites, with consequent reductions in the risk of human infections. In many but not all situations, this requires electricity, or sometimes natural gas or propane. There are many components of climate change, notably extreme events, which might interrupt, or in some situations terminate, access to these energy sources. Additionally, flooding can affect all types of food storage facilities, and higher or lower environmental temperatures resulting from climate change might affect energy-free types of food storage, for example, below-ground cellars. However, if these disruptions to the conditions of storage are prolonged and the food deteriorates, in many instances the affected foods and any parasites surviving in or on them would very probably be removed from the food supply. In some cultures traditional methods of meat storage, for example, air-drying or fermentation in buried pouches, cannot be guaranteed to kill all zoonotic parasites present. Examples include the possibility of viable *Trichinella* larvae in nikku (air-dried meat) and igunaq (walrus or other marine mammal meat and fat stored in buried sealskin bags), both important foods for northern residents in Canada (Forbes et al., 2003; Leclair et al., 2004). Additionally, infective larvae of *Trichinella nativa*, common in wildlife in northern latitudes, can survive long periods of low-temperature freezing and alternating freezing and thawing (Davidson et al., 2008).

3.12 Climate change and food processing

Many processing techniques are available for meat and other animal products, for example, cooking, smoking, pickling, drying, freezing, and mixing with other foods of animal or plant origin, and to a lesser extent for fruits and vegetables, for example, freezing, chilling, cooking, canning, drying, or juicing. In some regions of the world most food processing occurs in large commercial operations, but in probably every country some is done by small-scale operators, including producers and retailers, and by consumers in their homes. If done properly, many commercial processing techniques should kill any infecting or contaminating parasites, and quality control measures in place in most situations should ensure that any serious problems with the processing as a result of climate change would result in the removal of affected products from the food supply. The situation can be very different, however, with processing on a smaller scale, especially if it is done less carefully. Examples of the effects of climate change on food processing include altering the prevalence and abundance of foodborne parasites in the foods, disrupting the infrastructure supporting the processing (e.g., clean water and energy supplies), damaging the integrity of the processing systems (e.g., as a result of extreme climatic events), and causing stress and illness in those responsible for the processing, leading to reduced vigilance.

3.13 Climate change and food distribution

Food systems around the world are dependent on distribution, whether from the farm to the local market, by truck or train within a country, or by truck, train, ship, or plane across international boundaries. All these transportation networks, vital for bringing food to consumers, are vulnerable to many of the effects of the new climate, especially changes in temperatures, precipitation patterns, and extreme events. These vulnerabilities can be important locally, regionally, nationally, or internationally. Probably their major effect is delay or prevention of the movement of foods, for example, because of weather-driven damage to transportation systems or to energy supplies. For fruits and vegetables, these delays, together with warmer temperatures resulting from climate change or refrigeration failure could facilitate the development of the infective stages of contaminating protozoa (e.g., *Cyclospora* and *Toxoplasma* oocysts). For these foods and for meats, increases in temperatures during distribution could also render the foods unfit for human consumption and should result in their removal from the food supply.

3.14 Climate change and food retailing

The selling of foods to consumers takes many forms, from large supermarkets, through small retail outlets, to local markets and "farm gate" sales where meats, fish and other seafood, fruits, and vegetables are purchased directly from the producers. Large supermarkets are often part of national or international conglomerates and are sometimes vertically integrated with production and most or all of the other phases of the food supply system. Globally the majority of these supermarkets depend on inspection protocols following harvest to remove parasite-infected animals from the food supply, on production and inspection standards that at least minimize the likelihood of parasite contamination of foods of animal and plant origin and, for nonprocessed foods, on supply systems designed to prevent parasite contamination during all phases from inspection to retailing. In regions with fewer economic resources, however, food inspection might be less rigorous or absent, especially for foods of plant origin. In some countries, retailers might wash lettuce, celery, and other salad vegetables, and perhaps other vegetables and some fruits, prior to display for sale, but this practice is not universal and might be absent where these food items are produced close to where they are sold and consumed, or where the supply of clean water is uncertain.

In both large and small food retailers, shifts in the risk of contamination of previously parasite-free fruits and vegetables, and of human infections with foodborne parasites, could result from the frequent handling by customers as they make their selections. For example, if someone has viable parasites on their hands they could transfer them to the produce and thence to another person. The parasites could also be transmitted by direct contact between fruits and vegetables that are contaminated and others that are not. Climate change might affect these risks of contamination by altering the prevalence and abundance of the parasites in or on foods, customers, retail staff, people working in other phases of the food supply system, especially in the immediate environment of the foods as they progress through the system.

An additional possible consequence for retailers of climate change, and perhaps other factors, is reduction, interruption, or termination of shipments from long-term suppliers, in some cases because of changes in systems of production. This could cause the retailers to seek new sources for the missing foods. Some of these sources might not adhere to the same standards of production, harvest, inspection, processing, and distribution as the previous suppliers, at least initially, and this could lead to an increased risk for consumers of both infecting and contaminating parasites. It is also possible that cultural changes in food preferences and in food preparation techniques, increasing "exotic" tourism, and the effects of climate change on food production, and on food prices, could lead to changes in the animal and plant species produced and harvested for consumption by people, perhaps with changes in the risks of parasite infection and contamination (Broglia and Kapel, 2011).

3.15 Climate change and food in the home and in food services: Storage, preparation, and consumption

Around the world, the home, restaurant, or other types of food service is the final stop for foods before consumption. Contamination of foods with parasites can occur in all these locations, even if all previous phases of the food supply system are working effectively in preventing parasite infection and contamination, and in dealing with any parasites detected. Fruits and vegetables are often eaten raw, and for these the most important parasite contaminants are the infective life-cycle stages of gastrointestinal protozoa and helminths of people and animals in the home. This contamination can occur as a result of increased parasite prevalence and abundance in people and animals, problems with storage similar to those in earlier phases of the supply system, inadequate washing of the vegetables and fruits, washing them with contaminated water, contaminated cutting surfaces and kitchen equipment, and probably most importantly, inadequate personal hygiene, especially hand washing, by the people handling and preparing the food. Infection and contamination of these individuals is a particular risk when they have been or are in close contact with either people or animals known or likely to be infected with foodborne parasites, or with other contaminated foods. The risk of human infections in the home could also be affected by social factors, most notably stress which might be a direct or indirect consequence of climate change, and which might lead to a reduction in the vigilance of food preparation.

In addition to fruits and vegetables, some fish, meats, and meat products are also eaten without cooking; these include sushi and sashimi (possibly infected with anisakids, *Diphyllobothrium*, or larval trematodes), seal and walrus (*Trichinella*), and steak tartare (*Cysticercus bovis*). This consumption of raw meats and fish can increase the likelihood of human infection with foodborne parasites, although the risk varies with location, with cultural practices, and with production, inspection, and food preparation.

3.16 Conclusions: Some priorities

There are many uncertainties surrounding the causes and effects of climate change and the potential and actual linkages between the new climate and the occurrence of foodborne parasites in or on foods and in people. The primary goals of global interest in this group of parasites, however, remain detection and prevention of infection and contamination of foods and of infection of people. To help achieve these goals several key priorities can be identified, all of which can be vulnerable to the pervasive effects of climate change.

First is the education of all those involved in food supply systems, regardless of scale, from producers to consumers, about the foodborne parasites that might infect or contaminate their foods or infect them. This is especially true of sources of infection and contamination and means of prevention. Coupled with this is education about the new climate and its actual and potential effects on the occurrence of these parasites.

Second are effective public health programs, especially those for food safety. Another priority is optimization of the health and well-being of all those who work in food supply systems and of the animals and plants destined for human consumption. The role of the new climate in this health and well-being will vary and could result in reductions, improvements, or no change in health status, or shifts with place and time between these three possible outcomes. Fourth are reliable supplies of clean water to help maintain health and to minimize the contamination of meats and other animal products, especially fruits and vegetables, as they progress through the various phases of the food supply system. The ranking of these priorities will likely change with local needs and will depend on political drive, expertise, and resources. But they also apply to many other challenges faced by millions around the world, and this should mean that there is hope for successful implementation, certainly on local and regional scales, and eventually more broadly, and that foodborne parasites will not be forgotten, especially when and where they are major threats to human, animal, or plant health.

3.17 Possible future developments

Because of the often complex chain of events leading to infection or contamination of foods with parasites, and the complexity and spatial and temporal variations in climate change, teasing apart the linkages between the new climate and shifts in the occurrence of foodborne parasites is difficult. In many parts of the world layered over these difficulties is frequent sympatry of several different impacts of climate change, relatively limited economic resources, and endemic foodborne parasites (e.g., *T. solium*, *T. saginata*, fish- and plant borne trematodes, and intestinal protozoa). Also often important in these areas are long-standing cultural practices that can affect dietary choices and food preparation techniques, and thus the occurrence of these parasites in people. In many parts of the world, very sadly human and animal infections with foodborne parasites are part of life, and despite many efforts to reduce their occurrence and health impacts are likely to remain so for many people.

Understanding how the new climate can affect the occurrence of foodborne parasites will depend on bringing together long-term data for climate and for the occurrence of the parasites and of parasitic disease in people and in animals, and for parasite occurrence on plants consumed by people, together with epidemiological analysis and observational and experimental studies on the effects of the new climate on parasite ecology. The occurrence data depend on well-designed and accurate surveillance which, even on a small scale, might be beyond the resources of many of those most affected by foodborne parasites. A possibly useful first step is to explore the climate–parasite linkages associated with significant human disease in multiple settings over time to develop insights into the linkages, as is beginning for *Cryptosporidium* and rainfall (e.g., Nichols et al., 2009; Lal et al., 2013), and then to explore the use of this information in the development of predictive models.

The life cycles of many foodborne parasites are relatively well known in that many of the source host species have been identified, as have many of the possible routes of human infection. This knowledge means that breaking the life cycle to prevent human infection with many of the foodborne parasites should be possible, and that these breaks can occur at several of the phases of food supply systems, but especially during production, inspection, retailing, and preparation and consumption in the home or in a food service location. In some circumstances climate change might reduce the risk of infection with foodborne parasites, for example, by increasing mortality of life-cycle stages free-living in the environment. It is also possible, however, that its disruptive effects on animal and human hosts, and on food supply systems (whatever their operating standards, efficiency, or scale) could increase the importance of these parasites as causes of human disease, especially in areas of the world with limited economic resources. Any increases should be met with resources for exploration of all relevant aspects of the parasites' ecology, for public education, and for the prevention of infection and disease in animals and people.

Climate change is a major challenge for life on earth and will be so probably long into the future. The reports published by the IPCC provide useful overviews of advancing knowledge of what, why, when, where, and with what consequences, but the overall picture they paint is far from complete, largely because of the complexity of the new climate and its effects on our biosphere. A key goal of the IPCC effort is to use data and other information from the past and present in attempts to foresee the future, both short and long terms, a task pervaded by many uncertainties. In a discussion of some of the characteristics of emerging diseases, Stephen et al. (2004) adopted some descriptors applied to emerging phenomena in business (Bonabeau, 2002) that can be applied to climate change, surely an emerging phenomenon, and to the ecosystems supporting foodborne parasites: climate change and its effects on ecosystems are often unpredictable and counterintuitive; small climate-driven changes in one component of an ecosystem can result in large changes in other components and sometimes the whole system; and it is often difficult to identify how a change in one component of the ecosystem can affect the whole system. These features produce many challenges in the prevention and management of foodborne parasites and, as is so often the case, many of the individuals and societies least able to overcome these challenges are those in greatest need.

Acknowledgments

Many discussions with my colleagues Eric Hoberg, Emily Jenkins, and Susan Kutz enhanced my understanding of the multiple links between parasitism and the new climate, as did the writings of those whose explorations of this area of parasitology have helped to generate many new and useful insights.

References

Alarcón de Noya, B., Diaz-Bello, Z., Colmenares, C., Ruiz-Guevara, R., Mauriello, L., Zavala-Jaspe, R., Suarez, J.A., Abate, T., Naranjo, L., Paiva, M., Rivas, L., Castro, J., Marques, J., Mendoza, I., Acquatella, H., Torres, J., Noya, O., 2010. Large urban outbreak of orally acquired acute Chagas disease at a school in Caracas, Venezuela. J. Infect. Dis. 201, 1308–1315.

Atkinson, J.M., Gray, D.J., Clements, A.C.A., Barnes, T.S., McManus, D.P., Yang, Y.R., 2013. Environmental changes impacting *Echinococcus* transmission: research to support predictive surveillance and control. Glob. Chang. Biol. 19, 677–688.

Bonabeau, E., 2002. Predicting the unpredictable. Harv. Bus. Rev. 80, 109–116.

Broglia, A., Kapel, C., 2011. Changing dietary habits in a changing world: emerging drivers for the transmission of foodborne parasitic zoonoses. Vet. Parasitol. 182, 2013.

Burek, K.A., Gulland, F.M.D., O'Hara, T., 2008. Effects of climate change on marine mammal health. Ecol. Appl. 18 (Suppl.), S126–S134.

Davidson, R., Handeland, K., Kapel, C.M.O., 2008. High tolerance to repeated cycles of freezing and thawing in different *Trichinella nativa* isolates. Parasitol. Res. 103, 1005–1010.

Davidson, R., Simard, M., Kutz, S.J., Kapel, C.M.O., Hamnes, I.S., Robertson, L.J., 2011. Arctic parasitology: why should we care? Trends Parasitol. 27, 238–244.

FAO/WHO, 2014. Multicriteria-Based Ranking for Risk Management of Foodborne Parasites. Microbiological Risk Assessment Series No. 23. Rome, Food and Agriculture Organization of the United Nations/World Health Organization, 302 pp.

Forbes, L.B., Measures, L., Gajadhar, A.A., Kapel, C., 2003. Infectivity of *Trichinella nativa* in traditional northern (country) foods prepared with meat from experimentally infected seals. J. Food Prot. 66, 1857–1863.

Fox, N.J., White, P.C.L., McClean, C.J., Marion, G., Evans, A., Hutchings, M.R., 2011. Predicting impacts of climate change on *Fasciola hepatica* risk. PLoS One 6, e16126.

Gesy, K.M., Schurer, J.M., Massolo, A., Liccioli, S., Elkin, B.T., Alisauskas, R., Jenkins, E.J., 2014. Unexpected diversity of the cestodes *Echinococcus multilocularis* in wildlife in Canada. Int. J. Parasitol. Parasites Wildl. 3, 81–87.

IPCC, 2014a. Climate change 2014: impacts, adaptation and vulnerability. Part A: global and sectorial aspects. In: Field, C.B., Barros, V.R., Dokken, D.J., Mach, K.J., Mastrandrea, M.D., Bilir, T.E., Chatterjee, M., Ebi, K.L., Estrada, Y.O., Genova, R.C., Girma, B., Kissel, E.S., Lvey, A.N., MacCracken, S., Mastrandrea, P.R., White, L.L. (Eds.), Contribution of Working Group II to the Fifth Assessment Report of the Intergovernmental Panel on Climate Change. Cambridge University Press, Cambridge, UK/New York, NY, USA.

IPCC, 2014b. Climate change 2014: mitigation of climate change. In: Edenhofer, O., Pichs-Madruga, R., Sokona, Y., Farahani, S., Kadner, K., Seyboth, A., Adler, I., Baum, S., Brunner, P., Eckermeier, B., Kriemann, J., Savolainen, S., von Stechow, C., Zwickel, T., Minx, J.C. (Eds.), Contribution of Working Group III to the Fifth Assessment Report of the Intergovernmental Panel on Climate Change. Cambridge University Press, Cambridge, UK and New York, NY, USA.

Jenkins, E.J., Schurer, J.M., Gest, K.M., 2011. Old problems on a new playing field: helminth zoonoses transmitted among dogs, wildlife, and people in a changing northern climate. Vet. Parasitol. 182, 54–69.

Jenkins, E.J., Castrodale, L.J., de Rosemond, S.J.C., Dixon, B.R., Elmore, S.A., Gest, K.M., Hoberg, E.P., Polley, L., Schurer, J.M., Simard, M., Thompson, R.C.A., 2013. Tradition and transition: parasitic zoonoses of people and animals in Alaska, Northern Canada, and Greenland. Adv. Parasitol. 82, 33–202.

Karesh, W.B., Cook, R.A., 2005. The human–animal link. Foreign Aff. 84, 38–50.

Kaschner, K., Tittensor, D.P., Ready, J., Gerrodette, T., Worm, B., 2011. Current and future patterns of global marine mammal biodiversity. PLoS One 6, e19653.

Kirby, R.M., Bartram, J., Carr, R., 2003. Water in food production and processing: quantity and quality concerns. Food Control 14, 283–299.

Kutz, S.J., Hoberg, E.P., Polley, L., Jenkins, E.J., 2005. Global warming is changing the dynamics of arctic host–parasite systems. Proc. Biol. Sci. 271, 2571–2576.

Lal, A., Baker, M.G., Hales, S., French, N.P., 2013. Potential effects of global environmental changes on cryptosporidiosis and giardiosis transmission. Trends Parasitol. 29, 83–90.

Leclair, D., Forbes, L.B., Suppa, S., Proulx, J.F., Gajadhar, A.A., 2004. A preliminary investigation on the infectivity of *Trichinella* larvae in traditional preparations of walrus meat. Parasitol. Res. 93, 507–509.

Lindsey, P.A., Balme, G., Becker, M., Begg, C., Bento, C., Bocchino, C., Dickman, A., Diggle, R.W., Eves, H., Henschel, P., Lewis, D., Marnewick, K., Mattheus, J., McNutt, J.W., McRobb, R., Midlane, M., Milanzi, J., Morley, R., Murphree, M., Opyene, V., Phadima, J., Purchase, G., Rentsch, D., Roche, C., Shaw, J., van der Westhuizen, H., Van Vliet, N., Zisadza-Gandiwa, P., 2013. The bushmeat trade in African savannas: impacts, drivers, and possible solutions. Biol. Conserv. 160, 80–96.

Marcogliese, D.J., 2008. The impact of climate change on the parasites and infectious diseases of aquatic animals. Rev. Sci. Tech. 27, 467–484.

Mas-Coma, S., Valero, M.A., Bargues, M.D., 2008. Effects of climate change on animal and zoonotic helminthiases. Rev. Sci. Tech. 27, 443–452.

Mas-Coma, S., Valero, M.A., Bargues, M.D., 2009. Climate change effects on trematodiases, with emphasis on zoonotic fascioliasis and schistosomiasis. Vet. Parasitol. 163, 264–280.

Miller, M.A., Miller, W.A., Conrad, P.A., James, E.R., Melli, A.C., Leutenegger, C.M., Dabritz, H.A., Packham, A.E., Paradies, D., Harris, M., Ames, J., Jessup, D.A., Worcester, K., Grigg, M.E., 2008. Type X *Toxoplasma gondii* in a wild mussel and terrestrial carnivores from coastal California: new linkages between terrestrial mammals, runoff and toxoplasmosis of sea otters. Int. J. Parasitol. 38, 1319–1328.

Morgan, E.R., Wall, R., 2009. Climate change and parasitic disease: farmer mitigation? Trends Parasitol. 25, 308–313.

Morley, N.J., Lewis, J.W., 2013. Thermodynamics of cercarial development and emergence in trematodes. Parasitology 140, 1211–1224.

Nichols, G., Lane, C., Asgari, N., Verlander, N.Q., Charlett, A., 2009. Rainfall and outbreaks of drinking water related disease in England and Wales. J. Water Health 7, 1–8.

Ollerenshaw, C.B., Rowlands, W.T., 1959. Forecasting the incidence of fascioliasis in Anglesey. Vet. Rec. 71, 591.

Patz, J.A., Vavrus, S.J., Uejio, K., McLellan, S.L., 2008. Climate change and waterborne disease risk in the Great Lakes region of the U.S. Am. J. Prev. Med. 35, 451–458.

Paull, S.H., Johnson, P.T.J., 2011. High temperature enhances host pathology in a snail–trematode system: possible consequences of climate change for the emergence of disease. Freshw. Biol. 56, 767–778.

Paull, S.H., Johnson, P.T.J., 2014. Experimental warming drives a seasonal shift in the timing of host–parasite dynamics with consequences for disease risk. Ecol. Lett. 17, 445–453.

Poulin, R., 2006. Global warming and temperature-mediated increases in cercarial emergence in trematodes parasites. Parasitology 132, 143–151.

Rapsch, C., Dahinder, T., Heinzmann, D., Torgerson, P.R., Braun, U., Deplazes, P., Hurni, L., Bar, H., Knubben-Schweizer, G., 2008. An interactive map to assess the potential spread of *Lymnaea truncatula* and the free-living stages of *Fasciola hepatica* in Switzerland. Vet. Parasitol. 154, 242–249.

Rausch, R.L., George, J.C., Brower, H.K., 2007. Effect of climate warming on the pacific walrus, and potential modification of its helminth fauna. J. Parasitol. 93, 1247–1251.

Rollo, C.D., 1991. Endogenous and exogenous regulation of activity in *Deroceras reticulatum*, a weather-sensitive terrestrial slug. Malacologia 33, 199–220.

Sadorus, L.L., Mantua, N.J., Essington, T., Hickey, B., Hare, S., 2014. Distribution patterns of pacific halibut (*Hippoglossus stenolepis*) in relation to environmental variables along the continental shelf waters of the US West Coast and southern British Columbia. Fish. Oceonogr. 23, 225–241.

Simon, A., Rousseau, A.N., Savary, S., Bigras-Poulin, M., Ogden, N.H., 2013. Hydrological modelling of *Toxoplasma gondii* oocysts transport to investigate contaminated snowmelt as a potential source of infection for marine mammals in the Canadian Arctic. J. Environ. Manage. 127, 150–161.

Stephen, C., Artsob, H., Bowie, W.R., Drebot, M., Fraser, E., Leighton, T., Morshed, M., Ong, C., Patrick, D., 2004. Perspectives on emerging zoonotic disease research and capacity building in Canada. Can. J. Infect. Dis. Med. Microbiol. 15, 339–344.

Thieltges, D.W., Jensen, K.T., Poulin, R., 2008. The role of biotic factors in the transmission of free-living endohelminth stages. Parasitology 135, 407–426.

Tirado, M.C., Clarke, R., Jaykus, L.A., McQuatters-Gollop, A., Frank, J.M., 2010. Climate change and food safety: a review. Food Res. Int. 43, 1745–1765.

Torgerson, P.R., de Silva, N.R., Fevre, E.M., Kasuga, F., Rokni, M.B., Zhou, X.-N., Sripa, B., Gargouri, N., Willingham, A.L., Stein, C., 2014. The global burden of foodborne parasitic disease: an update. Trends Parasitol. 30, 20–26.

Van Bressem, M.-F., Raga, J.A., Di Guardo, G., Jepson, P.D., Duignan, P.J., Siebert, U., Barrett, T., de Oliviera Santos, M.C., Moreno, I.B., Siciliano, S., Aguilar, A., Van Waerebeek, K., 2009. Emerging infectious diseases in cetaceans worldwide and the possible role of environmental stressors. Dis. Aquat. Organ. 86, 143–157.

van Dijk, J., Sargison, N.D., Kenyon, F., Skuce, P.J., 2010. Climate change and infectious disease: helminthological challenges to farmed ruminants in temperate regions. Animal 4, 337–392.

Vermeulen, S.J., Campbell, B.M., Ingram, J.S.I., 2012. Climate change and food systems. Annu. Rev. Environ. Resour. 37, 195–222.

Wang, Q.-P., Lai, D.-H., Chen, X.-G., Lun, Z.-R., 2008. Human angiostrongyliasis. Lancet Infect. Dis. 8, 621–630.

World Meteorological Organization, 2014. WMO statement on the status of the global climate in 2013. WMO report no. 1130. WMO, Geneva.

Role of society and culture in the epidemiology and control of foodborne parasites

4

C.N.L. Macpherson, S. Bidaisee
St. George's University, Grenada, West Indies

4.1 Introduction

4.1.1 Global context

Culture and society both play a fundamental role in the epidemiology, public health, economic importance, and control of foodborne parasites (Macpherson, 2005; Azim et al., 2008; Broglia and Kapel, 2011; Branden and Tauxe, 2013; Jenkins et al., 2013a,b). The increasing demand for food due to an expanding global population and sociocultural interfaces has had a profound effect on the epidemiology of foodborne parasitic diseases. Unprecedented changes in global population demographics are important contributors to socioculturally informed behaviors that determine the type, method of preparation, and consumption of foods. According to the United Nations Population Fund (UNFPA, 2014), the global population now stands at 7.18 billion and is growing at a rate of one birth every few seconds, with an international migrant changing location every 44 s. The UNFPA reports that 96% of the projected population growth will occur in developing countries with the 50 least developed countries expected to grow by 228% by 2050. The UN reports a global refugee population of 52.1 million; this means that 3% of the world's population do not live in the country in which they were born. Within countries the expanding population has migrated with their domestic animals and pests into new environments. The rural to urban migration, emigration, wars, and the resulting displacement of millions of people and tourists serve to introduce and mix cultural preferences, customs, and food-eating behaviors. Increasing populations have had to move into new habitats and require the production of more food and construction of dams to reduce water insecurity. Such environmental changes bring increased risks of parasitic infections (Patz et al., 2000).

4.1.2 Society and culture

Customs, traditions, and cultural and religious beliefs have an impact on the choices of foods that are consumed, choices that determine the potential exposure to different parasitic species. The customs and religious beliefs in different societies vary with differing attitudes regarding the role of animals. Eating habits alter with rising income, increasing the demand for animal protein and, in some areas, the demand for exotic foods. Consumption of exotic species (e.g., crocodile in Scandinavia), or products

Foodborne Parasites in the Food Supply Web. http://dx.doi.org/10.1016/B978-1-78242-332-4.00004-7

out of season (e.g., strawberries from different parts of the world), has expanded food choices as well as species of parasitic infection (Broglia and Kapel, 2011). Low socioeconomic regions are also disproportionately affected by foodborne parasites. The socioeconomic impacts are due to the burden of human disease and the economic losses caused to livestock populations (Torgerson, 2013).

Climatic variability and land use changes as well as social factors have been associated with human cryptosporidiosis and giardiasis (Lal et al., 2013). Climate change can also cause high vulnerability for those parasites with free-living life-cycle stages or that involve arthropod vectors. Climate change can serve to shift the boundaries and processes of parasitic transmission and parasites' distribution in animal-host species (Polley and Thompson, 2009; Jenkins et al., 2013a,b). The socioeconomic burden of most parasitic diseases is not well known, but foodborne trematode infections, cysticercosis, echinococcosis, and diarrhea resulting from zoonotic protozoan species have a significant global economic impact (Torgerson and Macpherson, 2011).

4.1.3 Human behavior

Foodborne parasitic diseases are cosmopolitan and ubiquitous. Human behavior impacts the distribution, prevalence, and intensity of foodborne parasites. Globalization has had the unintended consequence of establishing new niches and exposing new populations of humans and animals to infections (Robertson et al., 2013). Foodborne trematodiasis (syn. trematodiasis) is a cluster of zoonotic infections whose prevalence in Asia and Latin America is increasing because of the growth of fish farming and fish production (Furst et al., 2012). Foodborne infections are often reported in migrants, returning workers, and tourists. The rapid expansion of both human and accompanying animal populations has placed pressure on sanitation and waste management systems, resulting in the pathways for spreading foodborne parasites. The epidemiology of foodborne parasites through their emergence, frequency, and transmission is a result of the socioculturally determined consumption of meat, fresh and saltwater fish, plants, invertebrates, and environmental contamination (Jenkins et al., 2011).

4.2 Societal and cultural practices and the transmission of foodborne parasites

Ethnicity, culture, and religion are factors that influence the foods consumed, preparation methods, and transmission risks of parasites and their geographical distribution. There is a diversity of beliefs and rituals regarding food from various religious and cultural groups. The beliefs and practices are grounded on the availability of food types, spiritual essences, and traditions that have traversed the extent of time (Johnson et al., 2011). The integration of religion as a part of the cultural expression of society and individuals applies to the consumption practices of food and resulting foodborne parasites. Pork, a source of infection for *Toxoplasma gondii*, *Taenia solium*, and *Trichinella spiralis* is shunned by Jews, Orthodox Christians in Ethiopia, and Muslims whose religious teachings forbid the consumption of pigs. Beef, which may contain cystercerci of *Taenia saginata*, is forbidden in Hinduism. *T. gondii* is also being increasingly recognized from beef consumption (Matsuo et al., 2014).

4.2.1 Societal and cultural practices

Traditional practices of food consumption and risks of foodborne parasites are also a result of geographic locations and resident parasitic burdens in the particular region. Helminthiasis and high prevalence of *Opisthorchis viverrini*, hookworm, *Trichuris trichiura*, and *Ascaris lumbricoides* in Laos was associated with the consumption of raw fish, as well as inadequate personal and village hygiene practices (Phongluxa et al., 2013). Traditional North African culinary preparations, including fermentation of dairy products for preservation and consumption of large amounts of raw meat and offal, are also a culturally relevant influence toward the occurrence of *T. gondii, Sarcocystis* spp., *Cryptosporidium parvum*, *Fasciola hepatica*, and other trematode, cestode, and nematode species (Benkerroum, 2013). The indigenous residents of Northern Canada have higher occurrence of zoonotic parasites than the general population (Jenkins et al., 2013a,b). Parasitic zoonoses endemic in the Arctic include *Diphyllobothrium* spp. and cervid strains of *Echinococcus granulosus*, which pose direct and indirect threats due to the consumption of locally harvested fish and wildlife. The northern region of Canada is also in transition as there is an increase in the number of food products exported from the North even as tourists and workers enter the region. The movement of people, animals, and products has made foodborne parasites, such as *Trichinella* spp., *T. gondii*, Anisakid nematodes, and Diphyllobothrid cestodes increasingly important (Jenkins et al., 2013a,b). In western countries, there is also an increased demand by consumers to seek out ethnic foods to satisfy their curiosity to experience new foods. With globalization, the number of ethnically or culturally homogenous cuisines has dwindled, which also diversifies the transmission and distribution of foodborne parasites.

4.2.2 Transmission

In the United States and Europe, the trend has moved away from intensified, restricted animal rearing to organically raised free-ranging food animals, a trend that could increase the risk of infection with *T. gondii* (Jones and Dubey, 2012). The increased consumption of foods shipped around the world has caused the distribution and global burden of foodborne parasitic diseases to expand. The potential for transmission of nonautochthonous parasites from imported foods requires a greater awareness of parasitic infections to better diagnose, treat, and prevent such cases (McEntire, 2013).

The globalization of the food supply and changes in culinary habits coupled to a greater proclivity to consume raw or undercooked meats, such as beef, pork, reptiles, amphibians, fish, and crustaceans can result in exposure to a wide range of parasite species (*Opisthorchis* spp., *Clonorchis sinensis*, *Paragonimus* spp., *Diphyllobothrium* spp., *Spirometra* spp., *Gnathostoma* spp.) (Dorny et al., 2009). The ingestion of other parasitic cysts or larvae of *Sarcocystis* spp., *T. gondii*, *Trichinella* spp., and *Taenia* spp. has been described as having a high probability of human infection (Fazly et al., 2013). Trichinellosis caused by ingesting first stage (L1) larvae of *Trichinella* spp. in undercooked meat from a huge variety of host species is one of the most important, worldwide zoonotic meat borne parasites (Pozio and Murrell, 2006; Chandrawathani et al., 2010).

Opisthorchis spp. and *Clonorchis* spp. are highly endemic in the Mekong Basin countries of Thailand, Cambodia, Laos, and Vietnam. The consumption of *koi-pla*, a popular raw fish dish, has resulted in high transmission and prevalence of the diseases and are associated with human movement and settlement (Sithithaworn et al., 2012). The rising popularity of Japanese cuisine traditional dishes (*sushi, sashimi*) has been linked to the transmission of fish borne parasitic zoonoses, especially anisakiasis (syn. Anisikosis) (Nawa et al., 2005). Such fish borne parasites are endemic in many Asian countries and are also found in many countries outside of Asia where *sushi* and *sashimi* are consumed. The expansion of fish borne parasitic zoonoses into international markets has also led to the recognition of infections in developed countries and upper-income societies (Chai et al., 2005). The demographic changes of human populations and associated integration of sociocultural practices and culinary cuisines have also been accompanied by an increase in livestock population and wildlife as sources of food. Associated with these changes in animal population is the closer interaction between humans and animals, which results in foodborne parasitic diseases. The movements of livestock, changes in agricultural practices, and global climate change have enabled zoonotic parasites that are transmitted either directly or indirectly between animals and humans to emerge.

Water borne outbreaks of cryptosporidiosis occur globally. Prior to 2010 the majority of foodborne outbreaks of *C. parvum* were reported in the United States and in the United Kingdom, but since then an increase has been noted in Nordic countries (Robertson and Chalmers, 2013). These authors suggest that imported meat with elevated consumption and prolonged survival of the oocysts in the Nordic climate may be the main reasons for such outbreaks.

Livestock infection associated with human activities is not uncommon for bovine cysticercosis. For example, the source of the infection in Australian cattle was copra meal imported from Papua New Guinea, which had been contaminated with human feces with *T. saginata* (Jenkins et al., 2013a,b). The cycle of infection of fish borne zoonotic trematodes was also demonstrated in Vietnam where dogs serve as reservoir hosts for a number of species of trematodes, and dogs become reinfected after treatment with praziquantal (Nissen et al., 2014). Dogs then have access to raw fish remains discarded by humans.

Parasitic emergence and risk of transmission due to wildlife contact with humans or anthropogenic activities have been noted for *Giardia* spp., *Toxoplasma* spp., and *Echinococcus* spp. (Thompson et al., 2009). Wildlife, which links people and the ecosystems in which they coexist, can serve as drivers of parasitic disease emergence. Parasites such as *Angiostrongylus cantonensis* in the Caribbean and the southern United States, *Baylisascaris procyonis* in California and Georgia, and *Cryptosporidium* spp., *Giardia* spp., and *T. gondii* in marine ecosystems can be parasites of human interest through foodborne transmission (Polley, 2005).

Concomitant contamination of the environment with night soil along with the increase in human and animal populations have also expanded the distribution and intensity of foodborne parasites. *Cryptosporidium* spp. is an example of a parasite that is ideally suited for foodborne transmission as it has a high oocyst excretion rate, it is microscopic, and it is able to survive for long periods in the environment and only requires a low infectious dose. Preparation and cleaning of vegetables may result in *Cryptosporidium* spp. oocyst contamination (Robertson, 2014). An assessment of parasitic infestation of vegetable sources from markets in Manila, in the Philippines, found a 45% infection rate for protozoan parasites (Su et al., 2012). Contamination of vegetables sold in markets with helminth eggs in Zaria, Nigeria, was also reported as linked to increasing use of wastewater from human and animal wastes for irrigation of agricultural produce (Maikai et al., 2012). Ingestion of raw vegetables also represented an important mode of transmission of intestinal parasites in Alexandria, Egypt, where 31.7% of examined vegetable samples contained *A. lumbricoides Toxocara* spp., *Hymenolepsis nana* eggs, *Giardia* spp. cysts, *Cryptosporidium* spp., and *Cyclospora* spp. oocysts, and *Microsporidium* spp. spores (Said, 2012).

Environmental contamination also leads to aquatic dwellers, such as fish, crustaceans, mollusks, and plants that serve as sources of parasites, especially trematodes. It is estimated that more than 10% of the world population is potentially at risk of foodborne trematodiasis, and globally, more than 100 million people are infected with one or more fluke species (Khurana and Malla, 2014).

The expanding global human and livestock populations, the increased dependence on aquaculture for food production, and the increased human and animal waste generation creates a global burden of illness associated with foodborne parasitic diseases. The epidemiology of foodborne parasites is affected by the sociocultural elements of human behavior and the interactions that occur in a given environment, as well as the global scale of food production and consumption. This chapter reviews illustrations of the epidemiology and control of foodborne parasites that are transmitted in meat, freshwater fish, saltwater fish, plants, invertebrates, and through environmental contamination.

4.3 Foodborne parasites transmitted by meat

Animals are kept as pets, used for work, and especially used for food: their meat is an important source of protein. Changes in animal husbandry practices and farming of wild species (such as crocodiles, etc.) are changing the distribution and importance of a number of parasites. Animals can serve as reservoirs for a variety of parasites and, through meat consumption, can lead to infection in humans. The practice of eating raw or undercooked meat is a source for many parasitic infections. The customs of eating raw or partially cooked meat has also grown worldwide and has led to the emergence of parasitic diseases in population groups where eating raw or undercooked meat was not previously common.

4.3.1 Epidemiology

The epidemiology of foodborne parasites transmitted through meat consumption is influenced by the sociocultural aspects of human behavior. The emerging trend in foodborne diseases transmitted through meat is projected to continue to increase. The number of persons in a population at risk has increased, and the nature of sources of meat has changed. Branden and Tauxe (2013), referring to the 1565 outbreaks of foodborne illnesses reported to the CDC, identified poultry, beef, and pork as three (25%) of the 12 food sources associated with the outbreaks.

T. gondii is possibly the most prevalent protozoan parasite and infects humans through a variety of routes. Foodborne infection through ingestion of the tissue stages in undercooked meat (especially pork, goat, lamb, free-range poultry, and game animals) is thought to be the most important route of human infection in Europe and Central and South America where cultural preferences favor the use of raw and undercooked meat (Azim et al., 2008). The accidental ingestion of oocysts, shed by cats, from environmental sources (water, contamination of fruits and vegetables, gardening, ingesting soil, etc.) are also important (Jones et al., 2014). Human infection with *T. gondii* is most significant for immuno-compromised patients and in the children born to women who are infected for the first time just prior to or during pregnancy. Measures to reduce infection through meat consumption include thoroughly cooking all meat before eating, not handling raw meat, and not feeding raw meat to pet cats. Changes in the rearing of animals in the United States where free-range production is increasingly being preferred to confined production may increase the incidence of *T. gondii* there (Jones and Dubey, 2012).

Sarcocystis spp. also has a global distribution. The life cycle is heteroxenous with herbivores (domestic and wild) as intermediate hosts that contain sarcocysts, and carnivores, including humans, serve as definitive hosts. Humans acquire *Sarcocystis hominis* from cattle, *Sarcocystis sinensis* from water buffalo, and *Sarcocystis suihominis* from pigs through undercooked meat consumption (Chen et al., 2011). Infection with *Sarcocystis* spp. can cause stomach pains, nausea, and diarrhea in humans. There is no effective treatment available, but control is possible by avoiding eating raw meat.

Paragonimosis results from infection by a number of species of lung-dwelling flukes with more than 20 million people infected worldwide. The parasites include *Paragonimus westermani* (Far East), *Paragonimus miyazakii*, *Paragonimus skrjabini*, and *Paragonimus heterotrema* in Asia, *Paragonimus agurans* and *Paragonimus uterobilateralis* in Africa, and *Paragonimus mexicanus* and other species in Latin America (Macpherson et al., 2000). Several species of mammals such as dogs, cats, and wild carnivores act as the definitive hosts that are infected by eating encysted metacercariae from intermediate hosts such as crabs, crayfish, or shrimp (Yamamoto, 2009). Humans are infected through the consumption of definitive hosts such as the wild boar. Human infection is characterized by chronic, productive cough and chest pain. Control measures include education on avoiding the eating of definitive host animal species and treatment with the use of praziquantel.

Taeniasis and cysticercosis are caused by *T. solium* and *T. saginata*, which are zoonotic cestodes. *T. solium* is widespread in the pig-rearing rural areas of Latin America, Africa, and Asia; *T. saginata* occurs in the cattle-rearing areas worldwide. People become infected with tapeworms after ingesting cysticerci in undercooked pork or beef and may suffer mild clinical symptoms. The major burden of disease is human infection with cysticercosis due to *T. solium* and the losses in animal productivity and condemnation of infected cattle and pigs. The burden of neurocysticercosis due to infection with *T. solium* cysticerci represents more than 1% of all 76 million cases of epilepsy worldwide (Coyle et al., 2012; Ngugi et al., 2011). Control of taeniasis and cysticercosis is complicated by the low prevalence and low positive predictive values issues in the definitive hosts. Control measures include education, emphasizing the proper cooking of beef and pork, provision and proper use of sanitation, and mass or targeted treatment of humans. In some instances the treatment of pigs with a single dose of oxfendazole and use of a recombinant vaccine has proved successful in the control of *T. solium* (Jayashi et al., 2012; Lightowlers, 2013). The successful treatment of ocular and neurocysticercosis due to *T. solium* cysticercosis has to be individualized, depending on the location, number, and condition of the cysts; it may involve anthelmintics, antiinflammatory drugs, and/or minimalized surgery and remains challenging (Del Brutto, 2014).

Trichinellosis is a zoonotic disease with humans and animals infected through the ingestion of meat containing viable larvae. Trichinellosis provides a good example of a point source of infection that can result in spectacular outbreaks resulting from the consumption of meat from one infected animal. There are numerous species of *Trichinella* that are all propagated through the consumption of meat by carnivores, omnivores, scavenging, or cannibalistic behaviors. The three main species that are widespread in humans are *T. spiralis*, *Trichinella britovi*, and *Trichinella nativa*. *T. spiralis* occurs mainly in domestic cycles whereas *T. britovi* and *T. nativa* occur mainly in wild animals.

Among the Inuit Eskimos, traditional methods of preparing meat from seals, walruses, and polar bears, such as *ignuaq* (meat and blubber placed in a sealskin bag and allowed to ferment), *nikku* (air-dried meat), and sausage that is partially cooked have all been linked to infections with *T. nativa* (Forbes et al., 2003). In Papua New Guinea the feeding of wild pigs to saltwater crocodiles served to maintain the transmission of *Trichinella papuae* (Pozio et al., 2005). The farming of any scavenging or cannibalistic species, such as crocodiles (*Crocodylus niloticus*) or monitor lizards (*Varanus niloticus*) in Africa can lead to exposure to *T. zimbabwensis* (Pozio et al., 2007). Hunters who incompletely cook or air-dry meat in the field are also an important risk group for *Trichinella* spp. infection. Often part of the carcass is left at the site that can then be consumed by others, thus perpetuating the infection in the wildlife populations. *T. murrelli* is another species that caused an outbreak of trichinellosis in Northern California in 2008 (Hall et al., 2012). Thirty of thirty-eight attendees of an event where black bear meat was served became infected, which produced an attack rate of 78% for *T. murrelli* infection. Free-range pig rearing is also increasing the possibility of *Trichinella* spp. infection. In Nigeria a 40% seroprevalence among pigs from backyard farms was reported (Momoh et al., 2012).

4.3.2 Control

Mebendazole and albendazole are the anthelmintics of choice for the treatment of human trichinellosis. Control measures for interrupting the transmission of *Trichinella* spp. can be achieved through good animal husbandry practices and *postmortem* diagnosis through meat inspection, the proper disposal of infected carcasses, and the proper cooking of meat. The decline in trichinellosis in Europe and the United States was attributed to improved standards and regulations in the pig-rearing industry as well as in the promotion of proper cooking of meat. Consumption of raw horse meat imported from Eastern Europe caused outbreaks of *T. spiralis* in Western Europe as horses in this region are occasionally fed pork (Murrell et al., 2014).

Toxocariasis due to *Toxocara* spp. can be contracted in a variety of ways, such as from ingesting raw infected animal viscera (mostly liver) or from ingesting invertebrate paratenic hosts, such as earthworms, and most commonly from ingesting embryonated eggs from the environment (Macpherson, 2013a). Toxocariasis symptoms are based on the host's inflammatory responses to migrating larvae and by the mechanical damage to tissues and organs where larvae migrate. There are four main syndromes associated with *Toxocara* spp. infection in humans, including visceral, ocular, neurotoxocariasis, and covert toxocariasis (CDC, 2013). Controlling *Toxocara* infection in dogs and cats through treatment and population control through reproductive control measures will reduce the number of eggs that are shed into the environment and will reduce the potential for other animals that are used as a food source to become infected.

4.4 Foodborne parasites transmitted by freshwater fish

The global consumption of fish represents 16.6% of the total intake of animal protein and provides more than 4.3 billion people with their animal protein intake (Tacon and Metian, 2013). The significant fish consumption by the global population represents diversity in the types, preparation, and cuisines of fish food products. The traditions of consuming raw fish in different parts of the world and, in particular, in the Far East, is becoming increasingly common in many other countries as well. Foods such as *sushi*, *sashimi*, *koi-pla*, *kinilaw*, and *ceviche* have become very popular worldwide. This increase in the consumption of raw fish products has led to a rise in the incidence of a large number of fish borne parasitic infections (Wiriya et al., 2013). The consumption of uncooked fish is an ethnic or culinary preference and is not due to the lack of fuel to cook them. The increased demand for fish protein by the increasing human population has also established aquaculture as an important practice in fish production. Aquaculture, like catching fish from natural sources, is also a medium for high prevalence of fish borne parasites, in particular, zoonotic trematodes (Pitaksakulrat et al., 2013). It is estimated that 48.6% of freshwater fish originates from aquaculture, a number that is expected to rise and further increase the occurrence of fish borne parasites (FAO, 2010). The consumption of raw, undercooked, or pickled freshwater fish has been reported by Clausen et al. (2012) to have caused several hundred million human infections. The main fish borne parasites include *Clonorchis* spp., *Opisthorchis* spp., *Echinostoma* spp., *Heterophyes heterophyes*, *Metagonimus yokogawai*, *Diphyllobothrium latum*, *Gnathostoma* spp., and *Capillaria philippinensis*.

4.4.1 Epidemiology

C. sinensis, *O. viverrini*, and *Opisthorchis felineus* affect tens of millions of people, particularly in Southeastern Asia and Europe and more than 680 million people are at risk of infection. In highly endemic areas, such as the northeastern provinces of Thailand, the prevalence of *O. viverrini* may reach 35% (Mairiang et al., 2012). Infection occurs through the consumption of raw or undercooked fish that contains metacercariae encysted in the muscles. Raw fish dishes are a dietary habit and culinary tradition in all countries where these flukes are commonly found. Most light infections are thought to be asymptomatic, but moderately or heavily infected individuals with *C. sinensis* or *O. viverrini* may experience fever, fatigue, renal, and hepatobiliary pathologies including liver cirrhosis, hepatitis, and cholangiocarcinoma (Saichua et al., 2013; Sithithaworn et al., 2012, 2014). The International Agency for Research on Cancer upgraded *C. sinensis* from a probable carcinogen (group 2A) to a definite carcinogen (group 1) (Bouvard et al., 2009). Patients developing cholangiocarcinoma have a poor prognosis, thereby increasing the importance of prevention and control of these fish borne trematode zoonoses. Control is achieved through sanitation, education to discourage the consumption of raw fish, and discarding raw fish offal to dogs and cats that can also serve as definitive hosts; treatment, if possible, is done with praziquantel. Mass drug administration programs have had some success in Northeastern Thailand in reducing the incidence of these flukes.

Echinostomiasis is reported with high prevalence in endemic countries such as Korea, the Philippines, Indonesia, Malaysia, and Thailand. The species involved include *Echinostoma ilocanum*, *Echinostoma revolutum*, *Echinostoma malayanum*, *Echinostoma echinatum*, and *Echinostoma hortense* (Hung et al., 2013). Humans are infected by consuming freshwater fish that contain encysted metacercariae. Heavy infections can result in diarrhea and abdominal discomfort. For control, education on the risks of consuming raw or undercooked freshwater fish in endemic regions is important, and treatment is done with praziquantel. *M. yokogawai* and *Heterophes heterophes* are important heterophyids that can cause parasitic zoonotic diseases. These two species are intestinal flukes that are ingested as encysted metacercariae in raw or undercooked fish. Birds are also infected through their consumption of raw fish. These flukes are more commonly found in Japan, Laos, Thailand, Korea, Hawaii, the Balkan countries, the Philippines, China, Turkey, and Siberia (Dhaliwal and Juyal, 2013). Clinical manifestations are rare and, if present, are due to eggs trapped in various tissues. Treatment and control with praziquantel and discouragement of raw fish consumption has proven to be useful.

Diphyllobothriosis is caused by tapeworms of the genus *Diphyllobothrium* with *D. latun* being the predominant species affecting tens of millions of people worldwide. The global distribution of *D. latun* has foci in the freshwater lake areas of Europe, Asia, and North America. The life cycle includes copepods as the first intermediate hosts and freshwater fish as the second intermediate hosts harboring the plerocercoid larvae (Overstreet, 2013). Upon ingestion of the plerocercoid in raw fish by humans, and other domestic and wild carnivore species, as definitive hosts, the larva matures to adult tapeworms in the small intestine. Symptoms of infection include gastrointestinal obstruction, abdominal pain, and rarely diarrhea. Anemia also occurs among persons infected related to the high affinity of the tapeworms to vitamin B12 absorbed through its surface. A study of German travelers revealed 7.1% of people returned with anemia associated with *D. latum* infection emphasizing travel as an influence of foodborne parasitic infections (Herbinger et al., 2013). Control measures include appropriate cooking of fish and treatment with praziquantel. In areas where carnivores are in proximity and there is contact with freshwater fish, routine praziquantel administration to domestic carnivores can help to interrupt the life cycle of the parasite.

D. latum infection was also described in a nonendemic country where a case was confirmed in a 27-year-old Spanish male (Esteban et al., 2014). The patient expelled a 110-cm worm while not suffering from any apparent symptoms. Analysis of the patient's potential exposure revealed the possibility of consuming imported fish. The international exposure to fish borne parasites is increasingly becoming an issue as culinary habits and import/export of food products expand.

4.4.2 Transmission

Fish borne zoonoses also occur with several species of the nematode genus *Gnathostoma*. Copepods serve as the initial intermediate hosts that are eaten by fish that serve as secondary intermediate hosts. The infective third stage (L3) larvae develop in fish and infect humans who have consumed raw or undercooked fish. The majority of reported cases occur in Asia in which a cutaneous or visceral larval migrans condition may arise (Cui et al., 2013). Treatment is usually surgical removal for superficially occurring larvae, and control is based on the properly cooking fish. *C. philippinensis* is another nematode species responsible for intestinal infection. The geographical range includes the Phillipines, extending to Egypt where epidemics occur along rivers. The consumption of raw or undercooked fish leads to infection, which may persist over many years leading to chronic malabsorption syndrome. Thewjitcharoen et al. (2012) reported a fatal case of intestinal capillariasis in a construction worker with a 6-month history of chronic watery diarrhea. The control of capillariasis involves educating against the consumption of undercooked fish which, when discontinued, has greatly reduced the parasite in areas traditionally affected. Avoidance of the use of night soil as fertilizer for fish ponds is also an important method to reduce transmission.

4.5 Foodborne parasites transmitted by saltwater fish

Saltwater resources represent 82% of the edible fish supplied by capture fisheries (Tacon and Metian, 2013). The production and consumption of saltwater fish account for approximately 12% of the total seafood consumption globally (Raatz et al., 2013). The global consumption of saltwater fish provides a considerable contribution to the human diet. The incidence in human population has also placed an increased demand for saltwater fish supply. Unlike the diverse parasites of freshwater fish, only a few parasites are transmitted through the consumption of saltwater fish as saltwater is not directly linked to human, animal, or environmental mechanisms that support parasitic life cycles.

4.5.1 Epidemiology

Anisakiasis is a widespread parasitic infection whereby humans are infected by the consumption of raw or undercooked saltwater fish, squid, or pickled herring. A large number of cases of gastric anisakiasis have been reported in countries where eating of raw fish is customary, as in Japan, although the first case was noted in the Netherlands in 1960 (Kim et al., 2013). Subsequently, many cases have been reported in Western Europe where raw fish is also being consumed frequently (Mattiucci et al., 2013). The larvae consumed by humans do not develop further; however, they penetrate the gastrointestinal tract and form eosinophilic granulomas and potentially life-threatening allergic reactions when the live parasite penetrates the gastric mucosa. Greater awareness of the infection and a change in the tradition of eating raw fish would help to prevent transmission.

4.5.2 Transmission

Nanophyetus salmincola is another zoonotic trematode transmitted by the consumption of undercooked saltwater fish. Salmon are the most common fish host where the metacercariae reside in its kidneys (Romer et al., 2013). The fluke also serves as the transport host for the bacteria *Neorickettsia helminthoeca*, which causes "salmon poisoning" in dogs that consume discarded salmon carcasses.

4.6 Foodborne parasites transmitted by the consumption of plants

4.6.1 Epidemiology

Parasitic diseases caused by helminths and protozoa affect an estimated 3.5 billion people globally with 450 million developing clinical disease as a result of infection (Fentie et al., 2013). Plants, directly or through the infection by larvae from water contamination and through water consumption itself, are common routes for parasitic infection. Watercress (*Nasturtium officinale*) is consumed by many people and is a source of *F. hepatica*. Watercress is a member of the Brassicaceae family and is cultivated as a perennial, nutritionally valuable, and staple vegetable in a number of countries. Increasing prevalence in fascioliasis has been reported worldwide, and a prevalence of 13.3% was recently reported among schoolchildren in Puebla State, Mexico (Zumaquero-Rios et al., 2013). An outbreak of fascioliasis in Southwest China due to *F. gigantica* was reported in 2011, where 29 patients were infected by consumption of the herb *Houttuynia cordata* serving as the most likely source (Chen et al., 2013). South America is the most prevalent area for fascioliasis infection, accounting for more than half of the estimated 2.6 million people infected worldwide (Song et al., 2013). The animal reservoirs of *F. hepatica* include the ruminants: cattle, sheep, goats, and camels. The obligate intermediate host is the snail, and cercariae emerge from snails to form metacercariae on aquatic plants. In definitive hosts, embryos hatch and the excysted larvae penetrate the duodenal wall and migrate into the peritoneal cavity, the liver capsule, and the liver parenchyma. In the liver, the flukes migrate to the bile duct lumen where they mature and reside as adults. Control is achieved by preventing livestock from access to snail-infested areas and in countries that can afford it by the treatment of ruminant species with triclabendazole. In endemic areas, raw leaf vegetables should be carefully prepared and drinking possibly contaminated water should be avoided.

4.6.2 Transmission

In recent years, there have been several outbreaks of foodborne parasites associated with fresh ready-to-eat berries and leafy greens. The cultural practice of ready-to-eat foods is commonplace in the Western world as consumers have limited time to obtain their dietary requirements while meeting the needs of daily living. *Giardia* spp. cysts have been detected in fresh fruits and vegetables (Robertson, 2013), and *Cyclospora cayentanensis* was identified in several outbreaks associated with fresh produce in Canada (Kozak et al., 2013). *Cyclospora* spp., *Cryptosporidium* spp., and *Giardia* spp. were also identified in ready-to-eat packaged leafy green products in Ontario, Canada, as a part of the number of foodborne disease outbreaks investigations (Gendel et al., 2013). The significant increase in the incidence of foodborne outbreaks caused by contaminated ready-to-eat leafy greens and berries is a part of the current food safety challenge in applying minimal processing, nonthermal methods in preparing foods for consumption. The culture of Western society's demands for ready-to-eat foods while maintaining the freshness of food products is the practice promoting these foodborne parasitic infections.

4.7 Foodborne parasites from consumption of invertebrate hosts

4.7.1 Epidemiology

The practice of consuming undercooked meat, fish, fresh berries, and leafy greens also includes the consumption of undercooked crabs, crayfish, and shrimp. An estimated 21 million persons are currently infected with *Paragonimus* spp. with epidemiologic surveys from Cameroon and Nigeria reporting prevalence of up to 16.8% (Rothe, 2013). The lung fluke uses aquatic snails as its first intermediate host, from which cercariae are released; subsequently encysting as metacercariae on crabs, crayfish, or shrimp. Humans are infected by eating raw or undercooked invertebrate species. Macpherson et al. (2000) also noted that crabs, which are sometimes pickled in wine or brine, are also a major source of *Paragonimus* spp. Infection can lead to pulmonary conditions characterized by chronic productive cough. The flukes have also been found in the brain, giving rise to neurological conditions (Miranda et al., 2013). Control measures include education against consumption of raw and undercooked invertebrate species and treatment with praziquantel.

4.7.2 Transmission

The consumption of mollusks or food contaminated by snails is a common cause of eosinophilic meningitis due to infection with *Parastrongylus* spp., currently referred to as *Angiostrongylus* spp.; *A. cantonensis* is the causative organism for thousands of human infections as a result of consumption of infected mollusks or food contaminated by snails (Azim et al., 2008). In recent years the increased popularity of eating the large African land snail *Achatina fulica* has seen an increase in the incidence of angiostrongyliasis. In the United States, nonindigenous apple snails, *Pomacea maculate*, are currently spreading the parasite (Teem et al., 2013). *A. cantonensis* is established in Southeast Asia, Australia, the Pacific Islands, the Caribbean, and the Americas (Wang et al., 2008). Rats (*Rattus norwegicus*) serve as an accidental host, which is why *A. cantonensis* is sometimes referred to as rat lungworm. Control measures include education to change the practice of mollusk consumption and chemotherapy, which may include albendazole with concomitant medication with steroids. Control of rodent populations is also indicated.

Other foodborne parasites transmitted through the consumption of arthropods include the ingestion of beetles in flour, which is a source of infection with *Hymenolepis* spp. The flour beetle, *Tribolium castanean* is an intermediate host for the tapeworm *Hymenolepis diminuta*. Infection occurs by the accidental ingestion of infected intermediate host beetles or fleas. *H. diminuta* is commonly found in areas where rats are present such as in grain silos and storage facilities for harvested crops. The distribution of *H. diminuta* infection is mainly in warm, tropical countries such as Thailand, Singapore, and Indonesia. Currently, only a few hundred cases have been reported globally; however, prevalence studies have shown rates in excess of 8% in the Brazilian Amazon region of Mato Grosso (Malheiros et al., 2014). Symptoms are not usually present, and control is achieved through food safety measures to prevent the presence of beetles and moths in flour. Ingestion of fleas or lice containing the cysticercoids of *Dipylidium* spp. can result in infection in people and dogs with the adult tapeworm. Infection occurs most often in young children, and although infections are asymptomatic, the passing of proglottids is alarming to parents. Treatment is with niclosamide, and control must involve the concomitant treatment of pets and control of flea populations.

4.8 Environmentally transmitted parasites that can be accidentally ingested

4.8.1 Epidemiology

Contamination of food by free-living parasite stages is a significant route of transmission for many parasitic species. The World Health Organization (WHO) has embarked on an initiative to estimate the global burden of foodborne diseases including those of parasitic contamination of food (Havelaar et al., 2013). This initiative recognizes the determinants of foodborne diseases by age, sex, and region, which influences the socioeconomic, cultural characteristics and practices toward personal hygiene, water, and sanitary infrastructure influence. The growth and aging of the human population along with increasing poverty, malnutrition, environmental pollution, deforestation, crowding, inadequate infrastructure, poor sanitation, and water supply are all consequences of the socioeconomic status of various countries and determinants of environmentally transmitted parasites (Prasad, 2010). Poverty and the associated poor state of sanitation, unsafe water sources, low literacy, overcrowding, and the inability to pay for diagnostic and treatment services and lack of control of domestic pets and livestock all contribute to higher infection rates of parasites in low socioeconomic populations throughout the world (Torgerson and Macpherson, 2011). Polyparasitism is common and often include *Cryptosporidium* spp., *Cystoisospora belli*, *Microsporidium* spp., *Giardia intestinalis*, *Entamoeba* spp., and *Cyclospora* spp. owing to their ubiquitous nature (Mbae et al., 2013). The tropical climates and low altitudes in developing countries are also associated with more than 70 species of protozoan and helminthic parasites that infect humans through food and water contamination (Ishaku et al., 2013). The transmission route for most of the intestinal parasites is fecal-oral via contaminated food or water. Protozoan parasites, such as *Giardia* spp., *Cryptosporidium* spp., *Entamoeba* spp., *T gondii*, and *Cyclospora* spp., and Helminthic parasites, such as *A. lumbricoides*, along with *T. trichiura* are widespread in the environment, exposing humans through their contamination of food sources and water.

The symptoms of intestinal protozoan infections vary depending on the species involved but can generally include fatigue, watery and foul-smelling diarrhea, flatulence, abdominal distress with weight loss, and abdominal distension in chronic conditions. Children are more commonly affected, with higher age-specific prevalence due to associated risk factors of greater soil exposure from recreational behavior and lower nutritional and immune status. Malabsorptive syndromes and gastrointestinal morbidity due to at least one of the *G. intestinalis*, *Entamoeba histolytica/Entamoeba dispar*, or *Blastocystis hominis* was found in 48.7% of children in Pemba Island, Tanzania (Speich et al., 2013). This places a significant burden on their growth and development and forms part of the 100,000 people each year that die from infection with *Entamoeba histolytica* (Lozano et al., 2013). *G. intestinalis* also has a prevalence of 30% in developing countries and 3% in developed countries (Escobedo and Cimerman, 2007). *Cryptosporidium* spp. is another protozoan of global health importance especially due to its morbidity and mortality association with immune-compromised individuals such as those infected with human immunodeficiency virus (Davies and Chalmers, 2009; Jex et al., 2001). *B. hominis* is an additional anaerobic intestinal protozoan that is associated with lack of access to clean water and improper sanitation and hygiene.

4.8.2 Transmission

A study on the conditions of food establishments and the health status and personal hygiene among food handlers showed that poor hygienic practices were significantly associated with the presence of foodborne illnesses (Deshpande and Phalke, 2013). The study also linked the low socioeconomic status of the rural area of Western Maharashtra (India) with improper sanitary infrastructure, enforcement of hygienic provisions, and education of food handlers about food safety practices. Cryptosporidiosis, Entamoebiasis, and Giardiasis, which are routinely implicated in outbreaks of foodborne diseases, also occur in recreational waters, agricultural run-off, and wild animals, which are all sources of parasitic transmission via water. Outbreaks of waterborne parasitic infections have also been associated with *Ascaris suum* (Franco, 2013). These environmentally transmitted parasitic infections are based on the ability of the parasite to survive in the environment in soil and to withstand sewage and water treatment processes. Protozoan infection from food and water contamination occurs in both developed and developing countries and forms a significant part of the overall burden of illness. *T. gondii* is also noted for its survivability in the environment and ubiquitous presence worldwide. High concentrations of *T. gondii* oocysts in estuarine river outlets carried in snowmelt run-off present a source of infection for both humans and animals that drink those waters in the Arctic (Bowie et al., 1997; Simon et al., 2013). Municipal wastewaters also contain parasitic protozoan stages at varying levels. Among the protozoa, *Giardia* spp., *Entamoeba* spp., *Entamoeba coli*, *Endolimax nana*, *Idoamoeba butschlii*, and *Balantidium coli* were detected in wastewater treatment plants in Bangladesh (Khanum et al., 2012). The wastewater processing served to reduce the protozoan parasites, but it was not effective in their elimination. Pathogenic and commensal protozoa were also observed in 90% of water samples derived from deep wells in Aragua State, Venezuela (Guillen et al., 2013). Cysts of *G. intestinalis*, *E. coli*, and *E. nana* were identified and linked to human and animal excretion in the environment. *Cryptosporidium* spp., *E. histolytica/E. dispar*, and *G. intestinalis* were also found in stool samples of returning German soldiers from military deployment around the world (Frickmam et al., 2013). The soldiers' exposure to varying levels of hygiene in countries such as Afghanistan, Uzbekistan, the Balkans, Democratic Republic of Congo, and Sudan demonstrated chronic infections and colonization by the intestinal protozoa. Control of protozoan infections that contaminate water and food is based on practicing good personal hygiene, appropriate sanitary disposal, treatment of drinking water, and managing the exposure of wildlife, domestic, and livestock waste from contaminating water supplies. Education on food safety and measures for early detection and treatment of susceptible organisms using albendazole and nitazoxanide is also appropriate.

4.8.3 Human and animal interface

The close associations of humans with companion animals such as dogs and cats have substantial positive benefits, which are psychological and physiological (Beck, 2013). Companion animals serve as another example of social and cultural behaviors, which have determined the need for various companion animal species and the diverse role they play. Today, tens of millions of dogs and cats of a variety of breeds share our space as close companions or as stray or feral animals. Their ubiquitous distribution and close proximity to humans facilitate the transmission of several environmentally transmitted zoonotic parasites. The global distribution and importance of these environmentally transmitted zoonoses are influenced by a complex interplay of the heterogeneity of susceptibility to infection and behavior of the hosts (people and pets), the infectious agents, the environment, and socioeconomic conditions. The parasite agents involved include protozoan zoonoses *Giardia* spp., *B. coli*, *B. hominis*, and *Cryptosporidium* spp., cestodes including *Echinococcus* spp., especially *E. granulosus*, which has a global distribution and *E. multilocularis*, which is found throughout the northern hemisphere. *Taenia multiceps*, *Taenia serialis*, and *Taenia brauni* are rare zoonoses in humans and nematodes, in which humans are mostly aberrant accidental hosts in which the larval stages cause clinical symptoms. From a public health perspective the most important zoonotic nematode species is *Toxocara* spp., which is found throughout the warmer regions of the world. Visceral and ocular larva migrans are important common clinical outcomes of infection with *Toxocara* spp. larvae. Other nematode species of lesser importance globally include *Strongyloides stercoralis*, *Ancylostoma* spp. (causing cutaneous larval migrans and eosinophilic enteritis), *Gnathostoma* spp., *Thelazia callipaeda*, and *Dirofilaria immitis* (Macpherson, 2013a,b).

Dogs infected with *E. granulosus* and *E. multilocularis* are widely regarded as the main source of infection for human cystic and alveolar echinococcosis. These illnesses cause substantial morbidity and socioeconomic burden in several regions of the world (Carmena and Cardona, 2013). More than 90% of the estimated 18,000 annual new cases of alveolar echinococcus are reported from China, primarily in the Tibetan plateau where there is concomitant infections in dogs (Togerson et al., 2010). Cystic echinococcosis infects more than 3 million people globally, and there are an estimated 200,000 new cases diagnosed annually (Atkinson et al., 2013). Cystic echinococcosis has been established in vast endemic regions of Africa, as dogs are free to roam, scavenge, or deliberately feed on offal from infected animals resulting in high prevalence. There is also active transmission in Europe, Asia, and South America (Alvarez-Rojas et al., 2013). The route of transmission of eggs to humans include the adherence of taeniid eggs to fur, with which people can have direct contact, contamination of food, and contamination of drinking water. Management of both alveolar and cystic echinococcosis involves following WHO guidelines involving an individualized approach with chemotherapy and/or surgery. Control of alveolar and cystic echinococcosis is based on the veterinary concepts to manage the definitive host populations through appropriate population control, use of praziquantel and, in the case of *E. granulosus*, through the restriction of infection opportunities by the use of slaughterhouses for livestock.

4.8.4 Emerging issues

The emerging occurrences of parasitic diseases provide examples of current and future challenges to look out for. *B. procyonis,* a nematode of raccoons (*Procyon Iotor*) that can cause fatal, usually neurological, larval migrans disease in several bird and mammal species, including humans. The distribution and prevalence of *B. procyonis* is noted among raccoons in central and western North Carolina and counties bordering Tennessee (Hernandez et al., 2013). Beasley et al. (2013) has shown that habitat fragmentation through anthropogenic activities is altering the transmission dynamics of the parasite. *B. procyonis* was recently found in imported animals in Norway (Davidson et al., 2013).

4.9 Conclusions

This chapter examined parasites that are transmitted by the consumption of meat, fish, plants, invertebrates, as well as from environmental contamination of water, food, and other sources. The epidemiology of these parasitic diseases is affected by human behavior. The social and cultural aspects of human behavior determine the types and preparation of food cuisines, the species of animals with which we interact, and which foods are consumed. The exposures from environmental conditions, food processing, and infrastructure are also a reflection of the socioeconomic status of a region. Cultural practices of consuming undercooked meat and fish, the changing dietary patterns of ready-to-eat food products, together with the rapid expansion of the human population and migration promote improper sanitation and hygiene standards especially in developing countries. The spillover of parasitic infections from companion, livestock, and wildlife species of animals has emerged as the dynamics of society and culture, and the epidemiology and control of foodborne parasites have changed.

Educating how to properly cook foods, avoiding risky sources of food, and applying hygiene practices and sanitation standards is required if reductions in many parasitic species is to be achieved. Implementing the veterinary aspects of companion, livestock, and wildlife animal parasite management and surveillance is also essential, as is clinical care in using antiparasitic chemoprophylaxis and surgical interventions as a part of the control and management of foodborne parasites. The global sociocultural dynamics of the increasing human population, the increase in the demand for protein of animal origin, increasing culinary diversity, travel, and migration, waste management, and changing climates, together with the increasing socioeconomic divide, are contemporary realities, which ensure that foodborne parasitic diseases will remain and increase in their challenges to public health.

4.10 Future trends

4.10.1 Globalization

Global changes in the human population through continued growth, particularly in developing countries, rapid urbanization, migration both legal and illegal, wars and the vast numbers of refugees, currently estimated by the UN at 52.1 million, challenge our ability to control parasitic infection. This challenge is further complicated by increases in food production, export of meat and plants, and the infusion of different culinary traditions. The resultant changes in the environment, which include climate, agricultural practices of increased food production, and alterations in the population of domestic, livestock, and wildlife species, further promote the risk of foodborne parasitic diseases. The intensification of agriculture and environmental changes, driven by the expanding human population, is a consequence of human behavior (Jones et al., 2013). Another critical and related issue linked to the changing population demographics is the increased number of people living under water stress. The role of water in foodborne parasitic infections through aquatic and marine sources of food, environmental contamination, and only meat or only plant consumption will place pressure on the hygiene and sanitary standards for food safety. Pathogens may also be distributed in new niches and enable exposing new human and animal populations to infection (Robertson et al., 2014).

4.10.2 Zoonotic challenges

Zoonoses are gaining in importance globally due to the emergence of new foodborne parasites, which occur at the human–animal–environmental interface. However, the health status of populations, as it relates to foodborne parasitic infections, remains poorly defined despite the overall burden of parasitic diseases. Moving ahead, there is a need to update data on parasitic infections to address the gaps in knowledge (Bordier and Roger, 2013). This measure will require an allocation of funds for research, surveillance, and control programs, which include foodborne parasitic diseases as a part of the overall burden of disease. The human–animal–environmental interface that is relevant for addressing the burden of foodborne parasites requires a one-health approach. One-health interconnects zoonoses with agriculture and food safety and has enhanced the response by authorities to reorganize and respond to the majority of parasitic zoonoses (Bidaisee and Macpherson, 2014). The one-health approach must also recognize the social and cultural influences on the epidemiology of foodborne parasites and as such, implement a threefold measure toward prevention and control, which includes education, diagnostic, and public health measures.

4.10.3 Prevention and control

Educational programs for parasitic zoonoses have to contend with the social and cultural factors that favor the transmission of the infections. For example, the sociocultural traditions and values attached to food choices, preparation, and consumption challenge a system of beliefs and practices against health management. The educational efforts must therefore offer alternative, sustainable, and affordable solutions to inform relevant behavioral changes to traditional practices. Educational programs to effect behavioral changes suffer from the long prepatent periods and lack of association between behaviors, which resulted in infection and subsequent disease. An exception was the success of the prenatal educational program, which focused on reducing *T. gondii* exposure during pregnancy (Bresciani et al., 2013).

The development and implementation of new, affordable screening tools are required and should be routinely applied in the management of foodborne parasitic diseases. The new, cheaper, multispecies tests, which can be interpreted by minimally trained individuals, are required to confirm cases of foodborne parasitic infections. For these diagnostic aims to be achieved, the considerations of limited resources and expertise of staff at these facilities will require standardized interlaboratory test validation, intersectoral collaboration, and the establishment of an international one-health diagnostic platform (Johansen et al., 2013).

Public health measures are also necessary as foodborne parasitic infections continue to be a global health challenge for the future. Improvements to water supply and quality, hygiene, sanitation, and animal husbandry practices are all geared toward promoting food safety of consumed products. The protozoa and helminths of public health relevance require a global effort as the movements of animals and animal-derived products continue to promote the geographical transmission of foodborne parasites. The example from Jenkins et al. (2013a,b) illustrated the need for international health regulations to be inclusive as they relate to foodborne parasitic diseases. The priorities of globalization include development, security, and public health representation of the priorities for global health (De Cock et al., 2013). These priorities are reflected in the issues related to foodborne parasitic diseases. The role of community-based measures, such as screening, is also an essential tool to address the current and future trends of foodborne parasites. Detection of taeniasis carriers of *T. solium* using stool microscopy with direct smear and copro-PCR showed an overall parasitic burden of more than 80% in northwest Sichuan, Tibet (Li et al., 2013). A comprehensive epidemio-clinical picture of sporadic, domestically acquired cases of amoebiasis, cryptosporidiosis, and giardiasis in a Canadian community identified the exposure to risk factors and measures employed to manage the outbreak (Ravel et al., 2013). Epidemiological data and practices toward prevention and control at the community level will inform the global efforts in research programs and policy that are evidenced based on addressing the future trends of foodborne parasites.

References

Alvarez-Rojas, C.A., Romig, T., Lightowlers, M., 2013. *Echinococcus granulosus sensu lato* genotypes infecting humans-review of current knowledge. Int. J. Parasitol. 44 (1), 9–18.

Atkinson, J.A.M., Gray, D.J., Clements, A.C.A., Barnes, T.S., McManus, D.P., Yang, Y.R., 2013. Environmental changes impacting *Echinococcus* transmisison: research to support predictive surveillance and control. Glob. Chang. Biol. 19 (3), 677–688.

Azim, S., Dojki, F., Ahmad, S.S., Beg, M.A., 2008. Role of human behavior and parasitic diseases. Infect. Dis. J. Pak. 17 (4), 128–134.

Beasley, J., Egan, T.S., Page, K., Hennessy, C., Rhodes, O.E., 2013. *Baylisascaris procyonis* infection in white-footed mice: predicting patterns of infection from landscape habitat attributes. J. Parasitol. 99 (5), 743–747.

Beck, A.M., 2013. The human-dog relationship; a tale of two species. In: Macpherson, C.N.L., Meslin, F.X., Wandeler, A.I. (Eds.), Dogs, Zoonoses and Public Health. CAB International, Wallingford, Oxford, UK, pp. 1–12.

Benkerroum, N., 2013. Traditional fermented foods of North African countries: technology and food safety challenges with regard to microbial risks. Compr. Rev. Food Sci. Food Saf. 12, 54–89.

Bidaisee, S., Macpherson, C.N.L., 2014. Zoonoses and one health: a review of the literature. Int. J. Parasitol. Res. 2014. Article ID 874345, 8 pages. http://dx.doi.org/10.1155/2014/874345.

Bordier, M., Roger, F., 2013. Zoonoses in South-East Asia: a regional burden, a global threat. Anim. Health Res. Rev. 14, 40–67.

Bouvard, V., Baan, R., Straif, K., Grosse, Y., Secretan, B., El Ghissassi, F., Benbrahim-Tallaa, L., Guha, N., Freeman, C., Galichet, L., Cogliano, V., 2009. A review of human carcinogens—Part B: biological agents. Lancet Oncol. 10, 321–322.

Bowie, W.R., King, A.S., Werker, D.H., Isaac-Renton, J.L., 1997. Outbreak of toxoplasmasis associated with municipal drinking water. Lancet 350, 173–177.

Branden, C.R., Tauxe, R.V., 2013. Emerging trends in food-borne diseases. Infect. Dis. Clin. North Am. 27 (3), 517–533.

Bresciani, K.D.S., Galvao, A.L.B., de Vasconcellos, A.L., Soares, J.A., de Matos, L.V.S., Pierucci, J.C., Neto, L.D.S., 2013. Relevant aspects of human toxoplasmosis. Res. J. Infect. Dis. 1 (1), 7.

Broglia, A., Kapel, C., 2011. Changing dietary habits in a changing world: emerging transmission of food-borne parasitic zoonoses. Vet. Parasitol. 182 (1), 2–13.

Carmena, D., Cardona, G.A., 2013. Canine echinococcus: global epidemiology and genotypic diversity. Acta Trop. 128 (3), 441–460.

CDC, 2013. Parasites-Toxocariasis. Centers for Disease Control and Prevention (CDC), Atlanta, GA. Available from: http://www.cdc.gov/parasites/toxocariasis (accessed 26.11.13.).

Chai, J.Y., Darwin, M.K., Lymberg, A.J., 2005. Fishborne parasitic zoonoses. Int. J. Parasitol. 35 (11–12), 1233–1254.

Chandrawathani, P., Premaalathan, B., Zaini, M.Z., Adran, M., Nurulaini, R., Zawida, Z., Jamnah, O., Premila, M., Gajadhar, A., Ramlan, M., 2010. Seroprevalence of trichinellosis in pigs in northern states of Malaysia. Malays. J. Vet. Res. 1, 33–36.

Chen, X., Zuo, Y., Rosenthal, B.M., He, Y., Cui, L., Yang, Z., 2011. *Sarcocystis sinensis* in an ultrastructurally distinct parasite of water buffalo that can cause food-borne illness but cannot complete its life cycle in human beings. Vet. Parasitol. 178 (1–2), 35–39.

Chen, J.X., Chen, M.X., Ai, L., Xu, X.N., Jiao, J.M., Zhu, T.J., Su, H.Y., Luo, J.J., Guo, Y.H., Lu, S., Zhou, X.N., 2013. An outbreak of human *Fascioliasis gigantica* in Southwest China. PLoS One 8 (8), e71520.

Clausen, J.H., Madsen, H., Murrell, K.D., Van, P.T., Thu, H.N.T., Do, D.T., Thi, L.A.N., Manh, H.N., Dalsgaard, A., 2012. Prevention and control of fish-borne zoonotic trematodes in fish nurseries, Vietnam. Emerg. Infect. Dis. 18 (9), 1438.

Coyle, C.M., Mahanty, S., Zunt, J.R., Wallin, M.T., Cantery, P.T., White, A.I., O'Neal, S.E., Serpa, J.A., Southern, P.M., Wilkins, P., McCarthy, A.E., Higgs, E.S., Nash, T.E., 2012. Neurocysticersosis; neglected but not forgotten. PLoS Negl. Trop. Dis. 6 (5), e1500.

Cui, J., Wang, Y., Wang, Z.Q., 2013. Cutaneous Gnathostomiasis with recurrent migrating nodule and persistent eosinophilia: a case report from China. Korean J. Parasitol. 51 (4), 467–470.

Davidson, R.K., Oives, O., Hamnes, I., Schultz, J.E., 2013. Illegal wildlife imports more than just animals-*Baylisascaris procyonis* in Racoons (*Procyon Iotor*) in Norway. J. Wildl. Dis. 49 (4), 986–990.

Davies, A.P., Chalmers, R.M., 2009. Cryptosporidiosis. Br. Med. J. 339, b4168.

De Cock, K.M., Simone, P.M., Davison, V., Slutsker, L., 2013. The new global health. Emerg. Infect. Dis. 19 (8), 1192–1197.

Del Brutto, O.H., 2014. Clinical management of neurocysticercosis. Expert Rev. Neurother. 14 (4), 389–396. http://dx.doi.org/10.1586/14737175.2014.890892.

Deshpande, J.D., Phalke, D.B., 2013. The sanitary condition of food establishments and health status and personal hygiene among food handlers in a rural area of Western Maharashtra, India. Asian J. Med. Sci. 4 (2), 23–29.

Dhaliwal, B.B.S., Juyal, P.D. (Eds.), 2013. Trematode zoonoses. Parasitic Zoonoses. Springer, India, pp. 46–63.

Dorny, P., Praet, N., Deckers, N., Gabriel, S., 2009. Emerging food-borne parasites. Vet. Parasitol. 163 (3), 196–206.

Escobedo, A.A., Cimerman, S., 2007. Giardiasis: a pharmacotherapy review. Expert opinion. Pharmacotherapy 81, 1885–1902.

Esteban, J.G., Munoz-Antoli, C., Borras, M., Colomina, J., Toledo, R., 2014. Human infection by a "fish tapeworm", *Diphyllobothrium latum*, in a non-endemic country. Infection 42 (1), 191–194.

FAO, 2010. The State of World Fisheries and Aquaculture. The United Nations Food and Agriculture Organization (FAO), Rome. Available from: http://www.fao.org/docrep/013/i1820e/i1820e00.htm (accessed 27.11.13.).

Fazly, Z.A., Nurulaini, R., Shafarin, M.S., Fariza, N.J., Zawida, Z., Muhamad, H.Y., Adnan, M., Premaalatha, B., Erwanas, A.I., Zaini, C.M., Ong, C.C., Chandrawathani, P., 2013. Zoonotic parasites from exotic meat in Malaysia. Trop. Biomed. 30 (3), 535–542.

Fentie, T., Erqou, S., Gedefaw, M., Desta, A., 2013. Epidemiology of human fascioliasis and intestinal parasitosis among schoolchildren in Lake Tana Basin, Northwest Ethiopia. Trans. R. Soc. Trop. Med. Hyg. 107 (8), 480–486.

Forbes, L.B., Measures, L., Gajadhar, A., Kapel, C., 2003. Infectivity of *Trichinella nativa* in traditional northern (countries) foods prepared with meat from experimentally infected seals. J. Food Prot. 66, 1857–1863.

Franco, R.M.B., 2013. Environmental Contamination by Protozoa *Giardia* spp., *Cryptosporidium* spp., and *Ascaris summ*: Challenges of Detection, Removal and Inactivation of Infective Forms. Available from: http://www.bv.fapesp.br/auxilios/56139/environmental-contamination-by-protozoa (accessed 30.11.13.).

Frickmam, H., Schwartz, N.G., Wiemer, D.F., Fischer, M., Tannid, E., Scheid, D.L., Muller, M., Schotte, U., Bock, W., Hagen, R.M., 2013. Food and drinking water hygiene and intestinal protozoa in deployed German soldiers. Eur. J. Microbiol. Immunol. 3 (1), 53–60.

Furst, T., Sayasone, S., Odermatt, P., Keiser, J., Utzinger, J., 2012. Manifestation, diagnosis, and management of food-borne trematodiasis. Br. Med. J. 344, e4093.

Gendel, S.M., Khan, N., Yajnik, M., 2013. A survey of food allergen control practices in the US food industry. J. Food Prot. 2, 302–306.

Guillen, A., Gonzalez, M., Gallego, L., Suarez, B., Luz, H.H., Hernandez, T., Naranjo, M., Salazar, J., 2013. Presence of intestinal protozoans in water for consumption in “18 de Mayo Community”, Aragua State, Venezuela. Bol. Mal. Salud Amb. 53 (1), 29–36.

Hall, R.L., Lindsay, A., Hammond, C., Montgomery, S.P., Wilkins, P.P., da Silva, A.J., McAuliffe, I., de Almeida, M., Bishop, H., Mathison, B., Sun, B., Largensen, R., Jones, J.L., 2012. Outbreak of human Trichinellosis in Northern California caused by *Trichinella murrelli*. Am. J. Trop. Med. Hyg. 87 (2), 297–302.

Havelaar, A.H., Cawthorne, A., Angulo, F., Bellinger, D., Corrigna, T., Cravioto, A., Gibb, H., Hald, T., Ehiri, J., Kirk, M., Lake, R., Praet, N., Speybroeck, N., de Silva, N., Stein, C., Togerson, P., Kuchenmuller, T., 2013. WHO initiative to estimate the global burden of food-borne disease. Lancet 381, 559.

Herbinger, K.H., Metzner, M., Schmidt, V., Beissner, M., Nothdurft, H.D., von Sonneburg, F., Luscher, T., 2013. Infection induced anaemia: a cross sectional study of 14, 636 German travellers aged 20–49 years. Infection 41 (6), 1079–1087.

Hernandez, S.M., Galbreath, B., Riddle, D.F., Moore, A.P., Palamar, M.B., Levy, M.G., Deperno, C.S., Correa, M.T., Yabsley, M.J., 2013. *Baylisascaris procyonis* in racoons (*Procyon lotor*) from North Carolina and current status of the parasite in the USA. Parasitol. Res. 112 (2), 693–698.

Hung, N.M., Madsen, H., Froel, B., 2013. Global status of fishborne zoonotic trematodiasis in humans. Acta Parasitol. 58 (3), 231–258.

Ishaku, A.A., Asheojo, D., Habibu, T., Sunday, T.M., Amuto, E.A., Azua, A.T., 2013. Prevalence of intestinal parasitic infections among food vendors in Lafia Metropolis of Nasarawa State, Nigeria. Sch. J. Biotechnol. 2 (2), 21–25.

Jayashi, C.M., Gonzalez, A.E., Neyra, R.C., Kyngdon, C.T., Gauci, C.G., Lightowlers, M.W., 2012. Characterization of antobody responses in pigs induced by recombinant oncosphere antigens from *Taenia solium*. Vaccine 30 (52), 7475–7480.

Jenkins, E.J., Schwer, J.M., Gesy, K.M., 2011. Old problems on a new playing field: Helminth zoonoses transmitted among dogs, wildlife, and people in a changing northern climate. Vet. Parasitol. 182 (1), 54–69.

Jenkins, E.J., Castrodale, L.J., de Rosemond, S.J., Dixon, B.R., Elmore, S.A., Gesy, K.M., Hoberg, E.P., Polley, L., Schwer, J.M., Simard, M., Thompson, R.C., 2013a. Tradition and transition: parasitic zoonoses of people and animals in Alaska, Northern Canada and Greenland. Adv. Parasitol. 82, 33–204.

Jenkins, D.J., Brown, G.K., Traub, R.J., 2013b. 'Cysticercosis storm' in feedlot cattle in north-west New South Wales. Aust. Vet. J. 91 (3), 89–93.

Jex, A.R., South, H.V., Nolan, M.J., Campbell, B.E., Young, N.D., Cantacessi, C., Gasser, R.B., 2001. Cryptic parasite revealed improved prospects for treatment and control of human cryptosporidiosis through advanced technologies. Adv. Parasitol. 77, 141–173.

Johansen, M.V., Lier, T., Sithithaworn, P., 2013. Towards improved diagnosis of neglected zoonotic trematodes using a one health approach. Acta Trop. 141, 161–169. Available from: http://www.sciencedirect.com/science/article/pii/50001766X13001861 (accessed 2.12.13.).

Johnson, K.A., White, A.E., Boyd, B.M., Cohen, A.B., 2011. Matzah, meat, milk and mana, psychological influences on religio-cultural food practices. J. Cross Cult. Psychol. 42 (8), 1421–1436.

Jones, J.L., Dubey, J.P., 2012. Food-borne toxoplasmosis. Clin. Infect. Dis. 55 (6), 845–851.

Jones, B.A., Grace, D., Koch, R., Alonso, S., Ruston, J., Said, M.Y., McKeever, D., Mataa, F., Young, J., McDermott, J., Pfeiffer, D.U., 2013. Zoonosis emergence linked to agricultural intensification and environmental change. Proc. Natl. Acad. Sci. U.S.A. 110 (21), 8399–8404.

Jones, J.L., Parise, M.E., Fiore, A.E., 2014. Neglected tropical diseases in the United States: toxoplasmosis. Am. J. Trop. Med. Hyg. 90 (5), 794–799.

Khanum, H., Shanjida, K.S., Sultana, M., Uddin, M.H., Chandra, D.R., Islam, M.A., 2012. Protozoan parasites in a wastewater treatment plant of Bangladesh. Univ. J. Zool. Rajshahi Univ. 31, 5–8.

Khurana, S., Malla, N., 2014. Water and food-borne trematodiasis in humans. In: Singh, P. P., Sharma, V. (Eds.), Parasitic Zoonoses. Springer, India, pp. 219–227.

Kim, S.H., Park, C.W., Kim, S.K., Won, S., Park, W.K., Kim, H.R., Nam, K.W., Lee, G.S., 2013. A case of anisakiasis invading the stomach and the colon at the same time after eating anchovies. Clin. Endosc. 46 (3), 293–296.

Kozak, G.K., MacDonald, D., Landry, L., Faiter, J.M., 2013. Food-borne outbreaks in Canada linked to produce; 2001 through 2009. J. Food Prot. 1, 4–183.

Lal, A., Baker, M.G., Hales, S., French, N.P., 2013. Potential effects of global environmental changes on cryptosporidiosis and giardiasis transmission. Trends Parasitol. 29 (2), 83–90.

Li, T., Chen, X., Yanagida, T., Wang, H., Long, C., Sako, Y., Okamoto, M., Wu, T., Giraudoux, P., Raoul, F., Nkouawa, A., Nakao, M., Craig, P.S., Ito, A., 2013. Detection of human taeniasis in Tibetan endemic areas, China. Parasitology 140 (13), 1602–1607.

Lightowlers, M.W., 2013. Control of *Taenia solium* taeniasis/cysticercosis: past practices and new possibilities. Parasitology 140 (13), 1566–1577.

Lozano, R., Naghavim, M., Foreman, K., Lim, S., Shibuya, K., Aboyam, V., Abraham, J., Adair, T., Aggarwa, I.R., Ahn, S.Y., 2013. Global and regional mortality from 235 cases of death for 20 age groups in 1990 and 2010: a systematic analysis for the Global Burden of Disease Study. Lancet 380, 2095–2128.

Macpherson, C.N.L., 2005. Human behavior and the epidemiology of parasitic zoonoses. Int. J. Parasitol. 35 (11–12), 1319–1331.

Macpherson, C.N.L., 2013a. The epidemiology and public health importance of toxocariasis: a zoonosis of global importance. Int. J. Parasitol. 43 (12–13), 999–1008, Zoonoses special edition.

Macpherson, C.N.L., 2013b. Dogs, zoonoses and human health: a global perspective. CAB Mini Rev. 8, 1–2.

Macpherson, C.N.L., Gottstein, B., Geerts, S., 2000. Parasitic food-borne and waterborne zoonoses. Rev. Sci. Tech. 19 (1), 240–258.

Maikai, B.V., Elisha, I.A., Baba-Onoja, E.B.T., 2012. Contamination of vegetables sold in markets with helminth eggs in Zaria Metropolis, Kaduna State, Nigeria. Food Control 28 (2), 345–348.

Mairiang, E., Laha, T., Bethony, J.M., Thinkhemrop, B., Kaewkes, S., Sithithaworn, P., Tesana, S., Loukas, A., Brindley, P.J., Sripa, B., 2012. Ultrasonography assessment of hepatobiliary abnormalities in 3359 subjects with *Opisthorchis viverrini* infection in endemic areas of Thailand. Parasitol. Int. 61 (1), 208–211.

Malheiros, A.F., Matthews, P.D., Scalon Lemos, L.M., Braga, G.B., Shaw, J.J., 2014. Prevalence of *Hymenolepis nana* in indigenous Tapirapé ethnic group from the Brazilian Amazon. Am. J. Biomed. Res. 2 (2), 16–18.

Matsuo, K., Rika, K., Hirona, U., Hanyu, G., Yasuhiro, T., Kisaburo, N., 2014. Seroprevalence of *Toxoplasma gondii* infection in cattle, horses, pigs and chickens in Japan. Parasitol. Int. 63 (4), 638–639.

Mattiucci, S., Fazil, P., Nascetti, G., 2013. Anisakiasis and gastroallergic reactions associated with *Anisakis pegreffii* infection, Italy. Emerg. Infect. Dis. 19 (3), 496–499.

Mbae, C.K., Nokes, D.J., Mulinge, E., Nyambura, J., Waruru, A., Kariuki, S., 2013. Intestinal parasitic infections in children presenting with diarrohoea in outpatient and inpatient settings in an informal settlement of Nairobi, Kenya. BMC Infect. Dis. 13 (1), 243.

McEntire, J., 2013. Food-borne diseases: the global movement of food and people. Infect. Dis. Clin. North Am. 27 (3), 687–693.

Miranda, H.A., Castellar-Leones, S.M., Elzain, M.A., Moscote-Salazar, L.R., 2013. Brain abscess: current management. J. Neurosci. Rural Pract. 4 (2), 567–581.

Momoh, H.A., Bello, M., Inabo, H., Wada, Y., Adole, E.B., Madaiki, B.D., Aregbe, E.A., 2012. Prevalence and some risk factors associated with trichinellosis in backyard pig farms in Zaria, Nigeria. Trop. Anim. Health Prod. 45 (5), 1149–1152.

Murrell, K.D., Djordjevic, M., Cuperlovic, K., Sofronic, L.J., Savic, M., Djordjevic, M., Damjanovic, S., 2014. Epidemiology of *Trichinella* infection in the horse: the risk from animal product feeding practices. Vet. Parasitol. 123 (2–4), 223–233.

Nawa, Y., Hatz, C., Blum, J., 2005. Sushi delights and parasites. The risk of fishborne and foodborne parasitic zoonoses in Asia. Clin. Infect. Dis. 41 (9), 297–303.

Ngugi, A.K., Kariuki, S.M., Bottomley, C., Kleinschmidt, I., Sander, T.W., Newton, C.R., 2011. Incidemce of epilepsy. Neurology 77 (10), 1005–1012.

Nissen, S., Nguyen, L.A.T., Thamsborg, S.M., Dalsgaard, A., Johansen, M.V., 2014. Reinfection of dogs with fish-borne zoonotic trematodes in Northern Vietnam following a single treatment with praziquantel. PLoS Negl. Trop. Dis. 8 (1), e2625.

Overstreet, R.M., 2013. Waterborne parasitic diseases in the ocean. In: Kanki, P., Grimes, D. J. (Eds.), Infectious Diseases. Springer, New York, pp. 431–496.

Patz, J.A., Graczyk, T.K., Geller, N., Vittor, A.Y., 2000. Effects of environmental change on emerging parasitic diseases. Int. J. Parasitol. 30, 1395–1405.

Phongluxa, K., Xayaseng, V., Vonghachack, Y., Akkhavong, K., van Eeuwijk, P., Odermatt, P., 2013. Helminth infection in Southern Laos: high prevalence and low awareness. Parasit. Vectors 6, 328.

Pitaksakulrat, O., Sithithaworn, P., Laoprom, N., Laha, T., Petney, T.N., Andrews, R.H., 2013. A cross-sectional study on the potential transmission of the carcinogenic liver fluke *Opisthorchis viverrini* and other fishborne zoonotic trematodes by aquaculture fish. Foodborne Pathog. Dis. 10 (1), 35–41.

Polley, L., 2005. Navigating parasite webs and parasite flow: emerging and re-emerging parasitic zoonoses of wildlife origin. Int. J. Parasitol. 35 (11–12), 1279–1294.

Polley, C., Thompson, R.C., 2009. Parasite zoonoses and climate change: molecular tools for tracking shifting boundaries. Trends Parasitol. 25 (6), 285–295.

Pozio, E., Murrell, K.D., 2006. Systematics and epidemiology of Trichinella. Adv. Parasitol. 63, 367–439.

Pozio, E., Owen, I.L., Marucci, G., La Rosa, G., 2005. Inappropriate feeding practice favors the transmission of *Trichinella papuae* from wild pigs to saltwater crocodiles in Papua New Guinea. Vet. Parasitol. 127 (3–4), 245–251.

Pozio, E., Foggin, C.M., Gelanew, T., Marucci, G., Hailu, A., Rossi, P., Morales, M.A., 2007. Trichinella zimbabwensis in wild reptiles of Zimbabwe and Mozambique and farmed reptiles of Ethiopia. Vet. Parasitol. 143 (3–4), 305–310.

Prasad, K.J., 2010. Emerging and re-emerging parasitic diseases. J. Int. Med. Sci. Acad. 23 (1), 45–50.

Raatz, S.K., Silverstein, J.T., Jahns, L., Picklo, M.J., 2013. Issues of fish consumption for cardiovascular disease risk reduction. Nutrients 5, 1081–1097.

Ravel, A., Nesbitt, A., Pintar, K., MacArthur, A., Way, H.L., Marshall, B., Polleri, F., 2013. Epidemiological and clinical description of the top three reportable parasitic diseases in a Canadian community. Epidemiol. Infect. 141 (1), 431–442.

Robertson, L.J., 2013. Approaches to detecting giardia cysts in different food matrices. In: *Giardia* as a Foodborne Pathogen. Springer, New York, pp. 19–26.

Robertson, L., 2014. Cryptosporidium as a Food-Borne Pathogen. Springer Briefs in Food, Health, and Nutrition, Springer, New York. http://dx.doi.org/10.1007/978-1-4614-9378-5.

Robertson, L.J., Chalmers, R.M., 2013. Food-borne cryptosporidiosis: is there really more in Nordic countries? Trends Parasitol. 29 (1), 3–9.

Robertson, L.J., Sprong, H., Ortega, Y.R., van der Giessen, J.W.B., Fayer, R., 2013. Impacts of globalization on food-borne parasites. Trends Parasitol. 30 (1), 37–52. Available from: http://www.sciencedirect.com/science/article/pii/S14714922130015 (accessed 30 November 2013).

Robertson, L.J., Sprong, H., Ortega, Y.R., van der Giessen, J.W.B., Fayer, R., 2014. Impacts of globalisation on food-borne parasites. Trends Parasitol. 30 (1), 37–52.

Romer, J.D., Leblanc, C.A., Clements, S., Ferguson, J.A., Kent, M.L., Noakes, D., Schnech, C.B., 2013. Survival and behavior of juvenile steelhead trout (Oncorhynchus mykiss) in two estuaries in Oregon, USA. Environ. Biol. Fishes 96 (7), 849–863.

Rothe, C., 2013. Paragonimiasis. In: Mabey, D., Gill, G., Weber, M.W., Parry, E., Whithy, C.J.M. (Eds.), Principles of Medicine in Africa. Cambridge University Press, Cambridge.

Saichua, P., Sithithaworn, P., Jariwala, A.R., Diemert, D.J., Sithithaworn, J., Sripa, B., Laha, T., Mairiang, E., Pairojkul, C., Periago, M.V., Khuntikeo, N., Mulvenna, J., Bethony, J.M., 2013. Microproteinuria during *Opisthorchis viverrini* infection: a biomarker for advanced renal and hepatobiliary pathologies from chronic opisthorchiasis. PLoS Negl. Trop. Dis. 7 (5), e2228. http://dx.doi.org/10.1371/journal.pntd.0002228.

Said, D.E.S., 2012. Detection of parasites in commonly consumed raw vegetables. Alexandria J. Med. 48 (4), 345–352.

Simon, A., Rousseau, A., Savary, S., Bigras-Poulin, M., Ogden, N.H., 2013. Hydrological modelling of *Toxoplasma gondii* oocysts transport to investigate contaminated snowmelt runoff as a potential source of infection for marine mammals in the Canadian Arctic. J. Environ. Manage. 127, 150–161.

Sithithaworn, P., Andrews, R.H., van De, N., Wongsaroj, T., Sinuon, M., Odermatt, P., Nawa, Y., Brindley, P.J., Banchob, S., 2012. The current status of opisthorchiasis and clonorchiasis in the Mekong Basin. Parasitol. Int. 61 (1), 10–16.

Sithithaworn, P., Yongvanit, P., Duenngai, K., Kiatsopit, N., Pairojkul, C., 2014. Roles of liver fluke infection as risk factor for cholangiocarcinoma. J. Hepatobiliary Pancreat. Sci. 21 (5), 301–308. http://dx.doi.org/10.1002/jhbp.62.

Song, K.D., Lim, J.H., Kim, M.J., Jang, Y.J., Kim, J.W., Cho, S.H., Kwon, J.H., 2013. Peritoneal manifestation of fascioliasis on CT images: a new observation. Abdom. Imaging 38 (4), 839–843.

Speich, B., Marti, H., Ame, S.M., Bogon, I.I., Utzinger, J., Albonico, M., Keiser, J., 2013. Prevalence of intestinal protozoa infections among school aged children on Pemba Island, Tanzania, and effects of single dose albendazole, nitazoxanide and albendazole-nitazoxanide. Parasit. Vectors 6 (1), 1–8.

Su, G.L.S., Mariano, C.M.R., Matti, N.S.A., Ramos, G.B., 2012. Assessing parasitic infestation of vegetables in selected markets in Metro Manila, Philipines. Asian Pac. J. Trop. Dis. 2 (1), 51–54.

Tacon, A.G.T., Metian, M., 2013. Fish matters: importance of aquatic foods in human nutrition and global food supply. Rev. Fish. Sci. 21 (1), 22–38.

Teem, J.L., Qvarnstrom, Y., Bishop, H.S., da Silva, A.J., Carter, J., White Mclean, J., Smith, T., 2013. The occurrence of the rat lungworm, *Angiostrongylus cantonensis*, in non-indigenous snails in the Gulf of Mexico region of the United States. Hawaii J. Med. Public Health 72 (6 Suppl. 2), 11–14.

Thewjitcharoen, Y., Medhajirapat, S., Sanprasert, V., Saksirisampant, W., Nuchprayoon, S., 2012. A fatal case of intestinal Capillariasis due to misleading investigations. Asian Biomed. Clin. Rep. 6 (5), 781–785.

Thompson, R.I., Kutz, S.J., Smith, A., 2009. Parasitic zoonoses and wildlife: emerging issues. Int. J. Environ. Res. Public Health 6 (2), 678–693.

Togerson, P.R., Keller, K., Magnotta, M., Rayland, N., 2010. The global burden of alveolar echinococcosis. PLoS Negl. Trop. Dis. 4, e722.

Torgerson, P.R., 2013. One world health. Socioeconomic burden and parasitic disease control priorities. Vet. Parasitol. 195 (3–4), 223–232.

Torgerson, P.R., Macpherson, C.N., 2011. The socioeconomic burden of parasitic zoonoses: global trends. Vet. Parasitol. 182 (1), 79–95.

UNFPA, 2014. The ICPD Beyond 2014 Global Report. Available from: www.unfpa.org (accessed 23.06.14.).

Wang, Q.P., Lai, D.H., Zhu, X.Q., Chen, X.G., Lun, Z.R., 2008. Human angiostrongyliasis. Lancet Infect. Dis. 10, 621–650.

Wiriya, B., Clausen, J.H., Inpankaew, T., Thaenkhan, U., Jittapalapong, S., Satapornvanit, K., Dalsgaard, A., 2013. Fishborne trematodes in cultured *Nile tilapia* (*Oreochromis niloticus*) and wild caught fish from Thailand. Vet. Parasitol. 198 (1–2), 230–234.

Yamamoto, N., 2009. Waterborne and foodborne infectious diseases. J. Food Hyg. Soc. Jpn. 50 (3), 215–220.

Zumaquero-Rios, J.L., Sarracent-Perez, J., Rojas-Garcia, R., Rojas-Rivero, L., Martinez-Tovilla, Y., Valero, M.A., Mas Coma, S., 2013. Fascioliasis and intestinal parasites affecting schoolchildren in Atlixco, Puebla State, Mexico: epidemiology and treatment with nitazoxanide. PLoS Negl. Trop. Dis. 7 (11), e2553.

Socioeconomic burden of foodborne parasites

5

J. Conlan[1], *A. Lal*[2]
[1]Food Standards Australia New Zealand, Barton, ACT, Australia; [2]Australian National University, Canberra, ACT, Australia

5.1 Introduction

Governments and health agencies around the world are constrained by limited resources with which to address the competing health needs of their populations. Decision makers at all levels of government are therefore required to allocate these limited resources in the most efficient and effective manner possible to maximize the public health benefit across the population as a whole. To do this requires the complex analysis of clinical, epidemiological, and socioeconomic health data to compare and contrast the competing priorities and make evidence-based decisions.

The World Health Organization (WHO) defines *burden of disease* as "the incidence and prevalence of morbidity, disability, and mortality associated with acute and chronic manifestations of diseases" (WHO, 2007). Monetary economic estimates and nonmonetary measures of disease burden can quantify the burden of a given disease on a nation, a population subgroup, or on a global scale. Estimates of disease burden can serve multiple purposes with the primary objective of improving the health and well-being of a given population. These estimates can be used to compare the overall health of communities and to identify which diseases and risk factors contribute most to a loss of good health in a given population, and they allow an assessment of the relative strength of a health system. In addition, these estimates enable costs associated with disease to be evaluated and, from a policy perspective, used to assess the cost-effectiveness of a regulatory or nonregulatory intervention to prevent foodborne disease transmission (Buzby, 2011). Finally, burden estimates complement biomedical surveillance methodologies to monitor foodborne disease trends and help decision makers, researchers, and the general public to identify the most important pathogens in a given population, region, or country and whether conditions are improving or worsening over time.

This chapter provides a summary of the methods used to estimate economic costs and the burden of foodborne parasites and reviews the current body of knowledge with respect to the socioeconomic burden of important foodborne parasites at national and global levels. The chapter concludes with a brief discussion of some epidemiological limitations and knowledge gaps.

Foodborne Parasites in the Food Supply Web. http://dx.doi.org/10.1016/B978-1-78242-332-4.00005-9

5.1.1 Methods of estimating socioeconomic burden

The socioeconomic burden of disease can be measured in terms of monetary costs or nonmonetary measures related to a healthy quality of life. Monetary methods are used to estimate the costs associated with treating, recovering from, or preventing ill health due to a particular infection and nonmonetary methods estimate the burden of disease by calculating the quality-of-life years gained by avoiding infection or the quality-of-life years lost due to acquiring an infection (Buzby, 2011).

5.1.1.1 Monetary methods

The *cost of illness* (COI) and the *willingness-to-pay* methods are commonly used models to estimate the economic burden of a foodborne disease (Buzby, 2011). This chapter presents data, where available, on the monetary cost of foodborne parasites based on the COI methodology. The COI in essence is the sum total of direct medical costs such as medical treatment and hospitalization, direct nonmedical costs such as transportation and relocation and indirect costs such as lost productivity, losses to future earnings through an inability to work or premature death. The COI method first estimates the annual number of cases due to foodborne exposure and categorizes these cases in terms of disease severity, ranging from mild to requiring medical attention, hospitalization, long-term sequelae, and, in the most severe cases, death. The costs for each group are tallied to achieve an overall estimate of economic costs associated with a foodborne disease (Buzby, 2011). Recently, methods have been developed to monetize quality-of-life measures to enable costings on pain and suffering measures that would not otherwise be calculated in a basic COI model (Scharff, 2012).

In the case of zoonotic diseases, costing models can also be used to estimate the economic losses experienced by the agricultural sector (Torgerson and Macpherson, 2011). Costs to the agricultural sector may be calculated by summing the losses resulting from decreased productivity, animal culling, or quarantine, carcass condemnation, or downgrading and post-slaughter treatments. Additionally, it is possible to account for costs resulting from food aversion and subsequent decreased market value for an implicated product.

The COI method provides real-world estimates of the financial costs to a society, region, or country. Yet the method is disadvantaged by the difficulty of estimating direct medical costs and accounting for losses to productivity and future earnings for populations where a substantial proportion of people are in an unsalaried working role, for example, care givers or children in farming communities in low-income countries. From a global perspective, an important limitation of the COI approach is that the costs associated with treatment and recuperation in a high-income country are higher than comparable costs in a low-income country due to differences in medical and wage costs. A disease with low incidence in a wealthy country may therefore have a greater total cost than the same disease with high incidence in a low-income country (Carabin et al., 2005; Torgerson and Macpherson, 2011). This raises important equity and value-of-a-human-life issues (Murray et al., 2012b) and thereby diminishes the utility of the COI approach for comparing burden between countries. As a consequence of the problems that exist with monetary estimates of disease burden, nonmonetary burden estimates are preferred by many organizations, including the WHO.

5.1.1.2 Nonmonetary methods

Disability-adjusted life years (DALYs) and quality-adjusted life years (QALYs) are two common methods used to measure the burdens of disease and injury. The DALY metric is the nonmonetary measure reported throughout this chapter and is the measure used by the Global Burden of Diseases, Injuries, and Risk Factors (GBD) enterprise (Murray et al., 2012a), the WHO Global Health Estimates (WHO, 2013), and the WHO Foodborne Disease Burden Epidemiology Reference Group (FERG). DALYs measure both the morbidity and mortality associated with a particular disease or injury and is calculated as a sum of years of life lost (YLL) and years lived with disability (YLD). YLLs are years lost due to premature mortality and correspond to the number of deaths in a given population multiplied by the standard life expectancy at the age at which death occurs for a particular disease. YLDs for people living with a health condition or sequelae resulting from illness are calculated by multiplying the number of incident cases by the mean duration of illness and a disability weight (DW) that reflects the severity of the condition, ranging from perfect health (0) to death (1). WHO (2013) provides a detailed description of the methods used to calculate DALYs.

For diseases with high morbidity but low mortality, the DALY estimate is one of the few metrics that is versatile enough to elucidate the burden of chronic disease conditions (Hotez et al., 2014). The DALY estimate, does, however, have limitations. When applied to parasitic diseases, DALYs do not accurately reflect the nonlinear pathology of infections and do not necessarily account for comorbidities associated with polyparasitism (Payne et al., 2009). Further, DALYs do not reflect losses to future well-being or earning potential for diseases that may impact on normal development once the disability has resolved, such as school absenteeism. DALYs do not account for agricultural losses through lost labor and lost animal productivity, nor do they capture the costs borne by the state for costs associated with surveillance and disease control interventions (Hotez et al., 2014).

5.2 The foodborne cestode zoonoses

5.2.1 *Taenia solium*

The zoonotic tapeworm *Taenia solium* is widely distributed globally with a concentration of disease burden in low-income countries where poor hygiene practices are common and sanitation systems are lacking. *T. solium* transmission is wholly dependent on a two-host life cycle involving pigs and humans. Humans are the only natural definitive host acquiring the adult tapeworm (*T. solium* taeniasis) following ingestion of pork containing the larval stage of the parasite (cysticerci). Tapeworm carriers are then a source of infection for pigs and humans who become infected with cysticerci after ingesting eggs shed in feces (Conlan et al., 2009). Neurocysticercosis is the most severe and burdensome form of disease in humans and occurs when cysticerci become established in the central nervous system, causing serious neurological sequelae such as epilepsy, seizures, headaches, and increased intracranial pressure (Carabin et al., 2011). Socioeconomic losses are therefore seen in the health sector due to the disease burden and attendant costs associated with neurocysticercosis and the agricultural sector due to carcass condemnation (Carabin et al., 2005).

The Global Burden of Disease 2010 (GBD 2010) study estimated the burden of cysticercosis to be 503,000 DALYs lost globally or seven DALYs lost per 100,000 person-years (Murray et al., 2012b). In endemic countries, the burden can be far greater. In West Cameroon, for example, the burden of disease in the human population in 2009 was estimated to be 900 DALYs lost per 100,000 person-years (Praet et al., 2009), some 130 times greater than the global estimate. Other country-specific estimates include 25 DALYs lost per 100,000 person-years in Mexico (Bhattarai et al., 2012) and 54 DALYs lost per 100,000 person-years in Nepal (Devleesschauwer et al., 2014). Caution should, however, be exercised when comparing individual study results with the GBD 2010 study owing to differences in model inputs and assumptions. Notably, the GBD 2010 study used DWs for treated and untreated epilepsy that ranged from 0.072 for treated epilepsy to 0.657 for severe epilepsy (Murray et al., 2012a; Salomon et al., 2012). The West Cameroon, Nepal, and Mexico studies, on the other hand, used DWs ranging from 0.041 for treated epilepsy in patients 0–4 years old through to 0.150 for untreated epilepsy in patients older than 5 years (Bhattarai et al., 2012; Devleesschauwer et al., 2014; Praet et al., 2009). The number of epilepsy cases ascribed to cysticercosis in the GBD 2010 study was not clear, and regional extrapolation of data may have diluted burden estimates for endemic countries (Devleesschauwer et al., 2014; Torgerson et al., 2014). Furthermore, the GBD 2010, Nepal and West Cameroon studies measured only the burden associated with epilepsy, meaning the burden associated with other nonseizure-related neurological sequelae was not adequately addressed. Seizure-related illness, including epilepsy, accounts for between 70% and 80% of symptomatic neurocysticercosis cases (Bern et al., 1999; Carabin et al., 2011) and the DALYs lost from nonseizure-related illness would undoubtedly increase the global burden estimate and that for Nepal and West Cameroon. In Mexico, severe chronic headache prevalence data was available, which was used in combination with epilepsy and death data to calculate DALY estimates for neurocysticercosis; these headaches accounted for more than 9% of the overall DALYs lost (Bhattarai et al., 2012). Overall, the GBD 2010 study and the country-specific estimates may have underestimated the nonmonetary burden of disease associated with neurocysticercosis.

In the Eastern Cape Province of South Africa, the costs associated with human disease were estimated to be between US$18.6 and US$34.2 million (US$2.6 to US$4.8 per capita) depending on how productivity losses from illness were calculated. The cost to the agricultural sector was estimated to be US$5 million (Carabin et al., 2006). In West Cameroon, the monetary burden of cysticercosis was estimated at US$14.4 million (€10.3 million) (US$2.8 per capita), 95% of which was attributed to human illness and 5% attributed to losses in pig production (Praet et al., 2009).

In nonendemic high-income countries, the cost can also be substantial. In Los Angeles County, the cost of neurocysticercosis hospitalizations was estimated to be US$136.2 million for the period 1991–2008 (Croker et al., 2010). The cost model excluded other costs associated with the illness, such as losses to work time and productivity, and the overall cost to the economy would likely be far greater. Locally acquired neurocysticercosis has been documented in the United States (Sorvillo et al., 2011), but the vast majority of cases are due to travel to or immigration from endemic countries in Central and South America (Croker et al., 2010; Sorvillo et al., 2011).

5.2.2 Taenia saginata *and* Taenia asiatica

Human taeniasis caused by an infection with the adult tapeworms *T. saginata* or *T. asiatica* occurs through the consumption of viable cysticerci in undercooked beef or pork, respectively. The clinical signs associated with taeniasis, irrespective of taeniid species, are generally moderate or not observed, and the burden of disease in terms of DALYs lost are expected to be negligible (Torgerson and Macpherson, 2011). Few attempts have been made to estimate the cost burden of *T. saginata* or *T. asiatica*, and studies, where they exist, tend to report on the costs associated with losses due to carcass condemnation.

In areas of Asia where *T. asiatica* is endemic, crude costs associated with infection have been calculated taking into account food expenditure losses, treatment costs, and work losses (Fan, 1997). Fan (1997) calculated an annual economic loss of US$11.3 million in aboriginal communities of the mountainous regions of Taiwan, US$13.6 million on the Cheju Island of Korea, and US$2.4 million on Samosir Island of Indonesia. In all cases, loss of work time made the greatest contribution to economic loss, followed by treatment costs and food expenditure losses. In Ethiopia, the cost of treating taeniasis has been estimated to be US$0.08 to US$0.18 per dose of drug (niclosamide, mebendazole, or praziquantel) and taeniasis prevalence estimates range from 60% to 70% (Abunna, 2013; Abunna et al., 2007; Tesfaye et al., 2012). Abunna (2013) noted that 85% of interview respondents reported using "modern" anthelminthic drugs to treat their taeniasis. With such high overall prevalence in some areas, and the possibility that multiple doses may be required to treat taeniasis, the resulting costs to the economy could be substantial.

In Europe, the economic burden of *T. saginata* taeniasis has been estimated to be low in the human population, with the vast majority of the costs associated with the control of bovine cysticercosis at slaughter, including meat inspection and testing, carcass condemnation, chilling, and storage (Dorny and Praet, 2007). The costs associated with bovine cysticercosis control and carcass condemnation undoubtedly will vary for different countries. In England, for example, the losses due to condemnation, carcass downgrading, and the facilities for chilling, handling, and storage has been estimated to cost on average US$160 (£100) per infected carcass (Gracey et al., 1999). In Iran, costs have been estimated to be US$394 per condemned carcass equating to an annual loss of US$410,000 due to a prevalence of 0.25% (Khaniki et al., 2010). Differences in the cost of carcass contamination are possibly due to differences in the post slaughter treatments applied. Additional costs are borne by producers and the agricultural and food regulatory agencies that investigate and implement control measures on farm.

5.2.3 Echinococcosis

Human echinococcosis is caused by an infection with the larval stage of several species of the genus *Echinococcus* after consuming viable eggs shed in the feces of its canine or feline definitive host (Bowman et al., 2006). This chapter will consider the two species where significant information regarding the socioeconomic burden of disease is available, namely *Echinococcus granulosus*, which is the causative agent of cystic echinococcosis (CE), and *Echinococcus multilocularis*, which is the causative agent of alveolar echinococcosis (AE). Exposure to eggs shed in the feces of infected canids, the primary definitive hosts, is critical for transmission and foodborne exposure is one of the several potential modes of transmission. Other modes include contact with fur, soil, surfaces, and water contaminated with feces of infected definitive hosts (Bowman et al., 2006). In addition, the length of time between exposure and the development of clinical disease for both CE and AE can range from 5 to 15 years (Bowman et al., 2006), indicating that source attribution may be difficult to determine (Torgerson et al., 2014). As a consequence, the proportion of the burden that can be attributed to food is not well defined.

The GBD 2010 study reported a combined estimate of global burden for AE and CE (referred to generically as echinococcosis) of 144,000 DALYs lost or two DALYs lost per 100,000 human years (Murray et al., 2012b). Considering the different life cycles, geographic distribution, and clinical outcomes, the merit of this decision has since been questioned (Hotez et al., 2014). The GDB 2010 estimate contrasts with Torgerson et al. (2010) in which the global burden of AE alone was estimated to be greater than 666,000 DALYs lost, of which 95% of the YLL were estimated to occur in China. The global incidence of AE was estimated to be 18,235 new cases per year of which 91% were assumed to occur in China with just 1606 occurring outside of China (Torgerson et al., 2010).

With respect to CE, the global burden of disease was estimated in 2006 to be 285,000 DALYs lost without accounting for underreporting and increased to 1 million DALYs lost when underreporting was factored in. The corresponding cost estimates were US$193 million, assuming no underreporting, and US$764 million when underreporting was factored in. The greatest burden of CE was observed in China and countries of the Middle East (Budke et al., 2006). In Nepal, the country-specific estimate for CE was 251 DALYs lost or one DALY lost per 100,000 person-years (Devleesschauwer et al., 2014).

The DWs assigned to echinococcosis in the GBD 2010 study were conservative in comparison to the global burden estimates for AE and CE. The GBD 2010 study assigned DWs 0.015 for mild chronic respiratory disease, 0.123 for moderate abdominopelvic disease, and 0.072–0.657 for epilepsy cases linked to echinococcosis (Murray et al., 2012a; Salomon et al., 2012). The Nepalese study and the other global burden estimates for AE and CE used DWs of 0.200–0.809 for mild disease through to terminal liver cancer (Budke et al., 2006; Devleesschauwer et al., 2014; Torgerson et al., 2010).

Global livestock production losses due to CE are also substantial as a result of carcass condemnation; losses have been estimated to be approximately US$1.4 million to US$2.2 million annually for liver condemnation alone, increasing to greater than US$2 billion when production factor losses such as poor weight gain and decreased milk production were taken into account (Budke et al., 2006).

5.3 The foodborne nematode zoonoses

5.3.1 Trichinellosis

Trichinellosis is a direct zoonosis, and infection occurs after consuming infective larvae in meat. The parasite has a global distribution and occurs in areas where cultural food habits involve the consumption of raw or partially cooked meat. Pork from domestic pigs and wild boars is the most common source of human trichinellosis. Horsemeat may also be an uncommon source of *Trichinella spiralis* infection (Murrell and Pozio, 2011). A wide range of wild animal species have also been a source of human trichinellosis caused by sylvatic *Trichinella* species (Pozio, 2007).

Little published data describe the disease burden or cost of *Trichinella* infection in humans and livestock or the incidence of clinical disease. In the period 1986–2009, there were 65,818 cases and 42 deaths from trichinellosis reported from 41 countries (Murrell and Pozio, 2011). Europe accounted for approximately 87% of these cases and Romania, in particular, accounted for approximately 50% of these European cases. Underreporting of nonsevere cases in many European countries may also lead to an underrepresentation of incidence (Murrell and Pozio, 2011).

The true global incidence of trichinellosis is currently unknown, but there are an estimated 10,000 cases annually, of which 0.2% are fatal (Pozio, 2011). The concentration of reported cases in Europe also suggests substantial underreporting in other endemic regions and where meat consumption habits and livestock production practices support *Trichinella* spp. transmission to humans. This is supported by recent evidence from Southeast Asia that indicates raw pork consumption is common and trichinellosis may be more widespread than the reported numbers indicate (Conlan et al., 2014; Vu Thi et al., 2013) with the potential for substantial underreporting (Vu Thi et al., 2013). Even though current estimates of global cases may be underestimated, the global burden of disease due to trichinellosis will most likely be low because of the acute nature of disease and the small number of fatalities (Torgerson and Macpherson, 2011).

Burden estimates based on DALY calculations, however, do not consider the substantial cost borne by the pork and game meat industries globally. In the European Union, approximately 167 million pigs are tested for *Trichinella* spp. every year at a cost of US$35 to US$560 million (€25 to €400 million) (Alban et al., 2011; Murrell and Pozio, 2011), even though a recent report indicates that *Trichinella* spp. have not been detected in domestic pigs raised in controlled production systems for the past 10–20 years (Pozio, 2014). This has raised concerns that the cost of universal testing is not proportionate to the public health benefit and that a move to risk-based surveillance concentrating on uncontrolled production systems is warranted (Alban et al., 2011; Pozio, 2014; Torgerson et al., 2014). In many countries, post slaughter testing and treatments, such as freezing and cooking, are not reliably applied to control trichinellosis (Thompson, 2014), and so there are no cost burdens associated with testing. The occurrence of trichinellosis can, however, have substantial impact on localized pork sales with consequent financial impacts on pig producers and traders. In northern Laos, for example, pork was not sold in a local market for more than 3 months following several trichinellosis outbreaks in 2005 (Barennes et al., 2008), but the economic losses were not estimated.

5.3.2 Anisakiosis

Anisakiosis in humans is caused by accidentally ingesting the third-stage larvae of parasites belonging to the family Anisakidae in infected saltwater fish, squid, and eels, which act as the second intermediate host in the parasites' life cycle. Most human infections are attributed to *Anisakis simplex*, *Anisakis physeteris*, and *Pseudoterranova decipiens*, and occasionally *Contracaecum* spp. Clinical disease in humans is caused by penetration of the larvae into the wall of the stomach or small intestine and is characterized by mild to severe abdominal pain, indigestion, nausea, vomiting, and, on occasion, allergic hypersensitive reactions such as urticaria, angioedema, and anaphylaxis (Nash, 2010; Torgerson and Macpherson, 2011). Gastric anisakiosis is commonly associated with *Pseudoterranova* and intestinal anisakiosis with *Anisakis*. Intestinal masses associated with anisakiosis can be mistaken for cancers, enteritis, and diverticulitis, and the acute pain and signs of obstruction can be mistaken for appendicitis (Nash, 2010). Consumption of dead parasites in cooked fish can also cause allergic hypersensitive reactions in individuals sensitive to the *Anisakis* antigen (Audicana et al., 2002).

Anisakiosis has a global distribution, but approximately 95% of cases have been reported from Japan and most have involved *A. simplex* (Audicana et al., 2002). Anisakiosis has recently been considered to be a rare foodborne disease, and the global burden is expected to be low (Torgerson et al., 2014). There are currently no published estimates of disease burden due to anisakiosis.

5.3.3 Angiostrongyliosis

Angiostrongyliosis, caused by the rat lung worm *Angiostrongylus cantonensis*, occurs after ingesting third-stage larvae in infected intermediate hosts. Infective larvae are found in a number of molluscs including slugs and snails, and paratenic transport hosts such as prawns, crabs, frogs, toads, freshwater fish, and monitor lizards may also harbor infective larvae (Cowie, 2013; Torgerson et al., 2014). Humans can become infected as an accidental host after consuming unwashed contaminated vegetables (Torgerson et al., 2014). After the larvae migrate to the central nervous system in humans, development beyond the subadult stage is stalled, and subadults cannot migrate out of the brain and back into the bloodstream. Clinical disease ensues from the physical damage caused by the worms moving and the inflammation caused by the immune reaction to dead and dying worms (Cowie, 2013). Clinical manifestations vary and with massive infections, fatalities can occur. Symptoms range from mild illness including abdominal pain, headache, and stiff neck to eosinophilic meningitis. Most patients have a relatively uncomplicated illness that can last from several weeks to several months (Nash, 2010).

Epidemics and sporadic infections occur most commonly in East and Southeast Asia and the South Pacific, and more recently the geographic distribution has expanded to the Caribbean, South America, Africa, Japan, Australia, and the United States (Cowie, 2013; Odermatt et al., 2010). Although there is no question that angiostrongylosis is a clinically significant disease and of public health importance in endemic areas, no estimates of disease burden have been published. Further still, there is no evidence that clearly demonstrates that the expanding geographic distribution is causing substantial increases in disease burden.

5.4 The foodborne trematode zoonoses

Clinically important foodborne trematodes include the liver flukes *Opisthorchis* spp., *Clonorchis sinensis*, *Fasciola* spp., and the lung fluke *Paragonimus* spp. (Sripa et al., 2010; Waikagul, 2015). The most prevalent trematodes with severe clinical complications are the small foodborne liver flukes *Opisthorchis viverrini* and *Clonorchis sinensis*. These two species have a complex life cycle, and the final definitive hosts, including humans, dogs, and cats, become infected after eating raw or inadequately cooked fish harboring infective metacercariae. Infection with *Fasciola* spp. arises from ingestion of metacercariae found on contaminated water plants such as watercress, and infection with *Paragonimus* spp. occurs after consuming inadequately cooked freshwater crabs and other crustaceans that act as intermediate hosts (Sripa et al., 2010). *Opisthorchis* spp., *C. sinensis*, and *Paragonimus* spp. are exclusively foodborne parasites, and although *Fasciola* spp. are potentially waterborne, the vast majority of cases are foodborne (Torgerson et al., 2014).

The life cycle of foodborne trematodes is complex, and transmission is restricted to areas where the first and the second intermediate hosts coexist and where food habits enable transmission to people (Keiser and Utzinger, 2005). The geographical distribution of the foodborne trematodes is diverse and the spatially focal occurrence presents methodological challenges in estimating incidence and disease burden (Furst et al., 2012). Globally, approximately 56 million people were infected with a foodborne trematode in 2005 (Furst et al., 2012), and an estimated 750 million people were at risk of infection (Keiser and Utzinger, 2009; Sripa et al., 2010). Of those infected, approximately 8 million cases with severe sequelae resulted in more than 7000 deaths annually. *C. sinensis* and *O. viverrini* induce the most severe disease, and infection may result in cholangiocarcinoma, a debilitating cancer of the bile duct (Sripa et al., 2007). The potential for *Opisthorchis felineus* to cause cancer of the bile duct is currently subject to debate, but the infection does result in severe disease in endemic regions of Central Asia and Eastern Europe (Furst et al., 2012; Hotez and Alibek, 2011).

The global burden of foodborne trematodes was estimated to be 665,000 DALYs in 2005 with the vast majority of the burden borne by people residing in spatially focal areas of endemicity (Furst et al., 2012). Greater than 440,000 DALYs were lost in China alone (including Hong Kong and Macau), predominantly due to clonorchosis (231,547 DALYs) and paragonimosis (188,439 DALYs). The burden of opisthorchosis caused by *O. viverrini* is restricted primarily to endemic regions of Thailand and Laos in Southeast Asia resulting in 74,070 DALYs lost. The estimated burden of opisthorchosis caused by *O. felineus* in Central Asia and Eastern Europe was relatively small in comparison with an estimated 297 DALYs lost. The global burden of fasciolosis was predominantly borne by Bolivia, Ecuador, and Peru in Latin America (17,318 DALYs lost), and Egypt and Iran in North Africa and the Middle East (17,275 DALYS lost) (Furst et al., 2012).

The incidence estimates for the foodborne trematodes are conservative and most likely represent an underestimate of the true incidence (Furst et al., 2012). In contrast, the GBD 2010 study estimated the global burden of foodborne trematodoses to be approximately 1.9 million DALYs lost or 27 DALYs lost per 100,000 population (Murray et al., 2012b). The Furst et al.(2012) study used DWs of 0.099 for heavy paragonimiasis; 0.100 for cerebral paragonimiasis; 0.104 for heavy clonorchiasis, heavy opisthorchiasis, and heavy fascioloiasis; and 0.116 for heavy intestinal fluke infection. Whereas the GBD 2010 study used DWs for moderate abdominopelvic disease of 0.123 for all conditions (Murray et al., 2012a; Salomon et al., 2012). Importantly, however, the Furst et al. (2012) study ascribed deaths to opisthochiasis and clonorchiasis and the GBD 2010 study did not (Lozano et al., 2012), despite strong evidence to the contrary (Hotez et al., 2014). Methodological and disease weighting differences can account for the different estimates, but it is clear that the foodborne trematodoses cause substantial loss in quality of life globally. In addition, the focal nature of occurrence means that the burden of disease estimates would be substantial in endemic areas if smaller geographic units were used to calculate DALYs lost per 100,000 person-years.

5.5 The foodborne protozoa

5.5.1 *Toxoplasmosis*

Toxoplasmosis is caused by an infection with the protozoan parasite *Toxoplasma gondii*. It is a very common parasitic infection in humans and other warm-blooded animals. The principal modes of *T. gondii* transmission are environmental exposure to fecal oocysts or foodborne exposure to tissue cysts present in the muscle of meat-producing animals or fecal oocysts in contaminated shellfish or on vegetables (Pereira et al., 2010a). The proportion of cases attributed to these foods has not been well established and is likely to vary greatly across the world.

Most human infections with *T. gondii* are asymptomatic, but infection may result in severe clinical disease including fetal death, congenital toxoplasmosis, toxoplasmic encephalitis, toxoplasmic retinochoroiditis, or less severe, acute self-limiting disease (Montoya and Liesenfeld, 2004). Congenital toxoplasmosis, which occurs as a result of maternal infection for the first time during pregnancy, can cause congenital defects or spontaneous abortion. These congenital defects can result in neonatal death, toxoplasmic retinochoroiditis, hydrocephalus, mental retardation, and intracranial calcifications (Hill et al., 2007; Zhou et al., 2011). Both congenitally and postnatally acquired toxoplasmosis may result in lifelong disability; however, the majority of cases of toxoplasmic retinochoroiditis in regions endemic for highly virulent *T. gondii* genotypes are postnatally acquired (Dubey et al., 2012).

Disease burden estimates so far have been limited to congenital toxoplasmosis (Devleesschauwer et al., 2014; Havelaar et al., 2007; Torgerson and Mastroiacovo, 2013). The global burden of congenital toxoplasmosis has been estimated to be 1.2 million DALYs or 960 DALYs lost per 100,000 live births, arising from 190,000 incident cases (Torgerson and Mastroiacovo, 2013). Country-specific estimates have been calculated for Nepal and the Netherlands. The estimated burden in Nepal was 35 DALYs lost per 100,000 live births, and in the Netherlands 319 DALYs were estimated to be lost per 100,000 live births (Devleesschauwer et al., 2014; Havelaar et al., 2007). The global burden study ascribed a DW of one for fetal loss of more than 24 weeks gestation and neonatal deaths and ascribed DWs of 0.010 for intracranical calcifications, 0.033 for retinochoroiditis, and 0.360 for hydrocephalus, and central nervous system abnormalities (Torgerson and Mastroiacovo, 2013). The Nepalese and Netherlands studies ascribed a DW of 0.08 and 0.17 for retinochoroiditis, respectively (Devleesschauwer et al., 2014; Havelaar et al., 2007). The DWs for intracranial calcifications (0.010), hydrocephalus, and central nervous system abnormalities (0.360) were the same for all studies.

The global burden study took into account the severity of disease depending on the genotype to which a pregnant woman may have been exposed, using a higher incidence of eye lesions in South American countries. The diagnostic performance of IgM testing was also corrected using a relatively small number of studies to estimate the sensitivity of IgM testing at birth to be 53%. The incidence of congenital toxoplasmosis at birth as reported in the global burden study (Torgerson and Mastroiacovo, 2013) were substantially higher than country-specific estimates in the industrialized countries of the Western Pacific region such as Australia (FSANZ, 2013; Jayamaha et al., 2012). The global estimate may require further validation as data become available. Notwithstanding any potential limitations, the burden of disease associated with congenital toxoplasmosis is substantial.

Estimating disease burden for postnatally acquired toxoplasmosis is complicated by the fact that severe clinical disease typically manifests in immunocompromised individuals with underlying conditions such as those with HIV infection or organ transplant recipients. The disease burden in these cases are assigned to the primary condition (Torgerson and Macpherson, 2011). In countries endemic for highly virulent *T. gondii* genotypes, retinochoroiditis, and severe illness requiring hospitalization are well-described conditions in otherwise healthy individuals (Carme et al., 2009; Demar et al., 2012; Dubey et al., 2012) and may significantly increase the burden of disease estimates in those affected countries.

In the United States, an estimated 86,686 foodborne incident cases of toxoplasmosis occur annually resulting in 4428 hospitalizations and 327 deaths (Scallan et al., 2011).

From these estimates, the cost of toxoplasmosis in the United States, excluding sequelae associated with congenital toxoplasmosis, was estimated to be US$3.1 billion using a basic COI model and US$3.5 billion when pain and suffering were also considered in the COI model (Scharff, 2012).

Losses to the agricultural industry globally may also be substantial, although no estimates are currently available. In sheep, in particular, infection with *T. gondii* may cause embryonic and fetal death, mummification, abortion, stillbirth, and neonatal death (Dubey, 2009b). In pigs, neonatal deaths may occur but are becoming less common with improved management of pig production practices (Dubey, 2009a).

5.5.2 Cryptosporidiosis

Cryptosporidiosis is a gastrointestinal illness caused by an infection with the protozoan parasite *Cryptosporidium*. Species of this genus are transmitted via the fecal–oral transmission route, and infection occurs after consuming cysts in contaminated water or food or via person-to-person or animal-to-person contact. A global systematic review of the proportion of diarrheal cases in patients over 5 years old indicated that *Cryptosporidium* was identified as the cause of diarrhea in a median of 1.3% of patients admitted to hospitals and 6.9% of patients in the community (Fischer Walker et al., 2012). However, the proportion of diarrheal episodes due to cryptosporidiosis is markedly different in high- and low-income countries. About 20% of diarrheal episodes in low-income countries have been attributed to *Cryptosporidium*, compared to approximately 9% in high-income nations (Slifko et al., 2000). In high-income countries, the infection is usually self-limiting with few long-term consequences (Torgerson and Macpherson, 2011). In contrast to the relatively low impact in high-income nations, *Cryptosporidium* infections in infants in low-income countries may be associated with long-term conditions such as stunting, impaired cognitive function, and mortality due to chronic malnutrition (Berkman et al., 2002; Chalmers and Davies, 2010; Guerrant et al., 1999; Putignani and Menichella, 2010).

The 2010 GBD study reported the global burden of cryptosporidiosis for the first time and estimated a burden of 8.4 million DALYs lost or 122 DALYs lost per 100,000 person-years (Murray et al., 2012b). DWs of 0.061, 0.202, and 0.281 corresponding to mild, moderate, and severe diarrhea were used by the GDB 2010 study (Murray et al., 2012a; Salomon et al., 2012). The large burden estimate was largely attributed to severe disease and death in young children in the South Asian region (Lozano et al., 2012; Vos et al., 2012), but the burden attributed to food has not been estimated.

In the United States, an estimated 57,616 foodborne incident cases of cryptosporidiosis occur annually resulting in 210 hospitalizations and four deaths (Scallan et al., 2011). From these estimates, the cost of cryptosporidiosis in the United States was estimated to be US$118 million using a basic COI model and US$168 million when pain and suffering were also considered in the COI model (Scharff, 2012).

The pathogen is easily transmitted through water, and a lack of sanitation, hygiene, and clean drinking water supplies in impoverished areas plays a major role in the spread of infection (Checkley et al., 2004). Importantly, *Cryptosporidium* infection causes severe, chronic diarrhea in HIV positive patients (Rao Ajjampur et al., 2007), although disease burden is assigned to the primary condition (Torgerson and Macpherson, 2011). Despite its obvious importance, the underestimation of *Cryptosporidium* in low-income countries is a serious impediment to accurately estimating the socioeconomic burden of cryptosporidiosis (Putignani and Menichella, 2010).

Cryptosporidium has been identified as one of the top five foodborne parasites globally (Robertson et al., 2013), and the proportion of cryptosporidiosis cases attributed to food has been estimated to be 8% in the United States (Scallan et al., 2011) and 10% in Australia (Kirk et al., 2014). Foodborne outbreaks are less commonly reported than waterborne outbreaks (Gherasim et al., 2012; Rose, 1997). The lack of appropriate diagnostic tools to isolate the parasite along with piecemeal testing of food sources is a key constraint to estimating the foodborne burden of disease due to *Cryptosporidium* (Slifko et al., 2000). However, recent advances in molecular techniques and superior reporting systems (Gherasim et al., 2012) have resulted in increased detection of *Cryptosporidium* transmission through food handlers (Ethelburg et al., 2009), imported produce (Insulander et al., 2008), ready-to-eat salads (Amoros et al., 2010), shellfish (Potasman et al., 2002), meat (Budu-Amoako et al., 2011), and milk (Robinson et al., 2014).

5.5.3 Giardiosis

Giardiosis is a gastrointestinal illness caused by an infection with the microscopic protozoan parasite *Giardia duodenalis*. *Giardia* is transmitted via the fecal–oral transmission route, and infection occurs after consuming cysts in contaminated water or food or via person-to-person or animal-to-person contact. A systematic literature review commissioned by WHO Foodborne Disease Burden Epidemiology Reference Group (FERG) found that compared to *Cryptosporidium* spp. and *Entamoeba*, *Giardia* was globally the most prevalent of the three parasites (Torgerson et al., 2014). Similar to cryptosporidiosis, infection is associated with growth impairment in children. A study in an urban area in the Brazilian Amazon found that children infected with *Giardia* had lower averages for all anthropometric measurements taken (Carvalho-Costa et al., 2007).There is also some evidence to suggest that *Giardia* infection may result in chronic gastrointestinal conditions (Hanevik et al., 2009). Of interest are the results from a longitudinal cohort study conducted from 2001 to 2006 in Peru, where the association between indices of wealth and giardiosis was significant, with higher wealth indices apparently providing protection against acute and persistent *Giardia* infections (Nundy et al., 2011). A Brazilian study that looked at sociodemographic and nutritional status as covariates for *Giardia* infection in children under 6 years old found that living in a two-bedroom or smaller house, living in a family of five or more, and living with the lack of a sewage system were significant risk factors for infection. Conversely, inadequate animal protein intake according to the Dietary Reference Intake recommendation and low hemoglobin concentration were only weakly associated with infection (Silva et al., 2009). This suggests that poverty-driven factors such as inadequate housing and sanitation facilities are key drivers of *Giardia* infection in low-income countries.

The global burden of disease associated with giardiosis has not been calculated; however, the 2010 GBD study estimated that 89.5 million DALYs are lost annually due to diarrheal diseases and, of these, 21.9 million DALYs (24.5%) are lost due to diarrheal diseases other than cholera, salmonellosis, shigellosis, enterotoxigenic and enteropathogenic *E. coli* infection, campylobacteriosis, entamoebosis, cryptosporidiosis, and rotaviral enteritis (Murray et al., 2012b). The burden attributed to giardiosis is likely to be substantial and comparable to the other diarrheal protozoan pathogens, particularly in regions with inadequate sanitation and water infrastructure.

In the United States, an estimated 76,840 foodborne incident cases of giardiosis occur annually resulting in 225 hospitalizations and two deaths (Scallan et al., 2011). From these estimates, the cost of giardiosis in the United States was estimated to be US$185 million using a basic COI model and US$282 million when pain and suffering were also considered in the COI model (Scharff, 2012).

Foodborne outbreaks of giardiosis have largely been attributed to infected food handlers (Mintz et al., 1993; Porter et al., 1990; Quick et al., 1992), with only one outbreak explicitly linked to the consumption of sheep tripe soup contaminated with *Giardia* cysts (Karabiber and Aktas, 1991). In another sandwich-related outbreak in a combined nursing home–child care center, 57% of the food handlers were infected with *Giardia* (White et al., 1989). Cold noodle salad made with dirty hands was the cause of another foodborne giardiosis outbreak (Petersen et al., 1988). These data suggest that contaminated food can be an important transmission route. Although the proportion of giardiosis cases attributed to food has been estimated to be 7% in the United States (Scallan et al., 2011) and 6% in Australia (Kirk et al., 2014), the burden of disease attributed to food globally is an important data gap.

5.5.4 Entamoebosis

Entamoeba histolytica is a pathogenic amoeba that can cause the intestinal and extraintestinal disease entamoebosis (amoebiasis or amebiasis). *E. histolytica* is transmitted via the fecal–oral route, and infection occurs after consuming mature cysts in contaminated water, food, soil, or on hands. This protozoan parasite is recognized as the second-leading cause of death from parasitic disease globally (Stanley, 2003) and is prevalent in tropical low-income nations; at times 50% of the general population may be infected, and globally the disease is estimated to cause 100,000 deaths annually (WHO, 2014c). In industrialized countries, *E. histolytica* infections are frequently reported from travelers returning from overseas and from recent immigrants and homosexual men (Nagata et al., 2012; Weinke et al., 1990; Ximenez et al., 2009). However, domestically acquired infections in indigenous populations in Northern Australia have also been reported (McCarthy et al., 2002). Rates of *E. histolytica* infections are generally higher where unsanitary conditions and high population densities prevail (Ximenez et al., 2009).

Like cryptosporidiosis, the GBD 2010 study reported the global burden of entamoebosis for the first time and estimated a burden of 2.2 million DALYs lost or 32 DALYs lost per 100,000 person-years (Murray et al., 2012b). DWs of 0.061, 0.202, and 0.281 corresponding to mild, moderate, and severe diarrhea were used by the GDB 2010 study (Murray et al., 2012a; Salomon et al., 2012). Like cryptosporidiosis, deaths attributed to entamoebosis in the South Asian region made a substantial contribution to the global burden estimate (Lozano et al., 2012). The burden attributed to food has not been estimated.

Ingestion of food and water contaminated with *E. histolytica* is the most common route of infection. In Brazil, age, place of residence, quality of drinking water, and consumption raw vegetables were identified as important determinants of infection (Benetton et al., 2005). However, socioeconomic and personal hygiene were also significant risk factors for infection with *E. histolytica* in an agricultural community in Hanan, Vietnam (Pham Duc et al., 2011). Indeed, the finding that food vendors in Abeokuta, Nigeria, recorded the highest prevalence of *E. histolytica* (72%) was attributed to inadequate personal hygiene (Idowu and Rowland, 2006). Reported outbreaks include an incident at a school that had its water supply contaminated by sewage (Chen et al., 2001), a family outbreak due to previous overseas travel to an endemic destination (Vreden et al., 2000), and a clinic outbreak from contamination of a colonic-irrigation machine (Istre et al., 1982). Although produce contaminated with wastewater used for irrigation has been identified as a source of human *E. histolytica* infection (Cifuentes et al., 1991; Do et al., 2007; Melloul et al., 2002), there is a lack of comprehensive evidence to link any specific food sources to human infection.

5.5.5 Cyclosporosis

Cyclosporosis is a gastrointestinal illness caused by infection with the protozoan parasite *Cyclospora cayetanensis*. This species is transmitted via the fecal–oral route, and infection occurs after consuming sporulated oocysts in contaminated water or food. Infections due to *C. cayetanensis* have been reported globally (Ortega et al., 1998), although endemic areas tend to be concentrated in tropical and subtropical regions (Herwaldt, 2000). In areas where the infection is endemic, asymptomatic cases are more frequent whereas in nonendemic areas infections nearly always show clinical symptoms (Ortega and Sanchez, 2010). In high-income countries, locally acquired infections have been reported in immunocompetent (Ooi et al., 1995) and immunosuppressed individuals, and in the latter group, the infection may result in prolonged illness and weight loss (Sifuentes-Osornio et al., 1995). The parasite has also been found in travelers returning from endemic regions (Drenaggi et al., 1998). Excreted oocysts need an extended period outside the host to sporulate and become infectious (Chacin-Bonilla, 2010; Ortega and Sanchez, 2010), suggesting that contaminated food and water are the most frequent transmission pathways for the parasite (Ortega and Sanchez, 2010).

C. cayetanensis is recognized as an important foodborne parasite (Robertson et al., 2013); however, the global burden of disease has not been estimated. About 99% of US cyclosporosis cases are estimated to be foodborne, resulting in an estimated 11,407 foodborne incident cases and 11 hospitalizations annually (Scallan et al., 2011). From these estimates, the annual cost of cyclosporosis in the United States has been estimated to be US$11 million using a basic COI model and US$17 million when pain and suffering were also considered in the COI model (Scharff, 2012).

5.5.6 Chagas disease

Chagas disease, also known as American trypanosomosis, is a chronic infection caused by the parasite *Trypanosoma cruzi* (Aufderheide et al., 2004). The disease is a zoonosis with placental and marsupial mammals serving as natural reservoirs for the parasite (Gurtler et al., 2008). Geographically, the disease is restricted to the Americas, from the southern United States to northern reaches of Chile and Argentina (Zeledon et al., 2006). Although it is widespread, it is largely restricted to rural, socioeconomically disadvantaged communities in Latin America (Torgerson and Macpherson, 2011). It is estimated that 60 million people are exposed to the risk of infection with the disease resulting in approximately 14,000 deaths annually (Schofield et al., 2006; Senior, 2007). *T. cruzi* parasites are predominantly transmitted by contact with the feces of infected blood-sucking triatomine bugs, and the parasite enters the host via the site of the bug bite site, or the eyes, mouth, or any breaks in the skin. Food contaminated with the feces of infected bugs can also result in infection (WHO, 2014a).

A recent evaluation of the global burden of Chagas disease estimated an annual loss of 806,170 DALYs. In economic terms, losses had been estimated to be about $7.19 billion per year when mortality from Chagas disease was converted into lost productivity (Lee et al., 2013). The GBD 2010 study and the 2012 WHO Global Health Estimates reported the burden of Chagas disease to be 546,000 and 528,000 DALYs lost, respectively (Murray et al., 2012b; WHO, 2014b). DWs of 0.012–0.186, corresponding to mild abdominopelvic disease to severe heart failure were used in the GBD 2010 study (Murray et al., 2012a; Salomon et al., 2012). In terms of DALYs lost, greater than 96% of the global burden is borne by low- and middle-income countries of the Americas (Lee et al., 2013; WHO, 2014b). The United States and Canada, in contrast, account for less than 4% of the global DALY estimate (Lee et al., 2013; WHO, 2014b), but 12% of the total global costs and 19% of the global health care costs (Lee et al., 2013).

The foodborne threat posed by this parasite has been recognized (Pereira et al., 2010b; Robertson et al., 2013; Rodriguez-Morales, 2008). The largest ever orally transmitted outbreak of Chagas disease was documented in Venezuela, where 128 confirmed cases were reported. Guava juice contaminated by vectors as a result of unhygienic processing was implicated as the source of illness (Alarcon de Noya et al., 2010). Similarly, in the Brazilian Amazon, the parasite was found to be transmitted to humans via inadequately prepared açaí juice (Xavier et al., 2014). Recent experimental evidence indicates that metabolic reactions within the host may increase the invasive capability of the parasite, and that if this reaction occurs in humans, it may partly explain the high mortality associated with outbreaks of the disease following oral infection (Yoshida et al., 2011). These findings suggest that oral ingestion of the parasite through contaminated food and water may be important; however, the burden attributed to food is unknown.

5.6 Conclusions and challenges

Estimating the socioeconomic burden of foodborne parasites is challenging and complex due to the multiple transmission pathways and the diversity of health outcomes that may result from an infection (Torgerson et al., 2014). Table 5.1 lists the DALY estimates from the 2010 GBD study (Murray et al., 2012b) for the exclusively foodborne and possibly foodborne parasites in comparison to malaria, HIV/AIDS, and tuberculosis. The data in Table 5.1 and that presented throughout this chapter suggest the socioeconomic burden of foodborne parasites will be considerable and will have an important impact on human health and productivity. Nevertheless, a number of challenges remain to estimating the socioeconomic burden of foodborne parasitic zoonoses.

For monetary and nonmonetary methods alike, source attribution will continue to be of critical importance to accurately estimate the burden of disease attributable to food for those pathogens with complex nonfood transmission pathways. Some of the parasites discussed in this chapter, such as the fishborne trematodes *Trichinella* spp., and adult stage *Taenia* spp. are exclusively transmitted through food, whereas others such as *Echinococcus* spp. and the foodborne protozoa have a variety of potential pathways including food contamination and nonfood pathways. The allocation of limited resources to control parasitic infections in food will need to be based on the reliable data to maximize the public health benefit in an affected region or community.

Table 5.1 Summary table of estimated DALYs (in millions) of tuberculosis, HIV/AIDS, and malaria and the exclusively foodborne and possibly foodborne parasites from the 2010 Global Burden of Disease Study

Disease	DALYs from 2010 GBD study in millions (95% confidence interval)
HIV/AIDS	81.5 (75.0–88.4)
Tuberculosis	49.4 (40.1–56.1)
Malaria	82.7 (63.4–109.8)
Exclusively foodborne parasites	
Foodborne trematodosis	1.9 (0.7–4.8)
Possibly foodborne parasites	
Cysticercosis	0.5 (0.4–0.7)
Echinococcosis	0.1 (0.07–0.3)
Chagas disease	0.5 (0.3–1.1)
Cryptosporidiosis	8.4 (6.5–10.4)
Entamoebosis (amoebiasis)	2.2 (1.7–2.8)
Total foodborne and possibly foodborne parasites	13.7 (9.6–20.1)

Source: Murray et al. (2012b).

For the foodborne parasitic diseases with a focal distribution, such as neurocysticercosis and the foodborne trematodes, there is a high degree of uncertainty in estimating populations at risk. The use of large geographic units for assessment does not accurately reflect the spatial heterogeneity of risk factors and disease incidence (Hotez and Kamath, 2009; Mathers et al., 2007). The use of spatially disaggregated burden estimates as described for human African trypanosomiosis in Uganda (Hackett et al., 2014) has the potential to greatly improve the spatial precision of burden estimates. The data requirements for such an approach would be high and a lack of high-quality data is currently a problem for calculating the burden of most of the parasites described in this chapter.

Despite the challenges faced and the data limitations that may exist, estimates of the economic costs and burden of foodborne parasites can enhance our understanding of the pathogens that are causing the greatest economic and social harm on a global and national level. Burden estimates are updated regularly, taking into account new data, updated methodologies, and refined DWs (Hotez et al., 2014). These burden estimates should guide decision making with a complete understanding of the caveats that influence the calculations. Furthermore, monetary and nonmonetary burden estimates may be incorporated into a cost-benefit analyses and cost-effectiveness analyses with other pathogens with similar risk factors to determine the most efficient and effective food safety scheme to maximize public health outcomes with the limited resources available.

References

Abunna, F., 2013. Prevalence, organ distribution, viability and socioeconomic implication of bovine cysticercosis/teniasis, Ethiopia. Rev. Elev. Med. Vet. Pays Trop. 66 (1), 25–30.

Abunna, F., Tilahun, G., Megersa, B., Regassa, A., 2007. Taeniasis and its socio-economic implication in Awassa town and its surroundings, Southern Ethiopia. East Afr. J. Public Health 4 (2), 73–79.

Alarcon de Noya, B., Diaz-Bello, Z., Colmenares, C., Ruiz-Guevara, R., et al., 2010. Large urban outbreak of orally acquired acute Chagas disease at a school in Caracas, Venezuela. J. Infect. Dis. 201 (9), 1308–1315.

Alban, L., Pozio, E., Boes, J., Boireau, P., et al., 2011. Towards a standardised surveillance for *Trichinella* in the European Union. Prev. Vet. Med. 99 (2–4), 148–160.

Amoros, I., Alonso, J.L., Cuesta, G., 2010. Cryptosporidium oocysts and Giardia cysts on salad products irrigated with contaminated water. J. Food Prot. 73 (6), 1138–1140.

Audicana, M.T., Ansotegui, I.J., de Corres, L.F., Kennedy, M.W., 2002. *Anisakis simplex*: dangerous—dead and alive? Trends Parasitol. 18 (1), 20–25.

Aufderheide, A.C., Salo, W., Madden, M., Streitz, J., et al., 2004. A 9,000-year record of Chagas' disease. Proc. Natl. Acad. Sci. U.S.A. 101 (7), 2034–2039.

Barennes, H., Sayasone, S., Odermatt, P., De Bruyne, A., et al., 2008. A major trichinellosis outbreak suggesting a high endemicity of Trichinella infection in northern Laos. Am. J. Trop. Med. Hyg. 78 (1), 40–44.

Benetton, M.L.F.N., Goncalves, A.V., Meneghini, M.E.F., Silva, E.F., et al., 2005. Risk factors for infection by the *Entamoeba histolytica/E. dispar* complex: an epidemiological study conducted in outpatient clinics in the city of Manaus, Amazon Region, Brazil. Trans. R. Soc. Trop. Med. Hyg. 99 (7), 532–540.

Berkman, D.S., Lescano, A.G., Gilman, R.H., Lopez, S.L., et al., 2002. Effects of stunting, diarrhoeal disease, and parasitic infection during infancy on cognition in late childhood: a follow-up study. Lancet 359 (9306), 564–571.

Bern, C., Garcia, H.H., Evans, C., Gonzalez, A.E., et al., 1999. Magnitude of the disease burden from neurocysticercosis in a developing country. Clin. Infect. Dis. 29 (5), 1203.

Bhattarai, R., Budke, C.M., Carabin, H., Proano, J.V., et al., 2012. Estimating the non-monetary burden of neurocysticercosis in Mexico. PLoS Negl. Trop. Dis. 6 (2), e1521.

Bowman, N., Donroe, J., Gilman, R., 2006. Cestodes. In: Ortega, Y.R. (Ed.), Foodborne Parasites. Springer, New York, pp. 197–230 (Chapter 8).

Budke, C.M., Deplazes, P., Torgerson, P.R., 2006. Global socioeconomic impact of cystic Echinococcosis. Emerg. Infect. Dis. 12 (2), 296–303.

Budu-Amoako, E., Greenwood, S.J., Dixon, B.R., Barkema, H.W., et al., 2011. Foodborne illness associated with *Cryptosporidium* and *Giardia* from livestock. J. Food Prot. 74 (11), 1944–1955.

Buzby, J.C., 2011. Determining the economic costs and global burden of foodborne disease. In: Tracing Pathogens in the Food Chain. Woodhead Publishing Limited, Philadelphia, pp. 114–138 (Chapter 6).

Carabin, H., Budke, C.M., Cowan, L.D., Willingham III, A.L., et al., 2005. Methods for assessing the burden of parasitic zoonoses: echinococcosis and cysticercosis. Trends Parasitol. 21 (7), 327–333.

Carabin, H., Krecek, R.C., Cowan, L.D., Michael, L., et al., 2006. Estimation of the cost of *Taenia solium* cysticercosis in Eastern Cape Province, South Africa. Trop. Med. Int. Health 11 (6), 906–916.

Carabin, H., Ndimubanzi, P.C., Budke, C.M., Nguyen, H., et al., 2011. Clinical manifestations associated with neurocysticercosis: a systematic review. PLoS Negl. Trop. Dis. 5 (5), e1152.

Carme, B., Demar, M., Ajzenberg, D., Darde, M.L., 2009. Severe acquired toxoplasmosis caused by wild cycle of *Toxoplasma gondii*, French Guiana. Emerg. Infect. Dis. 15 (4), 656–658.

Carvalho-Costa, F.A., Goncalves, A.Q., Lassance, S.L., Silva Neto, L.M.d., et al., 2007. *Giardia lamblia* and other intestinal parasitic infections and their relationships with nutritional status in children in Brazilian Amazon. Rev. Inst. Med. Trop. Sao Paulo 49 (3), 147–153.

Chacin-Bonilla, L., 2010. Epidemiology of *Cyclospora cayetanensis*: a review focusing in endemic areas. Acta Trop. 115 (3), 181–193.

Chalmers, R.M., Davies, A.P., 2010. Minireview: clinical cryptosporidiosis. Exp. Parasitol. 124 (1), 138–146.

Checkley, W., Gilman, R.H., Black, R.E., Epstein, L.D., et al., 2004. Effect of water and sanitation on childhood health in a poor Peruvian peri-urban community. Lancet 363 (9403), 112–118.

Chen, K.T., Chen, C.J., Chiu, J.P., 2001. A school waterborne outbreak involving both *Shigella sonnei* and *Entamoeba histolytica*. J. Environ. Health 64 (4), 9.

Cifuentes, E., Blumenthal, U., Ruiz-Palacios, G., Bennett, S., 1991. Health impact evaluation of wastewater use in Mexico. Public Health Rev. 19 (1–4), 243–250.

Conlan, J.V., Vongxay, K., Fenwick, S., Blacksell, S.D., et al., 2009. Does interspecific competition have a moderating effect on *Taenia solium* transmission dynamics in Southeast Asia? Trends Parasitol. 25 (9), 398–403.

Conlan, J.V., Vongxay, K., Khamlome, B., Gomez-Morales, M.A., et al., 2014. Patterns and risks of *Trichinella* infection in humans and pigs in northern Laos. PLoS Negl. Trop. Dis. 8 (7), e3034.

Cowie, R.H., 2013. Biology, systematics, life cycle, and distribution of *Angiostrongylus cantonensis*, the cause of rat lungworm disease. Hawaii J. Med. Public Health 72 (6 Suppl. 2), 6–9.

Croker, C., Reporter, R., Mascola, L., 2010. Use of statewide hospital discharge data to evaluate the economic burden of neurocysticercosis in Los Angeles County (1991–2008). Am. J. Trop. Med. Hyg. 83 (1), 106–110.

Demar, M., Hommel, D., Djossou, F., Peneau, C., et al., 2012. Acute toxoplasmoses in immunocompetent patients hospitalized in an intensive care unit in French Guiana. Clin. Microbiol. Infect. 18 (7), E221–E231.

Devleesschauwer, B., Ale, A., Torgerson, P., Praet, N., et al., 2014. The burden of parasitic zoonoses in Nepal: a systematic review. PLoS Negl. Trop. Dis. 8 (1), e2634.

Do, T.T., Bui, T.T., Molbak, K., Phung, D.C., et al., 2007. Epidemiology and aetiology of diarrhoeal diseases in adults engaged in wastewater-fed agriculture and aquaculture in Hanoi, Vietnam. Trop. Med. Int. Health 12 (Suppl. 2), 23–33.

Dorny, P., Praet, N., 2007. *Taenia saginata* in Europe. Vet. Parasitol. 149 (1–2), 22–24.

Drenaggi, D., Cirioni, O., Giacometti, A., Fiorentini, A., et al., 1998. Cyclosporiasis in a traveler returning from South America. J. Travel Med. 5 (3), 153–155.

Dubey, J.P., 2009a. Toxoplasmosis in pigs—the last 20 years. Vet. Parasitol. 164 (2–4), 89–103.

Dubey, J.P., 2009b. Toxoplasmosis in sheep—the last 20 years. Vet. Parasitol. 163 (1–2), 1–14.

Dubey, J.P., Lago, E.G., Gennari, S.M., Su, C., et al., 2012. Toxoplasmosis in humans and animals in Brazil: high prevalence, high burden of disease, and epidemiology. Parasitology 139, 1375–1424.

Ethelburg, S., Lisby, M., Vestergaard, L.S., Enemark, H.L., et al., 2009. A foodborne outbreak of *Cryptosporidium hominis* infection. Epidemiol. Infect. 137 (3), 348–356.

Fan, P.C., 1997. Annual economic loss caused by *Taenia saginata asiatica* taeniasis in East Asia. Parasitol. Today 13 (5), 194–196.

Fischer Walker, C.L., Perin, J., Aryee, M.J., Boschi-Pinto, C., et al., 2012. Diarrhea incidence in low- and middle-income countries in 1990 and 2010: a systematic review. BMC Public Health 12, 220.

FSANZ, 2013. *Toxoplasma gondii*. Agents of Foodborne Illness, second ed. Food Standards Australia New Zealand, Canberra, pp. 103–114.

Furst, T., Keiser, J., Utzinger, J., 2012. Global burden of human food-borne trematodiasis: a systematic review and meta-analysis. Lancet Infect. Dis. 12 (3), 210–221.

Gherasim, A., Lebbad, M., Insulander, M., Decraene, V., et al., 2012. Two geographically separated food-borne outbreaks in Sweden linked by an unusual *Cryptosporidium parvum* subtype, October 2010. Euro Surveill. 17 (46), pii:20318.

Gracey, J., Collins, D.S., Huey, R., 1999. Diseases Caused by Helminth and Arthropod Parasites, Meat Hygiene, tenth ed. W. B. Saunders Company Ltd, London, pp. 635–698.

Guerrant, D.I., Moore, S.R., Lima, A.A., Patrick, P.D., et al., 1999. Association of early childhood diarrhea and cryptosporidiosis with impaired physical fitness and cognitive function four-seven years later in a poor urban community in northeast Brazil. Am. J. Trop. Med. Hyg. 61 (5), 707–713.

Gurtler, R.E., Diotaiuti, L., Kitron, U., 2008. Commentary: Chagas disease: 100 years since discovery and lessons for the future. Int. J. Epidemiol. 37 (4), 698–701.

Hackett, F., Berrang Ford, L., Fevre, E., Simarro, P., 2014. Incorporating scale dependence in disease burden estimates: the case of human African trypanosomiasis in Uganda. PLoS Negl. Trop. Dis. 8 (2), e2704.

Hanevik, K., Dizdar, V., Langeland, N., Hausken, T., 2009. Development of functional gastrointestinal disorders after *Giardia lamblia* infection. BMC Gastroenterol. 9, 27.

Havelaar, A.H., Kemmeren, J.M., Kortbeek, L.M., 2007. Disease burden of congenital toxoplasmosis. Clin. Infect. Dis. 44 (11), 1467–1474.

Herwaldt, B.L., 2000. *Cyclospora cayetanensis*: a review, focusing on the outbreaks of cyclosporiasis in the 1990s. Clin. Infect. Dis. 31 (4), 1040–1057.

Hill, D.E., Sreekumar, C., Jones, J., Dubey, J.P., 2007. *Toxoplasma gondii*. In: Simjee, S. (Ed.), Foodborne Diseases. Humana Press, Totowa, pp. 337–353 (Chapter 12).

Hotez, P.J., Alibek, K., 2011. Central Asia's hidden burden of neglected tropical diseases. PLoS Negl. Trop. Dis. 5 (9), e1224.

Hotez, P.J., Kamath, A., 2009. Neglected tropical diseases in sub-Saharan Africa: review of their prevalence, distribution, and disease burden. PLoS Negl. Trop. Dis. 3 (8), e412.

Hotez, P.J., Alvarado, M., Basanez, M.G., Bolliger, I., et al., 2014. The global burden of disease study 2010: interpretation and implications for the neglected tropical diseases. PLoS Negl. Trop. Dis. 8 (7), e2865.

Idowu, O.A., Rowland, S.A., 2006. Oral fecal parasites and personal hygiene of food handlers in Abeokuta, Nigeria. Afr. Health Sci. 6 (3), 160–164.

Insulander, M., Jong, B.d., Svenungsson, B., 2008. A food-borne outbreak of cryptosporidiosis among guests and staff at a hotel restaurant in Stockholm county, Sweden, September 2008. Euro Surveill. 13 (51), 2.

Istre, G.R., Kreiss, K., Hopkins, R.S., Healy, G.R., et al., 1982. An outbreak of amebiasis spread by colonic irrigation at a chiropractic clinic. N. Engl. J. Med. 307 (6), 339–342.

Jayamaha, J.C., Robertson, P., Rawlinson, W.D., 2012. Congenital toxoplasmosis over 10 years in a low-incidence population. Med. J. Aust. 196 (7), 443–444.

Karabiber, N., Aktas, F., 1991. Foodborne giardiasis. Lancet 337 (8737), 376–377.

Keiser, J., Utzinger, J., 2005. Emerging foodborne trematodiasis. Emerg. Infect. Dis. 11 (10), 1507–1514.

Keiser, J., Utzinger, J., 2009. Food-borne trematodiases. Clin. Microbiol. Rev. 22 (3), 466–483.

Khaniki, G.R.J., Raei, M., Kia, E.B., Haghi, A.M., et al., 2010. Prevalence of bovine cysticercosis in slaughtered cattle in Iran. Trop. Anim. Health Prod. 42 (2), 141–143.

Kirk, M., Ford, L., Glass, L., Hall, G., 2014. Foodborne illness, Australia, circa 2000 and circa 2010. Emerg. Infect. Dis. 20 (11), 1857–1864.

Lee, B.Y., Bacon, K.M., Bottazzi, M.E., Hotez, P.J., 2013. Global economic burden of Chagas disease: a computational simulation model. Lancet Infect. Dis. 13 (4), 342–348.

Lozano, R., Naghavi, M., Foreman, K., Lim, S., et al., 2012. Global and regional mortality from 235 causes of death for 20 age groups in 1990 and 2010: a systematic analysis for the Global Burden of Disease Study 2010. Lancet 380 (9859), 2095–2128.

Mathers, C.D., Ezzati, M., Lopez, A.D., 2007. Measuring the burden of neglected tropical diseases: the global burden of disease framework. PLoS Negl. Trop. Dis. 1 (2), e114.

McCarthy, J.S., Peacock, D., Trown, K.P., Bade, P., et al., 2002. Endemic invasive amoebiasis in northern Australia. Med. J. Aust. 177 (10), 570.

Melloul, A., Amahmid, O., Hassani, L., Bouhoum, K., 2002. Health effect of human wastes use in agriculture in El Azzouzia (the wastewater spreading area of Marrakesh city, Morocco). Int. J. Environ. Health Res. 12 (1), 17–23.

Mintz, E.D., Hudson-Wragg, M., Mshar, P., Cartter, M.L., et al., 1993. Foodborne giardiasis in a corporate office setting. J. Infect. Dis. 167 (1), 250–253.

Montoya, J.G., Liesenfeld, O., 2004. Toxoplasmosis. Lancet 363 (9425), 1965–1976.

Murray, C.J., Ezzati, M., Flaxman, A.D., Lim, S., et al., 2012a. GBD 2010: design, definitions, and metrics. Lancet 380 (9859), 2063–2066.

Murray, C.J.L., Vos, T., Lozano, R., Naghavi, M., et al., 2012b. Disability-adjusted life years (DALYs) for 291 diseases and injuries in 21 regions, 1990–2010: a systematic analysis for the Global Burden of Disease Study 2010. Lancet 380 (9859), 2197–2223.

Murrell, K.D., Pozio, E., 2011. Worldwide occurrence and impact of human trichinellosis, 1986–2009. Emerg. Infect. Dis. 17 (12), 2194–2202.

Nagata, N., Shimbo, T., Akiyama, J., Nakashima, R., et al., 2012. Risk factors for intestinal invasive amebiasis in Japan, 2003–2009. Emerg. Infect. Dis. 18 (5), 717–724.

Nash, T.E., 2010. Visceral larva migrans and other unusual helminth infections. In: Mandell, G.L., Bennett, J.E., Dolin, R. (Eds.), Mandell, Douglas and Bennett's Principles and Practice of Infectious Diseases, seventh ed. Churchill Livingstone Elsevier, Philadelphia, pp. 3617–3623 (Chapter 291).

Nundy, S., Gilman, R.H., Xiao, L., Cabrera, L., et al., 2011. Wealth and its associations with enteric parasitic infections in a low-income community in Peru: use of principal component analysis. Am. J. Trop. Med. Hyg. 84 (1), 38–42.

Odermatt, P., Lv, S., Sayasone, S., 2010. Less common parasitic infections in Southeast Asia that can produce outbreaks. Adv. Parasitol. 72, 409–435.

Ooi, W.W., Zimmerman, S.K., Needham, C.A., 1995. Cyclospora species as a gastrointestinal pathogen in immunocompetent hosts. J. Clin. Microbiol. 33 (5), 1267–1269.

Ortega, Y.R., Sanchez, R., 2010. Update on *Cyclospora cayetanensis*, a food-borne and waterborne parasite. Clin. Microbiol. Rev. 23 (1), 218–234.

Ortega, Y.R., Sterling, C.R., Gilman, R.H., 1998. *Cyclospora cayetanensis*. Adv. Parasitol. 40, 399–418.

Payne, R.J., Turner, L., Morgan, E.R., 2009. Inappropriate measures of population health for parasitic disease? Trends Parasitol. 25 (9), 393–395.

Pereira, K.S., Franco, R.M., Leal, D.A., 2010a. Transmission of toxoplasmosis (*Toxoplasma gondii*) by foods. Adv. Food Nutr. Res. 60, 1–19.

Pereira, K.S., Schmidt, F.L., Barbosa, R.L., Guaraldo, A.M.A., et al., 2010b. Transmission of chagas disease (American trypanosomiasis) by food. Adv. Food Nutr. Res. 59, 63–85.

Petersen, L.R., Cartter, M.L., Hadler, J.L., 1988. A food-borne outbreak of *Giardia lamblia*. J. Infect. Dis. 157 (4), 846–848.

Pham Duc, P., Nguyen-Viet, H., Hattendorf, J., Zinsstag, J., et al., 2011. Risk factors for *Entamoeba histolytica* infection in an agricultural community in Hanam province, Vietnam. Parasit. Vectors 4, 102.

Porter, J.D., Gaffney, C., Heymann, D., Parkin, W., 1990. Food-borne outbreak of Giardia lamblia. Am. J. Public Health 80 (10), 1259–1260.

Potasman, I., Paz, A., Odeh, M., 2002. Infectious outbreaks associated with bivalve shellfish consumption: a worldwide perspective. Clin. Infect. Dis. 35 (8), 921.

Pozio, E., 2007. World distribution of *Trichinella* spp. infections in animals and humans. Vet. Parasitol. 149 (1–2), 3–21.

Pozio, E., 2011. Trichinellosis. In: Palmer, S., et al. (Eds.), Zoonoses. Oxford University Press, Oxford.

Pozio, E., 2014. Searching for *Trichinella*: not all pigs are created equal. Trends Parasitol. 30 (1), 4–11.

Praet, N., Speybroeck, N., Manzanedo, R., Berkvens, D., et al., 2009. The disease burden of *Taenia solium* cysticercosis in Cameroon. PLoS Negl. Trop. Dis. 3 (3), e406.

Putignani, L., Menichella, D., 2010. Global distribution, public health and clinical impact of the protozoan pathogen cryptosporidium. Interdiscip. Perspect. Infect. Dis. 2010, pii: 753512.

Quick, R., Paugh, K., Addiss, D., Kobayashi, J., et al., 1992. Restaurant-associated outbreak of giardiasis. J. Infect. Dis. 166 (3), 673–676.

Rao Ajjampur, S.S., Asirvatham, J.R., Muthusamy, D., Gladstone, B.P., et al., 2007. Clinical features & risk factors associated with cryptosporidiosis in HIV infected adults in India. Indian J. Med. Res. 126 (6), 553–557.

Robertson, L.J., van der Giessen, J.W.B., Batz, M.B., Kojima, M., et al., 2013. Have foodborne parasites finally become a global concern? Trends Parasitol. 29 (3), 101–103.

Robinson, T.J., Scheftel, J.M., Smith, K.E., 2014. Raw milk consumption among patients with non-outbreak-related enteric infections, Minnesota, USA, 2001–2010. Emerg. Infect. Dis. 20 (1), 38–44.

Rodriguez-Morales, A.J., 2008. Chagas disease: an emerging food-borne entity? J. Infect. Dev. Ctries. 2 (2), 149–150.

Rose, J.B., 1997. Environmental ecology of *Cryptosporidium* and public health implications. Annu. Rev. Public Health 18, 135–161.

Salomon, J.A., Vos, T., Hogan, D.R., Gagnon, M., et al., 2012. Common values in assessing health outcomes from disease and injury: disability weights measurement study for the Global Burden of Disease Study 2010. Lancet 380 (9859), 2129–2143.

Scallan, E., Hoekstra, R.M., Angulo, F.J., Tauxe, R.V., et al., 2011. Foodborne illness acquired in the United States—major pathogens. Emerg. Infect. Dis. 17 (1), 7–15.

Scharff, R.L., 2012. Economic burden from health losses due to foodborne illness in the United States. J. Food Prot. 75 (1), 123–131.

Schofield, C.J., Jannin, J., Salvatella, R., 2006. The future of Chagas disease control. Trends Parasitol. 22 (12), 583–588.

Senior, K., 2007. Chagas disease: moving towards global elimination. Lancet Infect. Dis. 7 (9), 572.

Sifuentes-Osornio, J., Porras-Cortés, G., Bendall, R.P., Morales-Villarreal, F., et al., 1995. *Cyclospora cayetanensis* infection in patients with and without AIDS: biliary disease as another clinical manifestation. Clin. Infect. Dis. 21 (5), 1092–1097.

Silva, R.R., da Silva, C.A.M., de Jesus Pereira, C.A., de Carvalho Nicolato, R.L., et al., 2009. Association between nutritional status, environmental and socio-economic factors and *Giardia lamblia* infections among children aged 6–71 months in Brazil. Trans. R. Soc. Trop. Med. Hyg. 103 (5), 512–519.

Slifko, T.R., Smith, H.V., Rose, J.B., 2000. Emerging parasite zoonoses associated with water and food. Int. J. Parasitol. 30 (12–13), 1379–1393.

Sorvillo, F., Wilkins, P., Shafir, S., Eberhard, M., 2011. Public health implications of cysticercosis acquired in the United States. Emerg. Infect. Dis. 17 (1), 1–6.

Sripa, B., Kaewkes, S., Sithithaworn, P., Mairiang, E., et al., 2007. Liver fluke induces cholangiocarcinoma. PLoS Med. 4 (7), e201.

Sripa, B., Kaewkes, S., Intapan, P.M., Maleewong, W., et al., 2010. Food-borne trematodiases in Southeast Asia epidemiology, pathology, clinical manifestation and control. Adv. Parasitol. 72, 305–350.

Stanley, S.L., 2003. Amoebiasis. Lancet 361 (9362), 1025–1034.

Tesfaye, D., Sadado, T., Demissie, T., 2012. Public health and economic significance of bovine cysticercosis in Wolaita Soddo, Southern Ethiopia. Global Veterinaria 9 (5), 557–563.

Thompson, R.C.A., 2014. Parasites and food: ripe for exploitation. Trends Parasitol. 30 (1), 1–3.

Torgerson, P.R., Macpherson, C.N.L., 2011. The socioeconomic burden of parasitic zoonoses: global trends. Vet. Parasitol. 182 (1), 79–95.

Torgerson, P.R., Mastroiacovo, P., 2013. The global burden of congenital toxoplasmosis: a systematic review. Bull. World Health Organ. 91 (7), 501–508.

Torgerson, P.R., Keller, K., Magnotta, M., Ragland, N., 2010. The global burden of alveolar echinococcosis. PLoS Negl. Trop. Dis. 4 (6), e722.

Torgerson, P.R., de Silva, N.R., Fevre, E.M., Kasuga, F., et al., 2014. The global burden of foodborne parasitic diseases: an update. Trends Parasitol. 30 (1), 20–26.

Vos, T., Flaxman, A.D., Naghavi, M., Lozano, R., et al., 2012. Years lived with disability (YLDs) for 1160 sequelae of 289 diseases and injuries 1990–2010: a systematic analysis for the Global Burden of Disease Study 2010. Lancet 380 (9859), 2163–2196.

Vreden, S.G., Visser, L.G., Verweij, J.J., Blotkamp, J., et al., 2000. Outbreak of amebiasis in a family in The Netherlands. Clin. Infect. Dis. 31 (4), 1101–1104.

Vu Thi, N., Trung, D.D., Litzroth, A., Praet, N., et al., 2013. The hidden burden of trichinellosis in Vietnam: a postoutbreak epidemiological study. Biomed Res. Int. 2013, 149890.

Waikagul, J., 2015. Foodborne trematodes. In: Gajadhar, A. (Ed.), Foodborne Parasites in the Food Supply Web: Occurrence and Control. Elsevier/Woodhead Publishing Ltd, Philadelphia (Chapter 10).

Weinke, T., Friedrich-Janicke, B., Hopp, P., Janitschke, K., 1990. Prevalence and clinical importance of *Entamoeba histolytica* in two high-risk groups: travelers returning from the tropics and male homosexuals. J. Infect. Dis. 161 (5), 1029–1031.

White, K.E., Hedberg, C.W., Edmonson, L.M., Jones, D.B., et al., 1989. An outbreak of giardiasis in a nursing home with evidence for multiple modes of transmission. J. Infect. Dis. 160 (2), 298–304.

WHO, 2007. The global burden of foodborne diseases: taking stock and charting the way forward. WHO Consultation to Develop a Strategy to Estimate the Global Burden of Foodborne Diseases. World Health Organisation, Geneva. Available at: http://www.who.int/foodsafety/publications/foodborne_disease/fbd_2006.pdf (accessed 07.04.14.).

WHO, 2013. WHO Methods and Data Sources for Global Burden of Disease Estimates 2000–2011. World Health Organization, Geneva. Available at: http://www.who.int/healthinfo/statistics/GlobalDALYmethods_2000_2011.pdf?ua=1 (accessed 08.08.14.).

WHO, 2014a. Chagas Disease (American Trypanosomiasis). Fact Sheet No. 340, World Health Organization, Geneva. http://www.who.int/mediacentre/factsheets/fs340/en/ (accessed 08.08.14.).

WHO, 2014b. Global Health Estimates 2014 Summary Tables: DALY by Cause, Age and Sex, by World Income Category and WHO Region, 2000–2012. World Health Organization, Geneva. Available at: http://www.who.int/healthinfo/global_burden_disease/en/ (accessed 26.09.14.).

WHO, 2014c. Initiative for Vaccine Research: Parasitic Disease. World Health organization, Geneva. Available at: http://apps.who.int/vaccine_research/diseases/soa_parasitic/en/index1.html (accessed 12.06.14.).

Xavier, S.C.d.C., Roque, A.L., Bilac, D., de Araujo, V.A.L., et al., 2014. Distantiae transmission of *Trypanosoma cruzi*: a new epidemiological feature of acute Chagas disease in Brazil. PLoS Negl. Trop. Dis. 8 (5), e2878.

Ximenez, C., Moran, P., Rojas, L., Valadez, A., et al., 2009. Reassessment of the epidemiology of amebiasis: state of the art. Infect. Genet. Evol. 9 (6), 1023–1032.

Yoshida, N., Tyler, K.M., Llewellyn, M.S., 2011. Invasion mechanisms among emerging foodborne protozoan parasites. Trends Parasitol. 27 (10), 459–466.

Zeledon, R., Marin, F., Calvo, N., Lugo, E., et al., 2006. Distribution and ecological aspects of *Rhodnius pallescens* in Costa Rica and Nicaragua and their epidemiological implications. Mem. Inst. Oswaldo Cruz 101 (1), 75–79.

Zhou, P., Chen, Z., Li, H., Zheng, H., et al., 2011. *Toxoplasma gondii* infection in humans in China. Parasit. Vectors 4, 165–173.

Part Two

Parasites

Foodborne apicomplexan protozoa: Coccidia

6

A.A. Gajadhar[1], L.F. Lalonde[1], B. Al-Adhami[1], B.B. Singh[2], V. Lobanov[1]
[1]Canadian Food Inspection Agency, Saskatoon, SK, Canada; [2]Guru Angad Dev Veterinary and Animal Science University, Ludhiana, India

6.1 Introduction

Protozoan parasites are some of the most cosmopolitan and ubiquitous foodborne parasites in the world. Many of them are members of the phylum Apicomplexa and produce environmentally resistant oocysts. Although they share many common features of life-cycle and transmission dynamics, some species have unique characteristics. Foodborne oocyst-producing apicomplexan parasites include *Cryptosporidium* spp. *Toxoplasma gondii, Cyclospora cayetanensis, Cystoisospora belli* (syn. *Isospora belli*), and *Sarcocystis* spp. and may be grouped as coccidian protozoa. They can be significant pathogens for animals and/or humans. *Cryptosporidium* spp. are prevalent in animals and humans globally, and *T. gondii* is considered to be the second leading cause of death attributed to foodborne illness in the United States (Scallan et al., 2011).

Apicomplexan parasites are responsible for some of the most important medical and veterinary diseases, including malaria and coccidiosis. Apicomplexan parasites use the environment as well as hosts to replicate and complete their life cycles. To control these parasites, it is necessary to understand their biology, transmission, and other features. In this chapter, we provide information on the basic biology, occurrence and distribution, ecology, epidemiology, disease, and control measures as they relate to these foodborne apicomplexan parasites.

6.2 Basic biology and phylogeny

As members of the Apicomplexa phylum, the protozoa included in this chapter have an apical complex, multiple life-cycle stages, and both sexual and asexual phases of reproduction. By producing oocysts in the definitive hosts, these parasites are considered coccidia, which comprise the families Eimeriidae, Sarcocystidae, and Toxoplasmatidae. Although *Cryptosporidium* spp. have many developmental features and other basic biological characteristics of coccidia, molecular phylogeny places them in a basal position relative to the group. However, for practical reasons and for the purpose of this chapter, *Cryptosporidium* spp. are included with the coccidian parasites. Genus classification within the coccidia is based on the structure of fully developed (sporulated) oocysts, specifically, the distribution of sporozoites and sporocysts within oocysts (Table 6.1). Traditionally, criteria used for the identification

Foodborne Parasites in the Food Supply Web. http://dx.doi.org/10.1016/B978-1-78242-332-4.00006-0

Table 6.1 **Characteristics of oocysts of foodborne coccidian protozoa of humans**

Species	Definitive host(s)	Sporulation period (days)	Oocysts at excretion	Sporulated oocyst	Size (range, μm)	Susceptible hosts	Period in days	
				Sporocysts/ sporozoites			Prepatent	Patent
Cyclospora cayetanensis	Humans	7–13	Unsporulated	Two sporocysts, each with two sporozoites	8.6×8.6 (7.7–9.9×7.7–9.9)	Humans	~7	7–>30
Cryptosporidium hominis	Humans	n/a	Sporulated	Zero sporocyst, four sporozoites	5.2×4.9 (4.4–5.9×4.4–5.4)	Humans	5–10	6–9 (>60)
Cryptosporidium parvum	Cattle, humans, other domestic and wild mammals	n/a	Sporulated	Zero sporocyst, four sporozoites	5.0×4.5 (4.5–5.4×4.2–5.0)	Cattle, humans, other domestic and wild mammals	2–22	1–20
Cystoisospora belli	Humans	1–10	Unsporulated	Two sporocysts, each with four sporozoites	30.0×12.0 (20.0–33.0×10.0–19.0)	Humans	3–14	≥15
Sarcocystis hominis	Humans	n/a	Sporulated	Two sporocysts, each with four sporozoites	19.3×14.9 sporocyst: 14.7×9.3 (14.0–15.0×9.0–11.0)	Cattle	9–10	>42
Sarcocystis suihominis	Humans	n/a	Sporulated	Two sporocysts, each with four sporozoites	18.5–20.0×12.3–14.6 sporocyst: 12.6×10.0 (11.6–13.9×9.1–10.8)	Pigs	12–14	≥18
Toxoplasma gondii	Felids	1–5	Unsporulated	Two sporocysts, each with four sporozoites	12.5×11.0 (11.0–14.0×9.0–11.0)	Mammals and birds (including humans)	3–>18	7–14

of species and genus of coccidian parasites relied on the morphometry (size, shape, and distribution of sporozoites) of oocysts, host susceptibility, and site of endogenous development. More recently, molecular analysis has enabled reliable characterization of species and genotypes and has revolutionized our understanding of the phylogeny and biological diversity of these coccidia.

Parasites such as *Cyclospora* spp. and *Cryptosporidium* spp., which require only a single host to complete their life cycles, can be considered as intestinal coccidia, whereas tissue coccidia such as *T. gondii* and *Sarcocystis* spp. require both definitive and intermediate hosts. Although the life cycle of *Cystoisospora* spp. is often completed in the intestine of a single host and the parasite can be considered as belonging to the intestinal coccidia, tissue stages have been found in the definitive host as well as in other host species. The life cycle of coccidia consists of multiple stages involving a sexual reproduction phase in the definitive host and two asexual phases of sporogony (usually in the environment) and merogony (also known as schizogony) within definitive and/or intermediate hosts (Figure 6.1). Endodyogeny and endopolygeny are rapid asexual replication of tachyzoites yielding two or more daughter cells. The number of host species required to complete a life cycle usually depends on the site of merogony of the coccidian

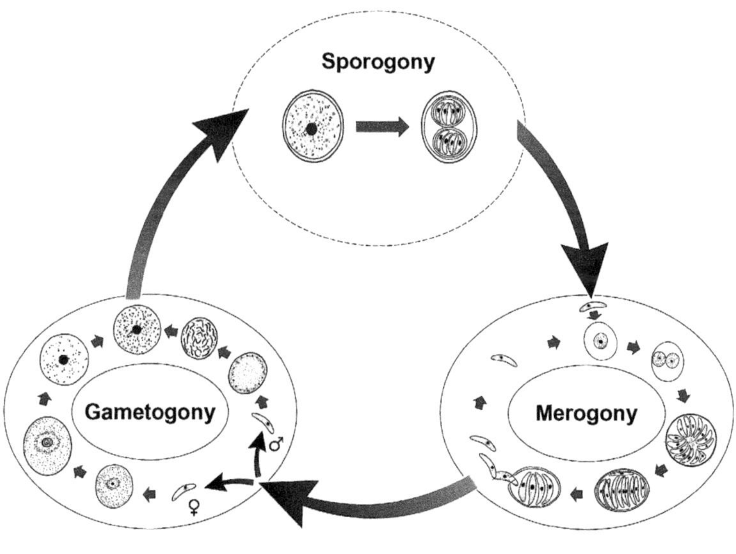

Canadian Food Inspection Agency Agence canadienne d'inspection des aliments

Figure 6.1 Life cycle pattern of apicomplexan coccidia showing the two asexual phases of reproduction (sporogony and merogony) and sexual reproduction (gametogony); however, endodyogeny may also occur as an additional form of replication in some coccidia. Depending on the genus of the coccidia, the parasite requires a single host or two hosts (intermediate and definitive) to complete its life cycle. Multiple cycles of merogony and a cycle of gametogony occur within hosts. Sporogony occurs exogenously for *Cyclospora, Cystoisospora,* and *Toxoplasma* and endogenously for *Cryptosporidium* and *Sarcocystis*. Details of the three phases of reproduction are provided in the text of the chapter.

genus. Furthermore, the predator–prey feeding behavior of the definitive hosts of tissue coccidia drives the transmission and life cycle of the parasite. For this reason, carnivores and omnivores, but not herbivores, serve as definitive hosts for tissue coccidia.

Oocysts excreted into the environment with the feces of definitive hosts are either already fully sporulated and infectious (e.g., *Cryptosporidium* spp. and *Sarcocystis* spp.), or immature, requiring sufficient time, humidity, and temperature to complete sporogony and produce sporocysts and sporozoites (e.g., *Cyclospora* spp., *T. gondii,* and *C. belli*). Once ingested by the appropriate host species, specific conditions in the gut cause the oocysts to rupture and/or sporocysts to excyst, releasing sporozoites. The sporozoites invade host cells, which typically are epithelial cells, and differentiate into trophozoites to begin the first of multiple generations of merogony; the number of generations of merogony varies according to the parasite species and the immunocompetence of the host. Each cycle of merogony generates numerous merozoites, so that the merogony phase of reproduction ultimately produces millions of merozoites, which are then destined for sexual reproduction (gametogony) in new host cells. Each merozoite differentiates into a female macrogamont that develops into a macrogamete or a male microgamont that divides into numerous microgametes. Following fertilization of the female macrogamete by a microgamete, a zygote is formed within the same host cell. The zygote coalesces proteins beneath its outer membrane and stores food granules in its depleting cytoplasm as it develops into an oocyst within a parasitophorous vacuole. Compromised by the growth and size of the oocysts, the host cell ruptures and releases oocysts into the lumen of the intestine, from which they are excreted with feces into the environment. As alluded to earlier, the oocysts of some coccidia species sporulate in the intestine and enter the environment immediately infectious for new hosts. The oocysts of *Cryptosporidium* spp. are also known to excyst *in situ* and reinfect the parasitized host without leaving the intestine (autoinfection).

The protective proteinaceous layers surrounding oocysts allow this stage of the parasite to survive most common disinfectants and adverse environmental conditions for long periods of time before and after sporulation. With less than optimal conditions, the sporulation period is often protracted, and oocysts can take several months to become infective. Oocysts can also sporulate and survive in seawater for long periods of time, especially at reduced temperatures. They can survive the various seasons and have been known to overwinter and remain infective. Additionally, the oocysts of some species may require a specific environmental stimulus, such as a sharp spike in temperature or specific durations of warm and cool temperatures to complete sporulation (Leighton and Gajadhar, 1986).

The minimum infectious dose for coccidian infection is very low, and this is due in part to the fact that a single oocyst consists of several infectious sporozoites, each of which undergo multiple cycles of reproduction in the life cycle, yielding tissue cysts each containing thousands of bradyzoites. Furthermore, each sporozoite or bradyzoite is capable of infecting a new host that could then excrete many millions of oocysts (definitive host) or generate billions of bradyzoites in tissues (intermediate host). The fecundity of coccidian species and the highly resistant oocysts are a few of the reasons that the protozoan species discussed in this chapter are exceedingly well adapted to the environment and their hosts, and as foodborne parasites are difficult to control.

6.3 *Cyclospora cayetanensis*

6.3.1 Taxonomy

Members of the *Cyclospora* genus are protozoan parasites in the Eimeriidae family of the subphylum Apicomplexa and belong to the coccidia group. *C. cayetanensis* is phylogenetically very closely related to *Eimeria* spp. and is indistinguishable by some molecular methods (Relman et al., 1996). The oocysts contain two sporocysts, each with two sporozoites (Ortega et al., 1993). *C. cayetanensis* is the only species in the genus known to infect humans; however, there are several other recognized species of *Cyclospora*, which may be differentiated morphologically and infect reptiles, insectivores, and other mammals, including nonhuman primates (Ortega et al., 1994). Beginning in 1979, there were reports describing a coccidian-like body, cyanobacterium-like body, large *Cryptosporidium*, or an *Isospora*-like organism associated with diarrhea in humans (Ashford, 1979; Mansfield and Gajadhar, 2004; Ortega and Sanchez, 2010). Following successful sporulation and excystation of the oocysts isolated from humans with chronic diarrhea, *C. cayetanensis* was described and named in the early 1990s (Ortega et al., 1993, 1994). Based solely on the finding of oocysts and 18S rRNA gene sequence analysis, three additional host-specific species have been described in nonhuman primates—*Cyclospora cercopitheci* (green monkeys), *Cyclospora colobi* (colobus monkeys), and *Cyclospora papionis* (baboons), but these species all had morphology similar to *C. cayetanensis* (Eberhard et al., 1999a). *Cyclospora*-like oocysts have been observed in dairy cattle feces, which were reported to be genetically distinct from both ruminant-associated *Eimeria* and *C. cayetanensis* (Li et al., 2007).

Different genes have been assessed for their utility in elucidating evolutionary relationships between *C. cayetanensis* strains to aid in molecular epidemiology. Analysis of 18S rRNA and HSP70 genes of *C. cayetanensis* isolates from humans in three distinct geographic regions (Nepal, Mexico, and Peru) revealed a fairly homogenous population at both loci (Sulaiman et al., 2013, 2014). Examination of 18S rRNA gene sequences of isolates from humans in China also revealed only minor sequence polymorphisms (Zhou et al., 2011). The internal transcribed spacer region I (ITS-1) is highly variable even within individual oocysts due to multiple divergent copies of the rRNA genes and is therefore not reliable for inferring relationships between strains. Efforts are underway to produce whole genome sequence data for *C. cayetanensis* to facilitate the development of reliable genetic markers for use in taxonomy, phylogeny, diagnostics, and tools for control strategies.

6.3.2 Host range, prevalence, and distribution

C. cayetanensis is endemic in many tropical and subtropical regions of the world but occurs worldwide. Humans are the only known host of the species. Although there have been speculations and assumptions that the parasite can complete its life cycle in various mammalian and avian livestock species, this seems unlikely considering its close phylogenetic status within the clade of coccidia with narrow host range at the species level, such as *Eimeria* spp. Large-scale surveillance studies in Peru,

Guatemala, Venezuela, Thailand, and Nepal reported *C. cayetanensis* oocysts in 1.1%, 2.3%, 6.1%, 0.5%, and 1.6% of human fecal specimens, respectively (Bern et al., 1999; Chacín-Bonilla et al., 2003; Madico et al., 1997; Tandukar et al., 2013; Thima et al., 2014). Young children are more likely to be infected than adults, and clinical symptoms are not always present, which suggests that immunity to cyclosporosis is acquired in endemic areas. Prevalence for *C. cayetanensis* seems to follow a seasonal pattern (Bern et al., 1999). *C. cayetanensis* is a common cause of traveler's diarrhea, incriminating endemic areas. Between 1997 and 2008, 33.5% of laboratory-confirmed cases of cyclosporosis in the United States were travel-related (Hall et al., 2011), whereas in Canada, 71% of reported cyclosporosis cases in 2006 were travel-related (Thomas et al., 2013), and the remainder were domestically acquired, presumably foodborne. *C. cayetanensis* is a cause of diarrhea in HIV-infected persons as well as in others who are immunocompromised or immunocompetent (Kurniawan et al., 2009; Mathur et al., 2013; Milord et al., 2012).

Surveys of domestic animal feces have been performed to determine if there is a reservoir host for *C. cayetanensis*. A survey of a total of 327 samples from pigs, cattle, horses, goats, dogs, cats, guinea pigs, chickens, ducks, turkeys, and pigeons in Haiti revealed no *Cyclospora* oocysts (Eberhard et al., 1999b). *Cyclospora*-like oocysts have been found in the feces of domestic animals in some endemic countries; however, these are likely to be spurious parasites passing through the gut (Ortega and Sanchez, 2010). Attempts to establish experimental infection of *C. cayetanensis* in both humans and laboratory animals have been unsuccessful (Alfano-Sobsey et al., 2004; Eberhard et al., 2000).

6.3.3 Life cycle and development

C. cayetanensis is an obligate intracellular parasite with a direct life cycle, completing both merogony and gametogony in the intestine of human hosts (Figures 6.1 and 6.2). Humans infected with *C. cayetanensis* excrete unsporulated, noninfective oocysts in their feces, within one to several weeks post infection or longer. Following 5–15 days in a warm (23–32 °C) humid environment, sporulation occurs yielding infective oocysts, containing two sporozoites within each of two sporocysts. Transmission entails ingestion of sporulated oocysts in contaminated water, food, or soil by a susceptible human host. The shedding and structure of oocysts of *C. cayetanensis* have specific characteristics that are shown in Table 6.1. They can remain viable in water or on fruits and vegetables for long periods of time. Following early patency when diarrhea and prolific oocyst shedding usually occur, oocysts may be shed intermittently and in low numbers depending on the host's immune status, treatment, and whether diarrhea symptoms persist.

6.3.4 Ecology and epidemiology

Because of the time required for sporulation, direct transmission from person to person is unlikely. Rather, ingestion of food, water, or soil contaminated with sporulated oocysts is the primary means of contracting the infection. Infection is more common in tropical and subtropical regions where the environmental conditions are favorable

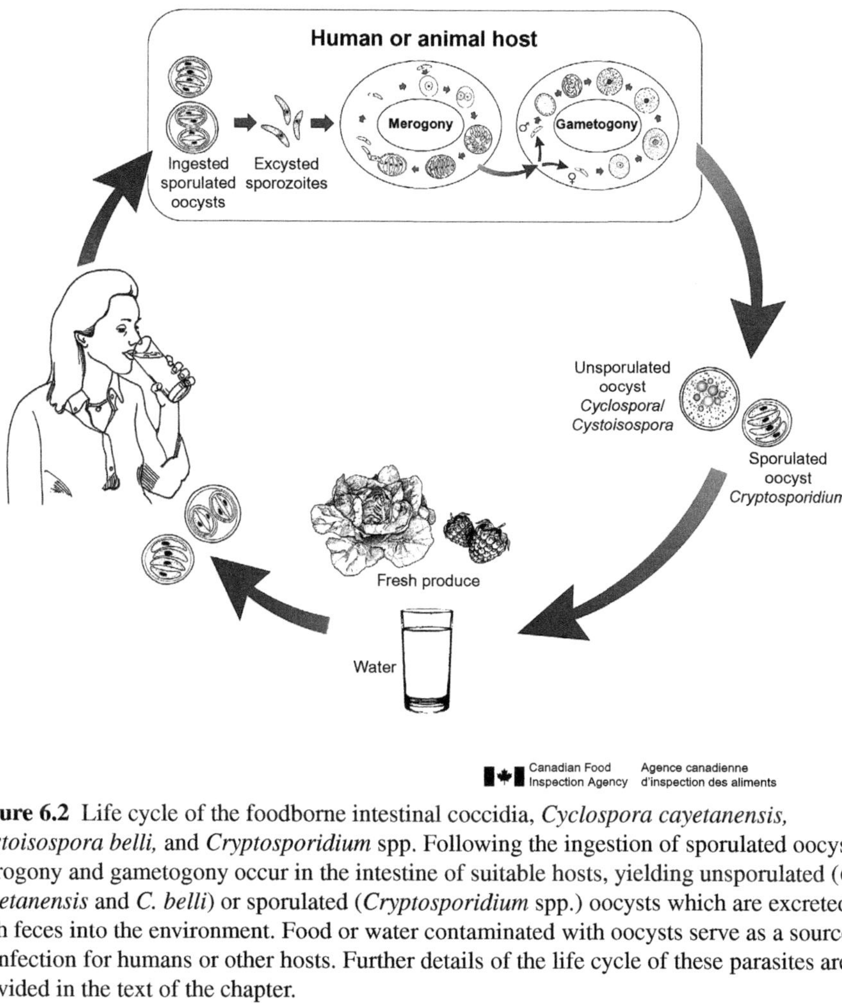

Figure 6.2 Life cycle of the foodborne intestinal coccidia, *Cyclospora cayetanensis, Cystoisospora belli,* and *Cryptosporidium* spp. Following the ingestion of sporulated oocysts, merogony and gametogony occur in the intestine of suitable hosts, yielding unsporulated (*C. cayetanensis* and *C. belli*) or sporulated (*Cryptosporidium* spp.) oocysts which are excreted with feces into the environment. Food or water contaminated with oocysts serve as a source of infection for humans or other hosts. Further details of the life cycle of these parasites are provided in the text of the chapter.

for rapid oocyst sporulation and long-term survival. Seasonality of infection is also apparent; however, peak seasons vary by region depending on the climate. In Haiti, infections peak during the cooler and drier periods (Eberhard et al., 1999c), whereas in Peru and Guatemala, infections are more common in warmer months and are lowest during the winter period (Bern et al., 2000, 2002). Changing weather and climate will undoubtedly impact the risk for the transmission of *C. cayetanensis* in endemic areas through altered patterns of rainfall, runoff, flooding, and drought, which could affect sporulation and survival of oocysts in the environment and contamination of water sources (Fletcher et al., 2012).

In developing countries where *C. cayetanensis* is endemic and water and sewage treatment systems are insufficient or lacking entirely, oocysts can spread readily through water supplies and distribution systems. Drinking unsafe water (not commercially bottled, boiled, chlorinated, or filtered) was more commonly linked to persons infected with *C. cayetanensis* in Nepal and Guatemala compared to controls (Bern et al., 1999; Sherchand and Cross, 2004). In Venezuela, the majority of cases of *C. cayetanensis* were clustered in the areas of extreme poverty where living in a hut, not having a toilet, and having contact with fecal-contaminated soil were strongly associated with infection (Chacín-Bonilla et al., 2007). In a survey of schoolchildren in Nepal, *C. cayetanensis* infection was more common where agriculture was the major family occupation, unboiled tap water was drunk, and hand washing was not practiced (Tandukar et al., 2013).

In nonendemic developed countries, outbreaks as well as individual cases of cyclosporosis are mostly linked to either international travel or consumption of contaminated imported produce, usually from endemic regions. Outbreaks have been reported regularly in North America since *C. cayetanensis* was first recognized in the early 1990s. Primarily berries, herbs, and other leafy green vegetables imported from endemic countries have been implicated as contaminated food sources in developed countries (Doller et al., 2002; Gibbs et al., 2013; Herwaldt and Ackers, 1997; Ho et al., 2002; Hoang et al., 2005; Insulander et al., 2010; Lopez et al., 2007). Fresh produce may become contaminated by food handlers or through irrigation with untreated water and is often consumed raw and with little or no washing. The oocysts are resistant to disinfectants commonly used in the food industry and water treatment. Washing of produce will not reliably remove oocysts, which may also have higher adhering affinities for certain produce types, such as raspberries, where they may become trapped in the fine hair-like structures on the berry's surface (Kniel et al., 2002).

6.3.5 Disease

Infection with *C. cayetanensis* can cause intermittent or sometimes prolonged watery diarrhea, mild to severe nausea, anorexia, abdominal cramping, fatigue, weight loss, body aches, and sometimes low-grade fever (Herwaldt, 2007). The infection is usually self-limiting, but symptoms can relapse for several weeks or months. Intestinal villi are shortened and widened due to diffuse edema and infiltration by inflammatory cells (Ortega et al., 1997). Loss of villar surface in the intestine can lead to severe dehydration. Oocysts are not shed during the first week of infection, but in heavy infections numerous oocysts are passed with loose feces, followed by intermittent shedding which can continue even when the host is asymptomatic. Frequent exposure in endemic areas may result in a gradual reduction in the severity of cyclosporosis in children as they age, and in the absence of symptomatic infection in adults (Madico et al., 1997). Those most susceptible to severe clinical symptoms include the very young, the very old who have subcompetent immune systems, immunocompromised individuals, and those without previous exposure. Although cyclosporosis may be considered to be a common infection in early childhood in developing regions, it is not without long-term negative consequences. Recent evidence suggests that early childhood diarrhea can have serious negative impacts on children's growth and cognitive development and may predispose them to chronic metabolic disease in later life (Guerrant et al., 2013).

C. cayetanensis oocysts can be identified in clinical or environmental samples by trained personnel using bright-field or phase contrast microscopy in wet-mount preparations or fecal smears, but they are not easily distinguished from other particles

(Mansfield and Gajadhar, 2004). The oocysts, like those of other coccidia, exhibit white-blue autofluorescence under epifluorescence microscopy using a 330–380 DM excitation filter, and stain variably with MZN acid-fast stain (Ortega and Sanchez, 2010). Concentration of the oocysts using ethyl acetate-formalin sedimentation, sucrose gradients, cesium chloride, or Percoll may be useful to improve sensitivity and specificity of detection solely by microscopy (Kimura et al., 2004; Ortega and Sanchez, 2010). Some molecular methods may have greater sensitivity and specificity than microscopy for detection and diagnosis of *C. cayetanensis*. However, they must be carefully designed and validated to ensure that closely related *Eimeria* species are not amplified and robust enough for use in clinical and environmental matrices containing polymerase chain reaction (PCR) inhibitors and high levels of background DNA. Conventional PCR, PCR-RFLP, and real-time qPCR with melt curve analysis have been developed for *C. cayetanensis* detection (Jinneman et al., 1998; Lalonde and Gajadhar, 2008, 2011; Lalonde et al., 2013; Shields and Olson, 2003; Varma et al., 2003). Application of a bead-based multiplex assay (Luminex) technology for detecting *C. cayetanensis* along with a few other eukaryotic enteropathogens has also been demonstrated (Taniuchi et al., 2011). No immunological detection methods are currently available for *C. cayetanensis*.

6.3.6 Control and prevention

Control and prevention strategies must exceed simple improvements to basic personal hygiene, as oocysts passed in the feces of humans are not infectious and require a minimum of several days of suitable environmental conditions to sporulate. Access to toilet facilities and proper disposal and treatment of human sewage in endemic areas are essential. Adequately treated (boiled or filtered) water must be used for drinking, food preparation, and growing and washing of any fruits and vegetables that are eaten raw. *C. cayetanensis* oocysts are resistant to many standard water and produce treatment methods such as chlorination or gaseous chloride dioxide (Ortega et al., 2008; Ortega and Sanchez, 2010). The oocysts can survive on basil leaves at 4 °C or room temperature for at least a week, but are susceptible to extreme temperatures (–70, 70, or 100 °C) (Sathyanarayanan and Ortega, 2006). Farmers should be educated regarding the risks of using sewage and contaminated water in fertilizing and irrigating crops of fruits and vegetables. Strict hygiene practices and toilet facilities should be in place for food pickers and handlers. Consumers should be aware of risks associated with consumption of raw, unwashed leafy greens and berries.

There are many challenges regarding tools for the control and prevention of *C. cayetanensis* infection in both developed and endemic developing regions. These problems arise from two major factors: (1) there is no animal model available for propagation of *C. cayetanensis* and (2) DNA sequence data for the parasite are limited to a few short conserved regions of its genome. The lack of parasite material and sequence data severely hamper the development and validation of suitable detection methods. Proficiency in identifying the oocysts by microscopy is a challenge, and pseudo-outbreaks have been reported as a result (Ortega and Sanchez, 2010). A specific immunofluorescent antibody test could improve detection by microscopy; however, it is difficult to develop without large numbers of oocysts. Oocysts are also necessary for test performance and validation studies, as controls for diagnostic testing of clinical samples, and for proficiency testing. Whole genome sequence data would contribute significantly to the development of reliable molecular typing methods for disease outbreak investigations. The combination of longer sporulation and prepatent periods makes it difficult to identify risk factors and foods that serve as transmission vehicles for *C. cayetanensis* infection. Some widely employed PCR methods, although sensitive, cannot reliably differentiate between *C. cayetanensis* and closely related *Eimeria* species, or are unsuitable for use on food or fecal samples, leading to the reporting of false-positive or false-negative results and further highlighting the need for reliable diagnostic tools.

6.4 *Cryptosporidium* spp.

6.4.1 Taxonomy

The genus *Cryptosporidium* was originally described from gastric glands of laboratory mice and the type species was established as *Cryptosporidium muris* (Tyzzer, 1907, 1910). Subsequently, Tyzzer (1912) described *Cryptosporidium parvum* from the small intestine of laboratory mice and having oocysts smaller than those of *C. muris* (Tyzzer, 1912). In the 1970s, *Cryptosporidium* emerged as an important pathogen of cattle and humans. In the 1980s, considerable interest emerged in the genus *Cryptosporidium* following reports of cases in patients with acquired immune deficiency syndrome (AIDS; Anonymous, 1982). Later, a massive waterborne outbreak of cryptosporidiosis in Milwaukee, WI, triggered concerns about *Cryptosporidium* as a significant waterborne pathogen (MacKenzie et al., 1995). More recently, studies on the basic biology of *Cryptosporidium* provided methods for detection, classification, prevention, and treatment. Oocysts of the genus are distinguished by having four sporozoites and no sporocysts.

Currently, a total of 20 valid species are recognized within the genus *Cryptosporidium*, and more than 40 genotypes have been described (Fayer, 2008, 2010; Ryan and Power, 2012; Xiao et al., 2004). Two species of *Cryptosporidium* (*Cryptosporidium hominis* and *C. parvum*) are most commonly detected in humans (Caccio et al., 2005). However, other species have also been detected in feces of both immunocompetent and immunocompromised humans (Table 6.2).

6.4.2 Host range, prevalence, and distribution

Cryptosporidium has recently emerged as an important enteric pathogen in a wide diversity of hosts. *Cryptosporidium* spp. infect a wide range of vertebrates, including humans, as well as domestic and wild animals. Affected hosts include mammals, reptiles, birds, amphibians, and fish (Fayer, 2010; Ryan and Power, 2012; Table 6.2). Oocysts excreted with feces can be transmitted to humans directly from infected persons or animals, and via contaminated food or water (Figure 6.2). In a study of *C. hominis* infection in human volunteers, the median dose required to infect 50%

Table 6.2 **Currently recognized *Cryptosporidium* species including those known to infect humans**

Species	Zoonosis reported	Primary host species	Other host species	Site of infection	Selected references
C. parvum	Yes	Cattle, sheep, goat, human	Deer, mice, pig	Small intestine	Leoni et al. (2006), Santin and Trout (2008a,b), Morse et al. (2007), Fayer (2010), and Santin (2013)
C. hominis	Yes	Human	Dugong, sheep, cattle	Small intestine	Morgan-Ryan et al. (2002), Leoni et al. (2006), Park et al. (2006), and Fayer (2010)
C. meleagridis	Yes	Turkey, human	Parrot	Small intestine	Slavin (1955), Leoni et al. (2006), and Morgan et al. (2000a)
C. muris	Yes	Rodents	Cattle, Bactrian camels, rock hyrax, human	Stomach	Fayer (2010), Morgan et al. (2000c), Palmer et al. (2003), and Tyzzer (1907)
C. canis	Yes	Dog	Human	Small intestine	Fayer (2010), Leoni et al. (2006), and Morgan et al. (2000b)
C. felis	Yes	Cat	Human, cattle	Small intestine	Bornay-Llinares et al. (1999), Iseki (1979), and Raccurt (2007)
C. suis	Yes	Pig	Human	Small and large intestine	Cama et al. (2007), Ryan et al. (2004)
C. andersoni	Yes	Cattle, Bactrian camel	Human	Abomasum	Leoni et al. (2006), Lindsay et al. (2000), Santin (2013), Santin and Trout (2008b), and Wang et al. (2008)
C. ubiquitum	Yes	Cattle	Human, lemur, domestic goat, sheep, deer, mouse, gerbil	Small intestine	Fayer et al. (2010)
C. cuniculus	Yes	European rabbit, human	Not known	Small intestine	Chalmers and Katzer (2013) and Robinson et al. (2010)
C. viatorum	Yes	Human	Not known	Not known	Elwin et al. (2012), Insulander et al. (2013)
C. fayeri	Yes	Kangaroo, koala, wallaby	Human	Small intestine	Ryan and Power (2012), Ryan et al. (2008), and Waldron et al. (2010)

Continued

Table 6.2 Continued

Species	Zoonosis reported	Primary host species	Other host species	Site of infection	Selected references
C. erinacei n. sp.	Yes	European hedgehog	Horse, human	Small intestine	Kvac et al. (2014a,b)
C. scrofarum n. sp.	Yes	Pig	Human, calf, wild boar	Small and large intestine	Kvac et al. (2009, 2013)
C. baileyi	Yes	Chicken	Turkey, duck, quail, human	Trachea, bursa of Fabricius, cloaca	Current et al. (1986) and Ryan and Xiao (2008)
C. bovis	No	Cattle	Sheep	Small intestine	Faye et al. (2005), Santin (2013), and Santin and Trout (2008b)
C. xiaoi	No	Sheep	Yak, goat	Not known	Fayer and Santin (2009), Feng et al. (2007), and Karanis et al. (2007b)
C. ryanae	No	Cattle	Not known	Not known	Fayer et al. (2008) and Santin (2013)
C. macropodum	No	Kangaroo	Wallaby, kangaroo	Intestine	Power and Ryan (2008)
C. galli	No	Chicken, Finch	Variety of exotic and wild birds	Proventriculus	Pavlasek (2001) and Ryan et al. (2003)
C. serpentis	No	Snake, lizard	Not known	Stomach	Fayer (2010), Levine (1980), and Tilley et al. (1990)
C. varanii (syn. *C saurophilum*)	No	Lizard	Snake	Stomach and small intestine	Pavlasek et al. (1995) and Pavlasek and Ryan (2008)
C. molnari	No	Fish	Not known	Stomach (and intestine)	Alvarez-Pellitero and Sitja-Bobadilla (2002)
C. scophthalmi	No	Fish	Not known	Intestine (and stomach)	Alvarez-Pellitero et al. (2004)
C. wrairi	No	Guinea pig	Not known	Small intestine	Fayer (2010), Jervis et al. (1966), and Vetterling et al. (1971)

of the population (ID50) was as low as 10 oocysts (range 10–83) (Chappell et al., 2006), whereas the range of ID50 for *C. parvum* was determined to be 9–1042 in healthy volunteers (Okhuysen et al., 1999). A mathematical model of the Milwaukee outbreak estimated that the ID50 might have been as low as one oocyst for some persons (MacKenzie et al., 1995). Over 90% of reported human infections with *Cryptosporidium* spp. are attributed to two species: the anthroponotic *C. hominis* and the zoonotic *C. parvum*. Prevalence of *C. hominis* and *C. parvum* in humans varies in different regions of the world. Both species are common in humans in European countries (Fayer, 2008; Leoni et al., 2006; Robertson and Chalmers, 2013). In the Middle East, *C. parvum* is the dominant species in humans (Al-Brikan et al., 2008; Alyousefi et al., 2013; Aslan et al., 2012). In the Americas, Australia, Africa, the Far East, and the Indian subcontinent, *C. hominis* is usually the predominant species in humans (Abd El Kader et al., 2012; Feng et al., 2014; Xiao, 2010). Geographic distribution of *C. parvum* and *C. hominis* seems to vary within countries; for example, in the United States and Ireland, *C. parvum* is more common than *C. hominis* in the rural regions (Feltus et al., 2006; Zintl et al., 2009). The distribution of *C. hominis* and *C. parvum* is also affected by temporal and demographic factors in different countries. In the United Kingdom, although the many hosts of both *C. parvum* and *C. hominis* were young, *C. hominis* was more prevalent in infants under 1 year and in females aged 15–44 years. In the Nordic countries, *C. hominis* was more commonly found in children, and *C. parvum* was more prevalent in adults (Wielinga et al., 2008). In developing countries (Guinea-Bissau), *C. parvum* was most prevalent during early childhood before the age of 2 years, and the pathogenicity was higher in boys than in girls (Valentiner-Branth et al., 2003). Seasonal variations in the disease burden between *C. parvum* and *C. hominis* have also been reported. *C. hominis* was more prevalent in autumn whereas *C. parvum* was more prevalent in spring, and there has been a decline in *C. parvum* cases in the United Kingdom since 2001, and an increase in reported cases in the Nordic countries (Chalmers et al., 2009; Robertson and Chalmers, 2013; Wielinga et al., 2008; Zintl et al., 2009). Other *Cryptosporidium* species (*Cryptosporidium meleagridis*, *Cryptosporidium felis*, *Cryptosporidium canis*, *Cryptosporidium suis*, *C. muris*, *Cryptosporidium andersoni*, and *Cryptosporidium ubiquitum*) have also been found in humans; in particular *C. meleagridis*, a parasite of turkeys that is now recognized as an emerging human pathogen. Although widespread geographically, *C. meleagridis* is responsible for ≤1% of *Cryptosporidium* cases among developed countries (Chalmers et al., 2009; Silverlas et al., 2012). This species has been reported in 10–12.6% of *Cryptosporidium* cases in both healthy children and HIV patients in Peru, where its prevalence was as high as that of *C. parvum* in HIV patients (Cama et al., 2003, 2007, 2008).

6.4.3 Life cycle and development

Infection with *Cryptosporidium* spp. begins with the ingestion of oocysts by a suitable host species followed by excystation and all three stages of reproduction (merogony, gametogony, and sporogony) occurring in the same host (Figures 6.1 and 6.2). The parasites penetrate the intestinal epithelial cell membrane without entering the cytoplasm (epicellular development) where they undergo multiple generations of merogony. The invading parasites cause the infected host cell membrane to enlarge and rupture after 48–72 h, releasing motile merozoites that follow either of two pathways: (a) infect fresh epithelial cells and repeat another generation of merogony or (b) differentiate into sexual gametes and fuse into zygotes, which mature into sporulated oocysts. These oocysts exit the infected cells and are excreted with feces from the host, or sporozoites are released from the oocysts in the epithelium or intestinal lumen of the host to infect fresh epithelial cells (autoinfection) and begin additional cycles of merogony and gametogony (Figure 6.2). Oocysts passed with feces into the environment do not undergo further replication or development until ingested by a new host (Figure 6.2).

6.4.4 Ecology and epidemiology

The epidemiology of *Cryptosporidium* spp., like other coccidia species, is influenced by the characteristics of the life cycle and oocysts, and transmission routes of the parasite species. Risk factors associated with cryptosporidiosis include contact with young children and elderly adults having diarrhea, traveling abroad, contact with farm animals, and swimming in freshwater or public swimming pools (Roy et al., 2004). Consumption of oocyst-contaminated water, drinks, and ready-to-eat fruits and vegetables represents a major risk factor for acquiring cryptosporidiosis. *Cryptosporidium* was responsible for 50.8% of water-associated outbreaks of parasitic protozoan diseases documented worldwide (Karanis et al., 2007a). In 23.7% of these outbreaks, *Cryptosporidium* oocysts contaminated water distribution systems and passed through filtered or unfiltered drinking water systems. Although cryptosporidiosis is generally considered a waterborne disease, several outbreaks of cryptosporidiosis have been documented to be associated with foodborne transmission (Robertson and Chalmers, 2013). Food contamination usually occurs via direct fecal contamination or via water used to process produce or prepare food. Traditional microscopic methods are not appropriate or sufficiently sensitive to detect *Cryptosporidium* oocysts in food. Recently developed molecular tools have facilitated the identification and characterization of *Cryptosporidium* at the species, genotype, and subtype levels. Molecular epidemiological studies have provided insights into the infection sources and transmission routes of the disease involving both humans and nonhuman sources, including livestock and wildlife. Molecular tools based on the small subunit (SSU) rRNA, oocysts wall protein, 70-kDa heat shock protein (HSP70), and actin genes are used in genotyping *Cryptosporidium.* SSU rRNA-based tools are now the preferred method for genotyping *Cryptosporidium.* Other genotyping tools have demonstrated fewer *Cryptosporidium* species and genotypes, which limited their application for molecular epidemiology (Xiao, 2010). Subtyping tools are used in epidemiological investigations involving *C. parvum* and *C. hominis* because they target genes with higher evolutionary rates than the more conserved sequences used for genotyping. The genetic targets used for subtyping include the 60-kDa glycoprotein (GP60) gene, microsatellites and minisatellites, double-stranded RNA element, and the internal transcribed spacer-2 (ITS-2) of the rRNA gene (Xiao and Ryan, 2008).

6.4.5 Disease

Cryptosporidium spp. are capable of causing mild to severe clinical illness in humans and animals. Infection with *Cryptosporidium* spp. can be sporadic and self-limiting or chronic. Although most infections with *Cryptosporidium* are asymptomatic, severe clinical illness manifested by diarrhea has been reported in humans, ruminants, dogs, cats, and horses. *C. hominis* is commonly found in humans; *C. parvum* is the primary zoonotic species. In livestock, it causes neonatal diarrhea and dehydration leading to death and economic loss (Santin, 2013). Oocysts of *C. parvum* are a major source of environmental contamination to pastures, crops, and water bodies. Self-limiting infections occur in individuals with a competent immune system and are asymptomatic or symptomatic, resolving in 1–2 weeks. Chronic infections with potentially life-threatening illness can occur in immunocompromised individuals, such as AIDS patients and those with malignancies and immunosuppressed transplant patients. Clinical symptoms of human infections with *C. parvum* and *C. hominis* are similar and most frequently associated with diarrhea, nausea, and abdominal discomfort, all of which resolve within 4–14 days (Warren and Guerrant, 2008). However, *C. hominis* appears to be more virulent than *C. parvum* as measured by the severity of clinical symptoms and output of oocysts (Cama et al., 2008). *C. hominis* is also associated with heavier infections and lower growth rates in children, even in the absence of symptoms, and an increased risk of nonintestinal sequelae in immunocompetent patients (Bushen et al., 2007; Hunter et al., 2004). Although a significant number of *Cryptosporidium* infections are asymptomatic, onset of clinical manifestations is influenced by the immune response, age, and nutritional status of the individual, among other factors. In immunocompetent individuals, diarrhea is generally self-limiting, but it can be more severe and even life-threatening in immunocompromised individuals, particularly those with low $CD4^+$ T-cell count (Assefa et al., 2009; Izadi et al., 2012). Age-related cryptosporidiosis most frequently involves children and the elderly. In developing countries, malnutrition as well as subsequent impaired physical and cognitive development are associated with *Cryptosporidium* infection in children (Guerrant et al., 1999).

6.4.6 Control and prevention

Oocysts of *Cryptosporidium,* which represent the transmission stage of the parasite, are highly resistant to external environmental conditions and to many physical and chemical disinfection methods routinely used as bactericides in water treatment plants, swimming pools, and irrigation systems (Gajadhar and Allen, 2004). At 5–15 °C *Cryptosporidium* oocysts remain viable for longer than 6 months (Fayer et al., 1998). Therefore, in mild weather conditions, oocysts in water may survive for long periods of time. However, survival time is shortened considerably as the temperature decreases below 5 °C or increases above 15 °C. Oocysts of *C. parvum* survive freezing temperatures at or above −15 °C for extended periods but are rendered nonviable when stored for 24 h or longer at −20 °C or lower (Fayer and Nerad, 1996). Desiccation and irradiation can also be lethal to *Cryptosporidium* oocysts. Air drying of oocysts at room temperature for slightly longer than 2 h resulted in complete inactivation of the parasite (Robertson et al., 1992). This probably explains the finding that most outbreaks associated with food are related to beverages and fresh produce (Insulander et al., 2008; Ponka et al., 2009). Ultraviolet (UV) irradiation from artificial sources can irreversibly inactivate *Cryptosporidium* oocysts, despite the presence of the UV repair genes in the parasite's genome (Smith et al., 2008). Oocysts are insensitive to commonly used disinfectants such as chlorine. Treatment of green peppers with chlorine followed by blast freezing did not significantly affect the viability of the oocysts (Duhain et al., 2012). Under experimental conditions, oocysts of *C. parvum* were shown to adhere strongly to the roots and leaves of spinach and resisted removal by vigorous washing. Oocysts can also be located within the leaves, negating any effectiveness of washing (Macarisin et al., 2010).

Because *Cryptosporidium* infection is contagious among persons, control measures aim to reduce or prevent transmission of oocysts that are shed in human and animal feces. Targeted areas include management and disposal of sewage from animals and humans, biosecurity, treatment and use of water, and education. Good sanitation as well as personal hygiene and food preparation hygiene are also important, including thorough washing of hands and uncooked food (e.g., fruits and vegetables).

There is no specific treatment for *Cryptosporidium* infection. In immunocompetent individuals, recovery usually occurs within a few weeks without medical intervention. Supportive therapy may be required in cases involving severe diarrhea (Leitch and He, 2012). In some countries, the antiprotozoan agent nitazoxanide (NTZ) has been approved for the treatment of cryptosporidiosis in immunocompetent children and adults (Rossignol, 2010). In immunocompromised patients, the combination of NTZ and highly active antiretroviral therapy has had a positive impact on reducing the prevalence of *Cryptosporidium* infection in patients with HIV/AIDS (Zardi et al., 2005). To date, there is no known control program for cryptosporidiosis; neither is there a commercially available vaccine.

Detection of oocysts in stool samples is the most common method for diagnosis of infection in humans and animals. Oocysts in samples may be concentrated using flotation/sedimentation techniques followed by microscopy or PCR, or isolated by immunomagnetic separation (IMS), and then detected by staining or immunofluorescence microscopy. Commercial IMS are available and widely used for the detection of *Cryptosporidium* and *Giardia* in water, but less so for fresh fruits, and vegetables. An ISO standard method to detect oocysts in produce has been developed and includes elution from the test product, concentration by IMS, and detection of oocysts by immunofluorescence microscope (AFNOR, 2013). Improved PCR-based methods are more sensitive than conventional and immunological methods for detecting oocysts and can provide reliable identification to species, genotype and subtype levels. Molecular assays also have to be designed and used to screen samples concurrently for *Cryptosporidium* and various other parasites such as *Toxoplasma*, *Cyclospora*, and *Sarcocystis* (Lalonde and Gajadhar, 2011; Lalonde et al., 2013).

6.5 *Cystoisospora* (syn. *Isospora*)

6.5.1 *Taxonomy*

C. belli is the only species of the genus that can complete its life cycle in humans. However, more than 300 species of *Cystoisospora* have been described, but since the identification of many was based primarily on morphometrics of the oocysts, their taxonomic status at the species as well as genus level is unclear. Oocysts that share the cystoisosporan configuration of two sporocysts, each with four sporozoites, may be the most misidentified and misnamed among the coccidia, and include *Cystoisospora hominis*, *Cystoisospora bigemina*, and *Cystoisospora bahiensis*. Furthermore, oocysts of *Cystoisospora* species can be morphometrically indistinguishable from those of the genera *Sarcocystis*, *Toxoplasma*, *Hammondia*, *Frenkelia*, and others. Cystoisosporan infections in humans are due primarily to *C. belli*. Because *Cystoisospora* spp. do not establish patent infection in herbivores, their occurrence in food animals is limited to a few species in pigs. However, many host species, including cattle, sheep, and other food animals could act as paratenic hosts for several *Cystoisospora* spp. (Fayer and Frenkel, 1979; Hendricks and Walton, 1974; Hilali et al., 1992; Lindsay et al., 1997). Paratenic hosts, including vertebrates and invertebrates, may be important vehicles of transmission and a significant source of foodborne infection.

6.5.2 Host range, prevalence, and distribution

Members of the genus *Cystoisospora* are usually host species-specific. For example, primates, apparently mostly humans, are the only suitable hosts for *C. belli*, and it has been shown that pigs, dogs, mice, rats, rabbits, guinea pigs, and rhesus monkeys are not (Foner, 1939; Jeffery, 1956; Lindsay et al., 1997). *C. belli* is globally distributed, but infections have been more commonly recorded from tropical and subtropical countries, and more commonly from Thailand, Haiti, Mexico, Brazil, El Salvador, and countries in the Middle East and Southeast Asia (Faust et al., 1961; Jongwutiwes et al., 2007; Junod et al., 1988; Lindsay et al., 1997; Sorvillo et al., 1995). Prevalence studies conducted on human populations in the United States and Japan showed no evidence of oocysts of *C. belli* (Obana et al., 2002; Ribes et al., 2004).

High prevalences of *C. belli* intestinal infections occur in immunocompromised individuals. In HIV-infected persons, prevalence rates of 15% (20/131), 9.9% (13/81), 5% (3/60), and 1% (127/16,351) were detected in Haiti (DeHovitz et al., 1986), Brazil (Sauda et al., 1993), Spain (Ros et al., 1987), and the United States (Los Angeles County) (Sorvillo et al., 1995), respectively. In France, *C. belli* infection among HIV-infected patients has been reported primarily in patients from sub-Saharan Africa (Guiguet et al., 2007), and in India, it was detected in 8% of 137 HIV-infected individuals with diarrhea (Kulkarni et al., 2009). Disseminated extraintestinal isosporosis due to *C. belli* has been rarely reported in AIDS patients (Michiels et al., 1994; Restrepo et al., 1987).

6.5.3 Life cycle and development

C. belli completes merogony and gametogony within a single host (Figures 6.1 and 6.2), usually in intestinal epithelial cells, and endodyogeny is also a feature of the asexual phase of reproduction. Similar to other species of *Cystoisospora,* extraintestinal infection in the form of monozoic tissue cysts has been observed (Lindsay et al., 1997, 2014); however, significant details of the life cycle of this parasite remain unknown. Unsporulated oocysts are excreted with the feces of infected hosts.

With sufficient temperature, humidity, and time, these oocysts sporulate, consisting of two sporocysts, each with four sporozoites. When oocysts are identified with concurrent knowledge of the host species, they may be distinguished based on the microscopic examination (Table 6.1). *C. belli* is transmitted via contaminated food and water. Infection consists of excystation of sporozoites followed by merogony and gametogony within epithelial cells and the shedding of unsporulated oocysts with feces (Figures 6.1 and 6.2).

The role of paratenic hosts, including both invertebrate and vertebrate species, can be important for completing the life cycle of the parasite, especially in areas where adequate sanitary conditions reduce the risk of direct transmission. Commonly infected sites in vertebrate paratenic hosts include extraintestinal sites such as lymph nodes, liver, and spleen (Lindsay et al., 1997).

6.5.4 Ecology and epidemiology

There is a dearth of information on the ecology and epidemiology of *I. belli*. The oocysts can remain viable in the environment for long periods of time. Although adverse conditions such as temperatures greater than 40 °C or less than 20 °C inhibit oocyst sporulation, development continues at a slower rate or when favorable conditions return, thus extending the period of survival in the environment.

C. belli is an important intestinal parasite in immunocompromised individuals especially AIDS patients. Recently, the parasite has been reported from a number of individuals with organ transplant or cancer (Koru et al., 2007; Marathe and Parikh, 2013; Meamar et al., 2009; Ud Din et al., 2012; Usluca et al., 2012; Yazar et al., 2006). *C. belli* oocysts have been reported from travelers and children with diarrhea in developing countries (Godiwala and Yaeger, 1987; Kochhar et al., 2007; Mirdha et al., 2002; Tavarez et al., 1991). Concomitant intestinal infection with other foodborne parasites may be present in such individuals. Poor sanitation, lack of clean drinking water, and absence of sewage disposal systems contribute to the transmission of this parasite in developing countries.

6.5.5 Disease

Immunocompetent individuals infected with *C. belli* are usually asymptomatic. The symptoms in infected infants and immunocompromised persons may include headache, fever, malaise, abdominal pain, diarrhea, vomiting, dehydration, weight loss, and rarely bloody diarrhea (Liebman et al., 1980). The infection can be chronic, and if not treated, oocysts may be shed for several months. Recrudescence of previously resolved infection may be possible by the reactivation and migration of zoites in monozoic tissue cysts to the intestine (Lindsay et al., 2014).

Individuals with low CD4+ lymphocyte counts (usually <200 cells/l) are at particular risk of being clinically infected (Certad et al., 2003; DeHovitz et al., 1986; Pape et al., 1989). In immunocompromised individuals, clinical illness due to *C. belli* infection appears to be more severe and of longer duration (Certad et al., 2003). *C. belli*-induced chronic diarrhea and wasting have been observed in AIDS patients receiving subtherapeutic plasma levels of antiretroviral drugs or none at all (Brantley et al., 2003; Maiga et al., 2002).

Infections of *C. belli* may be detected by demonstrating the oocysts in the feces using concentration methods followed by light microscopy, but identification of the species may not be possible without sporulation. Sheather's sugar flotation or sedimentation concentration is widely used method for the recovery of oocysts from fecal samples. These methods have a higher sensitivity compared to the examination of direct fecal smears (Faust et al., 1961). However, the reliability of microscopic examination and identification is dependent on the expertise and competence of the analyst. Staining techniques such as modified acid fast (Ng et al., 1984), auramine-rhodamine (Ma et al., 1983), and safranin-methylene blue (Bush and Markus, 1987) may be used to aid in the identification of oocysts. Parasitic stages may also be identified from duodenal aspirates or histopathology on biopsies.

Molecular techniques such as various PCR methods have been developed for the definitive identification of *Cystoisospora* spp. and may be used on virtually any stage of the parasite, including unsporulated oocysts (Lalonde and Gajadhar, 2011; Muller et al., 2000; Taniuchi et al., 2011; ten Hove et al., 2008).

6.5.6 Control and prevention

Adequate sanitation, including appropriate disposal of feces, proper personal hygiene, and thorough hand washing, should be practiced. To disrupt the life cycle of the parasite, contamination of food and water must be avoided to prevent new infections. Drinking water and fresh fruits and vegetables that are consumed raw should be treated by filtration, ozone, heating, or washing to remove or inactivate oocysts. Other aspects of control and prevention used for other coccidian infections may also be applicable to *I. belli*. There is no vaccine for humans or livestock to protect against *Cystoisospora* coccidian infections.

6.6 *Toxoplasma gondii*

6.6.1 Taxonomy

T. gondii is an apicomplexan protozoan parasite in the Sarcocystidae family. It can infect virtually all mammals and birds. Felid species serve as the only definitive hosts in which the parasite reproduces sexually and produces oocysts (Figure 6.3). Fully sporulated oocysts of *T. gondii* consist of two sporocysts each containing four sporozoites (Table 6.1). By virtue of the oocyst characteristics and life cycle, *T. gondii* is placed in the coccidia group of parasites and is most closely related to other cyst-forming tissue coccidia, including *Neospora caninum*, *Hammondia* spp., *Frenkelia* spp., and *Sarcocystis* spp. (Figure 6.1 and Table 6.1). *T. gondii* is the sole species of the genus *Toxoplasma*, and until recently, isolates were traditionally grouped by multilocus genotyping into three distinct clonal lineages (Types I, II, and III) with characteristics of low diversity within lineages and varying degrees of virulence. Type I isolates are highly virulent and found occasionally in South and Central America where various highly diverse genotypes also occur. Types II and III are less virulent and predominate in North America, Europe, and Africa, whereas Type III is most common in Asia. Ongoing sequence analyses of *T. gondii* isolates worldwide reveal highly complex and diverse population structures, consisting of multiple clonal groups (>3) and several haplogroups with varying virulence, and many atypical isolates that are too polymorphic to be grouped for any meaningful classification (Dubey, 2010b; Khan et al., 2011; Robert-Gangneux and Dardé, 2012).

6.6.2 Host range, prevalence, and distribution

T. gondii is widespread globally because of the cosmopolitan distribution of felids, and because of the diversity and abundance of suitable intermediate hosts in virtually all habitats. The infection rate in domestic and feral cats varies widely by region. Serological surveys report varying rates of prevalence of exposure in definitive and intermediate hosts. The seroprevalence of *T. gondii* in domestic animals and wildlife has been extensively reviewed by Dubey (2010b). In some populations, up to 100% of domestic and wild felids have antibodies to *T. gondii*. The prevalence in humans and food animals varies widely by region, with surveys reporting anywhere from 4% to 92% for humans, and similar variations for host species such as sheep (13–96%), cattle (0–76%), pigs (<1–90%), and chickens (13–96%). This wide variation in seroprevalence is likely due to both climatic and anthropogenic factors, many of the latter relating to food production and preparation practices, and association with cats; however, the different test methods used in the surveys could also have contributed to the variation. Infection rates may be influenced by environmental conditions affecting the survival and sporulation of oocysts. Low-lying regions and warmer climates typically have higher seroprevalences than higher regions and cooler climates (Dubey, 2010b). Socioeconomic level and cultural preferences in meat and vegetable selection and preparation appear to greatly influence infection rates.

Sheep, goats, cats, marsupials, and marine mammals can be infected with *T. gondii* and show mild to severe clinical signs of disease. Pigs, cattle, horses, dogs, chickens, deer, and rodents can also be infected but are less likely to show clinical signs. However, it should be noted that virulence can be influenced by many factors, including health status such as immune competence and stress of the host, parasite strain, or type, dose, and route of infection.

6.6.3 Life cycle and development

As an apicomplexan coccidian parasite, the *T. gondii* life cycle follows asexual forms of reproduction (sporogony, endodyogeny, and merogony) and a sexual phase (gametogony), as illustrated in Figures 6.1 and 6.3. *T. gondii* requires a felid definitive host for sexual reproduction and any warm-blooded vertebrate animal, such as a mammal or bird to complete its life cycle (Figure 6.3). Details of the parasite's transmission dynamics between humans, domestic animals, and wildlife involve various modes of transmission, including via food and water, and congenital transmission, and are illustrated in Figure 6.4 (Gajadhar et al., 2006). As with other tissue coccidia such as *Sarcocystis* spp., sexual replication in the felid definitive host is driven by ingestion

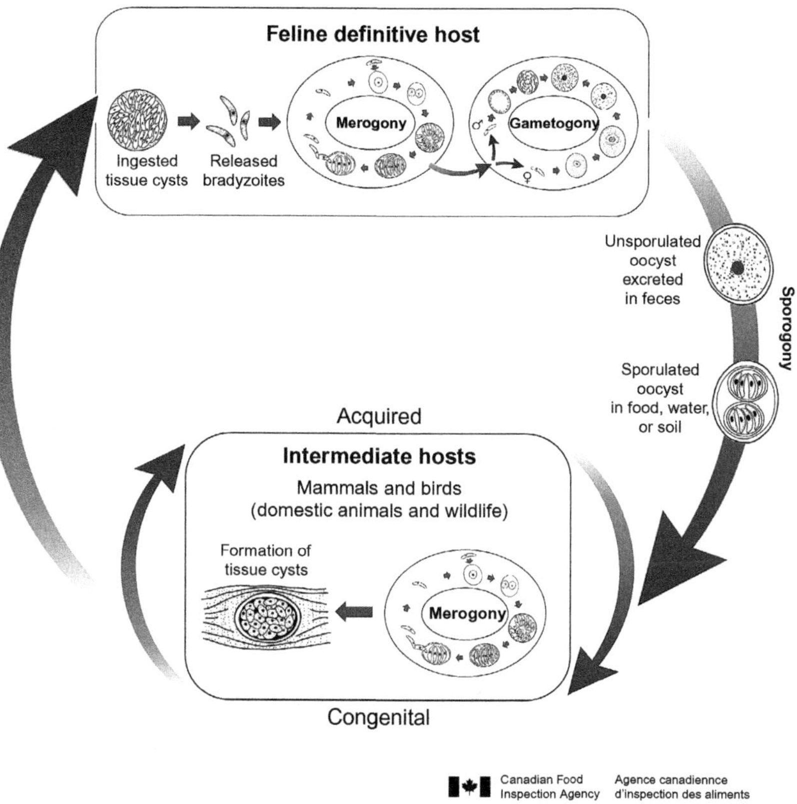

Figure 6.3 Life cycle of *Toxoplasma gondii*. Felid definitive hosts become infected by ingesting meat infected with tissue cysts or water or food contaminated with sporulated oocysts. Following merogony and gametogony in the intestine, oocysts are excreted with feces and sporulate in the environment. Intermediate hosts acquire the infection by ingesting oocysts or tissue cysts, or congenitally. The infection can be transmitted and maintained among intermediate hosts by acquired or congenital infection and serve as a source of infection for the definitive host.

of a prey species intermediate host-harboring tissue cysts containing bradyzoites, with the subsequent release of oocysts into the environment. Cats can also become infected by the ingestion of tachyzoites in tissues or fluids of infected hosts or less efficiently by oocysts shed by infected felids. The usual prepatent period before oocysts are excreted is 3–10 days after ingestion of bradyzoites, or more than 18 days after being infected with oocysts or tachyzoites (Dubey, 2010b). The oocysts are unsporulated when excreted and require a minimum of a few to several days to sporulate and become infective (Table 6.1). The *T. gondii* oocyst is basically similar in form, size, and shape to those of other coccidia genera such as *Neospora* and *Cystoisospora*, consisting of two sporocysts, each containing four sporozoites (Table 6.1). In the environment, oocysts are incredibly resistant to adverse conditions. Although most infected cats shed oocysts for only a little over a week during their lifetimes, many millions of resistant oocysts are released into the environment during this period of patency. Oocysts can survive in various matrices such as soil and water for up to 1 or 2 years. Various invertebrates such as earthworms, cockroaches, and bivalves can serve as biomagnifying transport hosts and harbor the parasites for long periods of time. *T. gondii* oocysts can survive in seawater at room temperature for up to 18 months (Lindsay and Dubey, 2009) and are highly resistant to chemical disinfectants (Dubey, 2010b).

Upon infection of the intermediate host, sporozoites or bradyzoites differentiate into tachyzoites and invade many types of host cells throughout the body and divide several times by endodyogeny until the parasitized cells rupture and release the newly formed tachyzoites that infect new host cells (Figure 6.3). This cycle of invasion, division, and release occurs rapidly over a period of several days until numerous tachyzoites are widely disseminated in leucocytes and most tissues, including the lamina propria, mesenteric lymph nodes, and various organs, with a predilection for the brain and less so for the heart and skeletal muscles. Multiple tachyzoites accumulate in each host cell, which eventually ruptures to release the parasites to invade new cells. Tachyzoites are fragile and do not survive long outside of the host. However, they have been found in milk, blood, and semen and are known to initiate infections by congenital transmission via the placenta and by organ or bone marrow transplantation (Dubey, 2010b).

The new tissue cysts develop a wall, grow in size within host cells, and accumulate tens of thousands or more bradyzoites. Tissue cysts can persist and remain infective throughout the lifetime of the host. In chronically infected hosts, tissue cysts are more prevalent in neural and muscular tissues, including brain, eyes, and cardiac and skeletal muscles, but may also be found in visceral organs, such as lungs, liver, and kidneys

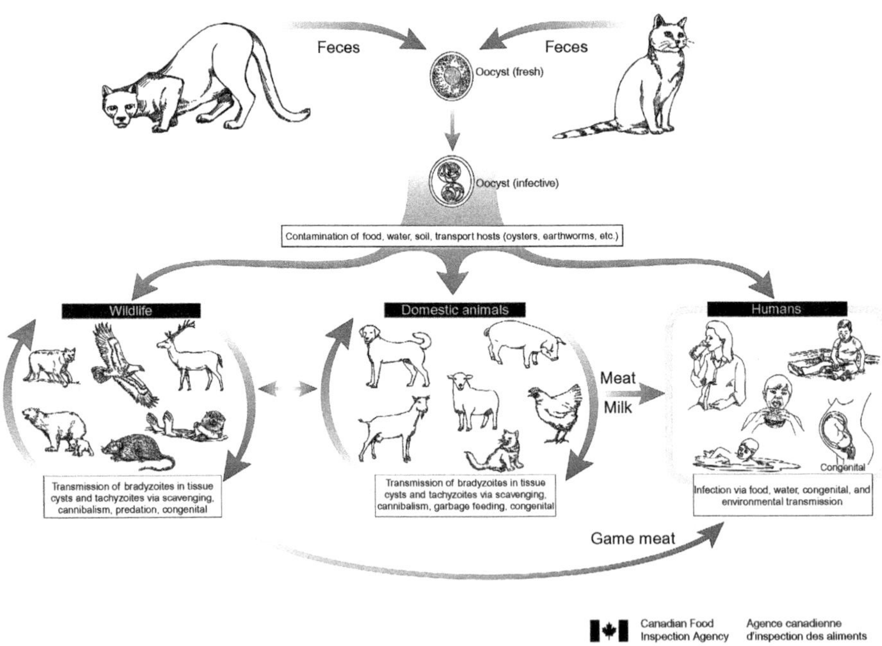

Figure 6.4 Diagram showing the epidemiology of *T. gondii* infection involving foodborne transmission from multiple sources and cycles.

(Dubey, 2010b). Foodborne transmission of *T. gondii* via bradyzoites in tissue cysts can occur by predation, scavenging, garbage feeding, and cannibalism in wildlife and in domestic animals (Figure 6.4). Humans can acquire infection by ingesting bradyzoites in undercooked meat containing tissue cysts, tachyzoites in milk, or sporulated oocysts contaminating water and foods such as fruits and vegetables. Congenital infection results from the transmission of tachyzoites via the placenta.

6.6.4 Ecology and epidemiology

The main sources of *T. gondii* as a leading cause of death in humans due to foodborne infection include tissue cysts in meat and oocysts in fresh fruits and vegetables. Transmission vehicles that are not foodborne include water and contaminants in the environment. Many factors contribute to acquired *T. gondii* infection in humans and animals. Climatic factors affecting the survival of oocysts in the environment are important for infection rates in humans, wildlife, and food animals. Oocysts of coccidia do not survive well in cold or dry environments, and generally, infection rates are higher in humid areas with warm temperatures (Farr and Wehr, 1949; Gajadhar and Allen, 2004). Infected cats can shed up to a billion or more oocysts in a short period of time, and, when covered with soil outdoors in a favorable climate, the oocysts can remain viable for months or longer, leading to a highly seeded environment and a source of contamination for surface and sea water through runoff (Dabritz et al., 2007). Oocysts remain viable for long periods in water and are not killed by chlorination, ozone, or most other treatments. In fact, extensive studies conducted in our laboratory showed that oocysts readily survive and develop to the sporulated stage while immersed for weeks in seawater or various chemical solutions, including ethanol, hydrogen peroxide, and iodine, and are capable of establishing fatal infection in mice. Experimental infections have demonstrated that marine and terrestrial mammals are also susceptible to *T. gondii* infection (Gajadhar et al., 2004). The presence of antibodies to the infection in wild marine mammals, such as sea otters, dolphins, seals, and walruses, suggests that oocyst-contaminated freshwater runoff is a source of infection because the diets of most of these animals do not include tissues of intermediate hosts (Dubey, 2010b). *T. gondii* oocysts can also accumulate in transport hosts such as marine bivalves, which can effectively remove and concentrate oocysts from seawater to potentially serve as a source of infection for marine mammals or humans (Lindsay et al., 2004). Multilocus PCR and DNA sequence analysis have shown that the unique Type X *T. gondii* strain commonly found in Californian sea otters is also found in coastal-dwelling felids and marine bivalves in the same area, which also supports the hypothesis that oocysts in feline feces are transmitted via runoff and transport hosts to marine mammals (Miller et al., 2008).

A recent study of risk factors associated with congenital toxoplasmosis in Brazil found that adverse socioeconomic conditions relating to the ingestion of oocysts were most significant (Carellos et al., 2014). Specifically, older mothers with higher levels of education and access to potable water and flush toilets had a lower probability of *T. gondii* infection. Living in a rural area, contact with cats, handling soil, and eating fresh unfrozen meat was associated with higher probability of infection. The *T. gondii* infection rate in cats is influenced mainly by their access to the outdoors and type of food sources (hunting versus sterile cat food). Cats in urban areas of developed countries are likely to be a lower risk to humans due to their controlled diet and management of their feces. As oocysts can contaminate fruits and vegetables either directly or indirectly through contaminated water or soil, cultural differences in which produce types are consumed, whether they are washed and if or how they are cooked will influence risk of infection for humans. Washing will not reliably remove *T. gondii* oocysts, which readily adhere to blackberries and raspberries and can remain viable for several weeks (Kniel et al., 2002), depending on the shelf life of the berries. Because fresh fruits and leafy vegetables are usually washed minimally and eaten raw, several produce types should be considered as potential sources of *T. gondii* infection.

Livestock production practices where animals are raised without access to rodents or cats are significant in reducing the risk of *T. gondii* infection in food animals. The recent upswing in demand for meat from free-range livestock contributes to the increased exposure of pigs, chickens, or other meat-producing animals to a contaminated environment. Increasing evidence of *T. gondii* infection has been found in free-ranging chickens and pigs, indicating exposure to oocysts through contact with cat feces or soil during rooting, scratching, and grazing or by scavenging infected rodents or other wildlife carcasses (Chumpolbanchorn et al., 2013; Dubey, 2010a; Dubey et al., 2012; Gebremedhin et al., 2015). Conversely, infection rates of *T. gondii* infection in pigs and chickens raised in controlled housing conditions are relatively low (Dubey, 2010b; van der Giessen et al., 2007). Sheep, goats, horses, and cattle are generally raised under free-ranging conditions worldwide, and thus at increased risk of infection with *T. gondii* (Dubey, 2010b; García-Bocanegra et al., 2012). The risk to humans from eating *T. gondii*-infected poultry is low because the meat is typically consumed thoroughly cooked; however, in some cultures pork, beef, lamb, horse, or game meat is sometimes consumed rare or prepared by methods such as smoking and barbecuing that does not ensure the uniform heating to at least 60 °C required to inactivate the parasite. The high human seroprevalence of *T. gondii* infection in some countries such as France is likely due to their tendency to consume undercooked meat, whereas in some Asian countries where seroprevalence is lower, meat is usually well cooked, and there is little contact with cats. The risk of accidental contamination of food with whole or ruptured tissue cysts during the processing of raw meat should not be underestimated, particularly involving home preparation of meat such as chicken, lamb, pork, and game.

Increasing urbanization has resulted in more interaction between humans, domestic and feral cats, and wildlife and has exposed previously underappreciated transmission routes for *T. gondii* (Singh and Gajadhar, 2014). Conversely, increased socioeconomic levels, improved hygienic conditions, intensive farming, frozen meat, and sterile cat food have reduced seroprevalence in many countries. Lower seroprevalence indicates less circulating *T. gondii* and reduced risk of primary infection during pregnancy, but a higher percentage of naive pregnant women who are at increased risk of infection and congenital transmission. However, immunity to one strain of *T. gondii* may not be protective against another (especially atypical) strain (Robert-Gangneux and Dardé, 2012).

6.6.5 Disease

T. gondii is a well-adapted parasite that can persist for many years in an immunocompetent host without causing any recognized illness in about 80% of infections. However, clinical toxoplasmosis can occur in all animals, including humans. In early infection, patients may experience fever, swollen cervical lymph nodes, headaches, muscle aches, fatigue, stiff neck, and sometimes rash. Ocular toxoplasmosis is likely the most common complication of acquired infection and is often associated with the ingestion of oocysts. An investigation of a cluster of retinitis cases in Canada revealed an outbreak of ocular toxoplasmosis that was linked to drinking water from a reservoir contaminated with oocysts, purportedly from a wild felid (Bowie et al., 1997). The immune status of the host and the life-cycle stage and strain of the parasite significantly influence the occurrence, symptoms, and severity of toxoplasmosis. In Western Europe and North America, the less virulent Type II strains are most common, and thus disease tends to be less severe. Although atypical and more diverse genotypes strains circulate in South America and Africa, they incur more serious disease manifestations (Carneiro et al., 2013; Robert-Gangneux and Dardé, 2012). For instance, congenitally infected children in Brazil were more likely to have serious ocular disease than those in Europe (Gilbert et al., 2008).

Toxoplasmosis is life-threatening in immunocompromised persons, where even previously acquired immune status does not prevent the rupture of tissue cysts and recrudescence of infection (Dubey, 2010b; Robert-Gangneux and Dardé, 2012). In nonimmune pregnant women infected with *T. gondii*, the occurrence, distribution, and severity of lesions in the fetus depends on the trimester of infection. The likelihood of congenital infection increases as the pregnancy progresses and the placenta degenerates and becomes more permeable to parasite transmission, but the consequences can be most severe for the development of the fetus if infection occurs in the first or the second trimester (Dunn et al., 1999). Abortion, stillbirth, and severe eye and brain abnormalities including intellectual disability, seizures, microcephalus, hydrocephalus, deafness, psychomotor deficiency, intracranial calcification, retinochoroiditis, and microphthalmia can result (Dubey, 2010b; Robert-Gangneux and Dardé, 2012) if the fetus is infected early in gestation. Fortunately, about 60–70% of babies born to infected mothers may not be infected, and approximately 50% of those infected do not have any clinical manifestation of toxoplasmosis (Dubey, 2010b; Dunn et al., 1999). The most common outcome for subclinically infected fetuses is the development of retinochoroiditis later in childhood (Robert-Gangneux and Dardé, 2012). However, there is increasing evidence linking otherwise unapparent congenital or acquired *T. gondii* infection to disturbances in mental development and behavior. For example, toxoplasmosis is increasingly associated with serious psychological disturbances, including schizophrenia, depression, anxiety, suicidal tendencies, and delayed response time (Dubey, 2010b). Thus, latent *T. gondii* infection may be the second most important latent parasitic infection, after malaria.

Clinical toxoplasmosis is of economic importance for ranchers of sheep and likely goats and other livestock species, due to abortions, stillbirth, neonatal deaths, and retarded development. Cats, marsupials, and marine mammals can also develop clinical toxoplasmosis. Although pigs, cattle, horses, dogs, chickens, deer, rodents, and other warm-blooded animals can act as intermediate hosts, most will only rarely develop the clinical disease.

6.6.6 Control and prevention

Because the eradication of *T. gondii* from the ecosystem is unlikely, strategies to control it from occurring in food and other sources of infection for humans should focus on measures to reduce exposure to the parasite. Key among these strategies are education, safe production and preparation of food, research for effective tests, treatments and vaccines, and the use of adequate detection and survey methods. Education is particularly important for people most at risk, including pregnant women and immunologically impaired individuals.

The control and prevention of *T. gondii* infection begins with limiting environmental contamination by oocysts from the felid definitive hosts. Domestic cats are less likely to be infected if they have limited access to rodents, the outdoors, other infected cats and are fed only dried, canned, or cooked foods. Litter should be removed daily to prevent any oocysts present from sporulating and should be stored away from kitchens and children. Any trays or utensils that contact cat litter should be washed thoroughly with hot (>60 °C) water. Avoid flushing cat feces in toilets since water treatments such as chlorination are ineffective in killing oocysts. As controlling fecal contamination of the environment by wild felids is impossible, measures should be taken to prevent their access to farms and residential areas, and surface water sources used for human consumption, recreation, or irrigation of crops. People, especially immunocompromised individuals and pregnant women, should thoroughly wash their hands after any contact with cats, cat litter, and soil and avoid uncooked meat, raw shellfish, unpasteurized milk, untreated or unfiltered water, and ingestion of recreational water. Vegetables, fruits, and herbs eaten raw should be washed thoroughly. Oral counseling and written information should be provided to pregnant women regarding all potential transmission routes of exposure for *T. gondii*.

Meat and meat products from virtually any animal species may be infected with *T. gondii*. Care should be taken to cook meats to well done (>67 °C) or freeze to at least −20 °C for 15 days. Other treatments such as irradiation and high pressure processing may be effective at specific conditions for inactivating tissue stages and oocysts. Hands, utensils, and containers should be adequately washed with hot water after contact with or handling of raw meat. Food animals such as sheep, goats, pigs, and chickens raised in free-range production systems are most at risk of infection with *T. gondii*. At the farm level, contact with cats and rodents should be limited for all animals.

Use of appropriate detection methods is important for the control of *T. gondii*. Various assays are available for the detection of the parasite or evidence of infection. Serological, bioassay, and molecular methods are used for the detection of *T. gondii* infection in humans and animals. Selection of an appropriate detection method is determined by the matrix of the sample and the purpose of the testing. Serological assays such as the modified agglutination test (MAT) and enzyme-linked immunosorbent assays (ELISAs) can be used on serum or meat juice to detect chronic infection but do not provide information about parasite viability. Infection of definitive and intermediate hosts with the many species of tissue coccidia that are closely related to *T.* gondii may result in serological cross reactivity. For example, *Hammondia* spp., which infect various species of livestock and wild animals, can serologically cross react with *T. gondii* in these hosts (Dubey and Sreekumar, 2003). There is no gold-standard serological test for the detection of *T. gondii* in all host species, and reference sera required to properly validate the assays for each host is lacking (Robert-Gangneux and Dardé, 2012). The MAT has been the most convenient and simple assay for detecting antibodies in various hosts without the requirement for species-specific reagents. Recently though, an ELISA using Protein A instead of specific anti-IgG has demonstrated similar versatility and efficiency in testing multiple host species for *T. gondii* infection (Al-Adhami and Gajadhar, 2014). Bioassay is a sensitive method for the detection of *T. gondii* tissue cysts and oocysts but is laborious, time consuming, expensive, and not suitable for screening large numbers of samples. PCR methods may be suitable for clinical samples (tachyzoites in amniotic fluid, blood, placenta, etc.), but the limited maximum sample size (usually ~50 mg) is unsuitable for detecting infected meat because cysts are not evenly distributed.

6.7 *Sarcocystis* spp.

6.7.1 Taxonomy

Sarcocystis was originally reported in 1843 as white thread-like structures (Meischer's tubules) in the muscle of mice. The type species of the genus was established in 1899 after sarcocysts of *Sarcocystis meischeriana* were found in the muscle of pigs, followed by ultrastructural evidence much later to demonstrate its taxonomic status as a tissue coccidia within the phylum Apicomplexa (Sénaud, 1967). The indirect predator–prey life cycle of this tissue coccidium was demonstrated by experimental transmission involving different intermediate and definitive hosts (Heydorn and Rommel, 1972; Rommel et al., 1972). *Sarcocystis* spp. tend to be species, genus, or family specific for hosts. Although intermediate hosts may be infected with multiple *Sarcocystis* spp., a definitive host species is usually infected by one or a few species of *Sarcocystis*. *Sarcocystis hominis* and *Sarcocystis suihominis* are the only species that use humans as definitive hosts. An unknown number of *Sarcocystis* spp. have been detected as sarcocysts in human muscle and probably represent aberrant intermediate host infections (Dubey et al., 1989; Fayer, 2004). Recently, *Sarcocystis nesbitti* was reported as the cause of tissue sarcocystosis in humans in Malaysia (Abubakar et al., 2013). *Sarcocystis* spp. tissue cysts identified from common food animals and humans are listed in Table 6.3.

6.7.2 Host range, prevalence, and distribution

All classes of vertebrate animals can serve as definitive or intermediate hosts for *Sarcocystis* spp., and several hundreds of *Sarcocystis* spp. have been described (Odening, 1998). Humans become infected with *S. hominis* and *S. suihominis* by consuming

Table 6.3 ***Sarcocystis* spp. found in the muscles of domestic food animals and humans**

Intermediate hosts	*Sarcocystis* species	Definitive host
Cattle (*Bos taurus*)	*S. cruzi* (syn. *S. bovicanis*)	Dog, coyote, red fox, racoon, wolf
	S. hirsuta (syn. *S. bovifelis*)	Cat
	S. hominis (syn. *S. bovihominis*)	Humans, other primates
	S. sinensis	Unknown
Pig (*Sus scrofa*)	*S. miescheriana* (syn. *S. suicanis*)	Dog, racoon, red fox, wolf, jackal
	S. suihominis	Humans, other primates
	S. porcifelis	Cat
Sheep (*Ovis aries*)	*S. arieticanis*	Dog
	S. gigantea (syn. *S. ovifelis*)	Cat
	S. medusiformis	Cat
	S. tenella (syn. *S. ovicanis*)	Dog, coyote, red fox
Goat (*Capra hircus*)	*S. capracanis*	Dog, coyote, red fox
	S. hiricancis	Dog
	S. moulei	Cat
Water buffalo (*Bubalus bubalis*)	*S. levinei*	Dog
	S. fusiformis	Cat
	S. dubeyi	Unknown
	S. buffalonis	Cat
Humans—aberrant host (*Homo sapien*)	*S nesbitti*	Unknown (possibly snake)

Further information, including references, are provided in the text of this chapter.

sarcocysts in raw or undercooked meat of the intermediate hosts, cattle and pigs, respectively. Although a number of aberrant cases of tissue sarcocystosis in humans have been reported, they do not contribute to maintaining the life cycle of the parasite.

6.7.2.1 *Zoonotic tissue* Sarcocystis *in cattle and pigs*

Sarcocysts of *S. hominis* in cattle have been reported primarily from European and Asian countries. The sarcocysts were first isolated and identified as *S. hominis* in Japan, based on the morphological and life-cycle studies on slaughtered cattle (Saito et al., 1998). A wide range of prevalences have been reported from the examination of beef samples in several countries, including Belgium (97.4%), Germany (63%), Italy (18.5%), and Argentina (1.8%) (Domenis et al., 2011; Fayer, 2004; More et al., 2011; Vangeel et al., 2007).

S. suihominis is believed to be widely distributed in Asia. The sarcocyst has been detected in pigs from many Asian countries including Japan and China (Li et al., 2004; Saito et al., 1998). Studies on pigs in India indicate high prevalences of *S. suihominis* at 49.5%, 53.6%, and 56.7% (Avapal, 2001; Devi et al., 1998; Solanki et al., 1991). However, these reported prevalences were based solely on the morphological identification by light microscopy examination. Among European countries, *S. suihominis* was found to be more prevalent in Germany than Austria, but little information is available from other countries (Fayer, 2004). The global prevalence of *Sarcocystis* spp. in pigs is estimated to vary between 3% and 36%.

6.7.2.2 Human intestinal sarcocystosis

Examination of human fecal samples from the Yunnan province of China revealed *Sarcocystis* sporocysts in 123 of 414 individuals who consumed raw pork (Zhou et al., 1990). In Thailand, Bunyaratvej et al. (1982) reported six cases of human intestinal sarcocystosis. Five patients recovered after intestinal resection, but one died due to extensive necrosis of the intestinal wall and leakage at the site of anastomosis. Although the prevalence of *S. hominis* in Thais has been reported as 1.5%, the incidence of intestinal sarcocystosis has been recorded as 23.2% (Nichpanit et al., 2010; Wilairatana et al., 1996). The sporocysts of *Sarcocystis* species were found in 1.1% (14/1228) of Vietnamese who were on an 18-month resident apprenticeship in Central Slovakia (Straka et al., 1991). In Tibet, the prevalence of *S. hominis* and *S. suihominis* in three counties of Tibet, as determined by fecal examination of 926 persons varied from 0% to 7%, respectively (Yu, 1991).

6.7.2.3 Human tissue sarcocystosis

There have been many cases of sarcocysts in the muscle of humans. Prior to 1990, 46 cases were reported from tropical and subtropical countries in Asia (Dubey et al., 1989). Later, an additional 46 cases from Africa (4), Europe (4), the United States (4), Central and South America (5), Malaysia (4), China (1), India (11), and other Southeast Asian countries (13) were also reported (Fayer, 2004). In addition to these case reports, an outbreak of human sarcocystosis involving the muscle of 7 of 15 military personnel has been reported in Malaysia (Arness et al., 1999), and more recently *S. nesbitti*-related infections have been reported as an emerging pathogen of humans in some regions (Abubakar et al., 2013). Sarcocysts of *S. nesbitti* were first identified in monkeys which, like humans, are probably aberrant intermediate hosts. The primary intermediate host(s) for the parasite is unknown, and snakes or birds are possible definitive hosts (Abubakar et al., 2013).

6.7.3 Life cycle and development

The parasite *Sarcocystis* has a two-host life cycle. Carnivorous or omnivorous animals serve as definitive hosts and typically herbivorous animals are the usual intermediate hosts. The predator–prey and feeding behavior of the hosts drives the transmission cycle and may be partly responsible for the selection of intermediate and definitive hosts and their unique combinations for the host specificity of the genus.

The definitive host becomes infected after ingesting sarcocysts in the muscles of the respective intermediate hosts. The sarcocyst's wall ruptures releasing numerous bradyzoites that penetrate cells of the intestinal lamina propria and undergo gametogony followed by oocyst formation and sporogony (Figure 6.1). The much-expanded host cell ruptures to release sporulated oocysts, which are excreted with the feces of the definitive host. Individual sporocysts often occur in the feces due to rupturing of the thin-walled oocysts. The intermediate host is infected by ingesting food or water contaminated with the sporocysts shed in the feces of the definitive host. In the stomach of the suitable intermediate host, sporocysts excyst and release sporozoites that migrate through the gut epithelium and penetrate endothelial cells of small arteries. Asexual replication involves multiple generations of merogony as well as endodyogeny in cells at different locations in the host (depending on the species of *Sarcocystis* and the immune status of the host) yielding numerous merozoites that subsequently enter muscle cells to initiate formation of tissue cysts (sarcocysts) with bradyzoites. Various characteristics of *S. hominis* and *S. suihominis*, including host species and shape, size, and structure of the various life-cycle stages, have been described and include those commonly used for diagnostic purposes (Fayer, 2004).

6.7.4 Ecology and epidemiology

Sarcocysts of various *Sarcocystis* spp. are commonly found in meat of animals raised outdoors, including beef, pork, and mutton. For example, the vast majority of muscle samples from livestock tested for the presence of *Sarcocystis* spp. have been positive (Gajadhar et al., 1987). However, in meat produced in most developed regions virtually all sarcocysts are those of nonzoonotic species. Tissue coccidia in meat, including sarcocysts, remain infectious for several days to weeks, especially at cool temperatures such as 4 °C. Viability is lost as the microenvironment in the infected meat is altered by decomposition.

Numerous oocysts and sporocysts are passed in the feces of definitive hosts whose diet includes infected meat and consist of mature sporozoites that are immediately infectious for suitable intermediate hosts (Table 6.1). These coccidian stages, as described elsewhere in this chapter, are resistant to a wide range of environmental conditions and treatments and are capable of surviving outdoors for long periods of time. Savini et al. (1996) found that sporocysts of *Sarcocystis cruzi* retained viability, as determined by excystation for at least 90 days after being subjected to temperatures of 4, 21, or 37 °C and relative humidities of 18%, 75%, or 100%. Heat treatment of sporocysts of *S. neurona* at 50 °C for 60 min or 55 °C for 5 min did not prevent the infection of "knock-out" mice, whereas 55 °C for 15 min and 60 °C for more than 1 min were effective (Dubey et al., 2002).

Consumption of raw or undercooked beef and pork is the mode of transmission for *S. hominis* and *S. suihominis*, respectively, to humans and represents the most important risk factors for zoonotic sarcocystosis. Poor hygiene between the handling of pork and preparation of food is also a risk factor. Young children playing in pork-processing areas at home have been known to become infected with *S. suihominis* by ingesting scraps of raw meat (Banerjee et al., 1994; Solanki et al., 1991). High frequency of consumption of raw or undercooked meat in some European countries could also be a significant risk factor for intestinal sarcocystosis in humans (Dubey and Lindsay, 2006).

Farm management practices can greatly influence the occurrence and transmission of zoonotic *Sarcocystis*. Free-ranging cattle and scavenging pigs are at risk of becoming infected when exposed to human sewage. Disposal of untreated human sewage in areas where cattle or pigs' roam facilitates the transmission of the zoonotic *Sarcocystis* spp. A review of the published literature concluded that *S. hominis* sporocysts in sewage applied to pasture survive environmental conditions and remain infectious for long periods of time (Bürger and Wilken, 1985). Incidence of infection was lowest in calves raised indoors and the highest sarcocyst burden was found in calves that had been kept in mountainous grasslands (Meshkov, 1975). Pasturing in mountainous areas has been found to be significantly associated with bovine sarcocystosis (Domenis et al., 2011). The prevalence of infection could also be associated with the age of the animals and seasonal variations. A survey of bovine fetuses and suckling calves did not reveal any sarcocysts, but the earliest cases *Sarcocystis* infection (18.3%) were recorded in calves being fed milk (Lukesova et al., 1986). As alluded to previously, virtually all muscle samples of adult cattle raised on pasture contained sarcocysts, but they were not considered zoonotic species. Studies in Western Australia demonstrated a positive correlation between the prevalence of infection and the age of the host up to 4 years old, and a drop in prevalence in older animals (Savini et al., 1992). Seasonal correlation with infection rates was also demonstrated in India, with lowest levels in May, and highest levels in August and September, during the rainy season (Jain and Shah, 1985). However, there have been no significant differences noted in *Sarcocystis* infection rates between male and female cattle raised under similar conditions (Meshkov, 1975).

6.7.5 Disease

6.7.5.1 Tissue sarcocystosis

The intensity and distribution of sarcocysts in the muscle of cattle and pigs vary for individual animals and are influenced by the number and viability of sporocysts ingested and the age and immune competence of the host. For *S. hominis* and *Sarcocystis hirsuta* in cattle, the esophagus and other muscles, but not myocardium, have been found to be the most affected, whereas *S. cruzi*, in addition to a carcasswide distribution, is most abundant in the heart.

Bovine sarcocystosis is manifested in many forms, varying from mild fever to abortion and occasionally death (Dubey et al., 1989). Condemnation of carcasses of cattle and sheep due to the unesthetic appearance of macroscopic sarcocysts or granulomatous reactions around the parasite in meat results in considerable economic losses. Bovine eosinophilic myositis is a common finding at slaughter inspection, and the associated sarcocysts have been identified as *S. hominis* or *S. cruzi* (Gajadhar et al., 1987; Jensen et al., 1986). Ultrastructural analysis and transmission studies have shown that sarcocysts associated with these granulomas are ruptured and noninfectious for the definitive host (Gajadhar and Marquardt, 1992). Little information is available on the pathogenesis of *S. suihominis*, but the parasite is considered pathogenic for pigs (Dubey and Lindsay, 2006).

Sarcocysts of unknown *Sarcocystis* spp. have been found in the muscle of humans and most were not associated with clinical illness. Nevertheless, fever, erythema, and swelling, limb pain, chronic myositis, and eosinophilia have been reported (McLeod et al., 1980; Mehrotra et al., 1996; Van den Enden et al., 1995). In an outbreak of human tissue sarcocystosis of unknown species, 7 of 15 American military personnel in Malaysia experienced acute fever, myalgia, bronchospasm, pruritic rashes, lymphadenopathy, and subcutaneous nodules concurrently with elevated levels of eosinophilia, erythrocyte sedimentation rate, and creatinine kinase (Arness et al., 1999). Also in Malaysia, 89 of 92 visitors on Pangkor Island were recently diagnosed with *S. nesbitti* tissue infection associated with fever, myositis, and myalgia (Abubakar et al., 2013). It appears that cases of clinical sarcocystosis acquired in parts of Asia are often associated with *S. nesbitti* infection.

6.7.5.2 Intestinal sarcocystosis

Intestinal sarcocystosis involves gametogony and sporogony in the definitive hosts which consume meat and include humans, dogs, and cats, but not food animals such as pigs, cattle, and sheep. Clinical illness is usually mild or asymptomatic (Dubey and Lindsay, 2006). Human volunteers who consumed raw beef infected with *S. hominis* cysts in Germany and China experienced abdominal pain, nausea, and diarrhea (Aryeetey and Piekarski, 1976; Chen et al., 1999; Rommel et al., 1972). In Thailand, six patients who had consumed raw beef and acquired a mixed infection of *Sarcocystis* and gram-positive bacilli required surgery for necrotizing enteritis (Bunyaratvej et al., 1982). Other volunteers who consumed raw pork infected with *S. suihominis* reported various symptoms including abdominal pain, nausea, vomiting, loss of appetite, bloat, and diarrhea (Fayer, 2004; Heydorn and Rommel, 1972; Kimmig et al., 1979; Rommel et al., 1972). The dearth of case reports of human intestinal sarcocystosis is probably because the infection is rarely diagnosed in endemic areas, and the infection seldom occurs elsewhere.

6.7.6 Control and prevention

Infections of tissue sarcocystosis can be confirmed by detecting sarcocysts in the muscle of infected hosts. Methods to demonstrate the sarcocysts include gross inspection of meat for macroscopic sarcocysts, and analysis of muscle samples by artificial digestion or histopathological examination. Reliable species identification requires the use of molecular or ultrastructural analysis; knowledge of the host species and histology of the sarcocyst wall may be sufficient for identification in some cases.

Infection with intestinal sarcocystosis can be detected by using flotation or sedimentation methods to recover *Sarcocystis* sporocysts or sporulated oocysts from feces. Morphometric and molecular analysis are useful tools for the differentiation of *Sarcocystis* species.

There is no recommended prophylactic or therapeutic treatment available for human infections. By virtue of the fact that the endogenous replication and development characteristics of *Sarcocystis* are coccidia-based, drugs such as sulfonamides and pyrimethamines may be helpful for treating sarcocystosis. Similar to many other coccidian infections, there is no effective vaccine to protect livestock or humans against this disease.

Prevention and control measures rely primarily on disrupting the life cycle of the parasite. A significant mitigating strategy is preventing contamination of food, water, and bedding with the feces of definitive hosts such as canids and felids, and particularly of humans to prevent zoonotic transmission of *S. hominis* and *S. suihominis* to cattle and pigs, respectively. Special precautions should be taken to ensure that human sewage is adequately treated and appropriately disposed. Contamination of human food and water with oocysts and sporocysts of any *Sarcocystis* spp. should be avoided to prevent the possibility of tissue sarcocystosis.

For preventing intestinal infection with *S. hominis* or *S. suihominis* in humans, freezing or cooking of beef and pork at recommended temperatures can render bradyzoites noninfectious. It has been reported that cooking pork at 60, 70, and 100 °C for 20, 15, and 5 min, respectively, or freezing at –4 or –20 °C inactivated *Sarcocystis meisheriana* (Saleque et al., 1990). Similar results have also been reported for *Sarcocystis* in beef and beef products (Leek and Fayer, 1978). However, it is important to note that these various treatment conditions may be ineffective when the meat portions are large or the temperature distribution is uneven.

6.8 Conclusions and future trends

Recently, there has been increased recognition of the significance of coccidian protozoa as foodborne parasites. Major contributing factors include the globalization of the food supply web, consumer demands for free-range animals, organic, and ready-to-eat foods and improved detection and diagnostic methods. The ecology and life cycle of coccidian parasites make them extremely well suited for foodborne transmission and difficult to prevent or control. Prolific three-phase reproduction occurs in all coccidian life cycles, and their oocysts survive for long periods of time in the environment where they are highly resistant to adverse conditions. The minimum infectious dose for oocysts contaminating fruits or vegetables or tissue cysts in meat is very low.

The burden of infection by both tissue and intestinal coccidian parasites is massive and has recently been recognized at various levels around the world, including consumers, governments, and standard-setting organizations. Toxoplasmosis is considered to be a leading cause of death attributed to foodborne illness in the United States, with about 20% of the population asymptomatically infected, according to the US CDC. The prevalence and associated disease burden are probably much higher in many other regions of the world. Recent reports of clinical cases of tissue sarcocystosis in humans as aberrant infections seem to indicate emergence of a new category of foodborne infections.

Foodborne intestinal coccidiosis continues to occur increasingly, and the long-term negative health implications of such infections are beginning to be recognized. Although *Cystoisospora* infections in humans are rarely detected and reported, the number of outbreaks of cyclosporosis due to the consumption of contaminated fruits and leafy vegetables has been fluctuating or increasing depending on the country. From the review in this chapter, it is clear that most species of *Cryptosporidium* can infect humans, although some more readily than others. Therefore, it is prudent to consider all *Cryptosporidium* spp. as potentially zoonotic, particularly those for which the primary host is a mammal. Much research is required to provide valuable information to understand, detect, and control foodborne coccidia.

References

Abd El Kader, N., Blanco, M.-A., Ali-Tammam, M., Abd El Ghaffar, A.E.R., Osman, A., El Sheikh, N., Rubio, J., de Fuentes, I., 2012. Detection of *Cryptosporidium parvum* and *Cryptosporidium hominis* in human patients in Cairo, Egypt. Parasitol. Res. 110, 161–166.

Abubakar, S., Teoh, B.T., Sam, S.S., Chang, L.Y., Johari, J., Hooi, P.S., Lakhbeer-Singh, H.K., Italiano, C.M., Omar, S.F., Wong, K.T., Ramli, N., Tan, C.T., 2013. Outbreak of human infection with *Sarcocystis nesbitti*, Malaysia, 2012. Emerg. Infect. Dis. 19, 1989–1991.

AFNOR, 2013. Microbiology of the food chain. Detection and enumeration of *Cryptosporidium* and *Giardia* in fresh leafy green vegetables and berry fruits.

Al-Adhami, B.H., Gajadhar, A.A., 2014. A new multi-host species indirect ELISA using protein A/G conjugate for detection of anti-*Toxoplasma gondii* IgG antibodies with comparison to ELISA-IgG, agglutination assay and Western blot. Vet. Parasitol. 200, 66–73.

Al-Brikan, F.A., Salem, H.S., Beeching, N., Hilal, N., 2008. Multilocus genetic analysis of *Cryptosporidium* isolates from Saudi Arabia. J. Egypt. Soc. Parasitol. 38, 645–658.

Alfano-Sobsey, E.M., Eberhard, M.L., Seed, J.R., Weber, D.J., Won, K.Y., Nace, E.K., Moe, C.L., 2004. Human challenge pilot study with *Cyclospora cayetanensis*. Emerg. Infect. Dis. 10, 726–728.

Alvarez-Pellitero, P., Sitja-Bobadilla, A., 2002. *Cryptosporidium molnari* n. sp. (Apicomplexa: Cryptosporidiidae) infecting two marine fish species, *Sparus aurata* L. and *Dicentrarchus labrax* L. Int. J. Parasitol. 32, 1007–1021.

Alvarez-Pellitero, P., Quiroga, M.I., Sitja-Bobadilla, A., Redondo, M.J., Palenzuela, O., Padros, F., Vazquez, S., Nieto, J.M., 2004. *Cryptosporidium scophthalmi* n. sp. (Apicomplexa: Cryptosporidiidae) from cultured turbot *Scophthalmus maximus*. Light and electron microscope description and histopathological study. Dis. Aquat. Organ. 62, 133–145.

Alyousefi, N.A., Mahdy, M.A., Lim, Y.A., Xiao, L., Mahmud, R., 2013. First molecular characterization of *Cryptosporidium* in Yemen. Parasitology 140, 729–734.

Anonymous, 1982. Cryptosporidiosis, assessment of chemotherapy of males with acquired immune deficiency syndrome (AIDS). Morb. Mortal. Wkly. Rep. 31, 89–102.

Arness, M.K., Brown, J.D., Dubey, J.P., Neafie, R.C., Granstrom, D.E., 1999. An outbreak of acute eosinophilic myositis attributed to human *Sarcocystis* parasitism. Am. J. Trop. Med. Hyg. 61, 548–553.

Aryeetey, M.E., Piekarski, G., 1976. Serological studies on *Sarcocystis* in man and rats (author's transl). Z. Parasitenkd. 50, 109–124.

Ashford, R.W., 1979. Occurrence of an undescribed coccidian in man in Papua New Guinea. Ann. Trop. Med. Parasitol. 73, 497–500.

Aslan, G., Bayram, G., Otag, F., Direkel, S., Taylan Ozkan, A., Ceber, K., Emekdas, G., 2012. Investigation of the presence of *Cryptosporidium* spp. in different water sources in Mersin province, Turkey. Mikrobiyol. Bul. 46, 93–100.

Assefa, S., Erko, B., Medhin, G., Assefa, Z., Shimelis, T., 2009. Intestinal parasitic infections in relation to HIV/AIDS status, diarrhea and CD4 T-cell count. BMC Infect. Dis. 9, 155.

Avapal, R.S., 2001. Prevalence and immunodiagnosis of *sarcocystis* spp. of public health significance in swine. M.V.Sc. Punjab Agricultural University, Ludhiana.

Banerjee, P., Bhatia, B., Pandit, B., 1994. *Sarcocystis suihominis* infection in human beings in India. J. Vet. Parasitol. 8, 57–58.

Bern, C., Hernandez, B., Lopez, M.B., Arrowood, M.J., de Mejia, M.A., de Merida, A.M., Hightower, A.W., Venczel, L., Herwaldt, B.L., Klein, R.E., 1999. Epidemiologic studies of *Cyclospora cayetanensis* in Guatemala. Emerg. Infect. Dis. 5, 766–774.

Bern, C., Hernandez, B., Lopez, M.B., Arrowood, M.J., de Merida, A.M., Klein, R.E., 2000. The contrasting epidemiology of *Cyclospora* and *Cryptosporidium* among outpatients in Guatemala. Am. J. Trop. Med. Hyg. 63, 231–235.
Bern, C., Ortega, Y., Checkley, W., Roberts, J.M., Lescano, A.G., Cabrera, L., Verastegui, M., Black, R.E., Sterling, C., Gilman, R.H., 2002. Epidemiologic differences between cyclosporiasis and cryptosporidiosis in Peruvian children. Emerg. Infect. Dis. 8, 581–585.
Bornay-Llinares, F.J., Da Silva, A.J., Moura, I.N., Myjak, P., Pietkiewicz, H., Kruminis-Lozowska, W., Graczyk, T.K., Pieniazek, N.J., 1999. Identification of *Cryptosporidium felis* in a cow by morphologic and molecular methods. Appl. Environ. Microbiol. 65, 1455–1458.
Bowie, W.R., King, A.S., Werker, D.H., Isaac-Renton, J.L., Bell, A., Eng, S.B., Marion, S.A., 1997. Outbreak of toxoplasmosis associated with municipal drinking water. Lancet 350, 173–177.
Brantley, R.K., Williams, K.R., Silva, T.M., Sistrom, M., Thielman, N.M., Ward, H., Lima, A.A., Guerrant, R.L., 2003. AIDS-associated diarrhea and wasting in Northeast Brazil is associated with subtherapeutic plasma levels of antiretroviral medications and with both bovine and human subtypes of *Cryptosporidium parvum*. Braz. J. Infect. Dis. 7, 16–22.
Bunyaratvej, S., Bunyawongwiroj, P., Nitiyanant, P., 1982. Human intestinal sarcosporidiosis: report of six cases. Am. J. Trop. Med. Hyg. 31, 36–41.
Bürger, H.J., Wilken, S., 1985. The infection risk of sarcosporidia in irrigating sewage (sludge). In: Block, J.C., Havelaar, A.H., L'Hermite, P. (Eds.), Epidemiological Studies of Risk Associated with the Agricultural Use of Sewage Sludge: Knowledge and Needs. Elsevier Applied Science, London.
Bush, J.B., Markus, M.B., 1987. Staining of *Isospora belli* oocysts. Trans. R. Soc. Trop. Med. Hyg. 81, 244.
Bushen, O.Y., Kohli, A., Pinkerton, R.C., Dupnik, K., Newman, R.D., Sears, C.L., Fayer, R., Lima, A.A., Guerrant, R.L., 2007. Heavy cryptosporidial infections in children in northeast Brazil: comparison of *Cryptosporidium hominis* and *Cryptosporidium parvum*. Trans. R. Soc. Trop. Med. Hyg. 101, 378–384.
Caccio, S.M., Thompson, R.C., Mclauchlin, J., Smith, H.V., 2005. Unravelling *Cryptosporidium* and *Giardia* epidemiology. Trends Parasitol. 21, 430–437.
Cama, V.A., Bern, C., Sulaiman, I.M., Gilman, R.H., Ticona, E., Vivar, A., Kawai, V., Vargas, D., Zhou, L., Xiao, L., 2003. *Cryptosporidium* species and genotypes in HIV-positive patients in Lima, Peru. J. Eukaryot. Microbiol. 50 (Suppl.), 531–533.
Cama, V.A., Ross, J.M., Crawford, S., Kawai, V., Chavez-Valdez, R., Vargas, D., Vivar, A., Ticona, E., Navincopa, M., Williamson, J., Ortega, Y., Gilman, R.H., Bern, C., Xiao, L., 2007. Differences in clinical manifestations among *Cryptosporidium* species and subtypes in HIV-infected persons. J. Infect. Dis. 196, 684–691.
Cama, V.A., Bern, C., Roberts, J., Cabrera, L., Sterling, C.R., Ortega, Y., Gilman, R.H., Xiao, L., 2008. *Cryptosporidium* species and subtypes and clinical manifestations in children, Peru. Emerg. Infect. Dis. 14, 1567–1574.
Carellos, E.V.M., de Andrade, G.M.Q., Vasconcelos-Santos, D.V., Januário, J.N., Romanelli, R.M.C., Abreu, M.N.S., Da Silva, F.M., Loures, I.R.C., de Andrade, J.Q., Caiaffa, W.T., Uctb Group, 2014. Adverse socioeconomic conditions and oocyst-related factors are associated with congenital toxoplasmosis in a population-based study in Minas Gerais, Brazil. PLoS ONE 9, e88588.
Carneiro, A.C.A.V., Andrade, G.M., Costa, J.G.L., Pinheiro, B.V., Vasconcelos-Santos, D.V., Ferreira, A.M., Su, C., Januário, J.N., Vitor, R.W.A., 2013. Genetic characterization of

Toxoplasma gondii revealed highly diverse genotypes for isolates from newborns with congenital toxoplasmosis in Southeastern Brazil. J. Clin. Microbiol. 51, 901–907.

Certad, G., Arenas-Pinto, A., Pocaterra, L., Ferrara, G., Castro, J., Bello, A., Nunez, L., 2003. Isosporiasis in Venezuelan adults infected with human immunodeficiency virus: clinical characterization. Am. J. Trop. Med. Hyg. 69, 217–222.

Chacín-Bonilla, L., Mejia de Young, M., Estevez, J., 2003. Prevalence and pathogenic role of *Cyclospora cayetanensis* in a Venezuelan community. Am. J. Trop. Med. Hyg. 68, 304–306.

Chacín-Bonilla, L., Barrios, F., Sanchez, Y., 2007. Epidemiology of *Cyclospora cayetanensis* infection in San Carlos Island, Venezuela: strong association between socio-economic status and infection. Trans. R. Soc. Trop. Med. Hyg. 101, 1018–1024.

Chalmers, R.M., Katzer, F., 2013. Looking for *Cryptosporidium*: the application of advances in detection and diagnosis. Trends Parasitol. 29, 237–251.

Chalmers, R.M., Elwin, K., Thomas, A.L., Guy, E.C., Mason, B., 2009. Long-term *Cryptosporidium* typing reveals the aetiology and species-specific epidemiology of human cryptosporidiosis in England and Wales, 2000 to 2003. Euro Surveill. 14, 1–9.

Chappell, C.L., Okhuysen, P.C., Langer-Curry, R., Widmer, G., Akiyoshi, D.E., Tanriverdi, S., Tzipori, S., 2006. *Cryptosporidium hominis*: experimental challenge of healthy adults. Am. J. Trop. Med. Hyg. 75, 851–857.

Chen, X., Zuo, Y., Zuo, W., 1999. Observation on the clinical symptoms and sporocyst excretion in human volunteers experimentally infected with *Sarcocystis hominis*. Zhongguo Ji Sheng Chong Xue Yu Ji Sheng Chong Bing Za Zhi 17, 25–27.

Chumpolbanchorn, K., Lymbery, A.J., Pallant, L.J., Pan, S., Sukthana, Y., Thompson, R.C.A., 2013. A high prevalence of *Toxoplasma* in Australian chickens. Vet. Parasitol. 196, 209–211.

Current, W.L., Upton, S.J., Haynes, T.B., 1986. The life cycle of *Cryptosporidium baileyi* n. sp. (Apicomplexa, Cryptosporidiidae) infecting chickens. J. Protozool. 33, 289–296.

Dabritz, H.A., Miller, M.A., Atwill, E.R., Gardner, I.A., Leutenegger, C.M., Melli, A.C., Conrad, P.A., 2007. Detection of *Toxoplasma gondii*-like oocysts in cat feces and estimates of the environmental oocyst burden. J. Am. Vet. Med. Assoc. 231, 1676–1684.

Dehovitz, J.A., Pape, J.W., Boncy, M., Johnson Jr., W.D., 1986. Clinical manifestations and therapy of *Isospora belli* infection in patients with the acquired immunodeficiency syndrome. N. Engl. J. Med. 315, 87–90.

Devi, P., Sarmah, P., Saleque, A., 1998. *Sarcocystis* spp. infection in carcasses of domestic pigs in Guwahati, Assam. J. Vet. Parasitol. 12, 56–57.

Doller, P.C., Dietrich, K., Filipp, N., Brockmann, S., Dreweck, C., Vonthein, R., Wagner-Wiening, C., Wiedenmann, A., 2002. Cyclosporiasis outbreak in Germany associated with the consumption of salad. Emerg. Infect. Dis. 8, 992–994.

Domenis, L., Peletto, S., Sacchi, L., Clementi, E., Genchi, M., Felisari, L., Felisari, C., Mo, P., Modesto, P., Zuccon, F., Campanella, C., Maurella, C., Guidetti, C., Acutis, P.L., 2011. Detection of a morphogenetically novel *Sarcocystis hominis*-like in the context of a prevalence study in semi-intensively bred cattle in Italy. Parasitol. Res. 109, 1677–1687.

Dubey, J.P., 2010a. *Toxoplasma gondii* infections in chickens (*Gallus domesticus*): prevalence, clinical disease, diagnosis and public health significance. Zoonoses Public Health 57, 60–73.

Dubey, J.P., 2010b. Toxoplasmosis of Animals and Humans, second ed. CRC Press, Taylor and Francis Group, Boca Raton, FL.

Dubey, J.P., Lindsay, D.S., 2006. Neosporosis, toxoplasmosis, and sarcocystosis in ruminants. Vet. Clin. North Am. Food Anim. Pract. 22, 645–671.

Dubey, J.P., Sreekumar, C., 2003. Redescription of *Hammondia hammondi* and its differentiation from *Toxoplasma gondii*. Int. J. Parasitol. 33, 1437–1453.

Dubey, J.P., Speer, C., Fayer, R., 1989. Sarcocystosis of Animals and Man. CRC Press, Inc., Boca Raton, FL.

Dubey, J.P., Saville, W.J., Sreekumar, C., Shen, S.K., Lindsay, O.S., Pena, H.F., Vianna, M.C., Gennari, S.M., Reed, S.M., 2002. Effects of high temperature and disinfectants on the viability of *Sarcocystis neurona* sporocysts. J. Parasitol. 88, 1252–1254.

Dubey, J.P., Hill, D.E., Rozeboom, D.W., Rajendran, C., Choudhary, S., Ferreira, L.R., Kwok, O.C.H., Su, C., 2012. High prevalence and genotypes of *Toxoplasma gondii* isolated from organic pigs in northern USA. Vet. Parasitol. 188, 14–18.

Duhain, G.L., Minnaar, A., Buys, E.M., 2012. Effect of chlorine, blanching, freezing, and microwave heating on *Cryptosporidium parvum* viability inoculated on green peppers. J. Food Prot. 75, 936–941.

Dunn, D., Wallon, M., Peyron, F., Petersen, E., Peckham, C., Gilbert, R., 1999. Mother-to-child transmission of toxoplasmosis: risk estimates for clinical counselling. Lancet 353, 1829–1833.

Eberhard, M.L., Da Silva, A.J., Lilley, B.G., Pieniazek, N.J., 1999a. Morphologic and molecular characterization of new *Cyclospora* species from Ethiopian monkeys: *C. cercopitheci* sp.n., *C. colobi* sp.n., and *C. papionis* sp.n. Emerg. Infect. Dis. 5, 651–658.

Eberhard, M.L., Nace, E.K., Freeman, A.R., 1999b. Survey for *Cyclospora cayetanensis* in domestic animals in an endemic area in Haiti. J. Parasitol. 85, 562–563.

Eberhard, M.L., Nace, E.K., Freeman, A.R., Streit, T.G., Da Silva, A.J., Lammie, P.J., 1999c. *Cyclospora cayetanensis* infections in Haiti: a common occurrence in the absence of watery diarrhea. Am .J. Trop. Med. Hyg. 60, 584–586.

Eberhard, M.L., Ortega, Y.R., Hanes, D.E., Nace, E.K., Quy Do, R., Robl, M.G., Won, K.Y., Gavidia, C., Sass, N.L., Mansfield, K., Gozalo, A., Griffiths, J., Gilman, R., Sterling, C.R., Arrowood, M.J., 2000. Attempt to establish experimental *Cyclospora cayetanensis* infection in laboratory animals. J. Parasitol. 86, 577–582.

Elwin, K., Hadfield, S.J., Robinson, G., Crouch, N.D., Chalmers, R.M., 2012. *Cryptosporidium viatorum* n. sp. (Apicomplexa: Cryptosporidiidae) among travellers returning to Great Britain from the Indian subcontinent, 2007–2011. Int. J. Parasitol. 42, 675–682.

Farr, M.M., Wehr, E.E., 1949. Survival of *Emeria acervulina*, *E. tenella*, and *E. maxima* oocysts on soil under various field conditions. Ann. N. Y. Acad. Sci. 52, 468–472.

Faust, E.C., Giraldo, L.E., Caicedo, G., Bonfante, R., 1961. Human isosporosis in the Western Hemisphere. Am. J. Trop. Med. Hyg. 10, 343–349.

Faye, R., Santi, M., Xia, L., 2005. *Cryptosporidium bovis* n. sp. (Apicomplexa: Cryptosporidiidae) in cattle (*Bos taurus*). J. Parasitol. 91, 624–629.

Fayer, R., 2004. *Sarcocystis* spp. in human infections. Clin. Microbiol. Rev. 17, 894–902, table of contents.

Fayer, R., 2008. General biology. In: Fayer, R., Xiao, L. (Eds.), *Cryptosporidium* and Cryptosporidiosis, second ed. CRC Press, Boca Raton, FL.

Fayer, R., 2010. Taxonomy and species delimitation in *Cryptosporidium*. Exp. Parasitol. 124, 90–97.

Fayer, R., Frenkel, J.K., 1979. Comparative infectivity for calves of oocysts of feline coccidia: *Besnoitia*, *Hammondia*, *Cystoisospora*, *Sarcocystis*, and *Toxoplasma*. J. Parasitol. 65, 756–762.

Fayer, R., Nerad, T., 1996. Effects of low temperatures on viability of *Cryptosporidium parvum* oocysts. Appl. Environ. Microbiol. 62, 1431–1433.

Fayer, R., Santin, M., 2009. *Cryptosporidium xiaoi* n. sp. (Apicomplexa: Cryptosporidiidae) in sheep (*Ovis aries*). Vet. Parasitol. 164, 192–200.

Fayer, R., Trout, J.M., Jenkins, M.C., 1998. Infectivity of *Cryptosporidium parvum* oocysts stored in water at environmental temperatures. J. Parasitol. 84, 1165–1169.

Fayer, R., Santin, M., Trout, J.M., 2008. *Cryptosporidium ryanae* n. sp. (Apicomplexa: Cryptosporidiidae) in cattle (*Bos taurus*). Vet. Parasitol. 156, 191–198.

Fayer, R., Santin, M., Macarisin, D., 2010. *Cryptosporidium ubiquitum* n. sp. in animals and humans. Vet. Parasitol. 172, 23–32.

Feltus, D.C., Giddings, C.W., Schneck, B.L., Monson, T., Warshauer, D., McEvoy, J.M., 2006. Evidence supporting zoonotic transmission of *Cryptosporidium* spp. in Wisconsin. J. Clin. Microbiol. 44, 4303–4308.

Feng, Y., Alderisio, K.A., Yang, W., Blancero, L.A., Kuhne, W.G., Nadareski, C.A., Reid, M., Xiao, L., 2007. *Cryptosporidium* genotypes in wildlife from a New York watershed. Appl. Environ. Microbiol. 73, 6475–6483.

Feng, Y., Tiao, N., Li, N., Hlavsa, M., Xiao, L., 2014. Multilocus sequence typing of an emerging *Cryptosporidium hominis* subtype in the United States. J. Clin. Microbiol. 52, 524–530.

Fletcher, S.M., Stark, D., Harkness, J., Ellis, J., 2012. Enteric protozoa in the developed world: a public health perspective. Clin. Microbiol. Rev. 25, 420–449.

Foner, A., 1939. An attempt to infect animals with *Isospora belli*. Trans. R. Soc. Trop. Med. Hyg. 33, 357–358.

Gajadhar, A.A., Allen, J.R., 2004. Factors contributing to the public health and economic importance of waterborne zoonotic parasites. Vet. Parasitol. 126, 3–14.

Gajadhar, A., Marquardt, W., 1992. Ultrastructural and transmission evidence of *Sarcocystis cruzi* associated with eosinophilic myositis in cattle. Can. J. Vet. Res. 56, 41.

Gajadhar, A.A., Yates, W.D., Allen, J.R., 1987. Association of eosinophilic myositis with an unusual species of *Sarcocystis* in a beef cow. Can. J. Vet. Res. 51, 373–378.

Gajadhar, A.A., Measures, L., Forbes, L.B., Kapel, C., Dubey, J.P., 2004. Experimental *Toxoplasma gondii* infection in grey seals (*Halichoerus grypus*). J. Parasitol. 90, 255–259.

Gajadhar, A.A., Scandrett, W.B., Forbes, L.B., 2006. Overview of food- and water-borne zoonotic parasites at the farm level. Rev. Sci. Tech. Off. Int. Epiz. 25, 595–606.

García-Bocanegra, I., Cabezón, O., Arenas-Montes, A., Carbonero, A., Dubey, J.P., Perea, A., Almería, S., 2012. Seroprevalence of *Toxoplasma gondii* in equids from Southern Spain. Parasitol. Int. 61, 421–424.

Gebremedhin, E.Z., Tesfamaryam, G., Yunus, H.A., Duguma, R., Tilahun, G., di Marco, V., Vitale, M., 2015. Seroepidemiology of *Toxoplasma gondii* infection in free-range chickens (*Gallus domesticus*) of Central Ethiopia. Epidemiol. Infect. 143, 608–617.

Gibbs, R.A., Nanyonjo, R., Pingault, N.M., Combs, B.G., Mazzucchelli, T., Armstrong, P., Tarling, G., Dowse, G.K., 2013. An outbreak of *Cyclospora* infection on a cruise ship. Epidemiol. Infect. 141, 508–516.

Gilbert, R.E., Freeman, K., Lago, E.G., Bahia-Oliveira, L.M.G., Tan, H.K., Wallon, M., Buffolano, W., Stanford, M.R., Petersen, E., European Multicentre Study On Congenital Toxoplasmosis, 2008. Ocular sequelae of congenital toxoplasmosis in Brazil compared with Europe. PLoS Negl. Trop. Dis. 2, e277.

Godiwala, T., Yaeger, R., 1987. Isospora and traveler's diarrhea. Ann. Intern. Med. 106, 908–909.

Guerrant, D.I., Moore, S.R., Lima, A.A., Patrick, P.D., Schorling, J.B., Guerrant, R.L., 1999. Association of early childhood diarrhea and cryptosporidiosis with impaired physical fitness and cognitive function four–seven years later in a poor urban community in northeast Brazil. Am. J. Trop. Med. Hyg. 61, 707–713.

Guerrant, R.L., Deboer, M.D., Moore, S.R., Scharf, R.J., Lima, A.A.M., 2013. The impoverished gut—a triple burden of diarrhea, stunting and chronic disease. Nat. Rev. Gastroenterol. Hepatol. 10, 220–229.

Guiguet, M., Furco, A., Tattevin, P., Costagliola, D., Molina, J.M., French Hospital Database on HIV Clinical Epidemiology Group, 2007. HIV-associated *Isospora belli* infection: incidence and risk factors in the French Hospital Database on HIV. HIV Med. 8, 124–130.

Hall, R.L., Jones, J.L., Herwaldt, B.L., 2011. Surveillance for laboratory-confirmed sporadic cases of cyclosporiasis—United States, 1997–2008. Morb. Mortal. Wkly. Rep. 60, 1–13.

Hendricks, L., Walton, B., 1974. Vertebrate intermediate hosts in the life cycle of an isosporan from a non-human primate. Proc. Int. Congr. Parasitol. 1, 96–97.

Herwaldt, B.L., 2007. *Cyclospora cayetanensis*: a review, focusing on the outbreaks of cyclosporiasis in the 1990s. Clin. Infect. Dis. 31, 1040–1057.

Herwaldt, B.L., Ackers, M.-L., 1997. An outbreak in 1996 of cyclosporiasis associated with imported raspberries. N. Engl. J. Med. 336, 1548–1556.

Heydorn, A.O., Rommel, M., 1972. Contributions on the life cycle of Sarcosporidia. II. Dog and cat as vectors of cattle Sarcosporidia. Berl. Munch. Tierarztl. Wochenschr. 85, 121–123.

Hilali, M., Nassar, A.M., El-Ghaysh, A., 1992. Camel (*Camelus dromedarius*) and sheep (*Ovis aries*) meat as a source of dog infection with some coccidian parasites. Vet. Parasitol. 43, 37–43.

Ho, A.Y., Lopez, A.S., Eberhart, M.G., Levenson, R., Finkel, B.S., Da Silva, A.J., Roberts, J.M., Orlandi, P.A., Johnson, C.C., Herwaldt, B.L., 2002. Outbreak of cyclosporiasis associated with imported raspberries, Philadelphia, Pennsylvania, 2000. Emerg. Infect. Dis. 8, 783–788.

Hoang, L.M., Fyfe, M.O.C., Harb, J., Champagne, S., Dixon, B., Isaac-Renton, J., 2005. Outbreak of cyclosporiasis in British Colombia associated with imported Thai basil. Epidemiol. Infect. 133, 23–27.

Hunter, P.R., Hughes, S., Woodhouse, S., Raj, N., Syed, Q., Chalmers, R.M., Verlander, N.Q., Goodacre, J., 2004. Health sequelae of human cryptosporidiosis in immunocompetent patients. Clin. Infect. Dis. 39, 504–510.

Insulander, M., de Jong, B., Svenungsson, B., 2008. A food-borne outbreak of cryptosporidiosis among guests and staff at a hotel restaurant in Stockholm county, Sweden, September 2008. Euro Surveill. 13, 1–2.

Insulander, M., Svenungsson, B., Lebbad, M., Karlsson, L., de Jong, B., 2010. A foodborne outbreak of *Cyclospora* infection in Stockholm, Sweden. Foodborne Pathog. Dis. 7, 1585–1587.

Insulander, M., Silverlas, C., Lebbad, M., Karlsson, L., Mattsson, J.G., Svenungsson, B., 2013. Molecular epidemiology and clinical manifestations of human cryptosporidiosis in Sweden. Epidemiol. Infect. 141, 1009–1020.

Iseki, M., 1979. *Cryptosporidium felis* sp. n. (Protozoa: Eimeriorina) from the domestic cat. Jpn. J. Parasitol. 28, 285–307.

Izadi, M., Jonaidi-Jafari, N., Saburi, A., Eyni, H., Rezaiemanesh, M.R., Ranjbar, R., 2012. Prevalence, molecular characteristics and risk factors for cryptosporidiosis among Iranian immunocompromised patients. Microbiol. Immunol. 56, 836–842.

Jain, P., Shah, H., 1985. Prevalence and seasonal variations of *Sarcocystis* of cattle in Madhya Pradesh. Indian J. Anim. Sci. 551, 29–31.

Jeffery, G.M., 1956. Human coccidiosis in South Carolina. J. Parasitol. 42, 491–495.

Jensen, R., Alexander, A.F., Dahlgren, R.R., Jolley, W.R., Marquardt, W.C., Flack, D.E., Bennett, B.W., Cox, M.F., Harris, C.W., Hoffmann, G.A., et al., 1986. *Eosinophilic myositis* and muscular sarcocystosis in the carcasses of slaughtered cattle and lambs. Am. J. Vet. Res. 47, 587–593.

Jervis, H.R., Merrill, T.G., Sprinz, H., 1966. Coccidiosis in the guinea pig small intestine due to a *Cryptosporidium*. Am. J. Vet. Res. 27, 408–414.

Jinneman, K.C., Wetherington, J.H., Hill, W.E., Adams, A.M., Johnson, J.M., Tenge, B.J., Dang, D.L., Manger, R.L., Wekell, M.M., 1998. Template preparation for PCR and RFLP of amplification products for the detection and identification of *Cyclospora* sp. and *Eimeria* sp. oocysts directly from raspberries. J. Food Prot. 61, 1497–1503.

Jongwutiwes, S., Putaporntip, C., Charoenkorn, M., Iwasaki, T., Endo, T., 2007. Morphologic and molecular characterization of *Isospora belli* oocysts from patients in Thailand. Am. J. Trop. Med. Hyg. 77, 107–112.

Junod, C., Nault, M., Copet, M., 1988. La coccidiose a *Isospora belli* chez les sujets immunocompétents. (Etude de 40 cas observés à Paris). Bull. Soc. Pathol. Exot. 81, 317–325.

Karanis, P., Kourenti, C., Smith, H., 2007a. Waterborne transmission of protozoan parasites: a worldwide review of outbreaks and lessons learnt. J. Water Health 5, 1–38.

Karanis, P., Plutzer, J., Halim, N.A., Igori, K., Nagasawa, H., Ongerth, J., Liqing, M., 2007b. Molecular characterization of *Cryptosporidium* from animal sources in Qinghai province of China. Parasitol. Res. 101, 1575–1580.

Khan, A., Dubey, J.P., Su, C., Ajioka, J.W., Rosenthal, B.M., Sibley, L.D., 2011. Genetic analyses of atypical *Toxoplasma gondii* strains reveal a fourth clonal lineage in North America. Int. J. Parasitol. 41, 645–655.

Kimmig, P., Piekarski, G., Heydorn, A.O., 1979. Sarcosporidiosis (*Sarcocystis suihominis*) in man (author's transl). Immun. Infekt. 7, 170–177.

Kimura, K., Kumar Rai, S., Takemasa, K., Ishibashi, Y., Kawabata, M., Belosevic, M., Uga, S., 2004. Comparison of three microscopic techniques for diagnosis of *Cyclospora cayetanensis*. FEMS Microbiol. Lett. 238, 263–266.

Kniel, K.E., Lindsay, D.S., Sumner, S.S., Hackney, C.R., Pierson, M.D., Dubey, J.P., 2002. Examination of attachment and survival of *Toxoplasma gondii* oocysts on raspberries and blueberries. J. Parasitol. 88, 790–793.

Kochhar, A., Saxena, S., Malhotra, V.L., Deb, M., 2007. *Isospora belli* infection in a malnourished child. J. Commun. Dis. 39, 141–143.

Koru, O., Araz, R.E., Yilmaz, Y.A., Erguven, S., Yenicesu, M., Pektas, B., Tanyuksel, M., 2007. Case report: *Isospora belli* infection in a renal transplant recipient. Turkiye Parazitol. Derg. 31, 98–100.

Kulkarni, S.V., Kairon, R., Sane, S.S., Padmawar, P.S., Kale, V.A., Thakar, M.R., Mehendale, S.M., Risbud, A.R., 2009. Opportunistic parasitic infections in HIV/AIDS patients presenting with diarrhoea by the level of immunesuppression. Indian J. Med. Res. 130, 63–66.

Kurniawan, A., Karyadi, T., Dwintasari, S.W., Sari, I.P., Yunihastuti, E., Djauzi, S., Smith, H.V., 2009. Intestinal parasitic infections in HIV/AIDS patients presenting with diarrhoea in Jakarta, Indonesia. Trans. R. Soc. Trop. Med. Hyg. 103, 892–898.

Kvac, M., Kvetonova, D., Sak, B., Ditrich, O., 2009. *Cryptosporidium* pig genotype II in immunocompetent man. Emerg. Infect. Dis. 15, 982–983.

Kvac, M., Kestranova, M., Pinkova, M., Kvetonova, D., Kalinova, J., Wagnerova, P., Kotkova, M., Vitovec, J., Ditrich, O., McEvoy, J., Stenger, B., Sak, B., 2013. *Cryptosporidium scrofarum* n. sp. (Apicomplexa: Cryptosporidiidae) in domestic pigs (*Sus scrofa*). Vet. Parasitol. 191, 218–227.

Kvac, M., Hofmannova, L., Hlaskova, L., Kvetonova, D., Vitovec, J., McEvoy, J., Sak, B., 2014a. *Cryptosporidium erinacei* n. sp. (Apicomplexa: Cryptosporidiidae) in hedgehogs. Vet. Parasitol. 201, 9–17.

Kvac, M., Sakova, K., Kvetonova, D., Kicia, M., Wesolowska, M., McEvoy, J., Sak, B., 2014b. Gastroenteritis caused by the *Cryptosporidium* hedgehog genotype in an immunocompetent man. J. Clin. Microbiol. 52, 347–349.

Lalonde, L.F., Gajadhar, A.A., 2008. Highly sensitive and specific PCR assay for reliable detection of *Cyclospora cayetanensis* oocysts. Appl. Environ. Microbiol. 74, 4354–4358.

Lalonde, L.F., Gajadhar, A.A., 2011. Detection and differentiation of coccidian oocysts by real-time PCR and melting curve analysis. J. Parasitol. 97, 725–730.

Lalonde, L.F., Reyes, J., Gajadhar, A.A., 2013. Application of a qPCR assay with melting curve analysis for detection and differentiation of protozoan oocysts in human fecal samples from Dominican Republic. Am. J. Trop. Med. Hyg. 89, 892–898.

Leek, R., Fayer, R., 1978. Infectivity of *Sarcocystis* in beef and beef products from a retail food store. In: Proceedings of the Helminthological Society of Washington (USA).

Leighton, F.A., Gajadhar, A.A., 1986. *Eimeria Fraterculase* sp. n. in the kidneys of Atlantic puffins (*Fratercula Arctica*) from Newfoundland, Canada: species description and lesions. J. Wildl. Dis. 22, 520–526.

Leitch, G.J., He, Q., 2012. Cryptosporidiosis—an overview. J. Biomed. Res. 25, 1–16.

Leoni, F., Amar, C., Nichols, G., Pedraza-Diaz, S., McLauchlin, J., 2006. Genetic analysis of *Cryptosporidium* from 2414 humans with diarrhoea in England between 1985 and 2000. J. Med. Microbiol. 55, 703–707.

Levine, N.D., 1980. Some corrections of coccidian (Apicomplexa: Protozoa) nomenclature. J. Parasitol. 66, 830–834.

Li, J.H., Lin, Z., Qin, Y.X., Du, J., 2004. *Sarcocystis suihominis* infection in human and pig population in Guangxi. Zhongguo Ji Sheng Chong Xue Yu Ji Sheng Chong Bing Za Zhi 22, 82.

Li, G., Xiao, S., Zhou, R., Li, W., Wadeh, H., 2007. Molecular characterization of Cyclospora-like organism from dairy cattle. Parasitol. Res. 100, 955–961.

Liebman, W.M., Thaler, M.M., Delorimier, A., Brandborg, L.L., Goodman, J., 1980. Intractable diarrhea of infancy due to intestinal coccidiosis. Gastroenterology 78, 579–584.

Lindsay, D.S., Dubey, J.P., 2009. Long-term survival of *Toxoplasma gondii* sporulated oocysts in seawater. J. Parasitol. 95, 1019–1020.

Lindsay, D.S., Dubey, J.P., Blagburn, B.L., 1997. Biology of *Isospora* spp. from humans, nonhuman primates, and domestic animals. Clin. Microbiol. Rev. 10, 19–34.

Lindsay, D.S., Upton, S.J., Owens, D.S., Morgan, U.M., Mead, J.R., Blagburn, B.L., 2000. *Cryptosporidium andersoni* n. sp. (Apicomplexa: Cryptosporiidae) from cattle, *Bos taurus*. J. Eukaryot. Microbiol. 47, 91–95.

Lindsay, D.S., Collins, M.V., Mitchell, S.M., Wetch, C.N., Rosypal, A.C., Flick, G.J., Zajac, A.M., Lindquist, A., Dubey, J.P., 2004. Survival of *Toxoplasma gondii* oocysts in eastern oysters (*Crassostrea virginica*). J. Parasitol. 90, 1054–1057.

Lindsay, D.S., Houk, A.E., Mitchell, S.M., Dubey, J.P., 2014. Developmental biology of cystoisospora (apicomplexa: sarcocystidae) monozoic tissue cysts. J. Parasitol. 100, 392–398.

Lopez, A.S., Dodson, D.R., Arrowood, M.J., Orlandi Jr., P.A., Da Silva, A.J., Bier, J.W., Hanauer, S.D., Kuster, R.L., Oltman, S., Baldwin, M.S., Won, K.Y., Nace, E.M., Eberhard, M.L., Herwaldt, B.L., 2007. Outbreak of *Cyclosporiasis* associated with basil in Missouri in 1999. Clin. Infect. Dis. 32, 1010–1017.

Lukesova, D., Nevole, M., Haidova, B., 1986. The extent of the incidence of sarcocystosis in cattle and pig farms. Vet. Med. (Praha) 31, 521–530.

Ma, P., Kaufman, D., Montana, J., 1983. *Isospora belli* diarrheal infection in homosexual men. AIDS Res. 1, 327–338.

Macarisin, D., Bauchan, G., Fayer, R., 2010. *Spinacia oleracea* L. leaf stomata harboring *Cryptosporidium parvum* oocysts: a potential threat to food safety. Appl. Environ. Microbiol. 76, 555–559.

Mackenzie, W.R., Schell, W.L., Blair, K.A., Addiss, D.G., Peterson, D.E., Hoxie, N.J., Kazmierczak, J.J., Davis, J.P., 1995. Massive outbreak of waterborne cryptosporidium infection in Milwaukee, Wisconsin: recurrence of illness and risk of secondary transmission. Clin. Infect. Dis. 21, 57–62.

Madico, G., McDonald, J., Gilman, R.H., Cabrera, L., Sterling, C.R., 1997. Epidemiology and treatment of *Cyclospora cayetanensis* infection in Peruvian children. Clin. Infect. Dis. 24, 977–981.

Maiga, M.Y., Dembele, M.Y., Traore, H.A., Kouyate, M., Traore, A.K., Maiga, I.I., Bougoudogo, F., Doumbo, O., Guindo, A., 2002. Gastrointestinal manifestations of AIDS in adults in Mali. Bull. Soc. Pathol. Exot. 95, 253–256.

Mansfield, L.S., Gajadhar, A.A., 2004. *Cyclospora cayetanensis*, a food- and waterborne coccidian parasite. Vet. Parasitol. 126, 73–90.

Marathe, A., Parikh, K., 2013. Severe diarrhoea due to *Cystoisospora belli* in renal transplant patient on immunosuppressive drugs. Indian J. Med. Microbiol. 31, 185–187.

Mathur, M.K., Verma, A.K., Makwana, G.E., Sinha, M., 2013. Study of opportunistic intestinal parasitic infections in human immunodeficiency virus/acquired immunodeficiency syndrome patients. J. Global Infect. Dis. 5, 164–167.

McLeod, R., Hirabayashi, R.N., Rothman, W., Remington, J.S., 1980. Necrotizing vasculitis and *Sarcocystis*: a cause-and-effect relationship? South. Med. J. 73, 1380–1383.

Meamar, A.R., Rezaian, M., Mirzaei, A.Z., Zahabiun, F., Faghihi, A.H., Oormazdi, H., Kia, E.B., 2009. Severe diarrhea due to *Isospora belli* in a patient with thymoma. J. Microbiol. Immunol. Infect. 42, 526–529.

Mehrotra, R., Bisht, D., Singh, P.A., Gupta, S.C., Gupta, R.K., 1996. Diagnosis of human sarcocystis infection from biopsies of the skeletal muscle. Pathology 28, 281–282.

Meshkov, S., 1975. Sarcosporidia and sarcosporidiosis in agricultural animals. II. Sarcosporidiosis in cattle. Vet. Med. Nauki 12, 55–61.

Michiels, J.F., Hofman, P., Bernard, E., Saint Paul, M.C., Boissy, C., Mondain, V., Lefichoux, Y., Loubiere, R., 1994. Intestinal and extraintestinal *Isospora belli* infection in an AIDS patient. A second case report. Pathol. Res. Pract. 190, 1089–1093, discussion 1094.

Miller, M.A., Miller, W.A., Conrad, P.A., James, E.R., Melli, A.C., Leutenegger, C.M., Dabritz, H.A., Packham, A.E., Paradies, D., Harris, M., Ames, J., Jessup, D.A., Worcester, K., Grigg, M.E., 2008. Type X *Toxoplasma gondii* in a wild mussel and terrestrial carnivores from coastal California: new linkages between terrestrial mammals, runoff and toxoplasmosis of sea otters. Int. J. Parasitol. 38, 1319–1328.

Milord, F., Lampron-Goulet, E., St-Amour, M., Levac, E., Ramsay, D., 2012. *Cyclospora cayetanensis*: a description of clinical aspects of an outbreak in Quebec, Canada. Epidemiol. Infect. 140, 626–632.

Mirdha, B.R., Kabra, S.K., Samantray, J.C., 2002. Isosporiasis in children. Indian Pediatr. 39, 941–944.

More, G., Abrahamovich, P., Jurado, S., Bacigalupe, D., Marin, J.C., Rambeaud, M., Venturini, L., Venturini, M.C., 2011. Prevalence of *Sarcocystis* spp. in Argentinean cattle. Vet. Parasitol. 177, 162–165.

Morgan, U.M., Xiao, L., Limor, J., Gelis, S., Raidal, S.R., Fayer, R., Lal, A., Elliot, A., Thompson, R.C., 2000a. *Cryptosporidium meleagridis* in an Indian ring-necked parrot (*Psittacula krameri*). Aust. Vet. J. 78, 182–183.

Morgan, U.M., Xiao, L., Monis, P., Fall, A., Irwin, P.J., Fayer, R., Denholm, K.M., Limor, J., Lal, A., Thompson, R.C., 2000b. *Cryptosporidium* spp. in domestic dogs: the "dog" genotype. Appl. Environ. Microbiol. 66, 2220–2223.

Morgan, U.M., Xiao, L., Monis, P., Sulaiman, I., Pavlasek, I., Blagburn, B., Olson, M., Upton, S.J., Khramtsov, N.V., Lal, A., Elliot, A., Thompson, R.C., 2000c. Molecular and phylogenetic analysis of *Cryptosporidium muris* from various hosts. Parasitology 120 (Pt 5), 457–464.

Morgan-Ryan, U.M., Fall, A., Ward, L.A., Hijjawi, N., Sulaiman, I., Fayer, R., Thompson, R.C., Olson, M., Lal, A., Xiao, L., 2002. *Cryptosporidium hominis* n. sp. (Apicomplexa: Cryptosporidiidae) from *Homo sapiens*. J. Eukaryot. Microbiol. 49, 433–440.

Morse, T.D., Nichols, R.A., Grimason, A.M., Campbell, B.M., Tembo, K.C., Smith, H.V., 2007. Incidence of cryptosporidiosis species in paediatric patients in Malawi. Epidemiol. Infect. 135, 1307–1315.

Muller, A., Bialek, R., Fatkenheuer, G., Salzberger, B., Diehl, V., Franzen, C., 2000. Detection of *Isospora belli* by polymerase chain reaction using primers based on small-subunit ribosomal RNA sequences. Eur. J. Clin. Microbiol. Infect. Dis. 19, 631–634.

Ng, E., Markell, E.K., Fleming, R.L., Fried, M., 1984. Demonstration of *Isospora belli* by acid-fast stain in a patient with acquired immune deficiency syndrome. J. Clin. Microbiol. 20, 384–386.

Nichpanit, S., Nak, W., Wongsaroj, T., Nithikathkul, C., 2010. First large scale of human *Sarcocystis hominis* in Thailand. Trends Res. Sci. Technol. 2, 1–5.

Obana, M., Sagara, H., Aoki, T., Kim, R., Takizawa, Y., Tsunoda, T., Irimajiri, S., Yamashita, K., 2002. The current status of infectious enteritis in Japan—reports of the "Research Group for Infectious Enteric Diseases, Japan" in the last 5 years (1996–2000). Kansenshogaku Zasshi 76, 355–368.

Odening, K., 1998. The present state of species-systematics in *Sarcocystis* Lankester, 1882 (Protista, Sporozoa, Coccidia). Syst. Parasitol. 41, 209–233.

Okhuysen, P.C., Chappell, C.L., Crabb, J.H., Sterling, C.R., Dupont, H.L., 1999. Virulence of three distinct *Cryptosporidium parvum* isolates for healthy adults. J. Infect. Dis. 180, 1275–1281.

Ortega, Y.R., Sanchez, R., 2010. Update on *Cyclospora cayetanensis*, a food-borne and waterborne parasite. Clin. Microbiol. Rev. 23, 218–234.

Ortega, Y.R., Sterling, C.R., Gilman, R.H., Cama, V.A., Diaz, F., 1993. *Cyclospora* species – a new protozoan pathogen of humans. N. Engl. J. Med. 328, 1308–1312.

Ortega, Y.R., Gilman, R.H., Sterling, C.R., 1994. A new coccidian parasite (Apicomplexa: Eimeriidae) from humans. J. Parasitol. 80, 625–629.

Ortega, Y.R., Nagle, R., Gilman, R.H., Watanabe, J., Miyagui, J., Quispe, H., Kanagusuku, P., Roxas, C., Sterling, C.R., 1997. Pathologic and clinical findings in patients with cyclosporiasis and a description of intracellular parasite life-cycle stages. J. Infect. Dis. 176, 1584–1589.

Ortega, Y.R., Mann, A., Torres, M.P., Cama, V., 2008. Efficacy of gaseous chlorine dioxide as a sanitizer against *Cryptosporidium parvum*, *Cyclospora cayetanensis*, and *Encephalitozoon intestinalis* on produce. J. Food Prot. 71, 2410–2414.

Palmer, C.J., Xiao, L., Terashima, A., Guerra, H., Gotuzzo, E., Saldias, G., Bonilla, J.A., Zhou, L., Lindquist, A., Upton, S.J., 2003. *Cryptosporidium muris*, a rodent pathogen, recovered from a human in Peru. Emerg. Infect. Dis. 9, 1174–1176.

Pape, J.W., Verdier, R.I., Johnson Jr., W.D., 1989. Treatment and prophylaxis of *Isospora belli* infection in patients with the acquired immunodeficiency syndrome. N. Engl. J. Med. 320, 1044–1047.

Park, J.H., Guk, S.M., Han, E.T., Shin, E.H., Kim, J.L., Chai, J.Y., 2006. Genotype analysis of *Cryptosporidium* spp. prevalent in a rural village in Hwasun-gun, Republic of Korea. Korean J. Parasitol. 44, 27–33.

Pavlasek, I., 2001. Findings of *Cryptosporidia* in the stomach of chickens and of exotic and wild birds. Veterinarstvi 51, 103–108.

Pavlasek, I., Ryan, U., 2008. *Cryptosporidium varanii* takes precedence over *C. saurophilum*. Exp. Parasitol. 118, 434–437.

Pavlasek, I., Lavickova, M., Horak, P., Kral, J., Kral, B., 1995. *Cryptosporidium varanii* n. sp. (Apicomplexa: Cryptosporiidae) in Emerald monitor (*Varanus prasinus* Schlegal, 1893) in captivity in Prague Zoo. Gazella 22, 98–108.

Ponka, A., Kotilainen, H., Rimhanen-Finne, R., Hokkanen, P., Hanninen, M.L., Kaarna, A., Meri, T., Kuusi, M., 2009. A foodborne outbreak due to *Cryptosporidium parvum* in Helsinki, November 2008. Euro Surveill. 14, 1–3.

Power, M.L., Ryan, U.M., 2008. A new species of *Cryptosporidium* (Apicomplexa: Cryptosporidiidae) from eastern grey kangaroos (*Macropus giganteus*). J. Parasitol. 94, 1114–1117.

Raccurt, C.P., 2007. Worldwide human zoonotic cryptosporidiosis caused by *Cryptosporidium felis*. Parasite 14, 15–20.

Relman, D.A., Schmidt, T.M., Gajadhar, A.A., Sogin, M., Cross, J., Yoder, K., Sethabutr, O., Echeverria, P., 1996. Molecular phylogenetic analysis of *Cyclospora*, the human intestinal pathogen, suggests that it is closely related to *Eimeria* species. J. Infect. Dis. 173, 440–445.

Restrepo, C., Macher, A.M., Radany, E.H., 1987. Disseminated extraintestinal isosporiasis in a patient with acquired immune deficiency syndrome. Am. J. Clin. Pathol. 87, 536–542.

Ribes, J.A., Seabolt, J.P., Overman, S.B., 2004. Point prevalence of *Cryptosporidium*, *Cyclospora*, and *Isospora* infections in patients being evaluated for diarrhea. Am. J. Clin. Pathol. 122, 28–32.

Robert-Gangneux, F., Dardé, M.-L., 2012. Epidemiology of and diagnostic strategies for toxoplasmosis. Clin. Microbiol. Rev. 25, 264–296.

Robertson, L.J., Chalmers, R.M., 2013. Foodborne cryptosporidiosis: Is there really more in Nordic countries? Trends Parasitol. 29, 3–9.

Robertson, L.J., Campbell, A.T., Smith, H.V., 1992. Survival of *Cryptosporidium parvum* oocysts under various environmental pressures. Appl. Environ. Microbiol. 58, 3494–3500.

Robinson, G., Wright, S., Elwin, K., Hadfield, S.J., Katzer, F., Bartley, P.M., Hunter, P.R., Nath, M., Innes, E.A., Chalmers, R.M., 2010. Re-description of *Cryptosporidium cuniculus* Inman and Takeuchi, 1979 (Apicomplexa: Cryptosporidiidae): morphology, biology and phylogeny. Int. J. Parasitol. 40, 1539–1548.

Rommel, M., Heydorn, A.O., Gruber, F., 1972. Life cycle of Sarcosporidia. 1. The sporocyst of *S. tenella* in cat feces. Berl. Munch. Tierarztl. Wochenschr. 85, 101–105.

Ros, E., Fueyo, J., Llach, J., Moreno, A., Latorre, X., 1987. *Isospora belli* infection in patients with AIDS in Catalunya, Spain. N. Engl. J. Med. 317, 246–247.

Rossignol, J.F., 2010. *Cryptosporidium* and *Giardia*: treatment options and prospects for new drugs. Exp. Parasitol. 124, 45–53.

Roy, S.L., Delong, S.M., Stenzel, S.A., Shiferaw, B., Roberts, J.M., Khalakdina, A., Marcus, R., Segler, S.D., Shah, D.D., Thomas, S., Vugia, D.J., Zansky, S.M., Dietz, V., Beach, M.J., Emerging Infections Program Foodnet Working Group, 2004. Risk factors for sporadic cryptosporidiosis among immunocompetent persons in the United States from 1999 to 2001. J. Clin. Microbiol. 42, 2944–2951.

Ryan, U., Power, M., 2012. *Cryptosporidium* species in Australian wildlife and domestic animals. Parasitology 139, 1673–1688.

Ryan, U.M., Xiao, L., 2008. Birds. In: Fayer, R., Xiao, L. (Eds.), *Cryptosporidium* and Cryptosporidiosis, second ed. CRC Press, Boca Raton, FL.

Ryan, U.M., Xiao, L., Read, C., Sulaiman, I.M., Monis, P., Lal, A.A., Fayer, R., Pavlasek, I., 2003. A redescription of *Cryptosporidium galli* Pavlasek, 1999 (Apicomplexa: Cryptosporidiidae) from birds. J. Parasitol. 89, 809–813.

Ryan, U.M., Monis, P., Enemark, H.L., Sulaiman, I., Samarasinghe, B., Read, C., Buddle, R., Robertson, I., Zhou, L., Thompson, R.C., Xiao, L., 2004. *Cryptosporidium suis* n. sp. (Apicomplexa: Cryptosporidiidae) in pigs (*Sus scrofa*). J. Parasitol. 90, 769–773.
Ryan, U.M., Power, M., Xiao, L., 2008. *Cryptosporidium fayeri* n. sp. (Apicomplexa: Cryptosporidiidae) from the Red Kangaroo (*Macropus rufus*). J. Eukaryot. Microbiol. 55, 22–26.
Saito, M., Shibata, Y., Ohno, A., Kubo, M., Shimura, K., Itagaki, H., 1998. *Sarcocystis suihominis* detected for the first time from pigs in Japan. J. Vet. Med. Sci./Jpn. Soc. Vet. Sci. 60, 307–309.
Saleque, A., Juyal, P., Bhatia, B., 1990. Effect of temperature on the infectivity of *Sarcocystis miescheriana* cysts in pork. Vet. Parasitol. 36, 343–346.
Santin, M., 2013. Clinical and subclinical infections with *Cryptosporidium* in animals. N. Z. Vet. J. 61, 1–10.
Santin, M., Trout, J., 2008a. Companion animals. In: Fayer, R., Xiao, L. (Eds.), *Cryptosporidium* and Cryptosporidosis, second ed. CRC Press, Boca Raton, FL.
Santin, M., Trout, J., 2008b. Livestock. In: Fayer, R., Xiao, L. (Eds.), *Cryptosporidium* and Cryptosporidiosis, second ed. CRC Press, Boca Raton, FL.
Sathyanarayanan, L., Ortega, Y., 2006. Effects of temperature and different food matrices on *Cyclospora cayetanensis* oocyst sporulation. J. Parasitol. 92, 218–222.
Sauda, F.C., Zamarioli, L.A., Ebner Filho, W., Mello Lde, B., 1993. Prevalence of *Cryptosporidium* sp. and *Isospora belli* among AIDS patients attending Santos Reference Center for AIDS, Sao Paulo, Brazil. J. Parasitol. 79, 454–456.
Savini, G., Dunsmore, J., Robertson, I., Seneviratna, P., 1992. The epidemiology of *Sarcocystis* spp. in cattle of Western Australia. Epidemiol. Infect. 108, 107–113.
Savini, G., Robertson, I., Dunsmore, J., 1996. Viability of the sporocysts of *Sarcocystis cruzi* after exposure to different temperatures and relative humidities. Vet. Parasitol. 67, 153–160.
Scallan, E., Hoekstra, R.M., Angulo, F.J., Tauxe, R.V., Widdowson, M.A., Roy, S.L., Jones, J.L., Griffin, P.M., 2011. Foodborne illness acquired in the United States—major pathogens. Emerg. Infect. Dis. 17, 7–15.
Sénaud, J., 1967. *Contribution à l'étude des sarcosporidies et des toxoplasmes (Toxoplasmea).* Protistologica 3, 167–232.
Sherchand, J.B., Cross, J.H., 2004. Parasitic epidemiological studies of *Cyclospora cayetanensis* in Nepal. Southeast Asian J. Trop. Med. Public Health 35, 12–19.
Shields, J.M., Olson, B.H., 2003. PCR-restriction fragment length polymorphism method for detection of *Cyclospora cayetanensis* in environmental waters without microscopic confirmation. Appl. Environ. Microbiol. 69, 4662–4669.
Silverlas, C., Mattsson, J.G., Insulander, M., Lebbad, M., 2012. Zoonotic transmission of *Cryptosporidium meleagridis* on an organic Swedish farm. Int. J. Parasitol. 42, 963–967.
Singh, B., Gajadhar, A., 2014. Role of India; wildlife in the emergence and re-emergence of zoonotic pathogens, risk factors and public health implications. Acta Trop. 138, 67–77.
Slavin, D., 1955. *Cryptosporidium meleagridis* (sp. nov.). J. Comp. Pathol. 65, 262–266.
Smith, H.V., Al-Adhami, B.H., Nichols, R.A.B., Kusel, J.R., O'Grady, J., 2008. Towards methods for detecting UV-induced damage in individual *Cryptosporidium parvum* and *Cryptosporidium hominis* oocysts by immunoflourescence microscopy. In: Ortega-Pierres, G., Cacciò, S., Fayer, R., Mank, T.G., Smith, H.V., Thompson, A. (Eds.), *Giardia* and *Cryptosporidium*: From Molecules to Disease. CAB International, United States.
Solanki, P., Shrivastava, H., Shah, H., 1991. Prevallence of *Sarcocystis* in naturally infected pigs in Madhya-Pradesh with an epidemiologic explanation for the higher prevalence of *Sarcocystis suihominis*. Indian Council of Agricultural Research, ICAR Bhawan, Pusa, New Delhi, India.

Sorvillo, F.J., Lieb, L.E., Seidel, J., Kerndt, P., Turner, J., Ash, L.R., 1995. Epidemiology of isosporiasis among persons with acquired immunodeficiency syndrome in Los Angeles County. Am. J. Trop. Med. Hyg. 53, 656–659.

Straka, S., Skracikova, J., Konvit, I., Szilagyiova, M., Michal, L., 1991. *Sarcocystis* species in Vietnamese workers. Cesk. Epidemiol. Mikrobiol. Imunol. 40, 204–208.

Sulaiman, I.M., Torres, P., Simpson, S., Kerdahi, K., Ortega, Y., 2013. Sequence characterization of heat shock protein gene of *Cyclospora cayetanensis* isolates from Nepal, Mexico, and Peru. J. Parasitol. 99, 379–382.

Sulaiman, I.M., Ortega, Y., Simpson, S., Kerdahi, K., 2014. Genetic characterization of human-pathogenic *Cyclospora cayetanensis* parasites from three endemic regions at the 18S ribosomal RNA locus. Infect. Genet. Evol. 22, 229–234.

Tandukar, S., Ansari, S., Adhikari, N., Shrestha, A., Gautam, J., Sharma, B., Rajbhandari, D., Gautam, S., Nepal, H.P., Sherchand, J.B., 2013. Intestinal parasitosis in school children of Lalitpur district of Nepal. BMC Res. Notes 6, 449.

Taniuchi, M., Verweij, J.J., Sethabutr, O., Bodhidatta, L., Garcia, L., Maro, A., Kumburu, H., Gratz, J., Kibiki, G., Houpt, E.R., 2011. Multiplex polymerase chain reaction method to detect *Cyclospora*, *Cystoisospora*, and *Microsporidia* in stool samples. Diagn. Microbiol. Infect. Dis. 71, 386–390.

Tavarez, L.A., Pena, F., Placencia, F., Mendoza, H.R., Polanco, D., 1991. Prevalence of protozoans in children with acute diarrheal disease. Arch. Domin. Pediatr. 27, 43–47.

Ten Hove, R.J., van Lieshout, L., Brienen, E.A., Perez, M.A., Verweij, J.J., 2008. Real-time polymerase chain reaction for detection of *Isospora belli* in stool samples. Diagn. Microbiol. Infect. Dis. 61, 280–283.

Thima, K., Mori, H., Praevanit, R., Mongkhonmu, S., Waikagul, J., Watthanakulpanich, D., 2014. Recovery of *Cyclospora cayetanensis* among asymptomatic rural Thai schoolchildren. Asian Pac. J. Trop. Med. 7, 119–123.

Thomas, M.K., Murray, R., Flockhart, L., Pintar, K., Pollari, F., Fazil, A., Nesbitt, A., Marshall, B., 2013. Estimates of the burden of foodborne illness in Canada for 30 specified pathogens and unspecified agents, Circa 2006. Foodborne Pathog. Dis. 10, 639–648.

Tilley, M., Upton, S.J., Freed, P.S., 1990. A comparative study on the biology of *Cryptosporidium serpentis* and *Cryptosporidium parvum* (Apicomplexa: Cryptosporidiidae). J. Zoo Wildl. Med. 21, 463–467.

Tyzzer, E.E., 1907. A sporozoan found in the peptic glands of the common mouse. Proc. Soc. Exp. Biol. Med. 5, 12–13.

Tyzzer, E.E., 1910. An extracellular coccidium, *Cryptosporidium muris* (Gen. Et Sp. Nov.), of the gastric glands of the common mouse. J. Med. Res. 23, 487–509.

Tyzzer, E.E., 1912. *Cryptosporidium parvum* (sp. nov.), a coccidium found in the small intestine of the common mouse. Arch. Protist. 26, 394–412.

Ud Din, N., Torka, P., Hutchison, R.E., Riddell, S.W., Wright, J., Gajra, A., 2012. Severe *Isospora* (*Cystoisospora*) *belli* diarrhea preceding the diagnosis of human T-cell-leukemia-virus-1-associated t-cell lymphoma. Case Rep. Infect. Dis. 2012, 640104.

Usluca, S., Inceboz, T., Unek, T., Aksoy, U., 2012. *Isospora belli* in a patient with liver transplantation. Turkiye Parazitol. Derg. 36, 247–250.

Valentiner-Branth, P., Steinsland, H., Fischer, T.K., Perch, M., Scheutz, F., Dias, F., Aaby, P., Molbak, K., Sommerfelt, H., 2003. Cohort study of Guinean children: incidence, pathogenicity, conferred protection, and attributable risk for enteropathogens during the first 2 years of life. J. Clin. Microbiol. 41, 4238–4245.

van den Enden, E., Praet, M., Joos, R., van Gompel, A., Gigasse, P., 1995. *Eosinophilic myositis* resulting from sarcocystosis. J. Trop. Med. Hyg. 98, 273–276.

van der Giessen, J., Fonville, M., Bouwknegt, M., Langelaar, M., Vollema, A., 2007. Seroprevalence of *Trichinella spiralis* and *Toxoplasma gondii* in pigs from different housing systems in The Netherlands. Vet. Parasitol. 148, 371–374.

Vangeel, L., Houf, K., Chiers, K., Vercruysse, J., D'Herde, K., Ducatelle, R., 2007. Molecular-based identification of *Sarcocystis hominis* in Belgian minced beef. J. Food Prot. 70, 1523–1526.

Varma, M., Hester, J.D., Schaefer, F.W., Ware, M.W., Lindquist, H.D.A., 2003. Detection of *Cyclospora cayetanensis* using a quantitative real-time PCR assay. J. Microbiol. Methods 53, 27–36.

Vetterling, J.M., Jervis, H.R., Merrill, T.G., Sprinz, H., 1971. *Cryptosporidium wrairi* sp. n. from the guinea pig *Cavia porcellus*, with an emendation of the genus. J. Protozool. 18, 243–247.

Waldron, L.S., Cheung-Kwok-Sang, C., Power, M.L., 2010. Wildlife-associated *Cryptosporidium fayeri* in human, Australia. Emerg. Infect. Dis. 16, 2006–2007.

Wang, R., Zhang, L., Ning, C., Feng, Y., Jian, F., Xiao, L., Lu, B., Ai, W., Dong, H., 2008. Multilocus phylogenetic analysis of *Cryptosporidium andersoni* (Apicomplexa) isolated from a bactrian camel (*Camelus bactrianus*) in China. Parasitol. Res. 102, 915–920.

Warren, C.A., Guerrant, R., 2008. Clinical disease and pathology. In: Fayer, R., Xiao, L. (Eds.), *Cryptosporidium* and Cryptosporidiosis, second ed. CRC Press, Boca Raton, FL.

Wielinga, P.R., De Vries, A., van der Goot, T.H., Mank, T., Mars, M.H., Kortbeek, L.M., van der Giessen, J.W., 2008. Molecular epidemiology of *Cryptosporidium* in humans and cattle in The Netherlands. Int. J. Parasitol. 38, 809–817.

Wilairatana, P., Radomyos, P., Radomyos, B., Phraevanich, R., Plooksawasdi, W., Chanthavanich, P., Viravan, C., Looareesuwan, S., 1996. Intestinal sarcocystosis in Thai laborers. SE Asian J. Trop. Med. Public Health 27, 43–46.

Xiao, L., 2010. Molecular epidemiology of cryptosporidiosis: an update. Exp. Parasitol. 124, 80–89.

Xiao, L., Ryan, U., 2008. Molecular epidemiology. In: Fayer, R., Xiao, L. (Eds.), *Cryptosporidium* and Cryptosporidiosis, second ed. CRC Press, Boca Raton, FL.

Xiao, L., Fayer, R., Ryan, U., Upton, S.J., 2004. *Cryptosporidium* taxonomy: recent advances and implications for public health. Clin. Microbiol. Rev. 17, 72–97.

Yazar, S., Tokgoz, B., Yaman, O., Sahin, I., 2006. *Isospora belli* infection in a patient with a renal transplant. Turkiye Parazitol. Derg. 30, 22–24.

Yu, S., 1991. [Field survey of sarcocystis infection in the Tibet autonomous region]. *Zhongguo yi xue ke xue yuan xue bao*. Acta Acad. Med. Sin. 13, 29–32.

Zardi, E.M., Picardi, A., Afeltra, A., 2005. Treatment of cryptosporidiosis in immunocompromised hosts. Chemotherapy 51, 193–196.

Zhou, Z., Li, W., Lian, Z., Xu, C., 1990. The prevalence of *S. suihominis* in the natives of Yunnan province, China. Chin. Sci. Bull. 36, 965–967.

Zhou, Y., Lv, B., Wang, Q., Wang, R., Jian, F., Zhang, L., Ning, C., Fu, K., Wang, Y., Qi, M., Yao, H., Zhao, J., Zhang, X., Sun, Y., Shi, K., Arrowood, M.J., Xiao, L., 2011. Prevalence and molecular characterization of *Cyclospora cayetanensis*, Henan, China. Emerg. Infect. Dis. 17, 1887–1890.

Zintl, A., Proctor, A.F., Read, C., Dewaal, T., Shanaghy, N., Fanning, S., Mulcahy, G., 2009. The prevalence of *Cryptosporidium* species and subtypes in human faecal samples in Ireland. Epidemiol. Infect. 137, 270–277.

Foodborne, enteric, non apicomplexan unicellular parasites

7

R.C.A. Thompson
Murdoch University, Murdoch, WA, Australia

7.1 Introduction

The non apicomplexan protozoa and fungi, in the case of the microsporidia (previously classified as protozoa), that form the subject of this chapter all share a number of characteristics (Table 7.1). The exception is the systemic, intracellular, vector borne flagellate *Trypanosoma cruzi*, which has been included here because of the emergence of foodborne transmission as a means of human infection in endemic regions.

Enteric unicellular parasites all have a global distribution, both in urban and rural environments, although some, such as *Entamoeba histolytica* and *Balantidium coli*, are more common in the developing world (Nichols, 1999; Thompson and Smith, 2011; Fletcher et al., 2012).

Apart from *T. cruzi*, they also have direct, one-host life cycles and, following asexual multiplication in the intestine, produce resistant cysts, or spores in the case of the microsporidia that are passed with the feces into the environment and are immediately infective. High temperatures and desiccation are the most important factors governing survival in the environment. In view of the importance of the environment for the survival and transmission of these parasites, they are considered to be susceptible to climate change (Polley and Thompson, 2009; Fletcher et al., 2012; FAO, 2014; Chapter 3).

E. histolytica and *B. coli* also can invade the mucosal tissues of the large intestine and reach other organs; this is discussed further below. *T. cruzi* does not colonize the intestine following the ingestion of infective stages but invades systemic organs and tissues following penetration of the intestine. The occurrence of *Blastocystis* and *Dientamoeba* has been principally reported in developed countries (Fletcher et al., 2012) although both parasites may be prevalent in developing countries but not sufficiently investigated in view of their recent emergence as pathogens. Often two or more of these parasites occur together as polyparasitic (mixed) infections (Thompson and Smith, 2011). The most commonly represented protozoa in polyparasitic infections are *Giardia*, *Blastocystis*, and *Entamoeba coli*, which are often also found with the cestode *Hymenolepis nana* (Chunge et al., 1991; Meloni et al., 1993; Nimri et al., 2004; Ouattara et al., 2008; Nematian et al., 2008). Depending on the endemic area, *E. histolytica* and *Entamoeba dispar* may also occur in mixed infections. In addition, other potentially zoonotic protozoa, such as *Chilomastix mesnili* and *Endolimax nana* that may have been dismissed as having no clinical consequence and not reported, are

Foodborne Parasites in the Food Supply Web. http://dx.doi.org/10.1016/B978-1-78242-332-4.00007-2

Table 7.1 Enteric foodborne protozoa

Parasite	Life cycle	Site[a]	Transmission stage	Zoonotic	Geographical distribution	Symptoms	Treatment
Giardia spp.	Direct	SI	Cyst	Yes	Worldwide	Diarrhea; failure to thrive	Albendazole; tinidazole; metronidazole
Entamoeba histolytica	Direct	LI	Cyst	No	Mainly tropical	Dysentery; liver abscess	Paromomycin; iodoquinol
Blastocystis spp.	Direct	SI	Cyst (possibly other LC stages)	Yes	Worldwide	Abdominal pain; diarrhea; bloating; etc.	Nitazoxanide; metronidazole[b]
Balantidium coli	Direct	LI	Cyst	Uncertain	Mainly tropical; rural	Dysentery	Tetracycline; metronidazole
Microsporida	Direct	SI	Spore	Yes	Worldwide	Diarrhea	Fumagillin; albendazole

[a]Small (SI) or large (LI) intestine; *E. histolytica* and *B. coli* are also invasive.
[b]But see text.

also probably common (e.g., Chunge et al., 1991) and in the context of polyparasitism should be considered (Thompson and Smith, 2011).

From a public health perspective, the enteric parasites featured here are all important as causes of outbreaks or ongoing chronic infections, often as a result of food or water contamination. In particular, this is often the case in endemic foci where the frequency of transmission is high as a result of poor hygiene. For example, in community settings in rural areas of the developing world or in disadvantaged communities, as well as in institutional settings such as child care centers and homes for the elderly (Thompson, 2011; Thompson and Smith, 2011).

All of the parasites listed in Table 7.1 can be transmitted by or with food (Nichols, 1999; Thompson and Smith, 2011; Fletcher et al., 2012). Infection is by the oral ingestion of the cysts, or spores, and can be initiated in most cases by very small infectious doses (Nichols, 1999; Robertson et al., 2014; Smith and Nichols, 2006). Cysts or spores can be transmitted directly from one host to another (fecal–oral route), or via the environment.

Food contamination can occur in a number of ways and by a variety of routes (Nichols, 1999; Cama and Ortega, 2006; Robertson et al., 2014). These routes include from an infected individual, via the fecal–oral route as a result of poor hygiene. This is when the individual who handles the food during harvesting or preparation transmits infection to one or multiple individuals, for example, family members. This scenario is considered to be especially common following contact with the feces of infected young children (Nichols, 1999). Alternatively, such poor hygiene may have a broader impact depending on who eats the contaminated food after it has been prepared, packed, and distributed. If the food is sold locally or distributed more widely, then outbreaks of varying size may occur. For example, food handlers are often considered to be a potential source of outbreaks of varying size (Nichols, 1999). Recent surveys in the Middle East and in Brazil that examined stool samples from food handlers in hotels and retail outlets found prevalences of intestinal protozoan infections ranging from 3% to 21%, which included *Blastocystis*, *Giardia*, *E. histolytica*, *E. coli*, and *Endolimax* (Abdel-Dayem et al., 2013; Colli et al., 2013; Kheirandish et al., 2014).

Food can also be contaminated indirectly, most commonly from contaminated irrigation water, soil, untreated manure, and biosolids used as fertilizer (Nichols, 1999; Dawson, 2005; Goodgame, 1996; Hamano et al., 2008). For example, vegetables from numerous countries have been found contaminated with protozoan cysts including *Giardia*, *E. histolytica*, *Blastocystis*, as well as microsporidian spores (Al-Binali et al., 2006; Jedrzejewski et al., 2007; Broglia and Kapel, 2011; Fletcher et al., 2012). Indirect transmission can also occur mechanically via the environment by vectors such as crawling and flying insects (Szostakowska et al., 2004; Karanis et al., 2007; Smith et al., 2007; Nyarango et al., 2008), and filter-feeding molluscs (see below), or animals such as dogs whose muzzle or coat can become contaminated following contact with infected feces or diapers. Infective stages can also be ingested by dogs, which then pass out in their feces and contaminate the environment. Such mechanical routes can enhance transmission and ensure a broader distribution and/or extend the range of transmission. In developed countries, large-scale food production, distribution, retailing, and importation of raw food ingredients increase the risk for the spread of foodborne infections and often result in costly recalls (Lynch et al., 2006).

As with most pathogens, rarely is infection likely to be exclusive to one transmission route (Thomas et al., 2013). It should also be noted that changing food habits contribute to the increased frequency of foodborne transmission of enteric protozoa (Chapter 4). Many foods, particularly vegetables, are more often eaten raw, or undercooked (Slifko et al., 2000; Pönka et al., 2009; Insulander et al., 2010; Broglia and Kapel, 2011; Robertson et al., 2014), thereby increasing the risks that protozoan cysts on contaminated food will remain viable and infective. The role of bivalve molluscs, which are filter feeders and thus have the potential to become contaminated with the infective stages of enteric protozoa from the environment, is of growing concern given that they are often eaten raw, pickled, or lightly cooked (Broglia and Kapel, 2011; Fletcher et al., 2012; Hohweyer et al., 2013). Their ability to trap and concentrate cysts from contaminated water has been demonstrated with *Giardia*, but other species of fecal borne protozoa, such as *Blastocystis*, are also likely to be concentrated from the environment by filter-feeding molluscs.

All of the aforementioned enteric parasites have zoonotic potential (see Table 7.1 and the following). However, the frequency and importance of zoonotic transmission vary between the different parasites, and the role that infected animals have in contaminating food is often not known.

7.2 Giardia

Following the ingestion of infective cysts, *Giardia* multiplies asexually in the small intestine as trophozoites which adhere to the mucosal surface but are not invasive. After 4–5 days, trophozoites pass posteriorly down the intestine and secrete a resistance cyst wall before being passed in the feces. *Giardia* has a broad host range, but it is those species that infect mammals that are of most relevance to public health. Taxonomic uncertainty over many years made it difficult to understand the host specificity of *Giardia* in mammalian hosts because of morphological uniformity of the parasite in the face of considerable evidence of phenotypic differences among isolates (Thompson, 2011). Genotyping techniques have now resolved the taxonomic issues, and it is clear that in addition to strains/assemblages that are host specific, some assemblages are capable of infecting a broad range of hosts and have zoonotic potential. The taxonomy has been recently clarified and revised with the use of species names that reflect those proposed by early taxonomists (Table 7.2).

The zoonotic species of *Giardia* and those infecting domestic animals and livestock are geographically widespread. In humans, *Giardia* causes an estimated 8×10^6 cases per year and is the most common enteric parasite of humans in many countries, both developed and developing (FAO, 2014). However, the infection rates are higher in developing countries, particularly in children (Thompson, 2011; Thompson and Smith, 2011). Children are more frequently infected than adults, particularly those from developing countries and those that are malnourished (FAO, 2014). In Asia, Africa, and Latin America, about 200 million people have symptomatic *Giardia* infections, with approximately 500,000 new cases reported each year (Lal et al., 2013). *Giardia* is also

Table 7.2 **Species of *Giardia***

Species	Assemblage	Host(s)
G. duodenalis	A	Humans and other primates, dogs, cats, livestock, rodents, and other wild animals
G. enterica	B	Humans and other primates, dogs, cats, and some species of wild animals
G. canis	C/D	Dogs and other canids
G. bovis	E	Catte and other hoofed animals
G. cati	F	Cats
G. simondi	G	Rats

From Thompson (2011).

the most common enteric parasite of dogs and cats in most developed countries and is frequently reported in dogs in other endemic areas (Palmer et al., 2008a; Thompson et al., 2008; Ballweber et al., 2010; Barutzki and Schaper, 2011; Covacin, et al., 2011). Numerous studies have shown that in urban or rural populations a proportion of the infected dogs will harbor zoonotic species of *Giardia* (Palmer et al., 2008b; Thompson et al., 2008; Covacin et al., 2011; Thompson, 2011).

The clinical impact of *Giardia* is the greatest in children, particularly in developing countries or disadvantaged communities where poor hygiene and the proximity of animal reservoirs sustain environmental contamination leading to a high frequency of transmission and the establishment of chronic infections (Thompson, 2008, 2009). In such situations, nutrition may be suboptimal, exacerbating the impact of *Giardia* infections that contribute to poor growth and development (failure to thrive) in early childhood, zinc and iron deficiency, poor cognitive function, and failure to thrive (growth retardation) as well as predispose to the development of allergic diseases (Berkman et al., 2002 and reviewed in Savioli et al., 2006; Thompson, 2008, 2009). Importantly, diarrhea is not necessarily a symptom in such chronic infections that are often shared with enteric parasites that contribute to the syndrome of failure to thrive such as *E. coli*, *Blastocystis*, and *H. nana* (Botero-Garcés et al., 2009; Thompson and Smith, 2011; FAO, 2014).

Giardia, along with *Cryptosporidium* and *Cyclospora*, are the main enteric protozoa associated with foodborne infections in developed countries (Nichols, 1999). Implicated foods have included canned salmon, sandwiches, noodle salad, fruit salad, salad items, raw vegetables, and ice (Nichols, 1999). Interestingly, *Giardia* was responsible for nearly half of the cases (total 53) from 1973 to 2006, of seafood-associated outbreaks (Iwamoto et al., 2010). An US report for the years 2000–2008 indicated that a significant proportion of lab-confirmed cases of foodborne parasitic diseases in the country were due to *Giardia* (Scallan et al., 2011). Most foodborne outbreaks of symptomatic *Giardia* infections have been related to direct contamination by a food handler (FAO, 2014). The estimated annual number of cases of domestically acquired foodborne illness due to *Giardia* infection in Canada in 2006, was 7776, representing 0.45% of 30 pathogens surveyed, an estimated 23.93 cases per 100,000 (Thomas et al., 2013).

7.3 Other flagellates

A variety of other flagellates are increasingly being reported infecting humans, not necessarily associated with any clinical symptoms but often associated with other parasites. These include *Dientamoeba fragilis*, *C. mesnili*, *Trichomonas hominis*, *Retortomonas intestinalis*, and *Enteromonas hominis* (Nichols, 1999; Fletcher et al., 2012). Evidence is now growing that *D. fragilis* is potentially pathogenic, but the other genera are usually considered as nonpathogenic. However, this probably needs to be reconsidered because they are often found in mixed infections with other enteric protozoa, and some such as *C. mesnili* is a frequent parasite of other mammals apart from humans. However, only *Chilomastix* is likely to be associated with contaminated food as the other flagellates mentioned above do not produce environmentally resistant cysts as the infective stage in their life cycles.

Outbreaks of acute Chagas disease following foodborne transmission of *T. cruzi* have been reported in several South American countries including Brazil, Colombia, and Venezuela (FAO, 2014). Infections by this route are most common in rural areas, particularly in the Amazonian region (Zingales et al., 2012). Infection by the oral route results from the ingestion of infected blood-sucking reduviid arthropod vectors, or their feces, on fruit, in juices, or in fermented fruit drinks (FAO, 2014). It is an emerging issue because control efforts have reduced the incidence of other modes of transmission, thus highlighting more recently recognized routes such as foodborne. Resultant disease tends to be acute, more severe, and with a high mortality as a result of foodborne transmission, frequently involving the heart. It is not known if only certain strains of *T. cruzi* are associated with the foodborne transmission of Chagas disease (Zingales et al., 2012).

7.4 Entamoeba

Numerous species of *Entamoeba* and related amoebae infect humans and other mammals, including: *E. histolytica*, *E. dispar*, *E. coli*, *Entamoeba moshkovskii*, *Entamoeba poleki* (syn. *Entamoeba chattoni*), and *Entamoeba hartmanii* (Thompson and Smith, 2011; Fletcher et al., 2012). All have a global distribution apart from *E. histolytica* and *E. dispar* that are principally restricted to tropical and subtropical regions, particularly South and Central America, Africa, India, and Southeast Asia, in areas with low socioeconomic conditions in which sanitation is likely to be compromised. However, *E. histolytica* is the only species considered to be of pathogenic significance. This is because of its invasive potential which can lead to amoebic dysentery and blood loss following mucosal invasion of the large intestine, a disease considered to be the third-leading cause of death from parasitic diseases worldwide (Haque et al., 2003; Mortimer and Chadee, 2010). In addition to amoebic dysentery and depending on the progression of infection, invasive disease associated with the formation of abscesses in the liver, lung, or brain may also occur. It should be emphasized that fewer than 10% of individuals infected with *E. histolytica* develop clinical disease within a year, and yet this represents approximately 5 million cases of invasive disease (Fletcher et al.,

2012). Mucosal invasion is a dead end for the parasite because cysts are not produced. Like *Giardia*, trophozoites multiply asexually in the large intestine secreting a cyst wall before being passed in the feces.

Transmission is via the fecal–oral route. The risk of zoonotic transmission of *E. histolytica* is minimal because although dogs may be coprophagic, the parasite rarely encysts (Barr, 1998; Eyles et al., 1954; Thompson and Smith, 2011). However, dogs may act as a mechanical means of transmitting cysts to food in community situations.

Because of the lack of any morphological differences between the more common and nonpathogenic *E. dispar*, as well as the less common *E. moshkovskii*, molecular tools are considered to be more accurate and sensitive than morphology for differentiating between the two species (Fletcher et al., 2012). However, clinical and local history, combined with microscopy, are often adequate in endemic foci and for travelers from such areas.

7.5 Other amoebae

Other amoebae that can occur in food are generally considered to be nonpathogenic commensals but are increasingly being reported in mixed infections, particularly *E. coli*, which has a wide host range apart from humans (Thompson and Smith, 2011).

7.6 Blastocystis

Blastocystis is a ubiquitous, globally distributed parasite of humans and numerous species of vertebrates. It is considered to be an emerging, genetically diverse pathogen in terms of its association with disease (Vassalos et al., 2008; Boorom et al., 2008; Parkar et al., 2010; Thompson and Smith, 2011).

A variety of morphological forms have been described in the life cycle, including a cyst stage that is thought to be the main agent of transmission (Singh et al., 1995; Fletcher et al., 2012). The developmental cycle of *Blastocystis* is not completely understood but appears to involve only asexual multiplication in the small intestine. It comprises a range of morphologically pleiomorphic stages, and it is not clear whether all are always represented or whether some are more pathogenic than others (Thompson and Smith, 2011). Transmission routes are presumed to be very similar to those of *Giardia*, involving contaminated food and water. Infection results from ingestion of cysts that give rise to colonization of the intestinal tract. *Blastocystis* is not invasive.

Humans are susceptible to infection with a variety of genetically distinct strains or subtypes, some of which also occur in domestic and wild animals (Parkar et al., 2007, 2010; Yoshikawa et al., 2008). The frequency of zoonotic transmission and risk factors still have to be clearly defined, but there is sufficient evidence that zoonotic transmission can occur (Thompson and Smith, 2011; Wang et al., 2014).

Blastocystis has the potential to cause illness but is more often associated with asymptomatic infection (Fletcher et al., 2012); it may not be recognized as causing chronic disorders. The association between sporadic, nonspecific symptoms such as flatulence, bloating, occasional cramps, and the like may not be linked with *Blastocystis* infection by infected individuals or physicians and thus is often overlooked in terms of *Blastocystis* being a possible etiology. The spectrum of disease manifestations associated with *Blastocystis* infections has yet to be clearly defined (Boorom et al., 2008). It is the most common enteric protozoan isolated from diarrheal patients in the most developed countries (Fletcher et al., 2012), but it is common without necessarily being associated with overt symptoms. It is also frequently reported in developing countries (Thompson and Smith, 2011) but likely to be overlooked in routine diagnostic surveillance using traditional microscopy. There is also a growing debate as to whether *Blastocystis* is associated with the etiology of inflammatory bowel disease (Boorom et al., 2008).

Clearly, the circumstances and mechanisms associated with disease as a result of *Blastocystis* infection are not understood (Boorom et al., 2008). As with *Giardia*, it is possible that some "strains" of *Blastocystis* are more often associated with overt disease than others (Boorom et al., 2008).

Treatment is not as straightforward as suggested in Table 7.1. Metronidazole has been the most frequently used drug, but treatment failures are common (Fletcher et al., 2012). There is, therefore, a need to consider whether the presence of *Blastocystis* warrants a treatment that may cause more problems in terms of its adverse effects on intestinal microflora than *Blastocystis* itself. Other drugs such as nitazoxanide are also considered useful (Fletcher et al., 2012). However, variation in drug sensitivity between strains is likely to be an emerging issue.

7.7 Balantidium

Balantidium is the only ciliate known to cause food- and waterborne infections in humans. It is uncommon in developed countries (Thompson and Smith, 2011; Fletcher et al., 2012). Like *E. histolytica*, *Balantidium* primarily occurs in rural, tropical regions where hygiene levels are poor and opportunities for person-to-person transmission via the fecal–oral route are high; under such conditions food contamination is also likely (Thompson and Smith, 2011).

Like *E. histolytica*, trophozoites of *Balantidium* proliferate asexually in the large intestine and are potentially invasive in humans. This can cause serious disease (Bellanger et al., 2013) taking the form of an ulcerative dysentery but seems to be a rare, sporadic occurrence (Nichols, 1999; Schuster and Visvesvara, 2004; Conlan et al., 2012).

Balantidium is most common in rural areas of tropical and subtropical regions (Zaman, 1998; Farthing et al., 2003; Owen, 2005). It is often stated that the risk of infection is in communities that have a close association with pigs (Schuster and Ramirez-Avila, 2008), but there is little evidence to support zoonotic transmission being common. For example, a recent survey of several villages in rural areas of Laos found that of 181 young pigs, 68.6% were infected with *Balantidium* although no cases of *Balantidium* were found in humans from the same villages from which the pigs were surveyed (Conlan et al., 2012). Similar results were also reported in Cambodian villages (Schär et al., 2014). These recent surveys thus confirm doubts expressed previously about the roles of pigs as reservoirs of human infection (Zaman, 1998; Owen, 2005).

7.8 Microsporidia

Two species of enteric microsporidia, *Encephalitozoon intestinalis* and *Enterocytozoon bieneusi*, commonly cause diarrhea in AIDS patients throughout the world (Nichols, 1999). Indeed, intestinal microsporidiosis was first identified in AIDS patients, with *E. bieneusi* being the more common of the two causative species (Dengjel et al., 2001; Stark et al., 2009). However, with increasing access to antiretroviral therapy, infection rates in HIV/AIDS patients have reduced significantly (van Hal et al., 2007; Stark et al., 2009). Infections have also been found in immunocompetent patients (Lores et al., 2002; Abreu-Acosta et al., 2005). Infections occur through ingestion of resistant spores that can be transmitted directly, via the fecal–oral route, or via the environment including food and water. Infection develops in the small intestine although the respiratory tract may be affected in infections with *Encephalitozoon*. In otherwise healthy individuals, infection has resulted in self-limiting diarrhea of up to approximately 1 month (Didier, 2005).

7.9 General discussion

7.9.1 Developed versus developing countries

In considering the etiology of foodborne enteric protozoan infections, a distinction must be made between the developed Western world and developing regions of the world. In developed countries, foodborne outbreaks are more often likely to be identified, reported, and their impact publicized compared to the developing world, where there is a situation, particularly in community settings, of chronic, long-term, continuing morbidity associated with enteric protozoan infections. Thus, trying to estimate a "global burden" of foodborne infections versus disease may not reflect the real situation (see below). Children are a particularly high-risk group, and the risk of infection appears greater within rural environments than within urban areas; presumably because of the increased opportunity for both direct and indirect transmission to occur in areas with poor sanitation (Thompson and Smith, 2011). For example, the predominant use of lakes and streams in Europe is recreational, whereas in Africa or Asia there is a much greater reliance on these water sources for drinking and in the preparation of food and personal hygiene (Thompson and Smith, 2011).

7.9.2 Sources of infection

Linking protozoan and microsporidian infections to a contaminated food source remains difficult for the majority of scenarios. Small-scale outbreaks, where the point of initial contamination may be the result of poor hygiene by an individual resulting in localized foodborne transmission to family members or the immediate community, are extremely common particularly in the developing world. Transmission resulting from contamination of food that leads to larger scale infections is a much less common event (Millard et al., 1994; Thompson and Smith, 2011). For example, the risk of becoming infected with *Blastocystis* from contaminated food appears low from the lack of reports in the literature, although infection arising through poor hygiene practices of food handlers has a potentially much higher infection rate. As an example, a survey of 150 apparently healthy food handlers in Bolivar State, Venezuela, showed that 25.8% ($n = 107$) were in fact positive for *Blastocystis* (Requena et al., 2003), whereas a review of 103 published reports concerning *Blastocystis* infection between 1990 and 2008 showed that none were able to conclusively ascribe infection to conventional foodborne transmission (Thompson and Smith, 2011). Enteric protozoan parasites are readily transmitted on food and, in some regions of the world, farming and agricultural practices such as the use of human waste for fertilization and inefficient or absent pasteurization techniques positively enhance transmission (FAO, 2014). Nonetheless, the majority of indirect transmission from contaminated food arises from more proximate sources of infection, such as infected food handlers and poor hygiene, often resulting from overcrowded living conditions where clean running water is scarce, and also from children and adults with little or no health education (Thompson and Smith, 2011).

Foodborne transmission, whether arising as a result of agricultural practices, poor hygiene within households, or infected food handlers, is undoubtedly responsible for a significant number of infections every year. For example, estimates derived from a literature review of published reports and case notes for *Giardia* occurrence suggest that the number of cases of foodborne transmission resulting in infection by *Giardia* range from 13 million in the World Health Organization-derived Eastern Mediterranean region to 76 million in the Western Pacific Rim region (Thompson and Smith, 2011).

7.9.3 Impact/burden of infection

Estimates of foodborne illness due to enteric protozoan infections are important for public health decision makers, but determining these estimates can be challenging given the large variability within foodborne illness in terms of pathogen, host, and environmental factors (Thomas et al., 2013). Cases of foodborne illness are underestimated by public health surveillance because of under-diagnosis (wherein subjects do not seek medical care or are not tested; Thomas et al., 2013), or, in some cases, overestimated due to presumptive diagnosis (e.g., of *Giardia* and prescribing metronidazole) or underreported because positive results not reported to surveillance systems (MacDougall et al., 2008). Difficulties of determining the health impact of enteric parasites are also exacerbated by the lack of a uniform standard for monitoring the incidence of foodborne illness directly attributed to parasitic infections (Broglia and Kapel, 2011).

Of the protozoa that could be transmitted by food to humans, *Giardia*, *Entamoeba*, and *Cryptosporidium* were identified as those that could produce a "substantial burden" (Torgerson et al., 2014), but these authors did not define what "substantial" means in this context. Trying to determine the global burden is therefore very difficult (Torgerson et al., 2014; FAO, 2014) and perhaps not realistic given the differences between developed and developing countries in terms of the impact enteric parasites can have. Trying to quantify the level of protozoan parasite infection using commonly applied metrics such as the DALY (e.g., Pruss et al., 2002) may be impractical unless gross nonspecific estimates are required as distinguishing between all possible sources of infection and the confounding impact of polyparasitism is rarely if ever possible (Payne et al., 2009; Thompson and Smith, 2011; Lymbery and Thompson, 2012). Poor sanitary conditions and the unavailability of effective water treatment will sustain conditions for their transmission in developing countries. The burden is not only likely to be greater in developing countries, but the chronic nature of these infections, the difficulty of estimating the burden of a particular parasite when polyparasitic infections are the norm, and determining the role of food as a vehicle compared to direct, mechanical, or water transmission, question the wisdom of trying to determine global estimates.

Epidemiological analysis of focal point contaminations caused by food contamination events can provide good estimates of the spread and impact of parasite infection. But on a global scale, due to the uncertainty caused by the scarcity of data (Payne et al., 2009), the impact of these occurrences remains poorly understood (Thompson and Smith, 2011). Statistical data of the economic costs of parasitic foodborne illness is mostly lacking or inaccurate (Orlandi et al., 2002). From an individual perspective, one has to take into account medical costs and lost wages. In outbreak situations, the costs could be very high, depending on the circumstances, and could involve industry recalls, litigation, and diminished reputation (Hellard et al., 2003; Imhoff et al., 2004; Buzby and Roberts, 2009).

7.10 Control and future trends

Food hygiene and management practices in food service and catering industries must be adequate, and hazard analysis plans need to be employed (FAO, 2014). People working in high-risk environments such as schools, day care centers, food-handling facilities, and senior care institutions must be educated properly on the risks of infection, and exclusion principles employed for anyone with diarrhea (Fletcher et al., 2012; FAO, 2014).

Given the importance of the fecal–oral route of transmission, areas of cultivation of fresh produce, particularly for raw consumption, need to be assessed in terms of their susceptibility to fecal contamination, whether via runoff from wild animals, farm animals, domestic animals, and/or humans, and the necessary measures taken to manage the identified risk (Nichols, 1999; FAO, 2014). It is important for on-farm sanitation and hygiene to be used to interrupt the life cycle of parasites and to minimize the opportunity for the fecal–oral route of transmission. This can be done with appropriate installation and use of the relevant facilities, for example, functional on-farm latrines and adequate hand-washing facilities. The use of organic fertilizer on produce should be monitored to ensure it is composted adequately to reduce the survival of parasites (FAO, 2014). The situation is exacerbated by the lack of efficient parasite detection methods for fresh produce, especially fruits and vegetables (Robertson et al., 2014).

Education and raising awareness are important components (Thompson and Smith, 2011; FAO, 2014) and may be the only feasible option available (FAO, 2014). Such education and training should be directed to all involved in the food chain, including farm and abattoir workers to food handlers (consumers and food retail outlets). Control strategies should address the whole chain from good animal husbandry practices to hygiene and sanitation (FAO, 2014). Consumers at high risk, such as the pregnant and immunocompromised, should be given particular consideration (Fletcher et al., 2012).

In endemic areas of the developing world, control is a far more difficult problem. Long-term freedom from infection requires education in terms of basic hygiene, but without improvement in sanitation it is difficult to see how the impact of enteric parasite infections can be improved. Drugs are not the answer as studies have shown that once drug pressure is removed without concurrent improvements in hygiene and sanitation, reinfection rapidly occurs (Thompson et al., 2001; Thompson, 2008). The situation is exacerbated by poor nutrition, which renders the clinical impact of enteric parasitic infections much greater than if nutrition levels were adequate.

References

Abdel-Dayem, M., Zou'bi, R.A., Hani, R.B., Amr, Z.S., 2013. Microbiological and parasitological investigation among food handlers in hotels in the Dead Sea area, Jordan. J. Microbiol. Immunol. Infect. 47, 377–380.

Abreu-Acosta, N., Lorenzo-Morales, J., Leal-Guio, Y., Coronado-Alvarez, N., Foronda, P., Alcoba-Florez, J., Izquierdo, F., Batista-Díaz, N., Del Aguila, C., Valladares, B., 2005. *Enterocytozoon bieneusi* (microsporidia) in clinical samples from immunocompetent individuals in Tenerife, Canary Islands, Spain. Trans. R. Soc. Trop. Med. Hyg. 99, 848–855.

Al-Binali, A.M., Bello, C.S., El-Shewy, K., Abdulla, S.E., 2006. The prevalence of parasites in commonly used leafy vegetables in south-western Saudi Arabia. Saudi Med. J. 27, 613–616.

Ballweber, L.R., Xiao, L., Bowman, D.D., Kahn, G., Cama, V.A., 2010. Giardiasis in dogs and cats: update on epidemiology and public health significance. Trends Parasitol. 26, 180–189.

Barr, S.C., 1998. Enteric protozoal infections. In: Greene, C.E. (Ed.), Infectious Diseases of the Dog and Cat. W.B. Saunders, Philadelphia, pp. 482–491.

Barutzki, D., Schaper, R., 2011. Results of parasitological examinations of faecal samples from cats and dogs in Germany between 2003 and 2010. Parasitol. Res. 109, S45–S60.

Bellanger, A.-P., Scherer, E., Cazorla, A., Grenouillet, F., 2013. Dysenteric syndrome due to *Balantidium coli*: a case report. New Microbiol. 36, 203–205.

Berkman, D.S., Lescano, A.G., Gilman, R.H., Lopez, S.L., Black, M.M., 2002. Effects of stunting, diarrhoeal disease, and parasitic infection during infancy on cognition in late childhood: a follow-up study. Lancet 359, 564–571.

Boorom, K.F., Smith, H., Nimri, L., Viscogliosi, E., Spanakos, G., Parkar, U., Li, L.-H., Zhou, X.-N., Ok, U.Z., Leelayoova, S., Jones, M.S., 2008. Oh my aching gut: irritable bowel syndrome, *Blastocystis*, and asymptomatic infection. Parasit. Vectors 1, 40.

Botero-Garcés, J.H., Garcéa-Montoya, G.M., Grisales-Patiéo, D., Aguirre-Acevedo, D.C., Alvarez-Uribe, M.C., 2009. *Giardia intestinalis* and nutritional status in children participating in the complementary nutrition program, Antioquia, Colombia, May to October 2006. Rev. Inst. Med. Trop. Sao Paulo 51, 155–162.

Broglia, A., Kapel, C., 2011. Changing dietary habits in a changing world: emerging drivers for the transmission of foodborne parasitic zoonoses. Vet. Parasitol. 182, 2–13.

Buzby, J.C., Roberts, T., 2009. The economics of enteric infections: human foodborne disease costs. Gastroenterology 136, 1851–1862.

Cama, V., Ortega, Y.R., 2006. Coccidian parasites: *Cyclospora cayetanensis*, *Isospora belli*, *Sarcocystis hominis/suihominis*. In: Ortega, Y.R. (Ed.), Foodborne Parasites. Springer, New York, NY, pp. 33–55.

Chunge, R.N., Karumba, P.N., Nagelkerke, N., Kaleli, N., Wamwea, M., Mutiso, N., Andala, E.O., Kinoti, S.N., 1991. Intestinal parasites in a rural community in Kenya: cross-sectional surveys with emphasis on prevalence, incidence, duration of infection, and polyparasitism. East Afr. Med. J. 68, 112–123.

Colli, C.M., Mizutani, A.S., Martins, V.A., Ferreira, E.C., Gomes, M.L., 2013. Prevalence and risk factors for intestinal parasites in food handlers, southern Brazil. Int. J. Environ. Health Res. 24, 450–458.

Conlan, J., Thompson, R.C.A., Blacksell, S., Fenwick, S., Vongxay, K., Khamlome, B., 2012. Final report for project AH/2006/161, Management of pig-associated zoonoses in Lao PDR. Report number FR2012-14. Australian Centre for International Agricultural Research, Canberra, Australia.

Covacin, C., Aucoin, D.P., Elliot, A., Thompson, R.C.A., 2011. Genotypic characterisation of *Giardia* from domestic dogs in the USA. Vet. Parasitol. 177, 28–32.

Dawson, D., 2005. Foodborne protozoan parasites. Int. J. Food Microbiol. 103, 207–227.

Dengjel, B., Zahler, M., Hermanns, W., Heinritzi, K., Spillmann, T., Thomschke, A., Löscher, T., Gothe, R., Rinder, H., 2001. Zoonotic potential of *Enterocytozoon bieneusi*. J. Clin. Microbiol. 39, 4495–4499.

Didier, E.S., 2005. Microsporidiosis: an emerging and opportunistic infection in humans and animals. Acta Trop. 94, 61–76.

Eyles, D.E., Jones, F.E., Jumper, J.R., Drinnon, V.P., 1954. Amebic infection in dogs. J. Parasitol. 40, 163–166.

FAO, 2014. In: Multicriteria-Based Ranking for Risk Management of Food-Borne Parasites. Microbiological Risk Assessment Series, vol. 23. Food Safety and Codex Unit, Food and Agriculture Organization of the United Nations, Rome, Italy.

Farthing, M.J.G., Cevallos, A.M., Kelly, P., 2003. Intestinal protozoa. In: Cook, G.C., Zumla, A. (Eds.), Manson's Tropical Diseases. W.B. Saunders, London, pp. 1373–1410.

Fletcher, S.M., Stark, D., Harkness, J., Ellis, J., 2012. Enteric protozoa in the developed world: a public health perspective. Clin. Microbiol. Rev. 25, 420–449.

Goodgame, R.W., 1996. Understanding intestinal spore-forming protozoa: cryptosporidia, microsporidia, *isospora*, and *cyclospora*. In: Merson, M., Black, R., Mills, A. (Eds.), Ann. Intern. Med. 124, 429–441.

Hamano, S., Petri Jr., W.A., Kris, H., 2008. Protozoan diseases: amebiasis. In: International Encyclopedia of Public Health. Academic Press, Oxford, United Kingdom, pp. 335–341.

Haque, R., Mondal, D., Kirkpatrick, B.D., Akther, S., Farr, B.M., Sack, R.B., Petri Jr., W.A., 2003. Epidemiologic and clinical characteristics of acute diarrhea with emphasis on *Entamoeba histolytica* infections in preschool children in an urban slum of Dhaka, Bangladesh. Am. J. Trop. Med. Hyg. 69, 398–405.

Hellard, M.E., Sinclair, M.I., Harris, A.H., Kirk, M., Fairley, C.K., 2003. Cost of community gastroenteritis. J. Gastroenterol. Hepatol. 18, 322–328.

Hohweyer, J., Dumetre, A., Aubert, D., Azas, N., Villena, I., 2013. Tools and methods for detecting and characterizing *Giardia*, *Cryptosporidiumi*, and *Toxoplasma* parasites in marine mollusks. J. Food Prot. 9, 1488–1657.

Imhoff, B., Morse, D., Shiferaw, B., Hawkins, M., Vugia, D., Lance-Parker, S., Hadler, J., Medus, C., Kennedy, M., Moore, M.R., Van Gilder, T., Emerging Infections Program FoodNet Working Group, 2004. Burden of self-reported acute diarrheal illness in FoodNet surveillance areas, 1998 and 1999. Clin. Infect. Dis. 38, S219–S226.

Insulander, M., Svenungsson, B., Lebbad, M., Karlsson, L., de Jong, B., 2010. A foodborne outbreak of *Cyclospora* infection in Stockholm, Sweden. Foodborne Pathog. Dis. 7, 1585–1587.

Iwamoto, M., Ayers, T., Mahon, B.E., Swerdlow, D.L., 2010. Epidemiology of seafood-associated infections in the United States. Clin. Microbiol. Rev. 23, 399–411.

Jedrzejewski, S., Graczyk, T.K., Slodkowicz-Kowalska, A., Tamang, L., Majewska, A.C., 2007. Quantitative assessment of contamination of fresh produce of various retail types by human-virulent microsporidiean spores. Appl. Environ. Microbiol. 73, 4071–4073.

Karanis, P., Kourenti, C., Smith, H., 2007. Waterborne transmission of protozoan parasites: a worldwide review of outbreaks and lessons learnt. J. Water Health 5, 1–38.

Kheirandish, F., Tarahi, M.J., Ezatpour, B., 2014. Prevalence of intestinal parasites among food handlers in Western Iran. Rev. Inst. Med. Trop. Sao Paulo 56, 111–114.

Lal, A., Baker, M.G., Hales, S., French, N.P., 2013. Potential effects of global environmental changes on cryptosporidiosis and giardiasis transmission. Trends Parasitol. 29, 83–90.

Lores, B., López-Miragaya, I., Arias, C., Fenoy, S., Torres, J., del Aguila, C., 2002. Intestinal microsporidiosis due to *Enterocytozoon bieneusi* in elderly human immunodeficiency virus negative patients from Vigo, Spain. Clin. Infect. Dis. 34, 918–921.

Lymbery, A.J., Thompson, R.C.A., 2012. The molecular epidemiology of parasite infections: tools and applications. Mol. Biochem. Parasitol. 181, 102–116.

Lynch, M., Painter, J., Woodruff, R., Braden, C., 2006. Surveillance for foodborne-disease outbreaks—United States, 1998–2002. Morb. Mortal. Wkly. Rep. 55, 1–48.

MacDougall, L., Majowicz, S., Doré, K., Flint, J., Thomas, K., Kovacs, S., Sockett, P., 2008. Under-reporting of infectious gastrointestinal illness in British Columbia, Canada: who is counted in provincial communicable disease statistics? Epidemiol. Infect. 136, 248–256.

Meloni, B.P., Thompson, R.C.A., Hopkins, R.M., Reynoldson, J.A., Gracey, M., 1993. The prevalence of *Giardia* and other intestinal parasites in children, dogs and cats from Aboriginal communities in the Kimberley. Med. J. Aust. 158, 157–159.

Millard, P.S., Gensheimer, K.F., Addiss, D.G., Sosin, D.M., Beckett, G.A., Houck-Jankoski, A., Hudson, A., 1994. An outbreak of cryptosporidiosis from fresh-pressed apple cider. J. Am. Vet. Med. Assoc. 272, 1592–1596.

Mortimer, L., Chadee, K., 2010. The immunopathogenesis of *Entamoeba histolytica*. Exp. Parasitol. 126, 366–380.

Nematian, J., Gholamrezanezhad, A., Nematian, E., 2008. Giardiasis and other intestinal parasitic infections in relation to anthropometric indicators of malnutrition: a large, population-based survey of schoolchildren in Tehran. Ann. Trop. Med. Parasitol. 102, 209–214.

Nichols, G.L., 1999. Food-borne protozoa. Br. Med. Bull. 55, 209–235.

Nimri, L.F., Elnasser, Z., Batchoun, R., 2004. Polymicrobial infections in children with diarrhoea in a rural area of Jordan. FEMS Immunol. Med. Microbiol. 42, 255–259.

Nyarango, R.M., Aloo, P.A., Kabiru, E.W., Nyanchongi, B.O., 2008. The risk of pathogenic intestinal parasite infections in Kisii Municipality, Kenya. BMC Public Health 8, 237.

Orlandi, P., Chu, D., Bier, J., Jackson, G., 2002. Parasites and the food supply. Food Technol. 56, 72–80.

Ouattara, M., Silue, K.D., N'Guessan, A.N., Yapi, A., Barbara, M., Raso, G., Utzinger, J., N'Goran, E., 2008. Prevalence and polyparasitism of intestinal protozoa and spatial distribution of *Entamoeba histolytica, E. dispar* and *Giardia intestinalis* from pupils in the rural zone in Cote d'Ivoire. Sante 18, 215–222.

Owen, I.L., 2005. Parasitic zoonoses in Papua New Guinea. J. Helminthol. 79, 1–14.

Palmer, C.S., Thompson, R.C.A., Traub, R.J., Rees, R., Robertson, I.D., 2008a. National study of the gastrointestinal parasites of dogs and cats in Australia. Vet. Parasitol. 151, 181–190.

Palmer, C.S., Traub, R.J., Robertson, I.D., Devlin, G., Rees, R., Thompson, R.C.A., 2008b. Determining the zoonotic significance of *Giardia* and *Cryptosporidium* in Australian dogs and cats. Vet. Parasitol. 154, 142–147.

Parkar, U., Traub, R.J., Kumar, S., Mungthin, M., Vitali, S., Leelayoova, S., Morris, K., Thompson, R.C.A., 2007. Direct characterisation of *Blastocystis* from faeces by PCR and evidence of zoonotic potential. Parasitology 134, 1–9.

Parkar, U., Traub, R.J., Vitali, S., Elliot, A., Levecke, B., Robertson, I.D., Geurden, T., Steele, J., Drake, B., Thompson, R.C.A., 2010. Molecular characterisation of *Blastocystis* isolates from zoo animals and their animal-keepers. Vet. Parasitol. 169, 8–17.

Payne, R.J., Turner, L., Morgan, E.R., 2009. Inappropriate measures of population health for parasitic disease? Trends Parasitol. 25, 393–395.

Polley, L., Thompson, R.C.A., 2009. Parasite zoonoses and climate change: molecular tools for tracking shifting boundaries. Trends Parasitol. 25, 285–291.

Pönka, A., Kotilainen, H., Rimhanen-Finne, R., Hokkanen, P., Hänninen, M.L., Kaarna, A., Meri, T., Kuusi, M., 2009. A foodborne outbreak due to *Cryptosporidium parvum* in Helsinki, November 2008. Euro Surveill. 14 (28), pii: 19269.

Pruss, A., Kay, D., Fewtrell, L., Bartram, J., 2002. Estimating the burden of disease from water, sanitation, and hygiene at a global level. Environ. Health Perspect. 110, 537–542.

Requena, I., Hernández, Y., Ramsay, M., Salazar, C., Devera, R., 2003. Prevalence of *Blastocystis hominis* among food handlers from Caroni municipality, Bolivar State, Venezuela. Cad. Saude Publica 19, 6.

Robertson, L.J., Sprong, H., Ortega, Y.R., van der Giessen, J.W.B., Fayer, R., 2014. Impacts of globalization on foodborne parasites. Trends Parasitol. 30, 37–52.

Savioli, L., Smith, H., Thompson, R.C.A., 2006. *Giardia* and *Cryptosporidium* join the 'Neglected Diseases Initiative'. Trends Parasitol. 22, 203–208.

Scallan, E., Griffin, P.M., Angulo, F.J., Tauxe, R.V., Hoekstra, R.M., 2011. Foodborne illness acquired in the United States—major pathogens. Emerg. Infect. Dis. 17, 7–15.

Schär, F., Inpankaew, T., Traub, R.J., Khieu, V., Dalsgaard, A., Chimnoi, W., Chhoun, C., Sok, D., Marti, H., Muth, S., Odermatt, P., 2014. The prevalence and diversity of intestinal parasitic infections in humans and domestic animals in a rural Cambodian village. Parasitol. Int. 63, 597–603.

Schuster, F.L., Ramirez-Avila, L., 2008. Current world status of *Balantidium coli*. Clin. Microbiol. Rev. 21, 626–638.

Schuster, F.L., Visvesvara, G.S., 2004. Amebae and ciliated protozoa as causal agents of waterborne zoonotic disease. Vet. Parasitol. 126, 91–120.

Singh, M., Suresh, K., Ho, L.C., Ng, G.C., Yap, E.H., 1995. Elucidation of the life cycle of the intestinal protozoan *Blastocystis hominis*. Parasitol. Res. 81, 446–450.

Slifko, T.R., Smith, H.V., Rose, J.B., 2000. Emerging parasite zoonoses associated with water and food. Int. J. Parasitol. 30, 1379–1393.

Smith, H.V., Nichols, R.A., 2006. Zoonotic protozoa-food for thought. Parassitologia 48, 101–104.

Smith, H.V., Cacciò, S.M., Cook, N., Nichols, R.A., Tait, A., 2007. *Cryptosporidium* and *Giardia* as foodborne zoonoses. Vet. Parasitol. 149, 29–40.

Stark, D., van Hal, S., Barratt, J., Ellis, J., Marriott, D., Harkness, J., 2009. Limited genetic diversity among genotypes of *Enterocytozoon bieneusi* strains isolated from HIV-infected patients from Sydney, Australia. J. Med. Microbiol. 58, 355–357.

Szostakowska, B., Kruminis-Lozowska, W., Racewicz, M., Knight, R., Tamang, L., Myjak, P., Graczyk, T.K., 2004. *Cryptosporidium parvum* and *Giardia lamblia* recovered from flies on a cattle farm and in a landfill. Appl. Environ. Microbiol. 70, 3742–3744.

Thomas, M.K., Murray, R., Flockhart, L., Pintar, K., Pollari, F., Fazi, A., Nesbitt, A., Marshall, B., 2013. Estimates of the burden of foodborne illness in Canada for 30 specified pathogens and unspecified agents, circa 2006. Foodborne Pathog. Dis. 10, 639–648.

Thompson, R.C.A., 2008. Giardiasis: modern concepts in control and management. Ann. Nestle 66, 29–35.

Thompson, R.C.A., 2009. The impact of *Giardia* on science and society. In: Ortega Pierres, G., Caccio, S.M., Fayer, R., Monk, T.G., Smith, H.V., Thompson, R.C.A. (Eds.), *Giardia* and *Cryptopsoridium*: from molecules to disease. CAB International, Wallingford, pp. 1–11.

Thompson, R.C.A., 2011. *Giardia* infections. In: Palmer, S.R., Soulsby, E.J.L., Torgerson, P., Brown, D. (Eds.), Zoonoses. Oxford University Press, Oxford, pp. 522–535.

Thompson, R.C.A., Smith, A., 2011. Zoonotic enteric protozoa. Vet. Parasitol. 182, 70–78.

Thompson, R.C.A., Reynoldson, J.A., Garrow, S.J., McCarthy, J.S., Behnke, J.M., 2001. Towards the eradication of hookworm in an isolated Australian community. Lancet 357, 770–771.

Thompson, R.C.A., Palmer, C.S., O'Handley, R., 2008. The public health and clinical significance of *Giardia* and *Cryptosporidium* in domestic animals. Vet. J. 177, 18–25.

Torgerson, P.R., de Silva, N.R., Fevre, E.M., Kasuga, F., Rokni, M.B., Zhou, X.-N., Sripa, B., Gargouri, N., Willingham, A.L., Stein, C., 2014. The global burden of foodborne parasitic diseases: an update. Trends Parasitol. 30, 20–26.

van Hal, S.J., et al., 2007. Declining incidence of intestinal microsporidiosis and reduction in AIDS-related mortality following introduction of HAART in Sydney, Australia. Trans. R. Soc. Trop. Med. Hyg. 101, 1096–1100.

Vassalos, C.M., Papadopoulou, C., Vakalis, N.C., 2008. Blastocystosis: an emerging or re-emerging potential zoonosis? Vet. Ital. 44, 679–684.

Wang, W., Owen, H., Traub, R.J., Cuttell, L., Inpankaew, T., Bielefeldt-Ohmann, H., 2014. Molecular epidemiology of *Blastocystis* in pigs and their in-contact humans in southeast Queensland, Australia, and Cambodia. Vet. Parasitol. 203, 264–269.

Yoshikawa, H., Wu, Z., Pandey, K., Pandey, B.D., Sherchand, J.B., Yanagi, T., Kanbara, H., 2008. Molecular characterization of *Blastocystis* isolates from children and rhesus monkeys in Kathmandu, Nepal. Vet. Parasitol. 160, 295–300.

Zaman, V., 1998. *Balantidium coli*. In: Cox, F.E.G., Kreier, J.P., Wakelin, D. (Eds.), Topley and Wilson's Microbiology and Microbial Infections. Arnold, London, pp. 445–450.

Zingales, B., Miles, M.A., Campbell, D.A., Tibayrenc, M., Macedo, A.M., Teixeira, M.M.G., Schijman, A.G., Llewellyn, M.S., Lages-Silva, E., Machado, C.R., Andrade, S.G., Sturm, N.R., 2012. The revised *Trypanosoma cruzi* subspecific nomenclature: rationale, epidemiological relevance and research applications. Infect. Genet. Evol. 12, 240–253.

Foodborne nematodes

8

E. Pozio
Istituto Superiore di Sanità, Rome, Italy

8.1 Introduction

Nematodes are roundworms belonging to the phylum Nemathelminthes. Of the more than half a million species identified so far, most are free-living organisms, and only 7000 are parasites of plants or animals. These worms complete their life cycle through four molts from fist-stage larvae (L1) to the adult stage. Typically, the infective stage for the final host is the L3. Notable exceptions are parasites of the genera *Trichinella* and *Bayliascaris*, which use infective L1 and L2, respectively. Most parasitic nematodes transmitted to humans by food are zoonotic in origin, and in some cases (*Ascaris* spp. and *Trichostrongylus* spp.) humans, in addition to animals, can act as reservoirs. Some of these pathogens have a cosmopolitan distribution (e.g., *Trichinella* spp., *Anisakis* spp., *Pseudoterranova* spp., *Ascaris* spp., *Toxocara* spp.); others are prevalent in the tropics (*Capillaria philippinensis*, *Gnathostoma* spp., *Angiostrongylus* spp., *Capillaria hepatica*, *Trichostrongylus* spp.). International travel to the tropics has increased over the past few decades, with a subsequent and significant increase in the number of patients presenting with tropical diseases in countries where such infections are not endemic. It is estimated that 50 million residents of developed countries travel annually to such areas, resulting in exposure to a broad range of pathogens rarely, if ever, encountered at home (Robertson et al., 2014). Such infections are rarely seen by physicians in temperate climates, and therefore diagnosis can prove elusive if these infections are not considered. Travelers are becoming increasingly adventurous in choice of country, and in the pursuit of remoteness and immersion in exotic cultures, which frequently include consuming local delicacies without consideration of pathogen risk. Migration has also increased substantially over the past few decades, with people from the tropics and subtropics to the West, and many unknowingly translocate harboring parasites (Herman and Chiodini, 2009). Humans harbor or become exposed to many of these pathogens due to conditions involving poverty and low socioeconomic status, poor sanitation, and lack of education. In fact, the transmission of the great majority of these nematode pathogens to humans can be easily prevented by cooking to a core temperature of at least 65 °C for meat, fish, and invertebrates. Nematode transmission by vegetables and other vehicles can also be prevented by improved sanitary and food production conditions and consumer and farmer education.

Foodborne Parasites in the Food Supply Web. http://dx.doi.org/10.1016/B978-1-78242-332-4.00008-4

8.2 Meat borne nematodes

8.2.1 *Trichinella spp.*

8.2.1.1 *Introduction*

Nematode worms belonging to the *Trichinella* genus are the etiological agent of trichinellosis (synonym: trichinosis), a zoonotic disease acquired by humans from the ingestion of raw or undercooked meat and meat-derived products of different animal origins (e.g., pork, horse, game) (Gottstein et al., 2009). These parasites are widespread in wildlife with carnivores and omnivores being the most important reservoirs on all continents but Antarctica, and in free-ranging and backyard pigs of many countries (Pozio, 2007, 2014). Within the genus, nine species and three genotypes are currently recognized: *Trichinella spiralis*, *Trichinella nativa*, *Trichinella britovi*, *Trichinella pseudospiralis*, *Trichinella murrelli*, *Trichinella nelsoni*, *Trichinella papuae*, *Trichinella zimbabwensis*, *Trichinella patagoniensis*, and genotypes T6, T8, and T9 (Pozio and Zarlenga, 2013). Members of all taxa can infect mammals including humans. Furthermore, *T. pseudospiralis* also infects birds, and *T. papuae* and *T. zimbabwensis* also infect some reptile species (crocodiles, monitor lizards, and possibly some turtle species). The infective stage is the L1, which occurs in the cells of striated muscles. As a role, the L1 can survive for several years in the muscle tissues of its hosts and for weeks to months in decaying tissues of dead hosts, depending on the environmental temperature and moisture. Muscle larvae of some species can survive freezing for long periods of time depending on the parasite and host species (Pozio and Murrell, 2006). The average yearly incidence of the disease in humans worldwide is several thousand cases with a mortality rate of about 0.2% (Murrell and Pozio, 2011). The global number of disability-adjusted life years due to trichinellosis was estimated to be 76 per billion per year (Devleesschauwer et al., 2015).

8.2.1.2 *Biology*

Nematodes of the *Trichinella* genus develop two generations of worms in the same host (Figure 8.1). Gravid female worms (1.26–3.35 mm × 29–39 μm) embedded in the intestinal mucosa produce newborn larvae (NBL, 110 μm × 7 μm) that migrate into the lymphatic vessels, then enter the blood vessels to reach and penetrate striated muscle cells. In the muscle cell, NBL develop to the infective L1 (the muscle larva measure 0.65–1.1 mm × 25–40 μm) in about 15 days (Despommier, 1998). In muscle cells, larvae are coiled and enclosed by a collagen capsule (encapsulated species: *T. spiralis*, *T. nativa*, *T. britovi*, *T. murrelli*, *T. nelsoni*, *T. patagoniensis*, and genotypes T6, T8, and T9), or appear to be free among the muscle fibers (nonencapsulated species: *T. pseudospiralis*, *T. papuae*, and *T. zimbabwensis*). The size of the collagen capsule is about 350–450 μm × 180–300 μm. In this ecological niche, larvae can survive for many years (over 20 years in polar bears and up to 40 years in humans) waiting to be ingested by a new host. When a new host ingests infected muscle tissues, the larvae are released from the muscle cells in the stomach by digestion. In the duodenum, they penetrate into the villa and within 2 days undergo four molts, and rapidly develop to the adult stage. Males and females copulate, and 6–7 days postinfection,

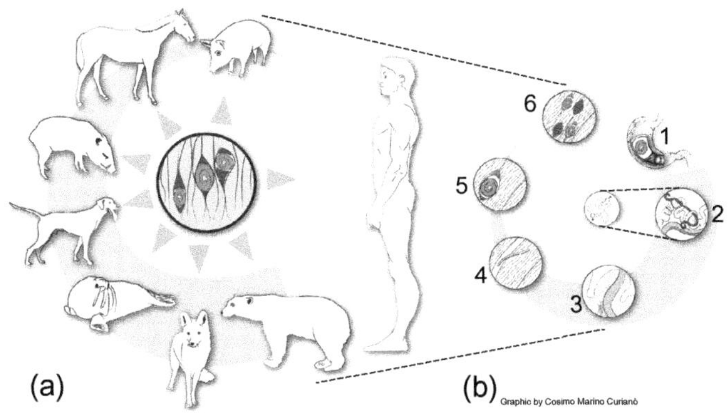

Figure 8.1 Life cycle of *Trichinella* spp. (a) Main domestic and sylvatic sources for *Trichinella* spp. infection in humans. (b) Developmental cycle that occurs within hosts: 1—ingested muscle tissues are digested in the stomach and first-stage larvae (L1) are released; 2—L1 penetrate the intestinal mucosa of the small intestine and develop to sexually active adult males and females within 48h; 3—female worms release NBL, which are transported by lymphatic and blood vessels; 4—NBL exit capillaries and enter cells of striated muscles; 5—the larvae grow to infective L1 within the muscle cell (nurse cell) and, depending on the species of *Trichinella*, may be enclosed by a capsule (encapsulated); 6—if the infected muscle is not ingested by a new host to repeat the cycle, the L1 die after a period of time ranging from weeks to years and are eventually calcified.

the females begin to produce NBL for at least 1–2 weeks or longer as influenced by the host's immune response at the gut level, which usually develops and results in the adult worm expulsion. The currently described 12 *Trichinella* taxa cannot be identified by their morphology at the species or genotype level. Each taxon can be reliably identified only by molecular methods (Pozio and La Rosa, 2010).

8.2.1.3 Epidemiology

Trichinella spp. are prevalent in wildlife. Spillover from wild animals to domestic animals can occur when there is improper management in segregating livestock and wildlife (Pozio and Murrell, 2006). There is no documented evidence of infection in pigs reared in herds kept under controlled management conditions. *T. spiralis* is the species more adapted to swine and, consequently, it is the species more frequently detected in domestic pigs. The domestic and the sylvatic cycles can function either independently from each other or interactively. The term *domestic cycle* refers to the transmission pattern where the focus is on a swine herd being fed, such as uncooked pork scraps, carrion, uncooked garbage (i.e., garbage-fed pigs), or the pigs can feed on carcasses that are not promptly removed from the farm; transmission can also become domestic via synanthropic animals (e.g., rats and mustelids) living near swine herds (Pozio, 2014). Horses fattened with pork scraps or with carcasses of carnivorous animals became infected with *Trichinella*. The use of *Trichinella*-infected meat of slaughtered crocodiles to feed other farmed crocodiles has been reported (Pozio and Murrell, 2006). The most common source of infection for humans is pork and pork-derived products from backyard and free-ranging pigs, wild boar, and wild pigs; other sources responsible for outbreaks include horses, bears, walruses, and dogs (Table 8.1).

Table 8.1 **Epidemiological information of foodborne nematodes and main clinical signs and symptoms in humans**

Parasite	Distribution	Hosts	Source of infection for humans	Main clinical signs and symptoms in humans
Trichinella spp.	Cosmopolitan	Domestic and wild swine, horses, wild carnivores and omnivores, including birds and reptiles	Raw meat and raw meat-derived products from domestic animals (e.g., swine, horse) and game (e.g., wild boar, walrus, bear)	Intestinal phase: loose stools or diarrhea, flatulence, abdominal pain, loss of appetite and sometimes vomiting Parenteral phase: general weakness, chills, headache, fever (up to 40 °C), excessive sweating, tachycardia, symmetrical eyelid and periocular edema (edema frequently affects the entire face), eosinophilia, leukocytosis, and alterations in muscle enzymes
Anisakis spp., *Pseudoterranova* spp.	Cosmopolitan	First intermediate hosts: marine fish or squid Final hosts: sea mammals	Raw or marinated sea fish	Gastric or intestinal anisakiosis: intermittent epigastric pain, nausea and vomiting Allergic reactions: isolated swelling to urticaria and life-threatening anaphylactic shock
Capillaria philippinensis	Philippines, Lao PDR, Japan, Taiwan, Korea, Indonesia, Iran, Egypt	First intermediate hosts: freshwater or brackish-water fish; final hosts: fish-eating birds, humans	Raw freshwater or brackish-water fish	Watery diarrhea weight loss, abdominal pain, borborygmi, muscle wasting, weakness, edema, malabsorption of fats and sugar, and low levels of potassium and albumin in blood
Gnathostoma spp.	Africa, Australia, China, Japan, India, Korea, Southeast Asia, Sri Lanka, Central and South America, Spain	First intermediate host: copepods Second intermediate hosts: fish, birds, amphibians, reptiles, and mammals Fish-eating mammals	Raw meat of catfish, eels, frogs, chickens, ducks, and snakes	Malaise, fever, urticaria, anorexia, nausea, vomiting, diarrhea, and epigastric or right upper quadrant pain and eosinophilia Cutaneous form: intermittent migratory swellings Gastrointestinal, genitourinary, CNS, ocular, or pulmonary manifestations

Angiostrongylus cantonensis	Africa, Asia, Australasia, Pacific and Caribbean islands, South Central and North America	First intermediate hosts: snails and slugs Paratenic hosts: shrimp, land crab, frog, lizard, and land planarian Final hosts: rats	Consumption of raw intermediate or paratenic hosts	Eosinophilic meningitis: headache, neck stiff, paresthesias, vomiting and nausea, face or limb paralysis Ocular angiostrongyliasis: photophobia, and diplopia
Angiostrongylus costaricensis	North, Central and South America	First intermediate hosts: slugs of Veronicellidae family Final hosts: rats, coati-mundi, marmoset, dog	Consumption of raw intermediate or paratenic hosts	Fever, anorexia, vomiting, diarrhea, constipation, and abdominal rigidity
Ascaris spp.	Cosmopolitan	Humans, pigs	Raw vegetables and other vehicles contaminated by infected human or pig feces	Lung inflammation, fever, abdominal pain, nausea, intestinal obstruction, and retarded growth and mental development in children
Toxocara spp.	Cosmopolitan	Dogs, cats, wild canides	Raw vegetables and other vehicles contaminated by dog or cat feces	Visceral larva migrant syndrome: weight loss, fever, asthmatic cough, wheezing, generalized lymphadenopathy Ocular syndrome: vision loss Neurological syndrome: meningitis, meningoencephalitis or transverse myelitis
Baylisascaris procionis	North America, Europe, Japan	Raccoons and other procyonid species	Raw vegetables and other vehicles contaminated by raccoon feces	Sudden lethargy, circling, ataxia, paralysis, tremor, seizures, torticollis, opisthotonus, nystagmus, dysphagia, and stupor progressing to coma
Capillaria hepatica	Cosmopolitan	Rats and other animals	Food and water contaminated by eggs	Fever, hepatomegaly, and leukocytosis with eosinophilia
Trichostrongylus spp.	Cosmopolitan	Humans, livestock	Eggs	Generally asymptomatic, but in highly infected persons (more than 100 worms), diarrhea, abdominal pain, nausea, mild anemia, and weight loss, have been documented

8.2.1.4 Infection in humans

The first signs of *Trichinella* infection commonly include diarrhea and abdominal pain due to intestinal invasion. This is usually followed by a few days of fever and myalgia (a flulike malaise) and then disappears in less than 1 week in mild infections. It has been observed that the shorter the duration between infection and the appearance of diarrhea and fever, the longer the duration of both fever and facial edema. In most persons, the acute stage begins with the sudden appearance of general discomfort and severe headaches, an increase in fever, chills, and excessive sweating. The major syndrome of the acute stage consists of persistent fever (39–40 °C for 8–10 days), periorbital or facial edema, myalgia, and severe asthenia. These signs and symptoms are always associated with high eosinophilia, leucocytosis, and increased muscle enzymes (Dupouy-Camet et al., 2002). In rare cases of severe infection, death may occur due to early cardiac insufficiency, encephalitis, or pneumonia. Sudden death resulting from the passage of NBL into the myocardium has also been described.

8.2.1.5 Diagnosis and treatment

The diagnosis of trichinellosis should be based on anamnesis (e.g., raw meat consumption), clinical signs and symptoms, and laboratory tests (immunodiagnosis or muscle biopsy). The diagnostic technique most used is enzyme-linked immunosorbent assay (ELISA) with excretory/secretory antigens, which have the highest ratio between sensitivity and specificity and is best used in combination with Western blot to confirm ELISA-positive results (Gómez-Morales et al., 2012). Seroconversion occurs between 12 and 60 days postinfection. To recover larvae for species identification or confirmation of infection, muscle biopsy (0.2–0.5 g of muscle tissue) should be collected preferentially from the deltoid muscle. *Trichinella* larvae can be detected in the biopsy by compressorium, HCl-pepsin digestion, or histological analysis. The collection of the muscle biopsy is seldom because it is an expensive, invasive, and very painful method. The two drugs of choice are mebendazole (25 mg/kg two to three times a day for 15 days) and albendazole (20 mg/kg two to three times a day for 15 days). Corticosteroids should be used for symptomatic treatment (e.g., prednisolone 30–60 mg/day) and always in combination with anthelmintic, but caution should be exercised due to the possibility of anaphylactic shock (Dupouy-Camet et al., 2002).

8.2.1.6 Infection in animals

Naturally infected animals are not known to show any clinical sign of the disease even when the worm burden has been very high (e.g., more than 8000 larvae/g in the diaphragm pillars of pigs) (Pozio, 2014). In experimentally infected pigs, dyspnea, periorbital edema, and reduced weight gain have been observed in some animals (Ribicich et al., 2007); however, these clinical signs cannot easily be detected in pigs reared in herds kept without controlled management conditions, that is, the only pigs at risk for *Trichinella* infections. The preferential muscles for infection can vary according to the host species (European Commission, 2005).

8.2.1.7 Detection, control, and prevention

To detect *Trichinella* infection in domestic or wild animals, samples of preferential muscles should be tested by artificial digestion (European Commission, 2005; Nöckler and Kapel, 2007; Table 8.2). The sensitivity of testing 1 g per carcass is about three to five larvae per gram (LPG) but it can reach one LPG when a sample of 5 g per carcass is tested. In field conditions, the compressorium method (trichinoscopy) can be used. This method shows a sensitivity of approximately three LPG when carried out properly by skilled personnel, but it usually misses *Trichinella* larvae belonging to nonencapsulated species. Once isolated from infected muscles, larvae can be identified to the species or genotype level by a molecular method (Pozio and La Rosa, 2010). Such identification of larvae is very useful for epidemiological and risk-based studies (Pozio, 2014). Since parasites of the genus *Trichinella* circulate mainly among wildlife, the main preventative measures for farmed animals are to (1) avoid access to wild animal carcasses, their scraps, and offal to domestic animals; (2) avoid the use of wild animal carcasses, their scraps, and offal for feeding domestic animals; (3) avoid access to pig carcasses, their scraps, and offal to domestic animals; and (4) avoid free range of domestic pigs in the wild (OIE, 2013; Pozio, 2014).

Table 8.2 Detection, control, and prevention of foodborne nematodes

Parasite	Detection	Control and prevention
Trichinella spp.	Detection of larvae in preferential muscle tissues of susceptible animals (mammals, birds, and reptiles) by pepsin–HCl digestion or by compressorium; the amount of digested muscles should be proportional to the risk of infection (e.g., 1 g from diaphragm pillars of fattening pigs, 2 g from diaphragm pillars of sows and boars; 10 g from diaphragm pillars of horses)	Search of larvae in all animals at risk for *Trichinella* intended for human consumption (backyards and free-ranging pigs, horses, game); improvement of pig-rearing practices; consumption of well-cooked meat; meat freezing
Anisakis spp., *Pseudoterranova* spp.	Detection of larvae in the coelomic cavity and in the muscle tissues of marine fish by visual inspection, candling, digestion, compressorium under UV light	Consumption of cooked fish; avoid waste elimination from fishing vessels; freezing treatment; salting
Capillaria philippinensis	Not feasible	Consumption of cooked fish, proper disposal of human feces, improvement of sanitary conditions

Continued

Table 8.2 Continued

Parasite	Detection	Control and prevention
Gnathostoma spp.	Not feasible	Consumption of well-cooked intermediate and paratenic hosts; drink only boiled or treated waters
Angiostrongylus spp.	Not feasible	Rodent and mollusc control, consumption of frozen and well-cooked snails; thorough washing of vegetables that are eaten raw
Ascaris spp.	Search of eggs in human and pig feces after concentration by a microscope	Improvement in sanitation, health education, and anthelminthic treatment of both human and pigs; improvement of pig herd systems and management practices
Toxocara spp.	Search of eggs in dog and cat feces	Anthelminthic treatment of dogs and cats; sandboxes should be steam sterilized or the sand should be replaced
Baylisascaris procionis	Search of eggs in pet raccoon feces	Elimination of raccoon defecation sites from backyards by burning; reduction of raccoon populations; deworming of pet raccoons
Capillaria hepatica	Not feasible	Rodent control and sanitary disposal of dead animals
Trichostrongylus spp.	Search of eggs in human and ruminant feces	Proper disposal of human and ruminant feces; periodic treatment of ruminant with anthelminthic; pasture rotation

8.3 Fish borne nematodes

8.3.1 Anisakis *spp. and* Pseudoterranova *spp.*

8.3.1.1 *Introduction*

Anisakidiosis (synonyms: anisakiasis, anisakiosis) is the result of accidental human infection with the larval stage of several nematode species found in raw or undercooked marine fish or squid. The first case of human infection by an Anisakidae worm was reported more than 50 years ago in the Netherlands by Van Thiel et al. (1960). Anisakidiosis has been increasingly identified as the cause of gastric, intestinal, and allergic syndromes in humans who consume uncooked seafood or have occupational exposure to seafood (Audicana and Kennedy, 2008). Most human infections of anisakidiosis are caused by worms of two genera of Anisakidae: *Anisakis* and *Pseudoterranova* (Pozio, 2013).

8.3.1.2 Biology

The eggs produced by the adult Anisakidae worms that are found mainly in the stomachs of cetaceans (e.g., whales, dolphins, and porpoises) or pinnipeds (e.g., seals, sea lions, and walruses) are excreted with the hosts' feces and hatch in the water. The hatched larvae are ingested by a wide variety of crustaceans in which the prevalence of infection is generally low (<1%). When infected crustaceans are eaten by fish and cephalopods, the larvae migrate to the coelomic cavity where they become encapsulated. When another fish or cephalopod ingests the infected fish, the new host acts as a paratenic host (i.e., the parasites do not develop further and remain at the L3 stage). Definitive hosts acquire the infection by eating infected fish, cephalopods, or crustaceans (Figure 8.2). Primary fish hosts are predominantly planktivores, such as herring, haddock, blue whiting, and juvenile plaice, mackerel and cod, which acquire the parasite directly from crustacean hosts. Secondary fish hosts are piscivorous, such as blue shark, barracuda, monkfish, and conger eel, which usually acquire the parasite from infected planktivorous fish (Pozio, 2013). Humans do not play a role in the life cycle of these parasites. Most of species of the genera *Anisakis* and *Pseudoterranova* are morphologically indistinguishable among them. Each taxon can be identified by polymerase chain reaction (PCR) methods (La Rosa et al., 2006).

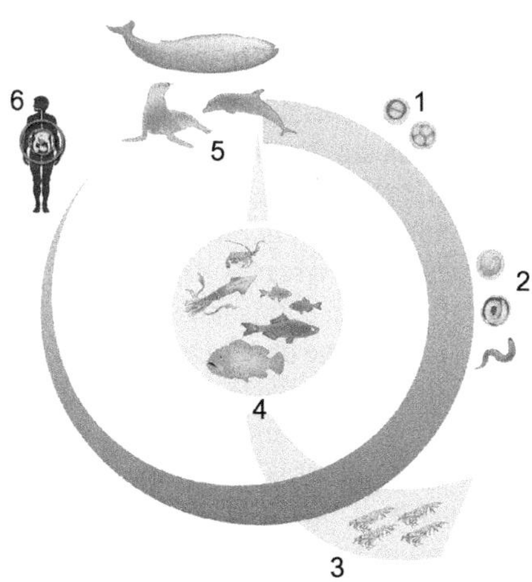

Figure 8.2 Life cycle of *Anisakis* spp. and *Pseudoterranova* spp. 1—Worm eggs are shed with the feces of marine mammals in seawater; 2—the embryo develops to the L1–L3 stages within the egg, after which the larvae are released into seawater; 3—krill and copepods ingest L1–L3 stages which develop to the L3 stage or remain at the L3 stage; 4—L3 are ingested by fish, crustaceans, and cephalopods, which act as paratenic hosts; 5—once an infected fish, crustacean, or cephalopod with L3 is ingested by a marine mammal (pinnipeds and cetaceans), the worms develop to adults in the gut; and humans become infected when they accidentally ingest infected fish, crustaceans, or cephalopods.

8.3.1.3 Epidemiology

A large number of fish and cephalopod species act as hosts for *Anisakis* spp. (200 fish and 25 cephalopod species) and *Pseudoterranova* spp. (75 fish species in the North Atlantic alone); it is believed that most species of fish and cephalopods can potentially harbor these parasites (Mattiucci and Nascetti, 2008). There is a higher prevalence and larval burden in larger and older fish and in carnivorous fish. The prevalence of infection in fish and cephalopods depends on their specific feeding behavior and biology and can range from less than 1% to nearly 100%. Factors favoring an increase of Anisakidae nematodes in fish and cephalopods are: (1) increasing attention focused on these zoonotic parasites and their impact on public health; (2) changes in food preferences with an increase of raw fish consumption; (3) expanding population size of the definitive hosts, due to the increasing public concerns for the protection of marine mammals; and (4) practice of untreated waste dumping from fishing vessels into the sea. The migration of larvae from the coelomic cavity to the muscles in fish is epidemiologically important, in that the muscles are the part of the fish that is consumed by humans (Table 8.1). In live fish, it is still unclear whether the migration of larvae is influenced by the Anisakidae species, or by the host species or fish age. When the fish dies, it is believed that larvae can migrate from the coelomic cavity to the muscles depending on the postmortem environmental conditions for example, the longer the time between death and evisceration, the higher the number of larvae in the muscles. Although the larvae can also reach distal muscles, most of them remain trapped in the abdominal muscles (belly flaps) of the fish.

8.3.1.4 Infection in humans

Of the approximately 20,000 cases of anisakidiosis reported to date worldwide, over 90% are from Japan (where ~2000 cases are diagnosed annually), with most of the remaining cases in Germany, Italy, the Netherlands, and Spain. When ingested, anisakid larvae invade the stomach or the intestinal wall. *Pseudoterranova decipiens* seems to be more often associated with gastric anisakiosis, whereas *Anisakis simplex* and *Anisakis pegreffii* are more often associated with intestinal anisakiosis. Most of the larvae remain in the gastric or intestinal submucosa and in the chronic stages cause the formation of a granuloma. Rarely, larvae may penetrate other sites (e.g., omentum, mesentery, lymph nodes, pancreas, ovaries, lungs, and liver). The clinical course of gastric anisakidiosis is characterized by an abrupt onset of symptoms (e.g., intermittent epigastric pain, nausea, and vomiting), usually within 6h of ingestion of the larvae. Epigastric pain is often very severe and may not respond to analgesics. In persons with intestinal anisakidiosis, symptoms usually begin 5–7 days after ingestion of the larvae. Anisakidiosis has often been reported to cause a strong allergic reaction within 2–6h of ingesting larvae. The clinical symptoms range from isolated swelling to urticaria and life-threatening anaphylactic shock. Most cases of allergic reactions have been reported in Spain, although cases have also been reported in Egypt, France, Italy, Japan, the Republic of Korea, Portugal, and South Africa. The *Anisakis* allergens that cause an allergic reaction appear to be highly resistant to heat and freezing. However, a priming infection with live parasites may be required to induce sensitisation (Audicana and Kennedy, 2008).

8.3.1.5 Diagnosis and treatment

Gastric anisakidiosis is often misdiagnosed as peptic ulcer, stomach tumor, or stomach polyps, and intestinal anisakidiosis can be misdiagnosed as appendicitis or peritonitis. The clinical diagnosis is usually made by performing endoscopy, or by radiological or ultrasound examination. Various immunological assays have been used for indirect diagnosis. Interpretation of the serological tests may be difficult because the sera of individuals with anisakidiosis cross-react with antigens from closely related nematode species (e.g., *Ascaris* spp., *Toxocara* spp.). For acute gastric anisakidiosis, it is necessary to remove the worm by an endoscope, which leads to the immediate improvement of symptoms. For all of the other forms of anisakidiosis, the choice of treatment depends on the specific complications (e.g., surgical removal of granuloma). For intestinal anisakidiosis, conservative treatment with isotonic glucose solution is recommended. The drugs of choice for treating anisakidiosis, albendazole, and ivermectin have been shown to be effective (Audicana and Kennedy, 2008; Hochberg and Hamer, 2010).

8.3.1.6 Detection, control, and prevention

The size of adult worms living in the stomach of cetaceans and pinnipeds varies according to the worm species (about 3–12 cm in length and about 0.3–0.5 cm in width; females are larger than males). Anisakidae larvae (white worms of 15–30 mm in length for those of the genus *Anisakis*; reddish worms of 20–40 mm in length for those of the genus *Pseudoterranova*) can be detected in fish by visual inspection of the coelomic cavity, slicing or candling of muscles that detect no more than 10% of larvae, pressing, HCl-pepsin digestion, and PCR. The compression method is considered as the method of choice for routine screening in fish inspection. This method uses the fluorescence of anisakid nematode larvae on flattened/pressed and frozen fish filets or viscera under UV light. More recently, a spectroscopic technique has been developed to overcome some of the disadvantages of traditional visual methods (Table 8.2). The critical control points for mitigation are fishing in areas believed to have a low prevalence of infection among fish and the application of physicochemical treatments to fish products to ensure the killing of larvae. Freezing or heat treatments remain the most effective processes guaranteeing the killing of parasitic larvae, under well-defined conditions. Treatments that provide an equivalent level of protection as freezing (−20 °C for not less than 24 h) for the killing of anisakid larvae include freezing at −35 °C for at least 15 h or at −15 °C for at least 96 h, at the core of the fish products and heat treatment at higher than 60 °C for at least 1 min. Many traditional marinating and cold-smoking methods are not sufficient to kill anisakid larvae (EFSA, 2010). Because Anisakidae allergens are highly resistant to heat and freezing, treatments that kill Anisakidae in fishery products may not protect consumers against allergic reactions. The freezing treatment must be applied to either the raw or the finished product. In the United States, the Food and Drug Administration requires that all fish and shellfish intended to be consumed raw or semi-raw (e.g., marinated or partially cooked) be blast frozen to −35 °C or below for 15 h, or be completely frozen to −20°C or below for 7 days (www.fda.gov/food/guidanceregulation/guidancedocumentsregulatoryinformation/seafood/default.htm).

A similar freeze treatment is required in Canada. Anisakidae larvae are sensitive to salt only under certain conditions. It has been estimated that 28 days of storage in brine with 6.3% salt and 3.7% acetic acid in the aqueous phase of the fish is the maximum survival time of the larvae in herring. Under industrial production conditions for dry salted herring, the total time needed to kill the parasites is 20 days. Studies showed that *A. simplex* larvae are resistant to traditional conditions of marinating and can survive for 25 days in a mixture of salt and vinegar; depending on the salt concentration, the survival of larvae can reach 35–119 days. A marinade of vinegar (6% acetic acid) and 10% sodium chloride applied for 24h to sardines, followed by the addition of sunflower seed oil and refrigeration for 13 days, inactivate *A. simplex* larvae. Factors that influence the effectiveness of freezing for inactivating anisakid larvae include the temperature, the time needed to reach the final temperature in the core fish tissues, the duration of freezing, and the fat content of the fish. Studies have shown that a core temperature of 60°C for 1 min is sufficient to kill any larva present in a fish product. However, reaching such a core temperature depends on the thickness and composition of the product. Hydrostatic pressure kills *A. simplex* larvae (200MPa for 10min at 0–15°C or 140MPa for 60min at 0–15°C). Larvae of *A. simplex* can be killed by an irradiation dose higher than 6–10kGy. Hot smoking at 70–80°C for 3–8h is sufficient to kill *A. simplex* larvae. By contrast, cold-smoking (<38°C) is not sufficient and these products must thus undergo an initial inactivation treatment. Freezing raw products prior to smoking remains the most effective way of ensuring that viable parasites are killed in cold-smoked products (www.efsa.europa.eu/en/search/doc/1543.pdf).

8.3.2 Capillaria philippinensis

8.3.2.1 Introduction

The discovery of *C. philippinensis*, a zoonotic nematode, dates back to 50 years ago when the first human case was discovered in Luzon, Philippines. *C. philippinensis* is the causative agent of intestinal capillariosis, a severe disease that may lead to death unless patients are treated. Infection can result from the consumption of raw freshwater or brackish-water fish (Cross, 1992).

8.3.2.2 Biology

The natural cycle occurs between fish-eating birds that act as final hosts and freshwater or brackish-water fish, which act as intermediate hosts, but adult worms develop also in the gut of experimentally infected gerbils and monkeys; it follows that the role of mammals in the natural cycle cannot be ruled out. In endemic areas, humans can play the role of final hosts by defecation in proximity to water resources (Figure 8.3). Adult worms develop in the gut mucosa of the final host (females are 2.3–5.3mm in length and 29–47μm in width; males are 1.5–3.9mm in length and 23–28μm in width) and release unembryonated eggs within 22–24 days. Eggs that reach water and embryonate can be ingested by the fish in which they hatch in a few hours. The larvae develop in the fish gut doubling in length in 3 weeks. When a fish-eating animal or human ingests the fish, the larvae develop at the adult stage in the host gut within

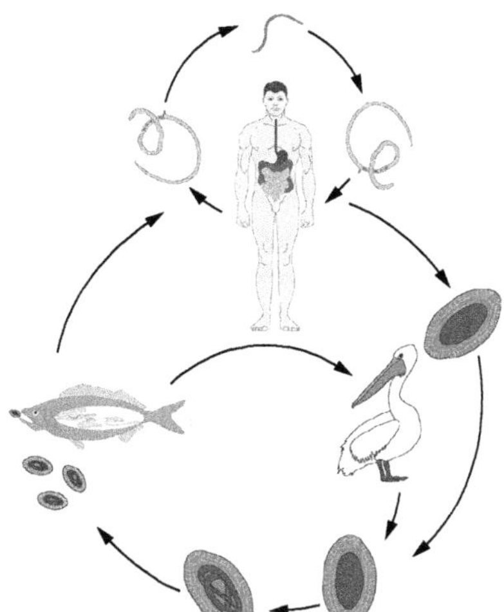

Figure 8.3 Life cycle of *Capillaria philippinensis*. 1—Adult worms develop in the gut mucosa of piscivorous birds and humans (the only known mammalian host); 2—shed eggs embryonate in water; 3—fish are infected by ingesting mature eggs; 4—when humans and fish-eating birds ingest infected fish, the larvae develop to the adult stage in the gut. In humans, adult females can produce larvae which develop to adult worms resulting in massive infections.

12–14 days. In humans and in experimentally infected gerbils and monkeys, adult females can produce larvae instead of eggs that develop to the adult stage causing massive infections.

8.3.2.3 Epidemiology

The most important focus of *C. philippinensis* infections in humans has been documented in the Philippines, where approximately 2000 cases and hundreds of deaths occurred since 1964. Since 1988, intestinal capillariosis in humans has also been documented in Egypt, Japan, Indonesia, Iran, India, Korea, Lao PDR, People's Republic of China, and Taiwan and in travelers who acquire the infection in one of these endemic countries and develop the disease when they return home (Lu et al., 2006; Saichua et al., 2008; Soukhathammavong et al., 2008; Fan et al., 2012; Jung et al., 2012; Vasantha et al., 2012). There are very few reports on *C. philippinensis* in naturally infected final or intermediate hosts, such as the bagsit, *Hypseleotris bipartita* (Table 8.1).

8.3.2.4 Infection in humans

Capillariosis is one of the few nematode diseases that can cause severe illness and death in untreated people. After an incubation period of about 3 weeks, the first symptoms of abdominal pain, diarrhea, and borborygmus appear. Within weeks, diarrhea increases, with 8–10 voluminous stools passed each day. Patients lose a great deal of body weight and suffer from malaise, anorexia, and, more rarely, vomiting. In addition, patients experience muscle wasting and weakness, distant heart sounds, hypotension, edema, gallop rhythm, pulsus alternans, abdominal distention and tenderness, and hyporeflexia. Laboratory findings include protein-losing enteropathy, malabsorption of fats and sugars, decreased excretion of xylose, and low serum levels of potassium, sodium, calcium, carotene, and total protein. Low levels of immunoglobulin G (IgG), IgM, and lgA with elevated levels of IgE present at the time of illness revert to normal on follow-up several months later. If treatment is not initiated soon enough, patients die because of the irreversible effects of the electrolyte loss, heart failure, or from septicaemia (Whalen et al., 1969).

8.3.2.5 Diagnosis and treatment

Parasitological diagnosis is made by microscopically detecting *C. philippinensis* eggs (36–45 by 20 μm), larvae (250–300 μm), or adults (female 2.3–5.3 mm in length and 29–47 μm in width; male 1.5–3.9 mm in length and 23–28 μm in width) in the feces after concentration by a sedimentation technique. Multiple stool examinations may be necessary, or small intestinal biopsy or intestinal aspiration also could reveal the parasites or eggs. In endemic areas, a clinical diagnosis can be made in patients presenting with abdominal pain, diarrhea, and gurgling stomach. Individuals with chronic infections experience weight loss, wasting, and an intractable diarrhea. Serology (ELISA) using heterologous antigens from *T. spiralis* can identify intestinal capillariosis cases in endemic areas where coproscopy has been negative for eggs, larvae, and adult stages (Intapan et al., 2010); however, the risk of cross-reactions with other helminthic antigens cannot be excluded. Albendazole is the drug of choice at 400 mg/day in two equal doses for 10 days.

8.3.2.6 Detection, control, and prevention

There is little information on intermediate and final hosts of *C. philippinensis*. Detection of this parasite in nature seems elusive, and efforts to control or prevent the transmission of this pathogen to human beings have not been effective. Intestinal capillariosis can be prevented by educating high-risk populations on the hazards of eating small freshwater fish whole and uncooked. Cooking for a short period of time is considered sufficient to kill larvae in the intestine. Human-to-human transmission most likely occurs during the outbreaks in endemic regions such as the Philippines and Thailand, because indiscriminate disposal of feces is common in these countries. In such cases, improvement of sanitary conditions would be beneficial. Treatment of infected persons with albendazole should be included in a control program. Because *C. philippinensis* is a parasite-infecting wild birds and fish, this zoonotic aspect of the pathogen impedes realistic control measures (Table 8.2).

8.3.3 Gnathostoma *spp.*

8.3.3.1 Introduction

Gnathostomosis (synonym: gnatostomiasis) is a disease caused by infection with the larval stage of nematodes of the genus *Gnathostoma* (Herman and Chiodini, 2009).

Adult parasites have been reported in canines, felines, and other carnivorous animals worldwide and in freshwater fish, amphibians, reptiles, rodents, and pigs as intermediate or paratenic hosts (Ando et al., 1992). Humans acquire the infection primarily from consuming raw fish, but infections can also arise from eating raw frogs, snakes, and wild boars and from drinking infected copepods in water. Skin penetration by L3 in food handlers and prenatal infections have been documented (Rusnak and Lucey, 1993). Human gnathostomosis has been reported in Africa, Asia, and Central America. Larval and immature *Gnathostoma* sp. adults cause migratory, often transitory, subcutaneous swellings in humans. The worms occasionally enter the internal organs and central nervous system (CNS), but they rarely reach sexual maturity in humans.

8.3.3.2 Biology

Adult worms of *Gnathostoma* spp. live in tumors in the stomach wall of fish-eating mammals. Females produce brownish ovoid eggs with a mucoid plug at one end (56–79 by 35–43 μm). The eggs pass in the animal feces, reach water, and embryonate in 7–10 days. The first-stage larva hatches from the egg and is eaten by a freshwater copepod, in which it develops into a second-stage larva. When the infected copepod is eaten by a second intermediate host, including fish, birds, amphibians, reptiles, and mammals, the parasite enters the tissue and grows to a third-stage larva. Paratenic hosts may eat a second intermediate host and the infective larva becomes encapsulated in the tissue and does not develop further. When a second intermediate host, or paratenic host, is eaten by a definitive host, the parasite is digested from the tissue, penetrates the stomach wall, and migrates to the liver and then to other organs, eventually returning to the peritoneal cavity and penetrating the stomach to form a tumor-like mass. The worms reach maturity and produce eggs in approximately 6 months (Figure 8.4). Felines and canines are definitive hosts for *Gnathostoma spinigerum*, and domestic and wild pigs are natural hosts for *Gnathostoma hispidium*. Infections are acquired by eating any of the many intermediate hosts. The main source of human infection is raw or poorly cooked meat of catfish, eels, frogs, chickens, ducks, and snakes. Infections occur in all age groups and both sexes.

8.3.3.3 Epidemiology

Gnathostomosis is acquired by eating one of the many intermediate hosts. The main source of human infection is raw or poorly cooked meat of catfish, eels, frogs, chickens, ducks, and snakes. Infections occur in all age groups and both sexes. Gnathostomosis has been reported prevalently in Japan and Southeast Asia (Cambodia, Indonesia, Laos, Malaysia, Myanmar, Philippines, Thailand, and Vietnam) (Herman and Chiodini, 2009; Sieu et al., 2009). Cases have also been documented in China, Korea, India, Sri Lanka, and Australia (Rusnak and Lucey, 1993; Kim et al., 2013; Jeremiah et al., 2011). In the last several years, it has become an increasing problem because of the consumption of raw fish marinated in lime (ceviche) in Mexico, Guatemala, Brazil, Ecuador, and Peru (Vargas et al., 2012). In Africa, the infection has been reported

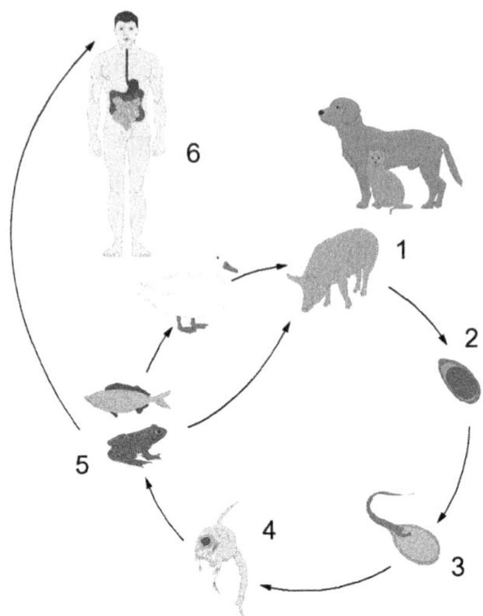

Figure 8.4 Life cycle of *Gnathostoma* spp. 1—Adult worms of *Gnathostoma* spp. live in tumors in the walls of the stomach of fish-eating mammals; 2—female worms produce ovoid eggs that are excreted in the feces; 3—eggs embryonate and hatch releasing L1; 4—L1 are ingested by freshwater copepods and develop to L2; 5—infected copepods are ingested by a second intermediate host (e.g., fish, amphibians), and the parasites enter the tissue where they become L3 paratenic, or transport hosts (e.g., birds) acquire the parasite by feeding on the second intermediate hosts; the infective stage larva becomes encapsulated in the host tissue and does not develop further; and 6—humans can acquire the infection by consuming one of the many intermediate hosts.

in Botswana, Namibia, Zambia, and Zimbabwe (Smith and Kok, 2006; Herman and Chiodini, 2009; Mukarati et al., 2013). In Spain, two persons have been diagnosed with gnathostomosis (Montero et al., 2001; Table 8.1). In addition, gnathostomosis has been reported in travelers who acquired the infection in one of these endemic countries and developed the disease when they returned to the home country, or in persons who acquired the infection consuming raw fish imported from endemic countries. Of the more than 12 species recognized by morphology in the genus *Gnathostoma*, six species have been detected in humans: *G. spinigerum* (in Asia and Africa), *Gnathostoma hispidum* (in Asia, Australia, Europe), *Gnathostoma doloresi* (in Asia), *Gnathostoma nipponicum* (in Asia), and *Gnathostoma binucleatum* (in America).

8.3.3.4 Infection in humans

Usually, only a single larva is involved in human infections. Clinical symptoms begin to occur shortly after the ingestion of infected food; the parasite enters the intestinal tissue, causing epigastric pain, nausea, vomiting, pruritus, urticaria, and low-grade fever. There is a leucocytosis with a marked eosinophilia. Acute pain is experienced as the larva migrates through abdominal and thoracic organs. The worm eventually makes its way to the subcutaneous tissue in about a month. The larva migrates through the tissues, causing edematous swellings up to 15 cm, usually on the chest, abdomen, or extremities. The lesion is red and warm and with pruritus lasts about a week. It may recur weeks or months later. At times, the larva may cause serpiginous tracks that are similar to but bigger than those caused by animal hookworm larvae. *Gnathostoma* larvae in the eye can cause exophthalmos, vitreous, corneal, or lenticular damage, impaired vision, and blindness. CNS invasion causes headache, nuchal rigidity, drowsiness, coma, and symptoms of a cerebral vascular accident. In the spinal cord, the worm may migrate along the nerve trunk, causing root pain and paralysis.

8.3.3.5 Diagnosis and treatment

Diagnosis of *Gnathostoma* infection in humans is made by the recovery and identification of larvae from surgical specimens, urine, sputum, or vaginal discharge. A presumptive diagnosis in endemic areas is based on the history, symptoms, or serology. Specific antigens are available for immunodiagnosis. On a Western blot, 24 and 21 kDa antigens of crude extract have been considered specific (Laummaunwai et al., 2007). More recently, a recombinant antigen has been successfully used for the serodiagnosis (Janwan et al., 2013). In differential diagnosis, other parasitic infections such as hookworms, cutaneous and visceral larval migrans, myosis, sparganosis, cutaneous paragonosis, loaosis, and meningitis caused by *Angiostrongylus cantonensis*, should be considered. Spontaneous recovery from cutaneous gnathostomosis is possible, but cutaneous migration could lead to complications of the CNS or ocular. The larva can be removed surgically from the eye. In cerebral gnathostomosis, albendazole is effective at the dose of 400 mg twice daily for 3 weeks and ivermectin at the dose of 200 μg/kg for 2 days (Nontasut et al., 2005). Repeat treatment is advised as relapses occur in 20–50% of patients.

8.3.3.6 Detection, control, and prevention

The most common species detected in humans is *G. spinigerum*, a short, stout nematode with a subglobose head armed with seven to nine transverse rows of hooklets. Spines also extend halfway down the body. Males measure 11–25 mm and females 25–54 mm in length. In addition to the morphological identification, the five zoonotic species of *Gnathostoma* can be identified among them by the molecular analysis of the cytochrome *c* oxidase subunit 1 of mitochondrial DNA and the internal transcriber spacer region 2 (Ando et al., 2006). Health education programs would be beneficial for control in endemic areas. Infections could be prevented by eating only well-cooked intermediate or paratenic hosts (e.g., fish, eels, snakes, frogs, and poultry) and drinking only boiled or treated waters that are potentially copepod infested. *Gnathostoma* spp. larvae are killed by freezing infected meat to −20 °C for 3–5 days. Marinating infected meat in various substances generally is not effective. Vinegar appears to kill the organism in approximately 6 h and soy sauce in 12 h; lime juice is not effective after 5 days at room temperature or after 30 days at +4 °C (Table 8.2).

8.4 Slug borne nematodes

8.4.1 Angiostrongylus cantonensis

8.4.1.1 Introduction

Nematodes of the genus *Angiostrongylus* are parasites of the vascular system of a variety of vertebrates. The intermediate hosts of these parasites are terrestrial molluscs. Of the more than 20 species occurring in nature, only two, *A. cantonensis* and *Angiostrongylus costaricensis*, are known to be zoonotic. Humans acquire the infection by ingesting raw terrestrial snails or slugs infected with third-stage larvae.

8.4.1.2 Biology

The adult worms of *A. cantonensis* undergo sexual maturity and lay eggs in pulmonary arteries of rats. Eggs hatch into first-stage larvae, which migrate up the bronchial tree, are swallowed, and are excreted out with the feces. Larvae ingested by intermediate snail and slug hosts, develop after two molts into third-stage larvae, which can be transmitted to paratenic hosts (e.g., shrimp, land crab, frog, lizard, and land planarian) or to the final hosts, that is, rats. The L3 penetrates the stomach of the rat, enters the hepatic portal system, and is carried to the liver, heart, and lungs. They pass through the alveoli into the veins, back to the heart, and enter the arterial circulation. The larvae reach the CNS and move into the neural parenchyma where they reach L4. The larvae move into the subarachnoid space and then invade the cerebral vein and migrate to the pulmonary arteries, where the worms reach sexual maturity (Wang et al., 2012; Figure 8.5).

8.4.1.3 Epidemiology

A. cantonensis has a widespread distribution, and it is transmitted via snails and rats. This parasite has been documented in many species of the genus *Rattus*, but it can develop partially in other rodents and mammals without reaching sexual maturity. Infection in humans is acquired by intentionally or accidentally eating uncooked intermediate hosts. Infection can also be acquired by drinking untreated water in which snails have died and released the infective larvae. Larvae may be also shed from slugs into mucus trails while crawling on vegetation. The infected planarians can then be eaten accidentally with vegetables (Table 8.1). Over 2800 cases of human angiostrongylosis have been reported in Asia (Cambodia, China, Japan, India, Indonesia, Malaysia, Sri Lanka, Taiwan, Thailand, Vietnam), the Pacific islands (Fiji, Hawaii, New Caledonia, Samoa, Tahiti, Vanuatu Republic), Caribbean islands (Cuba, Jamaica, Dominican Republic), South America (Brazil, Ecuador), Central America (Costa Rica), North America (United States), Africa (Egypt, Ivory Coast, Mayotte), and Australasia (Australia, New Zealand, Papua New Guinea). In addition, some travelers have acquired the infection in endemic countries and developed the disease upon returning home to places such as Belgium, Germany, Italy, Switzerland, the United Kingdom, and the United States (Wang et al., 2012).

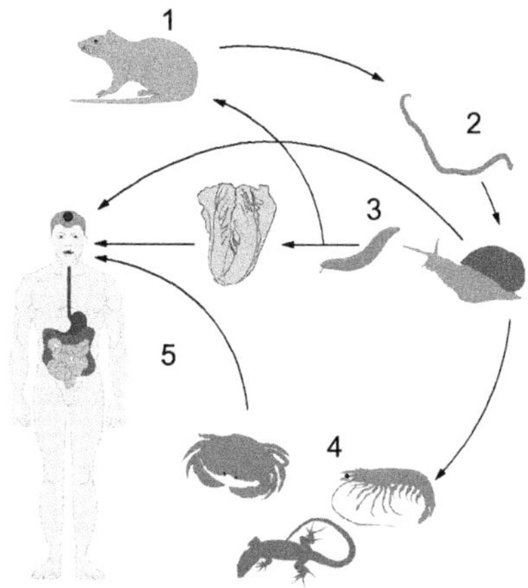

Figure 8.5 Life cycle of *Angiostrongylus* spp. 1—Adult worms live in pulmonary arteries of rats and produce eggs that deposit in the lungs, hatch to release L1 which pass through the respiratory tract to the gut; 2—L1 are excreted with the feces into the environment; 3—L1 are ingested by snail and slug intermediate hosts where they develop into L3; 4—paratenic hosts (e.g., shrimp, land crab, lizard) can ingest intermediate hosts and harbor the L3; and 5—humans acquire the angiostrongylosis by consuming intermediate or paratenic hosts or vegetables contaminated with snails and slugs.

8.4.1.4 Infection in humans

Humans are not natural definitive hosts of *A. cantonensis* but can acquire this parasite by eating either intermediate or paratenic hosts containing infective larvae. The worm is unable to complete its life cycle in a human but remains in the CNS to cause eosinophilic meningitis or moves to the eye chamber resulting in ocular angiostrongylosis. The average incubation period is 2 weeks but can range from 1 day to several months. The most frequent clinical symptom is headache, followed by neck stiffness, paraesthesia, vomiting, fever, nausea, and blurred vision of diplopia. The frequency of the clinical signs and symptoms is different between adults and children excluding headache and neck stiffness, which occur with a similar frequency in both adults and children (Wang et al., 2008).

8.4.1.5 Diagnosis and treatment

Diagnosis in humans is based primarily on clinical symptoms and medical history. A history of having eaten intermediate or paratenic hosts is very important for the diagnosis of the disease. The typical clinical manifestation of human angiostrongylosis is eosinophilic meningitis. Magnetic resonance imaging (MRI) and computed tomography (CT) are very useful for showing the lesions and for differencing the diagnosis from other parasitic infections. An ELISA has been developed to detect antigens of, or antibodies against, *A. cantonensis* in serum or cerebrospinal fluid (CSF). The detection of circulating antigens in serum or CSF provides a rapid confirmation of infection. Antigens from *A. cantonensis* can also be detected in sera by immuno-PCR.

However, no commercial tests are available (Wang et al., 2008). Patients can be treated successfully with albendazole (15–20 mg/kg/day for 2–4 weeks) or praziquantel (400–1200 mg/day for 2–3 weeks), always associated with corticosteroids (Chen et al., 2006).

8.4.1.6 Detection, control, and prevention

The body of the adult worms of *A. cantonensis* is filariform in shape and tapered at both ends. Males are 16–19 mm × 0.25 mm; females 21–25 mm × 0.30–0.36 mm. Eggs are of 21–25 µm. Larvae in the rat feces and in the snail and slug tissues can be detected by the Baermann method and identified by PCR (Qvarnstrom et al., 2007). Because of the worldwide distribution of rats and molluscs, which can act as final and intermediate hosts of *A. cantonensis*, it is impossible to eliminate this zoonotic parasite from the environment. However, rodent control in areas close to human settlements is recommended. Mollusc control near housing and vegetable gardens should be routine. Although changing established eating habits and customs is difficult to achieve, cooking the mollusc host would reduce or eliminate human infection with this parasite. Freezing snails at −15 °C for 12–24 h would also kill the larvae. Thorough washing of vegetables that are eaten raw helps to remove slugs, tiny snails, and mucus containing larvae from food. Children should be educated not to handle snails because hands could become contaminated with larvae. Paratenic host such as prawn, shrimp, crabs, and monitor lizards should be cooked before eating (Table 8.2). Travelers to endemic regions should be made aware of the dangers of eating raw terrestrial molluscs and vegetables. Also, importation of such food products from endemic areas may pose a risk to consumers. Washing hands frequently, particularly after gardening, is strongly recommended in endemic regions. Physicians should be aware of this parasite and know how to diagnose its infection in humans (Cross and Chen, 2007).

8.4.2 Angiostrongylus costaricensis

8.4.2.1 Biology

Several species of rats, coati-mundi, marmoset, and dogs have been reported as definitive hosts (Cross, 1998). Adult worms live in the mesenteric arteries of rats. Females deposit the eggs in the mesenteric arterioles from which they reach the intestinal wall where they embryonate and develop to first-stage larvae. These larvae migrate into the intestinal lumen and pass in the feces. Slugs of the family Veronicellidae eat the feces, and the larvae migrate into the fibro-muscular tissue where they reach the infective stage (L3). Larvae can remain in the tissue or emerge from the slug into the mucous secretion. When a rat or other definitive host ingests a slug or mucous trails, the larvae migrate to the lymphatic vessels where they develop to the adult stage. They then migrate to the mesenteric arteries and arterioles where sexual reproduction begins within 18 days. Ovoid eggs (90 µm) can be detected in the final host feces 22–24 days postinfection.

8.4.2.2 Epidemiology

A. costaricensis has been detected in rats in the Americas from Argentina to the United States. Human cases have been reported in these areas, with most cases in Costa Rica where the occurrence of 2116 human infections per 100,000 persons per year has been estimated (Morera, 1995). Human infections due to *A. costaricensis* have been also documented in the United States and in the former Republic of Zaire (Baird et al., 1987). The cotton rat, *Sigmodon hispidus*, is the most important definitive host with an infection rate of 43.2% in Costa Rica (Morera, 1995). Aquatic snails also act as intermediate hosts, and infected tiny slugs could be eaten on vegetables. Infective larvae excreted in mucous trails may also be ingested on unwashed leafy vegetables, and there are even reports of infants eating slugs (Table 8.1). The habit of children placing objects in their mouths may be responsible for the high number of cases of intestinal angiostrongylosis in children (Morera, 1995).

8.4.2.3 Infection in humans

Acute clinical symptoms involve the abdomen (Loria-Cortés and Lobo-Sanahuja, 1980). Patients also report fever, anorexia, vomiting, diarrhea, constipation, and abdominal rigidity. Leucocytosis and eosinophilia are reported. Clinical findings can be suggestive of appendicitis.

8.4.2.4 Diagnosis and treatment

The diagnosis of *A. costaricensis* infections in humans is difficult. Larvae are not found in the feces of infected persons. Radiological findings may show changes in the terminal ileum, caecum, appendix, and ascending colon. In radiographs the contrast medium shows incomplete filling and irritability of the involved area. The liver is usually involved, and laparoscopy reveals yellow spots on the liver surface (Morera, 1995). Parasitological diagnosis is generally made by histological examination of surgically removed specimens. Eggs, larvae, worms, and elevated eosinophilia are usually found in the tissue. Although serological tests have been developed, no kits are available on the market. The disease is often self-limiting, and specific treatment is not required. Anthelminthics such as albendazole (Morera, 1995) and mebendazole (Hulbert et al., 1992) have been used, but the results were not reliable. Chemotherapy is not recommended because the worms are known to become agitated when drugs are used in rodent infections (Morera, 1995). Surgery is the treatment of choice in most cases.

8.4.2.5 Detection, control, and prevention

The size and morphology of adult worms, eggs, and larvae are similar to that of *A. cantonensis*. The control and prophylactic measures are similar to those for *A. cantonensis* (Table 8.2).

8.5 Nematodes transmitted by fruits and vegetables via soil

8.5.1 Ascaris *spp.*

8.5.1.1 *Introduction*

Ascariosis (synonym: ascariasis) is a disease caused by the ingestion of soil, vegetables, fruits, and other ready-to-eat foods, contaminated by eggs of nematodes of the genus *Ascaris*, which became infectious after a maturation period on the soil. Human ascariosis is a helminthiosis infecting more than 1.2 billion people (Dold and Holland, 2011). Human and pig *Ascaris* spp. are two of the world's most common soil-transmitted parasites, and together they cause serious health and socioeconomic problems. Both *Ascaris lumbricoides*, the typical human parasite, and *Ascaris suum*, the typical pig parasite, and their hybrids, have been detected in humans with varying frequencies (Cavallero et al., 2013).

8.5.1.2 *Biology*

Hosts acquire *Ascaris* infection via the fecal-oral route. When infective eggs are ingested, eggs hatch in the small intestine, and L3 migrate to the caecum and proximal colon where they penetrate the mucosa (Crompton, 2001). The larvae then migrate via the portal blood to the liver reaching the lungs on days 6–8 p.i. The larvae penetrate the alveolar space and move to the pharynx where they are swallowed, resulting in returning to the small intestine 8–10 days p.i.; *Ascaris* spp. molt to L4 in the small intestine on day 10 p.i., where they develop to adult worms. Male and female adult worms measure 15–25 and 20–35 cm, respectively. The estimate of daily egg production per female is in the range of 200,000 eggs, but the number of eggs produced per female decreases with worm load. Unembryonated eggs enter the environment via feces and can remain viable in the soil for up to 15 years, and during embryonation, larvae undergo two molts in the egg (Geenen et al., 1999).

8.5.1.3 *Epidemiology*

Ascariosis occurs commonly in rural and impoverished urban areas and can facilitate poverty due to its high toll on children's health and development, pregnancy, and worker productivity (Crompton, 2001; Dold and Holland, 2011). Recent studies strongly suggest that *A. suum* acts as an important source of human ascariasis in endemic area such as China, where both *A. lumbricoides* and *A. suum* occur (Table 8.1). These parasites are distributed globally, as they have been detected in more than 150 countries of the world (Crompton, 2001).

8.5.1.4 *Infection in humans and pigs*

Although the majority of infections in pigs and humans are asymptomatic, clinical manifestations of human ascariosis can involve acute and chronic symptoms such as lung inflammation and fever due to larval migration; abdominal pain, nausea, retarded growth and mental development in children, and intestinal obstruction are due to the massive presence of adult worms (Crompton, 2001). Infection with *Ascaris* spp. may affect all age groups of pigs, but housing and management factors often determine which age group shows the highest prevalence.

8.5.1.5 Diagnosis and treatment

The detection of *Ascaris* eggs in fresh or fixed stool samples processed by a flotation or sedimentation method and examined by microscopy is the most reliable means of identifying cases of *Ascaris* spp. infection in both people and pigs. Humans can be successfully treated with albendazole (400 mg single dose), mebendazole (500 mg single dose), pyrantel embonate (11 mg/kg single dose), or levamisole (2.5 mg/kg single dose). Deworming of fattening pigs is not entirely effective and does not reduce the occurrence of liver white spots that are caused from migratory larvae.

8.5.1.6 Detection, control, and prevention

For the control of *Ascaris* spp., it is essential to reduce the parasite intensity by means of improvements in sanitation, health education, and anthelminthic treatment. The eradication of *Ascaris* spp. relies primarily on sanitation measures for the safe disposal of human feces to interrupt transmission, prevent reinfection, and gradually reduce and eliminate worm burdens. Transmission of *Ascaris* spp. among pig populations is dependent on housing systems, hygiene, management practices, and anthelminthic treatment (Table 8.2). The most important risk factors for ascarid infection in pigs include large fatteners and gilts (the age group with the highest infection intensity), country, weaning age (late weaning is associated with higher prevalence of infection), and water supply (drinking facilities located in the low-lying areas) (Roepstorff et al., 1998).

8.5.2 Toxocara *spp.*

8.5.2.1 Introduction

Toxocara canis is the main etiological agent of visceral and ocular larva migrans, covert toxocariosis (synonym: toxocariasis), and neurological toxocariosis in humans (Despommier, 2003). The dog and other canids (e.g., coyote, fox, jackal, wolf) act as hosts, whereas every species of mammals including humans and birds can serve as paratenic hosts by harboring the second-stage larvae in their tissues. *T. canis* has a cosmopolitan distribution. Two other nematodes of the superfamily Ascaridoidea, *Toxocara cati* of cats, and *Baylisascaris procyonis* of raccoons have occasionally been reported as agents of visceral and ocular larva migrans. Because the life cycle of *T. cati* is similar to that of *T. canis*, except that felids are definitive hosts, most of the information provided for *T. canis* is also applicable to *T. cati*.

8.5.2.2 Biology

The life cycle of *T. canis* is complex. When adult dogs ingest larvated eggs most of the larvae migrate to somatic tissues. In some dogs, larvae undergo tracheal migration, return to the intestine, and develop to adult worms. Those larvae in the tissues of dogs remain dormant for several years, and if a bitch becomes pregnant the somatic larvae become activated and migrate across the placenta to the fetus. The larvae then complete their migration to the intestine in the newborn pup, where they develop to adult worms and produce eggs. Adult worms in pups can also develop from larvae transferred from the bitch in her milk and from ingested eggs. Pups are often heavily infected. The lactating bitch can be reinfected with eggs from her pups while she is grooming them. Larvae in *T. canis* eggs eaten by any species of mammal or bird (paratenic hosts) hatch, migrate into the tissues, and remain viable for prolonged periods of time. Stray dogs, foxes, and others that scavenge rodents, lagomorphs and birds, and occasionally large animals (e.g., sheep, pigs, wild boars, and pets) that hunt or are fed with raw meat, ingest these larvae. The adults develop in the intestine without any further migration.

8.5.2.3 Epidemiology

Humans can become infected by ingesting *T. canis* eggs from dog feces by geophagia, poor hygiene, contact with dogs (mainly pups), contaminated food and water, and consumption of raw or undercooked meat of dogs and other animals harboring the larvae. Pups can shed up to 10^5 eggs per gram of feces, and a female worm can produce more than 10^5 eggs per day. Therefore, a heavily infected bitch and her pups can disseminate more than 10^7 eggs daily. The prevalence of infection in dogs varies widely. In most litters of puppies the prevalence is considered about 100%. Prevalence and fecundity of worms decline considerably in adult dogs, and the overall prevalence has declined in pets in developed countries in the last decade. The prevalence in pets also varies between treated and untreated animals and between adults and puppies. For example, 30% and 1–4% of untreated and treated (four times per year) dogs, respectively, were infected in the United Kingdom. In Poland, 58% of puppies and 2.5% of adult dogs were infected. The prevalence in pet dogs (both adults and pups) ranges from 0.4% in Australia, 3–5% in Canada, and 5% in United States (Palmer et al., 2008; Mohamed et al., 2009; Jenkins et al., 2011). Urban foxes are another source of infection with *T. canis* for gardens. In the European Union, the prevalence of infection ranges from 40% to 73% of urban and rural foxes (Table 8.1). Eggs begin to develop only at or above 10 °C and reach the L2 stage at 15–25 °C in 2–7 weeks, but they can remain viable at low temperatures protected by snow or feces. Only heat and desiccation is known to kill the embryo within eggs in the environment. In favorable conditions, eggs remain viable in large numbers for 6–12 months. Eggs can be common in soil samples (e.g., 0.1–23 eggs/g of soil), although most surveys do not differentiate *T. canis* and *T. cati* eggs. Because the egg surface is sticky, it could be carried long distances attached to objects. A number of invertebrates (e.g., slugs, earthworms, cockroaches, beetles) can ingest the eggs that pass intact through their gut, facilitating concentration and dissemination. Free-ranging farm animals and birds can ingest *Toxocara* eggs. Pigs and birds have been infected with L2 when fed raw viscera. The L2 of *T. canis* can persist in pigs for more than 1 month, but they have been described as dying relatively quickly in pigs. It has been reported that L2 persists for 7 months in lambs, 4.5 months in pigeons, and 3.5 years in chickens (Taira et al., 2004). Larvae can be detected in all host tissues, with the highest numbers in the liver. The viability of larvae declines after slaughter, but infective larvae can still remain after 4 days at 4 °C.

8.5.2.4 Infection in humans

Toxocariosis in humans can develop into visceral or ocular larva migrans, or asymptomatic form. The main clinical signs and symptoms of visceral toxocariosis (VT) are elevated eosinophilia, hepathosplenomegaly, fever, respiratory signs, lymphadenopathy, pallor, neurological manifestations (e.g., convulsions, strabismus), and myocarditis. Most of patients with VT are children 2–4 years of age. Ocular lesions can occur at any age. The inflammatory response involves granuloma, which can cause severe visual loss. Mild toxocariosis is characterized by highly variable signs and symptoms (e.g., weakness, abdominal pain, lymphadenopathy, skin lesions, pruritus, respiratory features, headache). Neurological signs and symptoms have also been documented. For example, a strong relationship between seropositivity and epilepsy has been documented in children with a diagnosis of ocular larva migrans (Quattrocchi et al., 2012).

8.5.2.5 Infection in animals

In newborn pups, the migration of an overwhelming larva burden can cause haemorrhagic pneumonia. Adult worms induce hypertrophy of the muscular layer of the gut, villous atrophy, and malabsorption. A heavy adult worm burden can be the cause of poor growth, emaciation, diarrhea, and constipation in pups.

8.5.2.6 Diagnosis and treatment

In humans, clinical signs and symptoms of toxocariosis are not pathognomonic. The diagnosis of choice is made by an ELISA using excretory/secretory larval antigens to detect circulating antibodies. However, this test has not been standardized or validated. The specificity and predictive values of this test are high in developed countries, but the values decrease in developing countries where cross-reactions with other nematode infections can occur (Fillaux and Magnavalc, 2013). Infections in dogs are diagnosed by the recovery of worm eggs on fecal flotation techniques using high specific gravity solutions. The test is sensitive for pups, whereas its sensitivity decreases to 50% for adult dogs due to the low levels of egg production. In humans, the treatment of choice is albendazole at 10–15 mg/kg bid for 5 days.

8.5.2.7 Prophylaxis

The eggshell confers considerable resistance from environmental conditions. On concrete exposed to sunlight, eggs will desiccate, but those in cracks will be protected. High concentrations of sodium hypochlorite solution (bleach), which can be a useful disinfectant for surfaces, are usually neutralized by organic matter or do not have sufficient contact time to be effective. A flame gun can be used to ensure destruction of the eggs. In damp, shaded soil, eggs could survive for years. Only severe measures can ensure disinfection of soil in gardens. It has been suggested that surface soil that is heavily contaminated with *B. procyonis* or *T. canis* should be thoroughly tilled and flamed several times or 10–20 cm of topsoil removed and replaced (Kazacos, 1991). Sand in sandboxes can be steam sterilized or replaced and sandboxes covered when not in use. Infection with *T. canis*, at least from pet dogs, can be prevented by treatment of the animals. Bitches should be treated with fenbendazole 50 mg/kg/day, every day for 3 weeks before parturition until 3 weeks after parturition. The treatment must be repeated for each pregnancy. Treatments at 1- or 2-month intervals for dogs and cats, respectively, should be appropriate (Table 8.2). Treatment of stray dogs and foxes is not practical. Stray populations should be excluded from gardens, play areas, and playgrounds by fencing. Removal of dirt from beneath fingernails and thorough hand washing are necessary. Vegetables eaten raw should be peeled or well washed, but as the eggs are sticky, vegetable gardens should be fenced to exclude all canids, although this will not keep out cats. Although the importance of larvae in meat is undetermined, meat, particularly liver, should be cooked well (Overgaauw and van Knapen, 2013).

8.5.3 Baylisascaris procionis

8.5.3.1 Biology

Raccoons and other procyonid species are the natural definitive hosts of *B. procyonis* (Kazacos et al., 2001). Adult male worms reach lengths of 7–12 cm and females14–28 cm. Domestic dogs are also suitable hosts for this parasite and can shed eggs. Unlike other *Baylisascaris* spp., *B. procyonis* is well documented as an important and frequent cause of visceral, ocular, and neural larva migrans in mammals, including humans, and in birds. Dogs, but not raccoons, also develop neural larva migrans following *B. procyonis* infection. Unlike most ascarid species in which the L3 is the infective stage within the egg, L2 in the eggs of *Baylisascaris* spp. are the infective stage, with the second molt occurring in the infected host animal (Bauer, 2013). Cubs acquire infection by ingesting embryonated eggs from the contaminated environment. The second-stage larvae penetrate the intestinal wall where they develop with the preadult stage returning to the intestinal lumen to mature. Adult raccoons may also become infected by ingesting third-stage larvae in prey intermediate hosts after which further development to mature worms occurs in the intestinal lumen. When an intermediate host ingests embryonated eggs, the second-stage larvae are released from hatched eggs, penetrate the intestinal wall, and migrate through the liver to the lungs and via blood to other tissues (Figure 8.6). A few larvae may invade the CNS and eyes (Bauer, 2013). In the tissues of intermediate hosts, the larvae grow, molt, and remain as L3 (Kazacos, 2001).

8.5.3.2 Epidemiology

B. procyonis is an indigenous parasite of North American raccoons. The prevalence of infection in raccoon populations varies by region according to the distribution of the host, but may be as high as 60% or more in some areas (Kazacos, 2001).

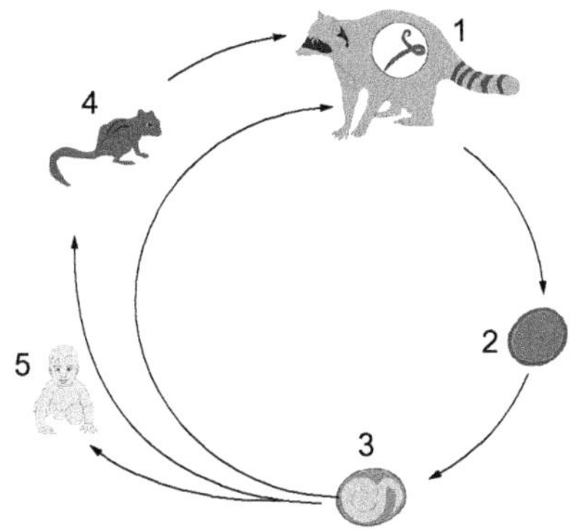

Figure 8.6 Life cycle of *Bayliascaris procionis*. 1—Adult worms live in the gut of raccoons and dogs following ingestion of embryonated eggs or intermediate hosts harboring L3; 2—unembryonated eggs are shed with the feces of infected hosts; 3—eggs embryonate in the environment and harbor L2; 4—various small mammals can act as intermediate hosts after ingesting fully embronated eggs which then develop to L3 in tissues; 5—humans can accidentally acquire the infection by ingesting embryonated eggs.

B. procyonis infection has also been identified in central Europe and Japan, following the introduction of raccoons from North America. Eggs remain infective for years and can survive freezing temperatures of −15 °C (Shafir et al., 2011). More than 100 animal species, both mammals, including humans, and birds, are known to act as intermediate hosts or "dead-end" hosts of *B. procyonis*, and commonly develop clinical signs of larva migrans. Pigs, small ruminants, and cats appear to be less susceptible to this parasite. Free-ranging raccoons habitually defecate at preferred sites where *B. procyonis* eggs can accumulate. These sites are commonly associated with raccoon resting and sleeping places. The number of documented infections in humans is limited, but most of them have been diagnosed in the United States (Table 8.1).

8.5.3.3 Infection in humans

Four clinical patterns of *B. procyonis* infection have been described in humans: neural, ocular, visceral larva migrans, and subclinical baylisascariosis. The intra vitam diagnosis of *B. procyonis* larva migrans is difficult and is based on clinical signs, history of exposure to raccoons, neuroimaging, laboratory findings, detection of specific serum antibodies, and detection of larvae in needle aspiration of brain biopsies (Gavin et al., 2005).

8.5.3.4 Diagnosis and treatment

An ELISA and an immunoblot assay (Dangoudoubiyam and Kazacos, 2009) that are based on excretory–secretory antigens from L2 of *B. procyonis* have been used for serological testing. A recombinant antigen from *B. procyonis* L3 has also been developed. In cases of ocular larva migrans, a single, motile larva may occasionally be detected in the retina by ophthalmoscopic examination. Postmortem diagnosis can be made by histopathological examination and detection of *B. procyonis* larvae or by PCR amplification of DNA in tissue samples. Clinical cases of neural larva migrans have been diagnosed in humans from North America (Haider et al., 2012). Patients were mainly toddlers, young children, and individuals with mental or developmental impairment, and nearly all were males. A significant number of the human cases of neural larva migrans caused by *B. procyonis* have been fatal or resulted in moderate to severe neurological sequelae. There is only one report in the literature of full recovery; it was preceded by early treatment using albendazole and high weekly doses of corticosteroid (Pai et al., 2007).

8.5.3.5 Prophylaxis

The most effective means of preventing infection in people and animals is to avoid exposure to raccoons and their feces. Practical control measurements include identification and rapid elimination of raccoon defecation sites from backyards (including the soil) by heat treatment such as burning using a flame or by steaming with boiling water (Vantassel, 2012). Heat is the most effective method of killing *B. procyonis* eggs, which become nonviable at temperatures above 62 °C (Shafir et al., 2011). Children should not be allowed to play in areas likely to be contaminated with raccoon feces. Raccoon populations should be controlled, particularly in residential areas and public parks. If raccoons are kept as pet animals or for public display in zoological gardens and other facilities, preventive measurements such as quarantine and deworming are essential to reduce the risk of transmission of *B. procyonis* to other animals and humans (Table 8.2).

8.5.4 Capillaria hepatica

C. hepatica is a cosmopolitan nematode parasitizing the liver of rodents, the primary host, and numerous other mammals including humans. It is the causative agent of hepatic capillariosis and spurious infections in humans. Adult female worms of *C. hepatica* lay eggs into the liver parenchyma. The eggs are released into the environment by the death and decomposition of its host, or by spurious release in the feces of a predator of the infected rodent. In humans, 72 cases of hepatic capillariosis have been documented worldwide (Table 8.1). Humans as well as animals acquire hepatic infections by ingesting embryonated eggs in food or drink. The eggs occur in the soil or on vegetation in areas especially where there is an abundance of rodents. Children more often than adults acquire the infection because of geophagy and placing contaminated objects in the mouth. Human hepatic capillariosis have been reported in Europe (Germany, Switzerland, Italy, England, Greece, former Czechoslovakia, former Yugoslavia, Turkey), North and South America (United States, Canada, Mexico, Brazil), Asia (India, Korea, Japan, Thailand), Africa (South Africa, Ivory Coast, Nigeria) and Australasia (New Zealand). Rodent control and sanitary disposal of dead animals, education, and improvement of hygiene are measures for the prevention and control of this zoonotic parasite (Fuehrer et al., 2011) (Table 8.2).

8.5.5 Trichostrongylus *spp.*

Members of the genus *Trichostrongylus* are common host-specific nematodes of the stomach or gut of ruminants worldwide, and human infections have been widely documented (Table 8.1). The infection is acquired while eating uncooked plants contaminated by infective L3. The most common source of infection is domestic animals that share living areas with humans. Furthermore, the use of animal feces as fuel has been implicated in the infection of people who gather and prepare the feces for this purpose (Ghadirian and Arfaa, 1975). The common source of infection in nonendemic areas is most likely the accidental ingestion of larvae acquired from livestock pasture or the ingestion of unwashed fruits and vegetables grown using animal manure fertilizer. A manure spreader has been implicated in the infection of people in Italy (Cancrini et al., 1982). The most common species detected in humans is *Trichostrongylus orientalis*, but other species such as *Trichostrongylus axei*, *Trichostrongylus capricola*, *Trichostrongylus colubriformis*, and *Trichostrongylus vitrinus* have also been identified (Nolan, 2011). In areas where *T. orientalis* is prevalent, uncooked vegetables are contaminated by human feces. In endemic areas where species of *Trichostrongylus* are found, hands should be washed before preparing or eating meals and vegetables should be thoroughly washed or cooked before eating. Animal manure can be composted to a high enough temperature to kill *Trichostrongylus* eggs and larvae before being used as a fertilizer. *T. orientalis* can be controlled by proper sanitation, removal of animal feces from areas occupied by humans, and the sterilization of feces before its use as a fertilizer. Infections with *Trichostrongylus* spp. of animal origin can be controlled by periodic treatment of domestic livestock with anthelmintics. The time between treatments should depend on the local conditions. Since well-nourished livestock is better able to reduce their parasite burdens, animals should be kept well fed and their diet supplemented with minerals. Particular care should be taken with animals under 1 year of age as they are still developing an immune response to the worms and therefore may have higher worm burdens than older animals. Because in warm weather larvae can survive on pasture for about 1 month, pasture rotation, with a period greater than 1 month, will help to reduce worm burdens in livestock (Table 8.2).

8.6 Future trends

The transmission of most foodborne nematodes to humans is linked to impoverished living conditions, lack of knowledge, inadequate sanitary conditions, and customary culinary practices, including consumption of raw or inadequately cooked meat and fish. Programs in public health and veterinary services are needed for the education of consumers, farmers, fishermen, and hunters to control these pathogens especially in developing regions of the world. Increasing number of tourists traveling from developed to endemic areas and the testing of locally produced and/or imported food are likely to occur over the next several years. An increasing amount of meat and fish products are being illegally translocated around the world by travelers, hunters, immigrants, and entrepreneurs. At the same time, developed countries are experiencing a reduction in the number of physicians specializing in parasitic diseases. There is a low interest in the industry to invest resources for the development of effective diagnostic tests, because of the lack of large markets. Many foodborne zoonotic parasites are directly or indirectly linked to wildlife. In the future, most meat and fish products will probably originate from animals farmed under controlled management conditions where transmission of these parasites are mitigated.

As a result of urbanization (more than 50% of the global population now lives in urban areas), demographic increases, and various market forces, food is now moving on a global scale, carried rapidly from continent to continent. The deployment of more efficient and rapid means of transporting perishable goods worldwide enable fresh products to be available nearly year-round. New technologies for food trade and transportation have allowed the spread of parasitic diseases in areas where they were not present before, both at the global and local levels. In South America, anisakiosis is associated with the increased consumption of "ceviche" not only in the coastal communities, but also in internal mountain regions, following the improved logistics in refrigerated transport of fresh food products.

Hunting and other outdoor activities may also be an exposure factor to eating inadequately cooked game (e.g., bear, wild boar, warthog), during or after hunting and shooting expeditions. Infection with sylvatic species of *Trichinella* are recurringly being associated with hunting activities in endemic areas, for example, infection acquired during hunting trips in the Arctic or tropical areas are diagnosed after the travelers return home (Houzé et al., 2009). It is estimated that 4.5 million tons of bushmeat are extracted from the Congo basin each year, and this meat is often consumed only partially cooked, thereby acting as a potential source of zoonotic pathogens (Wolfe, 2005).

There are emerging patterns of movements of migrants from less-developed parts of the world to developed countries in search of better opportunities. This mobility implies also importing different cultures, health beliefs, food preferences, and hence risk factors for foodborne transmission of parasites. For this reason, natural barriers for human infection with parasites, which were considered to be geographically limited because of parasites' adaptations to specific definitive and intermediate hosts, and particular environmental conditions, are slowly being breached (Orlandi et al., 2002; McPherson and Bidaisee, 2015).

In comparison to other classes of foodborne pathogens, particularly bacteria, the health impact of parasites is difficult to assess primarily because of the lack of uniform standards for monitoring the incidence of foodborne illness directly attributed to parasitic infections. Therefore, important efforts should be addressed for the standardization, implementation, and documentation of control measures to increase confidence in global food trade. Integration of veterinary and public health efforts in "One Health" is needed to monitor these foodborne parasites and to develop a comprehensive food safety program for these diseases, most of which are zoonotic (Murrell, 2013).

References

Ando, K., Tokura, H., Matsuoka, H., Taylor, D., Chinzei, Y., 1992. Life cycle of *Gnathostoma* nipponicum Yamaguti, 1941. J. Helminthol. 66, 53–61.

Ando, K., Tsunemori, M., Akahane, H., Tesana, S., Hasegawa, H., Chinzei, Y., 2006. Comparative study on DNA sequences of ribosomal DNA and cytochrome c oxidase subunit 1 of mitochondrial DNA among five species of gnathostomes. J. Helminthol. 80, 7–13.

Audicana, M.T., Kennedy, M.W., 2008. *Anisakis simplex*: from obscure infectious worm to inducer of immune hypersensitivity. Clin. Microbiol. Rev. 21, 360–379.

Baird, J.K., Neafie, R.C., Lanoie, L., Connor, D.H., 1987. Abdominal angiostrongyliosis in an African man: case study. Am. J. Trop. Med. Hyg. 37, 353–356.

Bauer, C., 2013. Baylisascariosis—infections of animals and humans with 'unusual' roundworms. Vet. Parasitol. 193, 404–412.

Cancrini, G., Boemi, G., Iori, A., Corselli, A., 1982. Human infestations by *Trichostrongylus axei*, *T. capricola* and *T. vitrinus*: 1st report in Italy. Parassitologia 24, 145–149 (in Italian).

Cavallero, S., Snabel, V., Pacella, F., Perrone, V., D'Amelio, S., 2013. Phylogeographical studies of *Ascaris* spp. based on ribosomal and mitochondrial DNA sequences. PLoS Negl. Trop. Dis. 7, e2170.

Chen, W.L., Zhong, J.M., Chen, H., Wu, S.Y., Ding, L., 2006. Eosinophilic meningitis: 31 case reports. Chin. J. Misdiagn. 6, 4668–4669.

Crompton, D.W., 2001. *Ascaris* and ascariasis. Adv. Parasitol. 48, 285–375.

Cross, J.H., 1992. Intestinal capillariasis. Clin. Microbiol. Rev. 5, 120–129.

Cross, J.H., 1998. Angiostrongylosis. In: Palmer, S.R., Soulsby, E.J.L., Simpson, D.I.H. (Eds.), Zoonoses. Oxford University Press, Oxford/New York/Tokyo, pp. 773–781.

Cross, J.H., Chen, E.R., 2007. Angiostrongyliasis. In: Murrell, K.D., Fried, B. (Eds.), Food-Borne Parasitic Zoonoses. Springer, New York, pp. 263–290.

Dangoudoubiyam, S., Kazacos, K.R., 2009. Differentiation of larva migrans caused by *Baylisascaris procyonis* and *Toxocara* species by Western blotting. Clin. Vaccine Immunol. 16, 1563–1568.

Despommier, D.D., 1998. How does *Trichinella spiralis* make itself at home? Parasitol. Today 14, 318–323.

Despommier, D., 2003. Toxocariasis: clinical aspects, epidemiology, medical ecology, and molecular aspects. Clin. Microbiol. Rev. 16, 265–272.

Devleesschauwer, B., Praet, N., Speybroeck, N., Torgerson, P.R., Haagsma, J.A., De Smet, K., Murrell, K.D., Pozio, E., Dorny, P., 2015. The low global burden of trichinellosis: evidence and implications. Int. J. Parasitol. 45, 95–99.

Dold, C., Holland, C.V., 2011. *Ascaris* and ascariasis. Microbes Infect. 13, 632–637.

Dupouy-Camet, J., Kociecka, W., Bruschi, F., Bolas-Fernandez, F., Pozio, E., 2002. Opinion on the diagnosis and treatment of human trichinellosis. Expert Opin. Pharmacother. 3, 1117–1130.

EFSA, 2010. Scientific Opinion on risk assessment of parasites in fishery products. EFSA J. 8, 1543.

European Commission, 2005. Regulation (EC) No 2075/2005 of 5 December 2005 laying down specific rules on official controls for *Trichinella* in meat. Off. J. EU L338, 60–82.

Fan, Z., Huang, Y., Qian, S., Lv, G., Chen, Y., Yang, B., Zhong, S., Lin, G., Yan, G., 2012. Serious diarrhea with weight loss caused by *Capillaria philippinensis* acquired in China: a case report. BMC Res. Notes 5, 554.

Fillaux, J., Magnavalc, J.F., 2013. Laboratory diagnosis of human toxocariasis. Vet. Parasitol. 193, 327–336.

Fuehrer, H.P., Igel, P., Auer, H., 2011. *Capillaria hepatica* in man—an overview of hepatic capillariosis and spurious infections. Parasitol. Res. 109, 969–979.

Gavin, P.J., Kazacos, K.R., Shulman, S.T., 2005. Baylisascaris. J. Clin. Microbiol. 18, 703–718.

Geenen, P.L., Bresciani, J., Boes, J., Pedersen, A., Eriksen, L., Fagerholm, H.P., Nansen, P., 1999. The morphogenesis of *Ascaris suum* to the infective third-stage larvae within the egg. J. Parasitol. 85, 616–622.

Ghadirian, E., Arfaa, F., 1975. Present status of trichostrongyliasis in Iran. Am. J. Trop. Med. Hyg. 24, 935–941.

Gómez-Morales, M.A., Ludovisi, A., Amati, M., Blaga, R., Zivojinovic, M., Ribicich, M., Pozio, E., 2012. A distinctive Western blot pattern to recognize *Trichinella* infections in humans and pigs. Int. J. Parasitol. 42, 1017–1023.

Gottstein, B., Pozio, E., Nöckler, K., 2009. Epidemiology, diagnosis, treatment, and control of trichinellosis. Clin. Microbiol. Rev. 22, 127–145.

Haider, S., Khairnar, K., Martin, D.S., Yang, J., Ralenvski, F., Kazacos, K.R., Pillai, D.R., 2012. Possible pet-associated baylisascariasis in child, Canada. Emerg. Infect. Dis. 18, 347–349.

Herman, J.S., Chiodini, P.L., 2009. Gnathostomiasis, another emerging imported disease. Clin. Microbiol. Rev. 22, 484–492.

Hochberg, N.S., Hamer, D.H., 2010. Anisakidosis: perils of the deep. Clin. Infect. Dis. 51, 806–812.

Houzé, S., Ancelle, T., Matra, R., Boceno, C., Carlier, Y., Gajadhar, A.A., Dupouy-Camet, J., 2009. Trichinellosis acquired in Nunavut, Canada in September 2009: meat from grizzly bear suspected. Euro Surveill. 14, 19383.

Hulbert, T.V., Larsen, R.A., Chandrasoma, P.T., 1992. Abdominal angiostrongyliasis mimicking acute appendicitis and Meckel's diverticulum: report of a case in the United States and review. Clin. Infect. Dis. 14, 836–840.

Intapan, P.M., Maleewong, W., Sukeepaisarnjaroen, W., Morakote, N., 2010. An enzyme-linked immunosorbent assay as screening tool for human intestinal capillariasis. Southeast Asian J. Trop. Med. Public Health 41, 298–305.

Janwan, P., Intapan, P.M., Yamasaki, H., Laummaunwai, P., Sawanyawisuth, K., Wongkham, C., Tayapiwatana, C., Kitkhuandee, A., Lulitanond, V., Nawa, Y., Maleewong, W., 2013. Application of recombinant *Gnathostoma spinigerum* matrix metalloproteinase-like protein for serodiagnosis of human gnathostomiasis by immunoblotting. Am. J. Trop. Med. Hyg. 89, 63–67.

Jenkins, E.J., Schurer, J.M., Gesy, K.M., 2011. Old problems on a new playing field: Helminth zoonoses transmitted among dogs, wildlife, and people in a changing northern climate. Vet. Parasitol. 182, 54–69.

Jeremiah, C.J., Harangozo, C.S., Fuller, A.J., 2011. Gnathostomiasis in remote northern Western Australia: the first confirmed cases acquired in Australia. Med. J. Aust. 195, 42–44.

Jung, W.T., Kim, H.J., Min, H.J., Ha, C.Y., Kim, H.J., Ko, G.H., Na, B.K., Sohn, W.M., 2012. An indigenous case of intestinal capillariasis with protein-losing enteropathy in Korea. Korean J. Parasitol. 50, 333–337.

Kazacos, K.R., 1991. Visceral and ocular larva migrans. Semin. Vet. Med. Surg. 6, 227–235.

Kazacos, K.R., 2001. *Baylisascaris procyonis* and related species. In: Samuel, W.M., Pybus, M.J., Kocan, A.A. (Eds.), Parasitic Diseases of Wild Animals, second ed. Manson, London, pp. 301–341.

Kim, J.H., Lim, H., Hwang, Y.S., Kim, T.Y., Han, E.M., Shin, E.H., Chai, J.Y., 2013. *Gnathostoma spinigerum* infection in the upper lip of a Korean woman: an autochthonous case in Korea. Korean J. Parasitol. 51, 343–347.

La Rosa, G., D'Amelio, S., Pozio, E., 2006. Molecular identification of nematode worms from seafood (*Anisakis* spp. and *Pseudoterranova* spp.) and meat (*Trichinella* spp.). In: Adley, C.C. (Ed.), Food-Borne Pathogens, Methods and Protocols. Humana Press Inc., Totowa, pp. 217–232.

Laummaunwai, P., Sawanyawisuth, K., Intapan, P.M., Chotmongkol, V., Wongkham, C., Maleewong, W., 2007. Evaluation of human IgG class and subclass antibodies to a 24 kDa antigenic component of *Gnathostoma spinigerum* for the serodiagnosis of gnathostomiasis. Parasitol. Res. 101, 703–708.

Loria-Cortés, R., Lobo-Sanahuja, J.F., 1980. Clinical abdominal angiostrongylosis. A study of 116 children with intestinal eosinophi!ic granuloma caused by *Angioslrongylus costaricensis*. Am. J. Trop. Med. Hyg. 19, 538–544.

Lu, L.H., Lin, M.R., Choi, W.M., Hsu, Y.H., Bair, M.J., Liu, J.D., Wang, T.E., Liu, T.P., Chung, W.C., 2006. Human intestinal capillariasis (*Capillaria philippinensis*) in Taiwan. Am. J. Trop. Med. Hyg. 74, 810–813.

MacPherson, C.N.L., Bidaisee, S., 2015. Role of society and culture in the epidemiology and control of food-borne parasites (Chapter 4 of this book).

Mattiucci, S., Nascetti, G., 2008. Advances and trends in the molecular systematics of anisakid nematodes, with implications for their evolutionary ecology and host–parasite coevolutionary processes. Adv. Parasitol. 66, 47–148.

Mohamed, A.S., Moore, G.E., Glickman, L.T., 2009. Prevalence of intestinal nematode parasitism among pet dogs in the United States (2003–2006). J. Am. Vet. Med. Assoc. 234, 631–637.

Montero, E., Montero, J., Rosales, M.J., Mascar6, C., 2001. Human gnathostomosis in Spain: first report in humans. Acta Trop. 78, 59–62.

Morera, P., 1995. Abdominal angiostrongylosis. In: Farthing, M.J.G., Keusch, G.T., Wakelin, D. (Eds.), Enteric Infection 2: Intestinal Helminths. Chapman & Hall, London, pp. 225–230.

Mukarati, N.L., Vassilev, G.D., Tagwireyi, W.M., Tavengwa, M., 2013. Occurrence, prevalence and intensity of internal parasite infections of African lions (*Panthera leo*) in enclosures at a recreation park in Zimbabwe. J. Zoo Wildl. Med. 44, 686–693.

Murrell, K.D., 2013. Zoonotic foodborne parasites and their surveillance. Rev. Sci. Tech. 32, 559–569.

Murrell, K.D., Pozio, E., 2011. Worldwide occurrence and impact of human trichinellosis, 1986–2009. Emerg. Infect. Dis. 17, 2194–2202.

Nöckler, K., Kapel, C.M.O., 2007. Detection and surveillance for *Trichinella* meat inspection and hygiene, and legislation. In: Dupouy-Camet, J., Murrell, K.D. (Eds.), FAO/WHO/OIE Guidelines for the Surveillance, Management, Prevention and Control of Trichinellosis. World Organization for Animal Health, Paris, pp. 69–97.

Nolan, T.J., 2011. Trichostrongylidosis. In: Palmer, S.R., Soulsby, E.J.L., Torgerson, P.R., Brown, D.W.G. (Eds.), Zoonoses Biology, Clinical Practice, and Public Health Control. Oxford University Press, Oxford, pp. 798–800.

Nontasut, P., Claesson, B.A., Dekumyoy, P., Pakdee, W., Chullawichit, S., 2005. Double-dose ivermectin vs albendazole for the treatment of gnathostomiasis. Southeast Asian J. Trop. Med. Public Health 36, 650–652.

OIE, 2013. Infection with Trichinella spp. In: Terrestrial Animal Health Code World Organization for Animal Health, Paris, pp. 452–455. (Chapter 8.14).

Orlandi, P., Chu, D., Bier, J., Jackson, G., 2002. Parasites and the food supply. Food Technol. 56, 72–80.

Overgaauw, P.A.M., van Knapen, F., 2013. Veterinary and public health aspects of *Toxocara* spp. Vet. Parasitol. 193, 398–403.

Pai, P.J., Blackburn, B.R., Kazacos, K.R., Warrier, R.P., Begue, R.E., 2007. Full recovery from *Baylisascaris procyonis* eosinophilic meningitis. Emerg. Infect. Dis. 13, 928–930.

Palmer, C.S., Thompson, R.C., Traub, R.J., Rees, R., Robertson, I.D., 2008. National study of the gastrointestinal parasites of dogs and cats in Australia. Vet. Parasitol. 151, 181–190.

Pozio, E., 2007. World distribution of *Trichinella* spp. infections in animals and humans. Vet. Parasitol. 149, 3–21.

Pozio, E., 2013. Integrating animal health surveillance and food safety: the example of *Anisakis*. Rev. Sci. Tech. 32, 487–496.

Pozio, E., 2014. Searching for *Trichinella*: not all pigs are created equal. Trends Parasitol. 30, 4–11.

Pozio, E., La Rosa, G., 2010. Trichinella. In: Liu, D. (Ed.), Molecular Detection of Foodborne Pathogens. CRC Press Taylor and Francis Group, Boca Raton/London/New York, pp. 851–863.

Pozio, E., Murrell, K.D., 2006. Systematics and epidemiology of *Trichinella*. Adv. Parasitol. 63, 367–439.

Pozio, E., Zarlenga, D.S., 2013. New pieces of the *Trichinella* puzzle. Int. J. Parasitol. 43, 983–997.

Quattrocchi, G., Nicoletti, A., Marin, B., Bruno, E., Druet-Cabanac, M., Preux, P.M., 2012. Toxocariasis and epilepsy: systematic review and meta-analysis. PLoS Negl. Trop. Dis. 6, e1775.

Qvarnstrom, Y., Sullivan, J.J., Bishop, H.S., Hollingsworth, R., da Silva, A.J., 2007. PCR-based detection of *Angiostrongylus cantonensis* in tissue and mucus secretions from molluscan hosts. Appl. Environ. Microbiol. 73, 1415–1419.

Ribicich, M., Gamble, H.R., Rosa, A., Sommerfelt, I., Marquez, A., Mira, G., Cardillo, N., Cattaneo, M.L., Falzoni, E., Franco, A., 2007. Clinical, haematological, biochemical and economic impacts of *Trichinella spiralis* infection in pigs. Vet. Parasitol. 147, 265–270.

Robertson, L.J., Sprong, H., Ortega, Y.R., van der Giessen, J.W., Fayer, R., 2014. Impacts of globalisation on foodborne parasites. Trends Parasitol. 30, 37–52.

Roepstorff, A., Nilsson, O., Oksanen, A., Gjerde, B., Richter, S.H., Örtenberg, E., Christensson, D., Martinsson, K.B., Bartlett, P.C., Nansen, P., 1998. Intestinal parasites in swine in the Nordic countries: prevalence and geographical distribution. Vet. Parasitol. 76, 305–319.

Rusnak, J.M., Lucey, D.R., 1993. Clinical gnathostomiasis: case report and review of the English-language literature. Clin. Infect. Dis. 16, 33–50.

Saichua, P., Nithikathkul, C., Kaewpitoon, N., 2008. Human intestinal capillariasis in Thailand. World J. Gastroenterol. 28, 506–510.

Shafir, S.C., Sorvillo, F.J., Sorvillo, T., Eberhard, M.L., 2011. Viability of *Baylisascaris procyonis* eggs. Emerg. Infect. Dis. 17, 1293–1295.

Sieu, T.P., Dung, T.T., Nga, N.T., Hien, T.V., Dalsgaard, A., Waikagul, J., Murrell, K.D., 2009. Prevalence of *Gnathostoma spinigerum* infection in wild and cultured swamp eels in Vietnam. J. Parasitol. 95, 246–248.

Smith, Y., Kok, O.B., 2006. Faecal helminth egg and oocyst counts of a small population of African lions (*Panthera leo*) in the southwestern Kalahari, Namibia. Onderstepoort J. Vet. Res. 73, 71–75.

Soukhathammavong, P., Sayasone, S., Harimanana, A.N., Akkhavong, A., Thammasack, S., Phoumindr, N., Choumlivong, K., Choumlivong, K., Keoluangkhot, V., Phongmany, S., Akkhavong, K., Hatz, C., Strobel, M., Odermatt, P., 2008. Three cases of intestinal capillariasis in Lao People's Democratic Republic. Am. J. Trop. Med. Hyg. 79, 735–738.

Taira, K., Saeed, I., Permin, A., Kapel, C.M., 2004. Zoonotic risk of *Toxocara canis* infection through consumption of pig or poultry viscera. Vet. Parasitol. 121, 115–124.

van Thiel, P.H., Kuiper, F.C., Roskam, R.T., 1960. A nematode parasitic to herring, causing acute abdominal syndromes in man. Trop. Geogr. Med. 2, 97–113.

Vantassel, S.M., 2012. A draft proposal for an industry protocol for the cleanup of raccoon latrines. In: Proceedings of the 14th Wildl Damage Manage Conference, Nebraska City, 18–21 April 2011, pp. 33–39.

Vargas, T.J., Kahler, S., Dib, C., Cavaliere, M.B., Jeunon-Sousa, M.A., 2012. Autochthonous gnathostomiasis, Brazil. Emerg. Infect. Dis. 18, 2087–2089.

Vasantha, P.L., Girish, N., Leela, K.S., 2012. Human intestinal capillariasis: a rare case report from non-endemic area (Andhra Pradesh, India). Indian J. Med. Microbiol. 30, 236–239.

Wang, Q.P., Lai, D.H., Zhu, X.Q., Chen, X.G., Lun, Z.R., 2008. Human angiostrongyliasis. Lancet Infect. Dis. 8, 621–630.

Wang, Q.P., Wu, Z.D., Wei, J., Owen, R.L., Lun, Z.R., 2012. Human *Angiostrongylus cantonensis*: an update. Eur. J. Clin. Microbiol. Infect. Dis. 31, 389–395.

Whalen, G.E., Rosenberg, E.B., Strickland, G.T., Gutman, R.A., Cross, J.H., Watten, R.H., 1969. Intestinal capillariasis–a new disease in man. Lancet 293, 13–16.

Wolfe, N.D., 2005. Bushmeat hunting deforestation, and prediction of zoonotic disease emergence. Emerg. Infect. Dis. 11, 1822–1827.

Foodborne cestodes

9

S. Geerts
Institute of Tropical Medicine, Antwerp, Belgium

9.1 Introduction

All foodborne cestode parasites that are covered in this chapter have complex indirect life cycles with at least one intermediate host. They are zoonotic, which means they are transmitted between animals and humans. Taeniosis[1] and cysticercosis are infections with adult and larval *Taenia* species, respectively. We will deal with three parasites causing taeniosis-cysticercosis: *Taenia solium*, *Taenia saginata*, and *Taenia asiatica*. Echinococcosis and cystic echinococcosis (or hydatidosis) are infections caused by adult and larval *Echinococcus granulosus*, respectively. Alveolar echinococcosis (or hydatidosis) is caused by the larval stages of *Echinococcus multilocularis*. Unlike the former cestode parasites, which are meat-borne, the last parasite we deal with in this chapter is the fish-borne tapeworm *Diphyllobothrium*. With the exception of *Diphyllobothrium* and *T. saginata*, all foodborne cestodes included in this chapter are considered by the World Health Organization (WHO) as neglected zoonotic diseases. "Neglected" means that these diseases affect mainly poor and marginalized populations in low resource settings (WHO, 2014). Over the past few years WHO, together with the Food and Agriculture Organization (FAO) of the United Nations and other strategic partners, has intensified their efforts to help reduce the burden of these diseases.

9.2 Taenia solium

9.2.1 Parasite biology and life cycle

The life cycle of *T. solium* is shown in Figure 9.1. Humans are the only definitive host in which the adult tapeworm develops after the ingestion of cysticerci (also called metacestodes) present in raw or undercooked pork. When the intermediate host ingests a *T. solium* egg, the oncosphere is liberated after its passage through the stomach, penetrates the intestinal wall, and is transported through the blood or lymphatics to the muscles where it develops into a cysticercus. In heavy infections the organs and brain can also be involved. Pigs are the most common intermediate hosts, but dogs and monkeys can also be infected. Humans may develop cysticercosis after the accidental ingestion of eggs, which are present in the environment (particularly in the vicinity of tapeworm carriers), in food or water contaminated by feces of a *T. solium* carrier, or by introduction of eggs from feces into the mouth by contaminated hands

[1] The term *taeniosis* is synonymous to *taeniasis*. In this chapter *taeniosis* is used according to the Standardised Nomenclature of Animal Parasitic Diseases (SNOAPAD).

Foodborne Parasites in the Food Supply Web. http://dx.doi.org/10.1016/B978-1-78242-332-4.00009-6

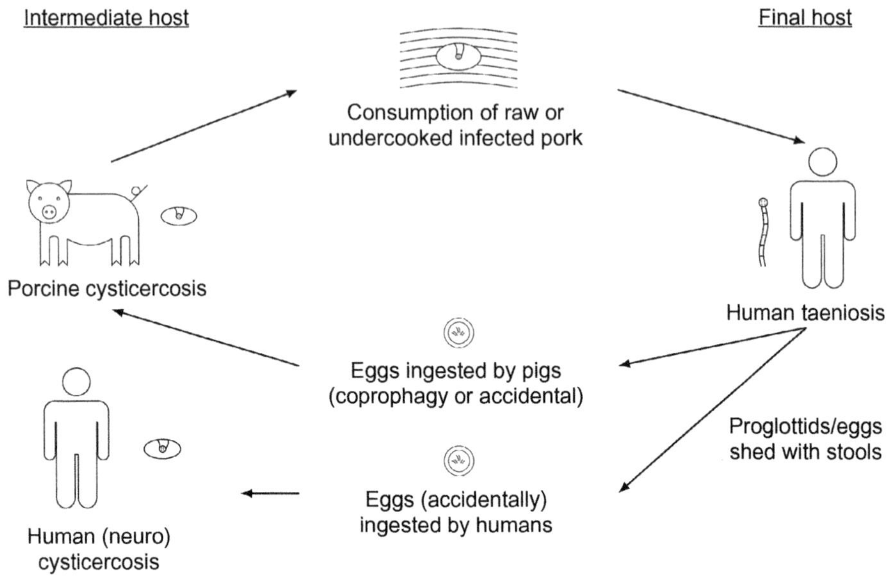

Figure 9.1 Life cycle of *Taenia solium*.
With permission of the author, Victor (2014).

(Flisser et al., 2005). The eggs of *T. solium* are quite resistant and may survive for long periods in the environment. After ingestion by a suitable intermediate host, the eggs develop into infective cysticerci within 8–10 weeks. These cysticerci usually survive during the average lifetime of a pig, which is about 1 year in the tropics. In the definitive host it takes 8–12 weeks for a cysticercus to develop into an adult tapeworm. Gravid proglottids are passively released with the feces daily or a few times a week. Although *T. solium* may survive up to 25 years in the human intestinal tract, its typical lifespan is probably less than 5 years (Garcia et al., 2003).

9.2.2 Geographical distribution and prevalence

T. solium taeniosis/cysticercosis is considered a neglected tropical disease (Budke et al., 2009). Porcine cysticercosis is widespread in the pig-rearing rural areas of Latin America, Africa, and Asia, whereas the disease has virtually disappeared in the industrialized countries (Murrell, 2005). However, imported cases of neurocysticercosis (NCC) in Europe and the United States are increasing in parallel to the increased number of migrations and amount of international travel (Serpa and White, 2012; Zammarchi et al., 2013). The prevalence of human cysticercosis is not well-known but is seriously underestimated due to (1) the wide range of clinical symptoms that can be confused with other diseases and (2) the absence of advanced diagnostic techniques in areas where the parasite is endemic. A systematic review of the literature showed that the proportion of NCC in people with epilepsy in Latin America, sub-Saharan Africa, and Southeast Asia was 29.6% (Ndimubanzi et al., 2010). Few data are available on prevalence and incidence of *T. solium* taeniosis in humans, as sensitive detection techniques are lacking and the *Taenia* species is often not identified. In general, the prevalence of *T. solium* is rather low, even in (hyper) endemic areas (<1%).

9.2.3 Epidemiology and risk factors

T. solium taeniosis/cysticercosis is a poverty-related disease. Porcine cysticercosis occurs where pigs are free ranging and have access to human feces. In modern, intensive pig husbandry, where pigs are confined for life, cysticercosis is absent. Consumption of pork containing cysticerci is the major risk factor for human *T. solium* taeniosis. Impoverished rural communities have the highest risk of exposure because in many developing countries only a small percentage of pig carcasses are inspected at slaughter. Tongue inspection is carried out before pigs are sold in many endemic areas, but this technique detects only the most heavily infected pigs (Dorny et al., 2004). Finally, a personal history of taeniosis or living in a household of a person with a history of, or currently with taeniosis, are the most important risk factors for human cysticercosis (Garcia et al., 2003).

9.2.4 Diagnosis

9.2.4.1 Taeniosis

It is well-known that the classical coprological techniques lack sensitivity for the detection of tapeworm ova in the feces, unless they are repeated several times. The eggs of *T. solium* and *T. saginata* or *T. asiatica* (or other taeniids) cannot be distinguished on morphological grounds. An enzyme-linked immunosorbent assay (ELISA) allowing for the detection of parasite antigens in stool samples (Allan et al., 1990), which is unfortunately not commercially available, has a relatively high sensitivity and specificity, but it does not distinguish between *T. solium* and the other human *Taenia* species. Differentiation between species is possible, however, using polymerase chain reaction (PCR) or copro-PCR assays (Praet et al., 2013). Specific serological identification of *T. solium* carriers is also possible using an immunoblot assay, but it is not known how long the antibodies persist after the expulsion of the tapeworm (Wilkins et al., 1999).

9.2.4.2 Porcine cysticercosis

Although cysticerci of *T. solium* may be found in any muscle or organ, the majority of the cysts are found in the so-called predilection sites such as the heart, diaphragm, masseters, tongue, neck, shoulder, intercostals, and abdominal muscles. Classical meat or tongue inspection has a very poor sensitivity for the diagnosis of *T. solium* cysticercosis in pigs (Dorny et al., 2004). Immunoblot assays using purified glycoproteins of *T. solium*, antibody and antigen-detection ELISAs (Ag-ELISA), are more sensitive and specific. The advantage of the Ag-ELISA is that it detects only pigs infected with living cysticerci (Dorny et al., 2005).

9.2.4.3 Human cysticercosis

Computed tomography (CT) scanning and magnetic resonance imaging (MRI) are the techniques of choice to confirm NCC. These sophisticated techniques, however, are usually not available in rural areas where most cases of NCC occur. Immunoblotting (or EITB: enzyme-linked immune-electrotransfer blot) using purified glycoproteins of *T. solium* is the most sensitive and specific serological test, but the Ag-ELISA is more appropriate to differentiate active from inactive NCC (Rodriguez et al., 2009). A QuickELISA™ using recombinant antigens has been developed with a similar sensitivity and specificity as the EITB (Lee et al., 2011).

A set of objective criteria has been proposed by Del Brutto et al. (2001) for the diagnosis of NCC, whereby the combination of various criteria offers different degrees of diagnostic certainty. Inclusion of the Ag-ELISA might improve the sensitivity of the Del Brutto criteria in resource-poor settings (Gabriel et al., 2012).

9.2.5 Disease and treatment

T. solium carriers usually show very mild symptoms or none at all. *T. solium* proglottids are generally eliminated with the feces and not outside the stools, as is the case for *T. saginata*. This could mean that *T. solium* infections are more likely to go unnoticed. Niclosamide and praziquantel are the treatment drugs of choice with a preference for the former because it causes no side effects when used in people with concurrent cysticercosis (Garcia et al., 2003).

In pigs, infection with cysticerci is generally asymptomatic. Only in massive infections have some clinical symptoms been described. Oxfendazole (30 mg/kg per os) is highly effective against porcine cysticercosis. However, it does not kill all the cysticerci in the brain (Mkupasi et al., 2013).

Symptoms due to NCC in humans vary considerably according to the number of cysticerci, their localization, the status of the cysticercus (living or dead), and the immune response of the host (Garcia et al., 2003). In many patients infection may remain asymptomatic despite long-term and even severe infections. The development of subcutaneous cysticerci seems to be more common in Asia and Africa than in Latin America. NCC is considered to be one of the most important causes of epilepsy, especially late-onset seizures, in developing countries (Ndimubanzi et al., 2010). The treatment of NCC depends on the number, location, and viability of the cysticerci (Garcia et al., 2002). Praziquantel or albendazole are commonly used for the antiparasitic treatment of NCC, with albendazole the preferred treatment (Abba et al., 2010).

9.2.6 Prevention and control

Taeniosis/cysticercosis due to *T. solium* is theoretically considered to be an eradicable disease for the following reasons: tapeworm infections in humans are the only source of infection for intermediate hosts; domestic animal intermediate host populations can be managed to avoid infection; no significant wildlife reservoir exists; and effective treatment is available for tapeworms (Schantz et al., 1993).

Meat inspection can help to prevent human taeniosis but is not sufficient alone because of its low sensitivity to detect infected pigs. Thorough cooking or deep freezing pork is the only way to avoid infection. A better strategy to prevent taeniosis in humans is to improve pig husbandry to the point where pigs have no access to human feces or contaminated feed or water.

Prevention of porcine cysticercosis is entirely possible by improved sanitation. In industrialized countries cysticercosis is virtually absent where pigs are kept in modern piggeries. A recombinant vaccine against *T. solium* cysticercosis in pigs has been developed and provides almost 100% protection under field conditions (Assana et al., 2010; Lightowlers, 2010). Unfortunately, it is not yet commercially available, and may not be economically feasible in some regions.

Human cysticercosis can be prevented by avoiding exposure to *T. solium* eggs. Therefore, tapeworm carriers need to be detected and treated as soon as possible, but unfortunately this is not always the case in many endemic regions.

9.3 Taenia saginata

9.3.1 Life cycle/parasite biology

The life cycle of *T. saginata* is very similar to that of *T. solium* except that the intermediate hosts include cattle, buffalo, and reindeer instead of pigs. Another important difference is that the eggs of *T. saginata*, contrary to those of *T. solium*, are not infective to humans. After ingestion of the egg by cattle it develops into an infective cysticercus in 8–12 weeks. Cysticerci are present in the muscles and, in case of heavy infections, also in the organs of the intermediate hosts. Although the heart, tongue, masseter muscles, esophagus, and diaphragm are usually considered to be predilection sites, several studies have shown that only the heart is a true predilection site (Dorny et al., 2004). Depending on the location and the intensity of the infection, cysticerci start to degenerate within a few months after infection and the majority are dead about 1 year after infection. Humans acquire the infection after consumption of raw or undercooked infected beef containing cysticerci. An adult tapeworm develops in about 3 months. Gravid proglottids containing 50,000–80,000 eggs are shed daily in the feces, but can also leave the host actively in between defecations. Eggs may survive for several months in sewage, water, or on pasture (Flisser et al., 2005).

9.3.2 Geographical distribution and prevalence

T. saginata has a worldwide distribution. The prevalence of adult *T. saginata* in humans varies widely. In some highly endemic countries such as Ethiopia and Turkey, the prevalence may reach 10% whereas in many regions of the world the prevalence is below 0.5% (Murrell, 2005). The prevalence figures should be interpreted with caution because of the poor sensitivity of coprological techniques. The distribution of bovine cysticercosis is related to that of taeniosis in humans and varies very widely. In some countries of East and Central Africa prevalence figures of bovine cysticercosis of >20% have been reported, whereas in most European countries the prevalence is <2% (Cabaret et al., 2002). However, since these figures are based on the meat inspection, which is known to lack sensitivity (see below), these figures seriously underestimate the true prevalence.

9.3.3 Epidemiology/risk factors

Transmission from cattle to humans occurs via the consumption of inadequately cooked or frozen beef that contains infective cysticerci. Taeniosis is particularly common in regions in which the people have a preference for raw or semi-raw beef dishes. Transmission from humans to cattle occurs via the contamination of pasture, fodder, or water with the eggs of *T. saginata*. Because proglottids actively leave the host in between defecations, and because a large proportion of the eggs are deposited around the anus and drop on the ground after some time, a tapeworm carrier disseminates *T. saginata* eggs wherever it goes. One infected farm worker or herdsman can thereby be responsible for a so-called cysticercosis storm, in which a large number of the herd or feedlot is infected. Because most conventional sewage treatment plants do not effectively remove taeniid eggs, bovine cysticercosis is often associated with cattle's access to wastewater effluent or surface water or with flooding of pastures (Murrell, 2005; Dorny and Praet, 2007).

9.3.4 Diagnosis

9.3.4.1 Taeniosis

Coprological techniques and copro-antigen detection ELISA do not enable distinguishing *T. solium* from *T. saginata* eggs. Gravid proglottids of both *Taenia* species can be distinguished by the number of unilateral uterine branches: between 14 and 32 for *T. saginata* and between 7 and 16 for *T. solium*. If the number of branches is between 14 and 16 it is advisable to confirm the identity of the tapeworm by molecular tools. Various PCR and copro-PCR techniques allow reliably identifying *T. saginata* (Dorny et al, 2005).

9.3.4.2 Bovine cysticercosis

Comparison of the efficacy of the classical meat inspection (incisions in the so-called predilection sites) with detailed examination of the carcass has shown that only 10–20% of the cysticercosis cases may be detected at the abattoir (Dorny and Praet, 2007; Eichenberger et al., 2013). As an alternative to these methods antigen detection techniques were developed. The Ag-ELISA is up to 10 times more sensitive than meat inspection. However, this technique detects only animals infected with living cysts and fails to detect a substantial number of light infections (Dorny and Praet, 2007). Because it is not always easy to correctly identify cysticerci at meat inspection, particularly the caseous and calcified ones, immunohistochemical techniques using specific monoclonal antibodies and various PCR techniques have been developed to improve the diagnosis (Geysen et al., 2007; Scandrett et al., 2012).

9.3.5 Disease and treatment

9.3.5.1 Taeniosis

Persons infected with *T. saginata* may suffer from abdominal pain, loss of appetite or increased appetite, constipation or diarrhea, but most often the infection is asymptomatic. The sensation generated when a proglottid actively exits the anus is the most commonly observed symptom. The drugs of choice to treat adult *T. saginata* are niclosamide and praziquantel.

9.3.5.2 Bovine cysticercosis

Even massive infections of cattle with cysticerci usually remain asymptomatic. Treatment should be considered for the reasons of public health. The treatment of choice for *T. saginata* cysticercosis in cattle is praziquantel at 50 mg/kg (preferably repeated twice). This dose kills all cysticerci, but it takes several months before the cysts are resorbed and disappear (Harrison et al., 1984).

9.3.6 Control and prevention

9.3.6.1 Human taeniosis

Because meat inspection is not reliable to detect all carcasses infected with cysticercosis at slaughterhouse, particularly lightly infected carcasses, people who want to avoid an infection with *T. saginata* should not eat raw or undercooked beef.

9.3.6.2 Bovine cysticercosis

The most important measures to prevent bovine cysticercosis are (1) early detection and treatment of tapeworm carriers and (2) avoiding exposure of cattle to the eggs of *T. saginata*. However, inasmuch as these eggs often appear to be widely dispersed in the environment, it is almost impossible to prevent cysticercosis in cattle that have access to pasture. Therefore, industrialized countries have not succeeded in eradicating bovine cysticercosis, contrary to the successful elimination of porcine cysticercosis. Imported feed and migrant farm laborers are important risk factors.

A recombinant vaccine has been developed to provide protection against *T. saginata* cysticercosis in more than 99% of the immunized animals (Lightowlers et al., 1996a). This vaccine, however, is not commercially available.

9.4 Taenia asiatica

9.4.1 Parasite biology and life cycle

Taenia asiatica was discovered at the end of the last century in Taiwan (Fan, 1988). Synonyms for this parasite include Asian *Taenia*, *Taenia saginata taiwanensis*, *Taenia saginata asiatica*, although now it is generally recognized as a distinct species (Eom, 2006). On morphological, biological, molecular, and epidemiological grounds the parasite is much closer to *T. saginata* than to *T. solium*. Morphologically the eggs of *T. asiatica* cannot be distinguished from those of other taeniids, including *T. saginata* and *T. solium*. The scolex and the proglottids of these three tapeworm species can be differentiated morphologically, but it is rather difficult (Table 9.1).

The cysticerci of *T. asiatica* are much smaller than those of *T. solium* and *T. saginata*. They are not present in the muscles but develop in the liver and, to a lesser extent, in the omentum, serosa, and lungs (Eom et al., 1992). The pig is the main

Table 9.1 Morphological differences between *T. solium*, *T. saginata*, and *T. asiatica*

	T. solium	*T. saginata*	*T. asiatica*
Adult worm			
• Length (m)	1.5–8	4–12	6 (4–8)
Scolex			
• Rostellum	Present	Absent	Present
• Hooks	22–32	Absent	Absent
Mature proglottids			
• Number of testes	375–575	800–1200	324–1216
• Ovary	Three lobes	Two lobes	Two lobes
• Vaginal sphincter	Absent	Present	Present
Gravid proglottids			
• Number of unilateral uterine branches	7–16	14–32	11–32
• Branching pattern	Dendritic	Dichotomous	Dichotomous
• Expulsion from host	Passively[a] (in groups)	Actively[b] (single)	Actively[b] (single)
Cysticercus	*C. cellulosae*	*C. bovis*	*C. viscerotropica*
• Localization	Muscles, brain, viscera	Muscles, viscera	Liver, (omentum, serosa, lungs)
• Dimensions (L/W, cm)	0.6–1.8/0.5	0.5–1/0.5	0.2–0.2
• Hooklets	Present	Absent	Rudimentary

L/W, length/width.
[a]Usually with feces.
[b]Outside defecation.
Source: Based on Fan (1988), Dorny et al. (2005), and Eom (2006).

intermediate host of *T. asiatica*, but cattle, goats, and monkeys can also harbor the cysticerci. People become infected by eating raw or undercooked pork liver, which seems to be a fairly widespread habit in some areas of the region. Whether or not the eggs of *T. asiatica* are also infective for humans is still unclear, but so far no cases have been reported (Ale et al., 2014).

9.4.2 Geographical distribution and prevalence

As indicated by its name, *T. asiatica* is currently believed to be limited to Asian countries. However, its real distribution is unknown because only molecular techniques, which are very often unavailable in endemic areas, are able to distinguish *T. asiatica* from *T. saginata* (Eom et al., 2009). In some countries, where raw pork liver is commonly consumed, a high prevalence of *T. asiatica* has been reported.

In a community in southeastern Nepal, Devleesschauwer et al. (2012) found a 13.5% prevalence of tapeworm carriers among the villagers and all tapeworms were identified as *T. asiatica.* In Bali, 23% of the pork livers were infected with *T. asiatica* (Simanjuntak et al., 1997).

9.4.3 Epidemiology and risk factors

Similar to *T. solium*, *T. asiatica* is a poverty-related parasite, and its epidemiology is very comparable. Transmission from pigs to humans occurs exclusively through consumption of raw or undercooked pork liver or viscera. Transmission from humans to pigs occurs where pigs are free ranging and have access to the eggs of *T. asiatica*, either within human feces (open defecation) or when the eggs, which are deposited around the anus, are disseminated in the environment when they drop on the ground wherever the tapeworm carrier goes (Devleesschauwer et al., 2012).

9.4.4 Diagnosis

Because the proglottids of *T. saginata* and *T. asiatica* are difficult to distinguish morphologically from each other, only molecular techniques (PCR-RFLP, multiplex PCR, or LAMP) are able to differentiate both tapeworms (Nkouawa et al., 2012). In endemic regions the presence of small cysticerci in the liver and viscera of pigs and not in the muscles is an indication of the presence of *T. asiatica* cysticercosis. Unfortunately, there is no specific immunodiagnostic test available to confirm the diagnosis. Only the postmortem molecular analysis of cysticerci using the abovementioned tests can identify the *Taenia* species responsible (Galán-Puchades and Fuentes, 2013).

9.4.5 Disease and treatment

The symptoms of an infection with adult *T. asiatica* are similar to those of *T. saginata* (Fan, 1988). Niclosamid and praziquantel are the preferred treatments for *T. asiatica.* To date, no cases of human cysticercosis due to *T.asiatica* have been reported. Porcine cysticercosis caused by *T. asiatica* generally remains asymptomatic (Eom et al., 1992).

9.4.6 Control and prevention

Measures for the prevention and control of *T. asiatica* are similar to those described for *T. saginata* and *T. solium*. Taeniosis can be prevented by avoiding the consumption of raw or undercooked liver or viscera infected with cysticerci. Porcine cysticercosis due to *T. asiatica* can be prevented by improving pig husbandry, whereby pigs have no access to human feces.

9.5 *Echinococcus* spp. causing cystic echinococcosis

9.5.1 *Parasite biology and life cycle*

Molecular studies have demonstrated that *E. granulosus* is a complex species of at least 10 distinct genotypes (G1-10): *E. granulosus* s.s. containings three genotypes (G1-3), *E. equinus* (G4), *E. ortleppi* (G5), and *E. canadensis* (G6-10), although the validity of the latter species is still controversial (Nakao et al., 2010) (see Table 9.2).

E. granulosus is a small tapeworm (<1 cm), of the small intestine of dogs and other canids. The adult tapeworm reaches sexual maturity within 5–6 weeks. Domestic and wild ungulates are intermediate hosts, and humans can accidentally get infected. Gravid proglottids, each containing several hundred eggs, and free eggs are excreted with the feces. After ingestion by a susceptible intermediate host, the oncosphere hatches from the egg and is subsequently transported to the liver and lungs, and less frequently to other organs. At these sites, hydatid cysts develop, which may result in the formation of protoscoleces. Once ingested by a definitive host, these protoscoleces grow into adult tapeworms.

9.5.2 *Geographical distribution and prevalence*

Although *E. granulosus* occurs worldwide, it is considered to be one of the neglected parasitic zoonoses. Human cystic echinococcosis (CE) is highly endemic in pastoral communities, particularly in regions of South America, the Mediterranean littoral, Eastern Europe, the Near and Middle East, East Africa, Central Asia, China, and Russia. In these regions the annual incidence varies from <1 to 200 per 100,000 inhabitants (Brunetti et al., 2010). Cystic echinococcosis in production animals is present in many rural areas of the world. Cardona and Carmena (2013) provide detailed information on the global prevalence of animal CE. Prevalence figures vary widely from one animal species to the other, but may reach very high levels in sheep and camels.

Table 9.2 Taxonomy of the *E. granulosus* complex

Species	Genotype	Intermediate host	Human infection
E. granulosus s.s.	G1	Sheep	Common
	G2	Sheep	Common
	G3	Cattle/buffalo	Common
E. equinus	G4	Horse	Unknown
E. ortleppi	G5	Cattle	Rare
E. canadensis	G6	Camel	Rare
	G7	Pig	Rare
	G8	Cervids	Rare
	G9	Pig	Rare
	G10	Cervids	Rare

Based on Nakao et al. (2010) and Thompson (2008).

In some countries in North Africa and South America, the prevalence of CE in sheep exceeds 50 percent. The main economic losses in domestic animals occur in cattle, sheep, goats, and camels and are due to condemnation of infected viscera, decreases in yield and quality of meat, milk, and wool, reduced hide value, reduced birth rate and fecundity, and delayed performance and growth (Torgerson, 2003).

9.5.3 Epidemiology and risk factors

Risk factors for the transmission of eggs to humans include close contact with infected dogs (taeniid eggs stick to the fur), contact with contaminated soil, especially at defecation sites of dogs, and consumption of food or water contaminated with *Echinococcus* eggs.

Factors associated with an increased risk for *E. granulosus* infection in dogs are access to raw infected viscera, the possibility of scavenging dead animals infected with fertile hydatid cysts, lack of anthelmintic treatment, and the poor health education of dog owners.

Key factors associated with CE in livestock are the ages of the animals and the intensity of environmental contamination with parasite eggs. Numerous studies have reported higher prevalence and intensity of infection in older animals as compared to young ones (Otero-Abad and Torgerson, 2013).

9.5.4 Diagnosis

9.5.4.1 Echinococcosis in dogs

The gold standard for the detection of *Echinococcus* spp. infections in definitive hosts is sedimentation and counting of worms in intestinal material performed at necropsy (Barnes et al., 2012). It has a sensitivity of 96–100%. Coprological examination has a low sensitivity and does not enable distinguishing the eggs of *Taenia* and *Echinococcus*. Arecoline hydrobromide purgation is used for mass surveillance in many control programs but has a sensitivity of only 39%. ELISA for copro-antigen detection is more specific and sensitive, but there is cross-reaction with *E. multilocularis* (Barnes et al., 2012).

9.5.4.2 Cystic echinococcosis in livestock

Diagnosis and monitoring of CE in domestic intermediate hosts is usually done by macroscopic examination of the viscera during the postmortem inspection at the slaughterhouse. However, a high rate of misclassification errors may occur if there is no confirmation by histology (Gatti et al., 2007).

9.5.4.3 Human cystic echinococcosis

Although a universal gold standard is lacking, ultrasonography (US) is the primary diagnostic procedure used for CE in abdominal locations (Brunetti et al., 2010). An international classification of US images is available to allow classifying each patient according to clinical status (WHO, 2003). CT, radiography, and MRI are the methods used for diagnosing CE in other anatomical locations.

Immunodiagnostic tests for the detection of serum antibodies are used to support the clinical diagnosis of CE. ELISA using *E. granulosus* hydatid fluid antigen is commonly used and has a high sensitivity for hepatic cases and for multiple organ localizations, but the diagnostic sensitivity is markedly lower for pulmonary cysts (Brunetti et al., 2010). Specificity is limited due to cross-reactions with other cestode infections and some other diseases. Aspiration cytology and *Echinococcus*-specific PCR are additional techniques which may also be used (Barnes et al., 2012).

9.5.5 Disease and treatment

The larval forms of the parasite (hydatid cysts) may occur in almost any organ, but lung and liver are most frequently affected. The cysts grow slowly and are usually well tolerated by the hosts. The course of CE in livestock is usually subclinical, but may cause important production losses. In humans, clinical symptoms usually appear when the cyst compresses or ruptures into neighboring structures (Brunetti et al., 2010). Cyst rupture may be a cause of anaphylactic or acute inflammatory pathology. Clinical manifestations are primarily determined by the site, size, and number of cysts.

For the treatment of CE, an image-based, stage-specific approach is followed to determine a choice of either percutaneous treatment, surgery, anti-infectious drug treatment or a "watch and wait" approach. Percutaneous treatments are carried out using PAIR (puncture, aspiration, injection, re-aspiration) to destroy the germinal layer of the cyst or by modified catheterization techniques to evacuate the entire endocyst (Brunetti et al., 2010). Albendazole is currently used to treat CE.

9.5.6 Prevention and control

In addition to education on hygiene, sanitation, and minimizing contact of dogs with slaughter offal, prevention of CE focuses primarily on regular treatment of definitive hosts with praziquantel and meat inspection to detect and destroy the hydatid cysts. Although the current gold standard for hydatid control programs is the treatment of all dogs every 4 weeks with praziquantel, this is almost impossible to realize because there are always some dogs missing at the time of dosing, and stray dogs are difficult to reach (Barnes et al., 2012). A recombinant vaccine (EG95) for ruminant intermediate hosts (Lightowlers et al., 1996b) has been shown to be very effective and is registered for use in China and Argentina (Craig et al., 2007). However, it needs two initial vaccinations followed by a booster to maximize the immune response, and the vaccination has no impact on existing cysts (Barnes et al., 2012). Research is currently ongoing to develop a vaccine against *E. granulosus* in dogs.

9.6 *Echinococcus multilocularis* (alveolar echinoccocosis)

9.6.1 Parasite biology and life cycle

The life cycle of *E. multilocularis* is similar to that of *E. granulosus*. The adult tapeworm occurs primarily in foxes and raccoon dogs, but domestic dogs and, more rarely, cats can also be involved as definitive hosts. Dogs can play a significant role in the transmission of the parasite to humans, because of their close contact. The eggs of *E. multilocularis* are resistant to cold and can survive for long periods in the environment. After a host ingests the eggs, alveolar hydatid cysts develop mainly in the liver of the intermediate hosts. More than 40 species of small mammals (microtine and arvicolid rodents and lagomorphs) can serve as intermediate hosts for *E. multilocularis.* In contrast to *E. granulosus*, *E. multilocularis* is predominantly maintained by a wildlife cycle.

9.6.2 Geographical distribution and prevalence

The geographical distribution of alveolar echinococcosis (AE) in humans is more restricted than that of CE. It is an important public health concern in parts of Central and Eastern Europe, Near East, Russia, China, and Northern Japan. The annual incidence is 0.03–1.2 per 100,000 inhabitants (Brunetti et al., 2010). However, there is accumulating evidence that *E. multilocularis* has considerably extended its range (Hegglin and Deplazes, 2013). In the past three decades, the parasite was reported in 17 previously nonendemic countries in Western and Northern Europe. This might be due to an increased awareness and better diagnostic tools, but certainly also to an increased fox population (Davidson et al., 2012). During the past two decades, the number of human cases has more than doubled in Switzerland and possibly also in France, Austria, and Germany. Although the prevalence of the parasite in wild carnivores is rather high in some regions of North America, the number of autochtonous human cases remains very low (Davidson et al., 2012).

9.6.3 Epidemiology and risk factors

The transmission dynamics of *E. multilocularis* depend on the densities and predator–prey relationships between definitive and intermediate hosts. Young and/or male foxes are most often infected, although hunting dogs and dogs that have access to rodents run the highest risk of infection (Otero-Abad and Torgerson, 2013).

The main risk factors for AE in humans are living in an endemic area and being a farmer (in a rural setting) or a gardener (in a nonrural setting) (Piarroux et al., 2013). Contact with fox and dog fur contaminated with *E. multilocularis* eggs is considered to be an important health hazard. Vegetables contaminated by fox or dog feces are considered to be an important source of infection for humans, but—contrary to what is often cited in other literature—this is not the case for consumption of raw wild berries (Piarroux et al., 2013).

9.6.4 Diagnosis

9.6.4.1 Diagnosis of AE in humans

Based on the imaging procedures (US, CT, and MRI), a classification system based on the parasitic mass in the liver, neighboring organs involvement, and metastasis (PNM) has been developed to enable classifying each patient according to clinical status (Kern et al., 2006).

Complementary to imaging, immunodiagnosis represents a secondary diagnostic tool useful in confirming the nature of the etiologic agent. Using *E. multilocularis*-purified or recombinant antigens, diagnostic sensitivities ranging between 91% and 100% and specificities of 98–100% can be obtained (Brunetti et al., 2010). Most of the purified antigens allow discrimination between AE and CE. Molecular techniques (e.g., PCR) can be used for a species-specific detection of *Echinococcus*.

9.6.4.2 *Diagnosis of* E. multilocularis *in carnivores*

Similar to *E. granulosus*, the gold standard for the detection of *E. multilocularis* is sedimentation, and counting of worms in intestinal material performed at necropsy. Arecoline hydrobromide purgation has an even lower sensitivity (21%) than it does for *E. granulosus*. The copro-antigen ELISA has a good sensitivity if the worm burden exceeds 100 but cross-reacts with *E. granulosus* (Barnes et al., 2012).

9.6.5 Disease and treatment

The primary location of AE is the liver, and in later stages, metastases may occur in lungs, brain, and other organs. Therefore, AE is often compared with a slow-growing liver cancer.

Clinical symptoms are usually nonspecific, with mild abdominal pain (in one-third of the cases) and/or cholestatic jaundice (in one-third of the cases). In the other third, fatigue, weight loss, and hepatomegaly are present. The average time between infection and occurrence of the first symptoms is between 5 and 15 years (Brunetti et al., 2010).

The primary treatment used is radical surgery followed by chemotherapy with albendazole. However, because the diagnosis of AE in most patients is confirmed only in later stages of the disease, radical surgery is usually not possible anymore, and continuous treatment with albendazole remains the only option (Brunetti et al., 2010).

9.6.6 Prevention and control

Using praziquantel for long-term anthelmintic baiting campaigns for foxes is the most effective tool to significantly reduce the infection pressure of *E. multilocularis*. Furthermore, monthly deworming of domestic dogs with access to rodents is very important given the high reproduction rate of the parasite in these animals (Hegglin and Deplazes, 2013). Finally, effective risk communication with high-risk groups (hunters, farmers, and dog owners) should emphasize simple protective actions such as frequent hand washing and proper handling of vegetables (Davidson et al., 2012; Piarroux et al., 2013).

9.7 *Diphyllobothrium* spp.

9.7.1 Parasite biology and life cycle

The life cycle of *Diphyllobothrium* spp. includes copepods as the first intermediate hosts in which procercoid larvae develop and freshwater, anadromous, and marine fish as the second intermediate hosts in which plerocercoid larvae develop. Following

Table 9.3 Most important *Diphyllobothrium* species

Species	Final host	Second intermediate host	Distribution
D. dendriticum	Fish-eating birds, mammals (incl. man)	Freshwater and anadromous fish, esp. salmonids	Circumboreal
D. latum	Humans, terrestrial mammals	Mainly pike, perch, burbot, char	Europe, North America, Asia
D. nihonkaiense	Brown bear, humans	Pacific salmon, Japanese huchen	Northern Pacific Ocean
D. pacificum	Sea lions, eared seals, occasionally humans	Marine fish	Pacific coast of South America, Japan

Adapted from Scholz et al. (2009) and Kuchta et al. (2013).

ingestion by definitive hosts, such as carnivore mammals, fish-eating birds, and also humans, these plerocercoids will mature to adult tapeworms that can reach 2–15 m or more and can contain several thousand proglottids. The prepatent period varies from 2 to 6 weeks according to the species. Typical operculate eggs and proglottids are eliminated with the feces. The most important features of *Diphyllobothrium dendriticum*, *Diphyllobothrium latum*, *Diphyllobothrium nihonkaiense*, and *Diphyllobothrium pacificum* are summarized in Table 9.3.

9.7.2 Geographical distribution and prevalence

Among the 50 valid species belonging to the genus *Diphyllobothrium*, 14 species are infective to humans. *D. latum* is the most frequently reported, whereas both *D. latum* and *Diphyllobothrium nikonhaiense* are considered to be the most pathogenic. It is estimated that about 20 million people are infected with *Diphyllobothrium* spp. worldwide (Scholz et al., 2009). Over the last decades there appears to be a decline of the infection rate in North America, Asia, and most of Europe. However, there is a re-emergence of the parasite in Russia, North Korea, Japan, Brazil, and some European countries, such as Switzerland, France, and Italy (Scholz et al., 2009). Owing to globalization and the increasing transport of fish around the globe, several outbreaks of *D. latum* have been reported since 2005 in Brazil, a country where this parasite was not endemic, from the consumption of raw salmon produced in southern Chile (Cabello, 2007). Similarly, human cases of *D. dendriticum* in some European countries where the parasite has not been reported previously show that *Diphyllobothrium* spp. have the potential to spread globally (Kuchta et al., 2013).

9.7.3 Epidemiology and risk factors

The fecundity of *Diphyllobothrium* spp. is extremely high (one worm produces up to 1 million eggs per day), and the eggs are disseminated by a variety of fish-eating birds and mammals. Furthermore, the plerocercoids survive in fish from several months to several years. All of these factors together make the parasite difficult to control (Scholz et al., 2009).

The major risk factor for human infection is the consumption of raw or undercooked fish. Research has convincingly demonstrated that the fish intermediate hosts are primarily nonsalmonid fish (e.g., perch and pike) for *D. latum* and salmonid and coregonid species for *D. dentriticum* (Chai et al., 2005). Because eating raw fish is becoming increasingly fashionable, principally with such foods as sushi, sashimi, koi-pla, kinilaw, and ceviche, it is not surprising that the parasite is emerging or reemerging in many countries (Macpherson, 2005).

9.7.4 Diagnosis

Routine diagnosis of diphyllobothriosis is based on the morphological characteristics of the eggs and proglottids in the feces. However, this allows only a genus-specific diagnosis. For a species-specific diagnosis, molecular tools are necessary. A multiplex PCR has been developed that allows for the differential identification of the most common *Diphyllobothrium* species infecting humans: *D. latum*, *D. dendriticum*, *D. nihonkaiense*, and *D. pacificum* (Wicht et al., 2010).

9.7.5 Disease and treatment

Intestinal infection with *Diplyllobothrium* spp. is usually mild or even asymptomatic. In some cases, diarrhea and abdominal pain may occur. Prolonged and heavy *D. latum* infection can cause a megaloblastic anemia due to the sequestration of vitamin B_{12} in the worm. Pernicious anemia with damage to the nervous system occurs rarely (Scholz et al., 2009). The drugs of choice for the treatment of diphyllobothriosis are praziquantel and niclosamide.

9.7.6 Prevention and control

Control measures include the prevention of water contamination by sewage treatment plants, the anthelmintic treatment of tapeworm carriers, and, of course, the prevention of transmission of infective larvae from fish to humans by the appropriate cooking or freezing of fish. Smoking of fish does not reliably kill the parasites (Scholz et al., 2009).

References

Abba, K., Ramaratnam, S., Ranganathan, L.N., 2010. Anthelmintics for people with neurocysticercosis (Review). Cochrane Database Syst. Rev. 1, CD000215.

Ale, A., Victor, B., Praet, N., Gabriël, S., Speybroeck, N., Dorny, P., Devleesschauwer, B., 2014. Epidemiology and genetic diversity of *Taenia asiatica*: a systematic review. Parasit. Vectors 7, 45.

Allan, J.C., Avila, G., Noval, J.G., Flisser, A., Craig, P.S., 1990. Immunodiagnosis of taeniasis by coproantigen detection. Parasitology 101, 473–477.

Assana, E., Kyngdon, T.C., Gauci, C.G., Geerts, S., Dorny, P., De Deken, R., Anderson, G., Zoli, A.P., Lightowlers, M.W., 2010. Elimination of *Taenia solium* transmission to pigs in a small-scale field trial of the TSOL18 vaccine in Cameroon. Int. J. Parasitol. 40, 515–519.

Barnes, T.S., Deplazes, P., Gottstein, B., Jenkins, D.J., Mathis, A., Siles-Luca, M., Torgerson, P.R., Ziadinov, I., Heath, D.D., 2012. Challenges for diagnosis and control of cystic hydatid disease. Acta Trop. 123, 1–7.

Brunetti, E., Kern, P., Vuitton, D.A., Writing Panel for the WHO-IWGE, 2010. Expert consensus for the diagnosis and treatment of cystic and alveolar echinococcosis in humans. Acta Trop. 114, 1–16.

Budke, C.M., White Jr., A.C., Garcia, H.H., 2009. Zoonotic larval cestode infections: neglected, neglected tropical diseases? PLoS Negl. Trop. Dis. 3 (2), e319. http://dx.doi.org/10.1371/journal.pntd.0000319.

Cabaret, J., Geerts, S., Madeline, M., Ballandonne, C., Barbier, D., 2002. The use of urban sewage sludge on pastures: the cysticercosis threat. Vet. Res. 33, 575–597.

Cabello, F.C., 2007. Salmon aquaculture and transmission of the fish tapeworm. Emerg. Infect. Dis. 13, 169–171.

Cardona, G.A., Carmena, D., 2013. A review of the global prevalence, molecular epidemiology and economics of cystic echinococcosis in production animals. Vet. Parasitol. 192, 10–32.

Chai, J.-Y., Murrell, K.D., Lymbery, A.J., 2005. Fish-borne parasitic zoonoses: status and issues. Int. J. Parasitol. 35, 1233–1254.

Craig, P.S., McManus, D.P., Lightowlers, M.W., Chabalgoity, J.A., Garcia, H.H., Gavidia, C.S., et al., 2007. Prevention and control of cystic echinococcosis. Lancet Infect. Dis. 7, 385–394.

Davidson, R.K., Romig, T., Jenkins, E., Tryland, M., Robertson, L.J., 2012. The impact of globalisation on the distribution of *Echinococcus multilocularis*. Trends Parasitol. 28, 239–247.

Del Brutto, O.H., Rajshekhar, V., White, A.C., Tsang, V.C.W., Nash, T.E., Takayanagui, O.M., Schantz, P.M., Evans, C.A.W., Flisser, A., Correa, D., Botero, D., Allan, J.C., Sarti, E., Gonzalez, A.E., Gilman, R.H., Garcia, H.H., 2001. Proposed diagnostic criteria for neurocysticercosis. Neurology 57, 177–183.

Devleesschauwer, B., Aryal, A., Joshi, D.D., Rijal, S., Sherchand, J.B., Praet, N., Speybroeck, N., Duchateau, L., Vercruysse, J., Dorny, P., 2012. Epidemiology of *Taenia solium* in Nepal: is it influenced by the social characteristics of the population and the presence of *Taenia asiatica*? Trop. Med. Int. Health 17, 1019–1022.

Dorny, P., Praet, N., 2007. *Taenia saginata* in Europe. Vet. Parasitol. 149, 22–24.

Dorny, P., Phiri, I.K., Vercruysse, J., Gabriel, S., Willingham III, A.L., Brandt, J., Victor, B., Speybroeck, N., Berkvens, D., 2004. A Bayesian approach for estimating values for prevalence and diagnostic test characteristics of porcine cysticercosis. Int. J. Parasitol. 34, 569–576.

Dorny, P., Brandt, J., Geerts, S., 2005. Detection and diagnosis. In: Murrell, K.D. (Ed.), WHO/FAO/OIE Guidelines for the Surveillance, Prevention and Control of Taeniosis/Cysticercosis. OIE, Paris, pp. 45–55.

Eichenberger, R.M., Lewis, F., Gabriël, S., Dorny, P., Torgerson, P.R., Deplazes, P., 2013. Multitest analysis and model-based estimation of the prevalence of *Taenia saginata* cysticercus infection in naturally infected dairy cows in the absence of a 'gold standard' reference test. Int. J. Parasitol. 43, 853–859.

Eom, K.S., 2006. What is Asian *Taenia*? Parasitol. Int. 55, S137–S141.

Eom, K.S., Rim, H.J., Geerts, S., 1992. Experimental infection of pigs and cattle with eggs of Asian *Taenia saginata* with special reference to its extrahepatic viscerotropism. Korean J. Parasitol. 30, 269–275.

Eom, K.S., Jeon, H.-K., Rim, H.-J., 2009. Geographical distribution of *Taenia asiatica* and related species. Korean J. Parasitol. 47, S115–S124.

Fan, P.C., 1988. Taiwan *Taenia* and taeniasis. Parasitol. Today 4, 86–88.

Flisser, A., Correa, D., Avilla, G., Marvilla, P., 2005. Biology of *Taenia solium, Taenia saginata* and *Taenia saginata asiatica*. In: Murrell, K.D. (Ed.), WHO/FAO/OIE Guidelines for the Surveillance, Prevention and Control of Taeniosis/Cysticercosis. OIE, Paris, pp. 1–9.

Gabriel, S., Blocher, J., Dorny, P., Abatih, E.N., Schmutzhard, E., et al., 2012. Added value of antigen ELISA in the diagnosis of neurocysticercosis in resource poor settings. PLoS Negl. Trop. Dis. 6 (10), e1851. http://dx.doi.org/10.1371/journal.pntd.0001851.

Galán-Puchades, M.T., Fuentes, M.V., 2013. *Taenia asiatica*: the most neglected human *Taenia* and the possibility of cysticercosis. Korean J. Parasitol. 51, 51–54.

Garcia, H.H., Evans, C.A., Nash, T.E., Takayanagui, O.M., White, A.C., Botero, D., Rajshekhar, V., Tsang, V.C., Schantz, P.M., Allan, J.C., Flisser, A., Correa, D., Sarti, E., Friedland, J.S., Martinez, S.M., Gonzalez, A.E., Gilman, R.H., Del Brutto, O.H., 2002. Current consensus guidelines for treatment of neurocysticercosis. Clin. Microbiol. Rev. 15, 747–756.

Garcia, H.H., Gonzalez, A.E., Evans, C.A.W., Gilman, R.H., Cysticercosis Working, G.P., 2003. *Taenia solium* cysticercosis. Lancet 362, 547–556.

Gatti, A., Alvarez, A.R., Araya, D., Mancini, S., Herrero, E., Santillan, G., Larrieu, E., 2007. Ovine echinococcosis. I. Immunological diagnosis by enzyme immunoassay. Vet. Parasitol. 143, 112–121.

Geysen, D., Kanobana, K., Victor, B., Rodriguez-Hidalgo, R., de Borchgrave, J., Brandt, J., Dorny, P., 2007. Validation of meat inspection results for *Taenia saginata* cysticercosis by PCR-restriction fragment length polymorphism. J. Food Prot. 70, 236–240.

Harrison, L.J.S., Gallie, G.J., Sewell, M.M.H., 1984. Absorption of cysticerci in cattle after treatment of *T. saginata* cysticerci with praziquantel. Res. Vet. Sci. 37, 378–380.

Hegglin, D., Deplazes, P., 2013. Control of *Echinococcus multilocularis*: strategies, feasibility and cost–benefit analyses. Int. J. Parasitol. 43, 327–337.

Kern, P., Wen, H., Sato, N., Vuitton, D.A., Gruener, B., Shao, Y., Delabrousse, E., Kratzer, W., Bresson-Hadni, S., 2006. WHO classification of alveolar echinococcosis: principles and application. Parasitol. Int. 55, S283–S287.

Kuchta, R., Brabec, J., Kubackova, P., Scholz, P., 2013. Tapeworm *Diphyllobothrium dendriticum* (Cestoda)—neglected or emerging human parasite? PLoS Negl. Trop. Dis. 7 (12), e2535. http://dx.doi.org/10.1371/journal.pntd.0002535.

Lee, Y.-M., Handali, S., Hancock, K., Pattabhi, S., Kovalenko, V.A., Levin, A., et al., 2011. Serologic diagnosis of human *Taenia solium* cysticercosis by using recombinant and synthetic antigens in QuickELISA™. Am. J. Trop. Med. Hyg. 84, 587–893.

Lightowlers, M.W., 2010. Eradication of *Taenia solium* cysticercosis: a role for vaccination of pigs. Int. J. Parasitol. 40, 1183–1192.

Lightowlers, M.W., Rolfe, R., Gauci, C.G., 1996a. *Taenia saginata*: vaccination against cysticercosis in cattle with recombinant oncosphere antigens. Exp. Parasitol. 84, 330–338.

Lightowlers, M.W., Lawrence, S.B., Gauci, C.G., Young, J., Ralston, M.J., Maas, D., Heath, D.D., 1996b. Vaccination against hydatidosis using a defined recombinant antigen. Parasite Immunol. 18, 457–462.

Macpherson, C.N.L., 2005. Human behaviour and the epidemiology of parasitic zoonoses. Int. J. Parasitol. 35, 1319–1331.

Mkupasi, E.M., Sikasunge, C.S., Ngowi, H.A., Johansen, M.V., 2013. Efficacy and safety of anthelmintics tested against *Taenia solium* cysticercosis in pigs. PLoS Negl. Trop. Dis. 7 (7), e2200. http://dx.doi.org/10.1371/journal.pntd.0002200.

Murrell, K.D., 2005. Epidemiology of taeniosis and cysticercosis. In: Murrell, K.D. (Ed.), WHO/FAO/OIE Guidelines for the Surveillance, Prevention and Control of Taeniosis/Cysticercosis. OIE, Paris, pp. 27–44.

Nakao, M., Yanagida, T., Okamoto, M., Knapp, J., Nkouawa, A., Sako, Y., Ito, A., 2010. State-of-the-art *Echinococcus* and *Taenia*: phylogenetic taxonomy of human-pathogenic tapeworms and its application to molecular diagnosis. Infect. Genet. Evol. 10, 444–452.

Ndimubanzi, P.C., Carabin, H., Budke, C.M., Nguyen, H., Qian, Y.-J., et al., 2010. A systematic review of the frequency of neurocyticercosis with a focus on people with epilepsy. PLoS Negl. Trop. Dis. 4 (11), e870. http://dx.doi.org/10.1371/journal.pntd.0000870.

Nkouawa, A., Sako, Y., Li, T., Chen, X., Nakao, M., Yanagida, T., et al., 2012. A loop-mediated isothermal amplification method for a differential identification of *Taenia* tapeworms from human: application to a field survey. Parasitol. Int. 61, 723–725.

Otero-Abad, B., Torgerson, P.R., 2013. A systematic review of the epidemiology of echinococcosis in domestic and wild animals. PLoS Negl. Trop. Dis. 7 (6), e2249. http://dx.doi.org/10.1371/journal.pntd.0002249.

Piarroux, M., Piarroux, R., Knapp, J., Bardonnet, K., Dumortier, J., Watelet, J., et al., 2013. Populations at risk for alveolar echinococcosis, France. Emerg. Infect. Dis. 19, 721–728.

Praet, N., Verweij, J.J., Mwape, K.E., Phiri, I.K., Muma, J.B., Zulu, G., van Lieshout, L., Rodriguez-Hidalgo, R., Benitez-Ortiz, W., Dorny, P., Gabriel, S., 2013. Bayesian modelling to estimate the test characteristics of coprology, coproantigen ELISA and a novel real-time PCR for the diagnosis of taeniasis. Trop. Med. Int. Health 18, 608–614.

Rodriguez, S., Dorny, P., Tsang, V.C.W., Pretell, E.J., Brandt, J., Lescano, A.G., Gonzalez, A.E., Gilman, R.H., Garcia, H.H., 2009. Detection of *Taenia solium* antigens and anti-T solium antibodies in paired serum and cerebrospinal fluid samples from patients with intraparenchymal or extraparenchymal neurocysticercosis. J. Infect. Dis. 199, 1345–1352.

Scandrett, W.B., Haines, D.M., Parker, S.E., Robinson, Y., Forbes, L.B., Gajadhar, A.A., Brandt, J., Geerts, S., Dorny, P., 2012. Validation of an immunohistochemical assay for bovine cysticercosis, with comparison to a standard histological method. Vet. Parasitol. 186, 301–311.

Schantz, P.M., Cruz, M., Sarti, E., Pawlowski, Z., 1993. Potential eradicability of taeniasis and cysticercosis. Bull. Pan Am. Health Organ. 27, 397–403.

Scholz, T., Garcia, H.H., Kuchta, R., Wicht, B., 2009. Update on the human broad tapeworm (genus *Diphyllobothrium*), including clinical relevance. Clin. Microbiol. Rev. 22, 146–160.

Serpa, J.A., White Jr., A.C., 2012. Neurocysticercosis in the United States. Pathog. Glob. Health 106, 256–260.

Simanjuntak, G.M., Margono, S.S., Okamoto, M., Ito, A., 1997. Taeniasis/cysticercosis in Indonesia as an emerging disease. Parasitol. Today 13, 321–323.

Thompson, R.C.A., 2008. The taxonomy, phylogeny and transmission of *Echinococcus*. Exp. Parasitol. 119, 439–446.

Torgerson, P.R., 2003. Economic effects of echinococcosis. Acta Trop. 85, 113–118.

Victor, B., 2014. Proteomic analysis of Taenia spp. excretion/secretion proteins: the search for Taenia solium-specific diagnostic antigens. Ph.D. Thesis. University of Ghent.

WHO, 2014. Neglected Zoonotic Diseases. Available from: http://www.who.int/neglected_diseases/zoonoses/en/ (accessed 09.05.14.).

WHO Informal Working Group, 2003. International classification of ultrasound images in cystic echinococcosis for application in clinical and field epidemiological settings. Acta Trop. 85, 253–261.

Wicht, B., Yanagida, T., Scholz, T., Ito, A., Jimenez, J.A., Brabec, J., 2010. Multiplex PCR for differential identification of broad tapeworms (*Cestoda*: *Diphyllobothrium*) infecting humans. J. Clin. Microbiol. 48, 3111–3116.

Wilkins, P.P., Allan, J.C., Verastegui, M., Acosta, M., Eason, A.G., Garcia, H.H., Gonzalez, A.E., Gilman, R.H., Tsang, V.C.W., 1999. Development of a serologic assay to detect *Taenia solium* taeniasis. Am. J. Trop. Med. Hyg. 60, 199–204.

Zammarchi, L., Strohmeyer, M., Bartalesi, F., Bruno, E., Munoz, J., et al., 2013. Epidemiology and management of cysticercosis and *Taenia solium* Taeniasis in Europe, systematic review 1990–2011. PLoS One 8 (7), e69537. http://dx.doi.org/10.1371/journal.pone.0069537.

Foodborne trematodes

10

J. Waikagul[1], *M. Sato*[2], *M.O. Sato*[3]
[1]Mahidol University, Bangkok, Thailand; [2]Niigata University, Niigata, Japan;
[3]Universidade Federal do Tocantins, Palmas, Brazil

10.1 Introduction

Humans can be infected with foodborne trematodes' helminths whose infective stages occur in animals or aquatic plants, by ingesting raw or insufficiently cooked food. Trematodes typically infect the intestines, lungs, or liver, but migrating species, such as *Fasciola* and *Paragonimus*, has been found outside these typical sites, in vital organs such as the eyes or brain, where severe manifestations are reported (WHO, 1995). The severity of these infections varies from asymptomatic to fatal depending on infection site, species, size, number of worms, duration and frequency of infection, and host tolerance. In this chapter we list the species according to their medical importance and the source of their infective stage and review their morphology, life cycle, pathogenesis, and symptoms. A summary of information on listed species of foodborne trematodes and hosts is provided in Table 10.1. The end of this chapter discusses the diagnosis, treatment, prevention, and control of trematodes.

10.1.1 General biology of trematodes

Trematodes are flatworms classified in the phylum Platyhelminthes, class Trematoda, subclass Digenea. In general, trematodes are dorso-ventrally flattened and leaflike in shape. Their bodies are covered with tegument, which is usually armed with scalelike spines. They have two suckers: one oral and one ventral. The mouth opens into the esophagus, which is accommodated with a small muscular body called the pharynx; the intestine has no distal opening and bifurcates into two ceca. Foodborne trematodes are hermaphroditic; male reproductive organs are composed of two testes (in some exceptional genera there are one or more testes), sperm ducts, seminal vesicle, prostatic glands, cirrus, and cirrus sac (in some genera); female reproductive organs include an ovary, oviduct, ootype, Mehlis' glands, vitelline glands, seminal receptacle, Laurer's canal, and uterus. Eggs or sperm are released through one (common) or two (male and female) genital pores. The shape and location of the ovary and testes, and the arrangement of other reproductive organs, form a basis for species identification. The excretory system consists of a bilateral group of flame cells, collecting tubules, excretory bladder, and pore, which are located at the posterior. The excretory bladder appears in various shapes (saccular, tubular, u-, v-, or y-shapes), which are useful in placing the trematodes at family or higher levels (Schell, 1970).

Foodborne Parasites in the Food Supply Web. http://dx.doi.org/10.1016/B978-1-78242-332-4.00010-2

Table 10.1 **Foodborne trematodes, hosts, distribution, and transmission vehicles for human infection**

Foodborne trematodes	Infection site (humans)	Geographic occurrence (humans)	Definitive hosts	Source of metacercariae/ intermediate hosts	Contaminated food items
Achillurbainia nouvelli	Mastoid bone	China, Thailand	Leopards (*Panthera pardus*)	Freshwater crabs (*Parathelphusa rugosa*, *Larnaudia beusekomae*)	Raw crabs
Achillurbainia recondita	Omentum, peritoneam	Hondurus	Opossums (*Didelphis marsupialis*)	Freshwater crabs	Raw crabs
Alaria americana	Eyes, lungs, and other organs	North America	Raccoons	Amphibians, reptiles, raccoons, opossums	Undercooked hosts
Amphimerus pseudofelineus	Bile duct	Ecuador	Cats, dogs	Freshwater fish	Sashimi, ceviche
Carneophallus breviceca	Small intestine	Philippines	Freshwater fish (*Glossogobius giurus*)	Freshwater shrimp (*Macrobrachium* sp.)	Jumping salad
Clinostoma complanatum	Throat, pharynx, larynx, eye	Japan, Israel, India, Korea, Thailand	Birds	Freshwater fish	Raw freshwater fish
Clonorchis sinensis	Bile duct	China, Japan, Korea, Russia, Taiwan, North Vietnam	Dogs, cats, hogs, martens, badgers, minks, weasels, rats	Freshwater fish (cyprinids)	Sashimi
Dicrocoelium dendriticum	Bile ducts	Worldwide	Ruminants	Ants	Salad
Echinochasmus spp.	Small intestine	Asia	Dogs, cats, rats, birds, pigs	Freshwater fish (loach)	Sashimi
Echinostoma spp.	Small intestine	Asia	Rats, cats, dogs, pigs, birds	Freshwater snails, clams	Undercooked snails
Eurytrema pancreaticum	Bile duct	Asia	Ruminants	Grasshoppers	Undercooked grasshopper

Fasciola spp.	Liver and ectopic foci	Worldwide	Ruminants	Aquatic plants	Salad
Fasciolopsis buski	Small intestine	Asia	Pigs, rabbits, monkeys	Water caltrop, chesnut, hyacinth, bamboo, lotus, lily, cress, morning glory	Salad
Fischoederius elongates	Large intestine	China	Ruminants	Aquatic plants	Salad
Gastrodiscoides hominis	Large intestine	Asia, Russia, Africa	Pigs, rodents, ungulates, primates	Aquatic plants, crustaceans, molluscs, amphibians	Salad, raw or undercooked contaminated hosts
Gymnophalloides seoi	Small intestine	Korea	Birds	Oysters	Raw oysters
Haplorchis spp.	Small intestine	Asia	Dogs, cats, fish-eating birds	Freshwater fish (cyprinids, gourami)	Koi Pla, raw or undercooked fish
Metorchis spp.	Bile duct	Canada, China, Russia	Dogs, cats, foxes, coyotes, minks, bears, raccoons, gray seals, eagles, ducks, beavers, otters, rats	Freshwater fish (white sucker, cyprinids)	Sashimi
Nanophyetus salmincola	Small intestine	United States, Siberia	Dogs, cats, foxes	Salmon, steelhead trout	Raw fish
Neodiplostomum soulense	Small intestine	Korea	Raccoons, rodents (*Apodemus agrarius*), cats	Frog tadpoles, grass snakes	Raw or undercooked frogs or snakes
Opisthorchis felineus	Bile duct	Eurasia	Dogs, cats, pigs, martens, foxes, chipmunks, beavers, seals, rats, minks, white-tailed eagles	Freshwater fish (ide, roach, minnow, tench, dace)	Raw or undercooked fish
Opisthorchis viverrini	Bile duct	Cambodia, Laos, Thailand, Vietnam	Cats, dogs	Cyprinids fish	Koi pla, Goi Ga

Continued

Table 10.1 Continued

Foodborne trematodes	Infection site (humans)	Geographic occurrence (humans)	Definitive hosts	Source of metacercariae/ intermediate hosts	Contaminated food items
Paragonimus spp.	Lungs	Worldwide	Tigers, cats, dogs, opossums, mongoose, minks, weasels, rats	Freshwater crabs, crayfish	Raw crabs or contaminated food
Phaneropsolus spp.	Small intestine	Indonesia, Laos, Thailand	Bats, monkeys, rats	Naiads of dragon fly	Jumping salad
Plagiorchis spp.	Small intestine	Korea, Thailand, Philippines,	Rats, dogs, birds	Nymphs of stone fly	Contaminated food
Poikilorchis congolensis	Mastoid bone	Cameroon, Nigeria, Malaysia	Weasels?	Freshwater crabs	Raw crabs
Prosthodendrium molenkampi	Small intestine	Indonesia, Laos, Thailand	Bats, monkeys, rats?	Naiads of dragon fly	Jumping salad
Watsonius watsoni	Intestine	Africa, eastern Asia	Primates	Aquatic plants	Salad

References for the information in the table are provided in the text of the chapter.

The trematode life cycle starts in a natural body of water (pond, lake, or river) after being contaminated with trematode eggs released by the definitive or reservoir hosts; snails and aquatic animals are infected and become the first and the second intermediate hosts; the infected aquatic animals are eaten raw by the definitive or reservoir hosts, completing their life cycle (Figure 10.1). With exception, trematodes in the family Dicrocoeliidae complete their life cycle on land, using land snails and insects as the first and the second intermediate hosts. The digenean trematodes have a complex life cycle; sexual reproduction occurs in the adult stage in the definitive host, and asexual multiplication occurs in the first intermediate host.

The typical life cycle of foodborne trematodes include three hosts and several stages. An adult lives in the definitive vertebrate host, producing eggs that are released together with the host's excreta. When in water, the fully developed embryo in the egg (miracidium) hatches and swims freely to find the first intermediate host—a specific aquatic snail species. Upon entering the snail, the miracidium develops into a sporocyst, which produces the next generation of sporocysts or rediae. The redia produces either another generation of rediae and/or cercariae, which leave the snail host and again swim freely in the water searching for the second intermediate host—aquatic animals. In the selected host, the cercariae encyst and develop into metacercariae, the infective stage to the final host. With exception, the metacercariae of trematodes in the family Fasciolidae encyst on substrates in the water, including plants. After the definitive hosts ingest infected animals or contaminated plants, the metacercariae excyst in the duodenum, migrate to the final site either in the intestine, liver, or lungs, and develop into adult stages (Schell, 1970).

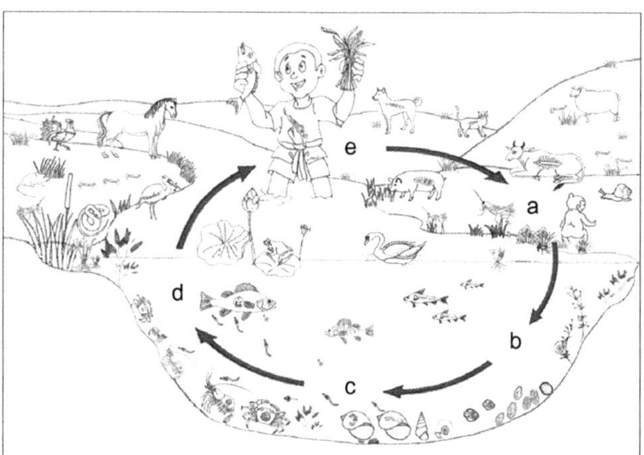

Figure 10.1 Schematic scenario depicting a typical life cycle of foodborne trematodes. (a) Trematode eggs in host excreta contaminating environment. (b) Fully developed miracidia hatch from trematode eggs. (c) Infected snail first intermediate hosts with miracidia, which develop into sporocysts, rediae, and cercariae. (d) Cercariae emerged from snails and infect the second intermediate hosts (fish, crustaceans) and develop to metacercariae. (e) Foodborne metacercariae are ingested by definitive hosts (humans and animals) and develop into adult trematodes.

10.2 Vegetable borne trematodes

Because of the transmission dynamics of these parasites, foodborne, and especially vegetable-transmitted trematodes deserve attention by health care professionals. There are two crucial reasons for this: vegetables are usually eaten raw in salads, and cultural and behavioral factors can increase the risk of infection. Vegetable borne flukes are normally parasites of animals and can eventually infect humans (zoonoses). They can be divided in to two groups: the liver flukes (*Fasciola hepatica*, *Fasciola gigantica*) and intestinal flukes (*Fasciolopsis buski*, *Gastrodiscoides hominis*, *Watsonius watsoni*, and *Fischoederius elongatus*).

10.2.1 Liver flukes

Fasciolosis (syn. fascioliasis) is a global disease caused by *F. hepatica* and *Fasciola gigantica*, affecting a large number of countries throughout the world. *F. hepatica* has an urban distribution, mainly in temperate zones, whereas *F. gigantica* is distributed in Africa and Asia. Together, the two *Fasciola* species are present in large geographical regions (Mas-Coma and Bargues, 1997). Sheep and cattle are natural hosts for *Fasciola* spp., but a wide range of other domestic animals may also be affected, for example, Bovidae, Equidae, and Camelidae species. Wild mammals may also contract the disease, and some are known to act as reservoir hosts, for example, Cervidae, Marsupialia, and Lagomorpha species (Boray, 1969). The World Health Organization (WHO) considers fasciolosis as one of the most important helminth diseases, with high importance for public health, and a significant impact on human development (WHO, 1995, 2004).

The liver flukes *F. hepatica* and *F. gigantica* are leaf-shaped flatworms; their body size varies from 20 to 50 mm in length and 10 to 15 mm in width. The foliate shape, oval in outline or considerably elongated and attenuated posteriorly, presents a cephalic cone in the anterior portion. The oral sucker is approximately 1 mm in diameter and lies in the anterior region and the ventral sucker with 1.5 mm diameter, is located at the base of the cephalic cone. The esophagus is well developed and divided into branched ceca extending to the posterior. The testes are noticeably dendritic and cover two-thirds of the posterior portion. The ovary is small and dendritic as well, situated anterior to the anterior testis, whereas the uterus is relatively short and located anterior to the ovary. The genital pore is located anterior to the ventral sucker. Vitellaria are dendritic and scattered in both lateral fields of the body. Eggs are large, ovoid, thin-shelled, and yellowish brown. The operculum is small and inconspicuous, and the cell inside is unsegmented (Belding, 1965).

The infective stage is the metacercaria, which encysts openly on aquatic plants or other materials in the water. The metacercarial cyst is round and thick-walled, composed of an outer cyst and an inner cyst. The inner cyst is formed by mucopolysaccharide and keratinized protein layers. These walls are important to the survival of the metacercaria. Even if the outer wall is removed, the cysts can survive for long periods and remain infective (Boray, 1969). The outer cyst is composed of layers of tanned protein and a fibrous mucoprotein, probably acting as a barrier against bacterial and fungal infections and an important component in the attachment to the substrate (Dixon, 1965). Mature metacercariae have a diameter of 0.215–0.256 mm (Hussein et al., 2010). The cyst is white when laid and is almost immediately infective to the definitive host. After a day or two, the cyst gradually becomes yellow in color due to the presence of quinine and gets darker as it hardens (Andrews, 1999). Metacercariae can survive for long periods in the environment and passively infect definitive hosts feeding on contaminated vegetables. The metacercaria excysts in the duodenum, where the juvenile worm migrates to the liver and develops into the adult stage in the bile duct (Reinhard, 1957; Andrews, 1999). The life span of *F. hepatica* in humans has been estimated to be 9–13 years, during which time it produces eggs (Esteban et al., 1997).

Fasciolosis in humans can appear in two distinct forms: acute and chronic. Acute disease is indicated by inflammatory lesions developing from an early infection, and signals of chronic disease include fibrosis in the tissues, a result of longstanding infection. Because the adult fluke has a long life span, the intensity of infection tends to increase by age group. In endemic areas, newly infected adult hosts are at an increased risk of acute disease, or if they acquire the parasites when young, they are at a higher risk of chronic disease (Esteban et al., 2002). Thus, acute lesions caused by repetitive infections, superimposed on chronic disease, can occur with relative frequency, prolonging and overlapping the acute phase with both the latent and the obstructive phases (Valero et al., 2000, 2003).

The presence and severity of symptoms are correlated with the number of infecting flukes and appear to be similar to the pathogenesis presented in animal fasciolosis (Mas-Coma and Bargues, 1997). The migration of the juvenile forms to the liver and the presence of the fluke in the circulatory system and biliary ducts are the main cause of the symptoms of fasciolosis, which depend on the location of the parasite. Pathological changes include inflammatory lesions, tissue injury, and damage to the infected organs, caused either directly through mechanical and chemical irritations by the parasites or indirectly through the host's immune response (Haswell-Elkins and Elkins, 1998; Sithithaworn et al., 2009). Signals of clinical fasciolosis include abdominal pain, frequently localized to the right hypochondrium, anorexia and weight loss, malaise, mild intermittent fever, mild hepatomegaly, jaundice, biliary abnormalities, traumatic and necrotic lesions in hepatic tissue, and fibrosis of the biliary ducts (Haswell-Elkins and Elkins, 1998; Mas-Coma et al., 2007). *Fasciola* can deviate substantially from their usual migratory route in human hosts and occur in ectopic locations, such as the skin, eyes, abdominal organs, heart, or central nervous system (CNS). In very rare cases, these infections can be fatal (Sithithaworn et al., 2009; Zhou et al., 2008; Xuan et al., 2005; WHO, 1995; Fried et al., 2004).

10.2.2 Intestinal flukes

10.2.2.1 *Fasciolopsis buski*

Fasciolopsiosis is present in many Asian countries (WHO, 1995). *F. buski* is one of the largest digeneans infecting humans, with a body 2–10 cm long, 0.8–3 cm wide, and

0.5–3 mm thick (Kumar, 1980). It differs from its relative, the *Fasciola* liver fluke, by having a rather thick body without a cephalic cone, and the ceca are unbranched. It inhabits the duodenum and jejunum, and in moderate and heavy infections it can also be found in the stomach (Graczyk et al., 2001). Pigs are important as definitive hosts and reservoirs for human disease—eggs laid by the adult worms contaminate the environment, increasing the risk of infection in humans. Rabbits and monkeys can also be reservoirs of *F. buski* in the wild (Kuntz and Lo, 1967; Hartman, 1961; Malviya, 1985).

F. buski produce a great number of eggs in humans (13,000–26,000, an average of 16,000 worms per day) (Hsieh, 1960). These eggs must reach freshwater to develop the miracidium and infect intermediate snail hosts, which are limited to small planorbids of different genera (Wang et al., 1977). Important vegetables for the transmission of fasciolopsiosis are: water caltrop (*Trapa natans* in China, *Trapa bispinosa* in Taiwan, and *Trapa bicornis* in Bangladesh and Thailand), water chestnut (*Eliocharis tuberosa*), water hyacinth (*Eichhornia* sp.), water bamboo (*Zizania* sp.), water lotus (*Nymphaea lotus*), water lily (*Nymphaea* sp.), watercress, gankola (*Otelia* sp.), and water morning glory (*Ipomoea aquatica*). Metacercarial cysts on plants are visible to the naked eye (average 3.9/2.1 mm) and are found on the surface of the vegetables. However, cercariae may also encyst on the water surface, contaminating the water (Weng et al., 1989). Definitive hosts are infected by ingesting plants or water-carrying metacercariae. The metacercariae excyst in the duodenum of definitive hosts and attach to the intestinal wall to grow into mature flukes within 3 months.

Fasciolopsiosis is usually benign in low worm burden cases, but morbidity in endemic areas can be high, and the disease can be fatal (Bunnag et al., 1983; Lee, 1972). Worms cause extensive intestinal and duodenal erosions, ulceration, hemorrhage, abscess, and catarrhal inflammation. Absorption of toxic and allergic worm metabolites causes ascites, which result in both general and facial edema (e.g., cheek and orbital edema). Pathological changes can be traumatic, obstructive, and toxic, especially in heavy infections (Fried et al., 2004). Light infections are usually asymptomatic, except for diarrheal episodes, alternating with periods of constipation and abdominal pain. Other common symptoms include anemia with eosinophilia, headache, dizziness, stomach ache, gastric pain, loose stools, asthenia, pallor, malnutrition, protuberant abdomen, and abdominal distention (Chandra, 1976). Moderate to heavy infection signals include malnutrition, severe epigastric and abdominal pain, diarrhea or bowel obstruction, poor appetite, mild abdominal colic, nausea and vomiting, fever, acute ileus, anasarca (extreme generalized edema), elevated eosinophilia and leukocytosis, and a significant lowering in serum vitamin B_{12} level (Jaroonvesama et al., 1986; Areekul et al., 1979). Heavy infections have general toxic and allergic symptoms, such as edema of the face, abdominal wall, and lower extremities. As well, abdominal pain and ascites are common signs, as are loss of appetite, bitemporal headache, giddiness, low-grade fever, nausea, and vomiting (Sadun and Maiphoom, 1953). Treated patients usually recover completely, although advanced, heavy infections can be fatal. Mortality has been reported in heavily infected children (Mas-Coma et al., 2005).

10.2.2.2 *Gastrodiscoides hominis*

G. hominis is a trematode of the cecum and colon of pigs and can infect humans. The adult worms are thick and conical in shape and reddish in color, 8–14 mm long, and 5.5–7.5 mm wide. The anterior portion of the parasite's body is short and conical-cylindrical, and the posterior portion is large, discoidal, up to 8.0 mm wide, and ventrally excavated (Kumar, 1980). Eggs are ovoid in shape, pale greenish-gray in color, and around 127–160 μm and 62–75 μm in size (Dutt and Srivastava, 1972). Domestic and wild pigs serve as definitive hosts (Dutt and Srivastava, 1972), but *G. hominis* has also been found in other species of animals, such as ungulates, rodents, and primates (Buckley, 1964; Fox and Hall, 1970; Herman, 1967; Pester and Keymer, 1968; Ivanov and Semenova, 2000). *G. hominis* is widely distributed in Asia (India, Pakistan, Burma/Myanmar, Thailand, Vietnam, the Philippines, China, and Kazakhstan), Russia, and Africa (Zambia, Nigeria) (Ahluwalia, 1960; Buckley, 1964; Kumar, 1980; Fried et al., 2004).

The life cycle of *G. hominis* is heteroxenous and similar to that of other digenetic flukes. The intermediate hosts are aquatic snail species *Helicorbis coenosus* (Dutt and Srivastava, 1966; 1972) or other planorbids, as reported from Africa. One important point of *G. hominis* biology is that encystation of cercariae generally takes place on the bottom of the pond. Encystation can occur on the shell of the snail host or any other available substrate such as a stalk of Nymphoea. The metacercaria is spherical and brownish, with a diameter of 201–227 mm. Definitive hosts are infected by ingesting metacercariae (Dutt and Srivastava, 1972). An important point in the transmission of gastrodiscoidosis is that the metacercariae are able to attach to different substrates. Thus, it has been suggested that human infection can occur by encysted metacercariae, contaminating not only vegetables or water but also raw or undercooked crustaceans, molluscs, or amphibians, as is the case in other species of the same family Gastrodiscidae (Surinthrangkul et al., 1965; Yu and Mott, 1994; Fried et al., 2004).

The pathology and symptomatology of *G. hominis* infection are not specific. In humans, the parasite causes inflammation of the mucosa of the cecum and ascending colon, resulting in diarrheal episodes. Deaths among untreated patients, especially children, have been attributed to this infection (Kumar, 1980). In pigs, a subacute inflammation of the cecum is usually present in gastrodiscoidiosis. Histopathologic studies of *G. hominis* lesions in the cecum show mucosal desquamation, mucosa/submucosa with cell infiltration (eosinophils, lymphocytes, and plasma cells), and a thick and edematous submucosa. Mucous diarrhea is an expected symptom in these cases (Ahluwalia, 1960; Yu and Mott, 1994). Marked desquamation of the epithelial lining, hypersecretion of mucus, and necrosis of the mucous glands are also the common findings in histopathological examinations. A similar picture might be expected in human infection (Mas-Coma et al., 2005).

10.2.2.3 Watsonius watsoni *and* Fischoederius elongates

There are few reports of *W. watsoni* and *F. elongates* infection among humans. *W. watsoni* is an intestinal trematode found in different species of primates in eastern Asia and Africa. Its life cycle is unknown, but the infection probably occurs by ingesting vegetables containing encysted metacercariae (Yu and Mott, 1994). Diarrhea is usually found in human infections with high worm burden (Pick, 1964, 1967). *F. elongatus* is a pouched amphistome of ruminants. Definitive hosts are infected by ingesting aquatic plants or snails carrying attached, encysted metacercariae. Lymnaeid snails are intermediate hosts. A reported case in China, where the parasite was expelled and identified, describes epigastric pain as the main symptom (Li, 1991).

10.3 Fish borne trematodes

This group comprises flukes of five families (Clinostomatidae, Echinostomatidae, Heterophyidae, Opisthorchiidae, and Troglotrematidae), with species known to cause disease in the human liver and intestine (Waikagul and Thaenkham, 2014).

10.3.1 Small liver flukes

Opisthorchids, small liver flukes, are the most common fish borne trematodes. They are small, 0.5–2.5 cm long, and 1–5 mm wide. Their body is slender, attenuated anteriorly, and transparent. Two testes are situated posterior to the ovary at the posterior end, and the uterus winds between the cecum, from the ventral sucker to the ovary. The vitelline follicles are situated on both lateral sides of the midsection of the body. The shape of the testes and the distribution of vitellariae vary between species. Eggs are small, 20–30 μm long, and 15–17 μm wide (Radomyos et al., 2004). Liver flukes of the family Opisthorchiidae comprise four genera distributed in America, Asia, and Europe.

10.3.1.1 *Amphimerus pseudofelineus*

Human infection with *Opisthorchis guayaquilensis* was first reported in Ecuador in 1949; however, the name of the parasite was subsequently changed to *A. pseudofelineus* (Artigas and Perez, 1962; Rodriguez et al., 1949). Recently, human infection with *Amphimerus* was reported in the northern coastal rainforest of Ecuador among the Chachi population. The infection rates of the three villages examined varied between 15.1% and 34.1%. Adult worms recovered after treatment of humans and those from infected domestic cats and dogs are morphologically similar, indicating that amphimeriasis is a foodborne zoonosis transmitted by domestic animals living with humans (Calvopina etal., 2011).

10.3.1.2 *Clonorchis sinensis*

Infection with *C. sinensis*, the Chinese or oriental liver fluke, has primarily been reported in humans in six countries: China, Japan, Korea, Russia, Taiwan, and North Vietnam (Figurnov et al., 2002; WHO, 2004). Recently, *C. sinensis* infection was also detected in central Thailand (Traub et al., 2009). Global estimations of *C. sinensis* infections indicate that more than 200 million people are at risk, with 15–20 million people infected and 1.5–2 million exhibiting symptoms or complications (Hong and Fang, 2012).

10.3.1.3 *Metorchis bilis*

Liver-fluke infections in Russia were mixed between *O. felineus* and *M. bilis*, especially in western Siberia. Metacercariae of *M. bilis* were found together with metacercariae of *O. felineus* in many kinds of freshwater fish, such as the ide (*Leuciscus idus*), dace (*Leuciscus leuciscus*), and minnow (subfamily Leuciscinae). *M. bilis* was also reported in Germany among white-tailed eagles (*Haliaeetus albicilla*), but not among humans. Wild animals, including otters, muskrats, and minks, were the natural definitive hosts of *O. felineus* and *M. bilis* in endemic areas of western Siberia (Mordvinov et al., 2012).

10.3.1.4 *Metorchis conjunctus*

Human infections of *M. conjunctus* are sporadically reported in Canada, primarily among native people (Watson et al., 1979). An outbreak of acute infection with *M. conjunctus* involved 19 cases of people who ate raw white suckerfish (*Catostomus commersoni*) caught from the north of Montreal. Metorchiosis has been described as an acute febrile illness with epigastric pain and eosinophilia (MacLean et al., 1996).

10.3.1.5 *Metorchis orientalis*

Natural infection of *M. orientalis* in humans was first reported in China, where the infection rate was estimated at 4.2%. It appears that human infection with *M. orientalis* was underestimated and reported as *C. sinensis*, in that both use the same second intermediate host fish, *Pseudorasbora parva*, and the same animal reservoir hosts, cats, dogs, and ducks (Lin et al., 2001).

10.3.1.6 *Opisthorchis viverrini*

The Mekong Basin is an endemic area for *O. viverrini*; southern Cambodia, central and southern Lao PDR, northern and northeastern Thailand, and central and southern Vietnam (Rim et al., 2003; De et al., 2003; Sohn et al., 2011; Yong et al., 2012; Sithithaworn et al., 2012). It is estimated that around 10 million Thai and Lao people are infected with *O. viverrini* (Sithithaworn et al., 2012).

10.3.1.7 *Opisthorchis felineus*

O. felineus is endemic in Eurasia; high human infection rates have been reported in the Ukraine and Russia. More recently, 45 cases of *O. felineus* in central Italy have been reported in humans who ate raw freshwater fish (Armignacco et al., 2008; Traverso et al., 2012). An investigation in the endemic area showed that only tench fish (*Tinca tinca*) were infected with metacercariae of *O. felineus*, and that infection rates ranged from 28% to 95%. Of cats, 24–40% were also found positive (De Liberato et al., 2011).

The pathologic effects of infection with small liver flukes are induced by the mechanical irritation caused by the worms' suckers, movement, toxic metabolic substances, immunologic response of the host, and secondary bacterial infection. These effects differ according to worm intensity and duration of infection. The early changes are mild, desquamation and adenomatous hypertrophy of the duct epithelium, progressing to glandular hyperplasia. Biliary obstruction, bile retention, periductal infiltration with eosinophils and round cells, fibrosis, and necrosis and atrophy of surrounding hepatic cells are observed in heavy and severe infections. Dilatation of the intrahepatic bile ducts is formed, accompanied by distal clubbing or cyst formation. The gallbladder frequently loses it function, contains white or muddy bile, and enlarges to 10–20 cm in length. Severe opisthorchiosis has been associated with cirrhosis, obstructive jaundice, cholangitis, pancreatitis, and cholangiocarcinoma (Bunnag et al., 2000). The association of liver-fluke infection and cholangiocarcinoma has been reported in two species: *C. sinensis* and *O. viverrini* (WHO, 1995; Mairiang and Mairiang, 2003; Koompirochana et al., 1978; Shin et al., 2010). The association of *O. felineus* infection and cholangiocarcinoma has not been reported; a recent report on the clinical manifestations of *O. felineus* suggested a febrile eosinophilic syndrome with cholestasis rather than a hepatitis-like syndrome (Traverso et al., 2012).

10.3.2 Intestinal flukes

10.3.2.1 Family Heterophyidae: Haplorchis taichui

Heterophyids are small flukes approximately 1 mm long. They are parasites of the small intestines of birds and mammals, rarely reported in fish and reptiles. Human infection occurs mostly in the small intestine; heterophyid flukes attach to the small bowel mucosa and may cause ulcers, mild inflammation, or superficial necrosis. Pathogenesis can depend on worm burden (Bunnag et al., 2000). In some cases, eggs and adult flukes can invade the blood vessels and reach the heart and central nervous system, causing embolism (Africa et al., 1940).

Over 25 heterophyid species have been found to parasitize humans around the world. The most common genera are *Heterophyes*, *Metagonimus*, and *Haplorchis*. Each genus has several species that reportedly infect humans, dogs, cats, and fish-eating birds, which play an important role as reservoir hosts. The most prevalent species in the Mekong Basin is *H. taichui*.

The adult worm of the *H. taichui* is elongated, oval, 1.1 mm long and 0.45 mm wide. Two-thirds of the body is covered with minute tegumental spines. The oral sucker is slightly subterminal. The ventral sucker is armed with 13–14 spines arranged in a fan shape, with the longest spines in the middle of the group. The egg provides with an operculum that fits into a rim of the egg shell. The shoulder is inconspicuous, but operculum is distinct (Radomyos et al., 2004).

10.3.2.2 Family Troglotrematidae: Nanophyetus salmincola

N. salmincola is known to cause "salmon-poisoning disease" in dogs. Salmon and steelhead trout are the second intermediate hosts carrying metacercaria, which acts as a vector of rickettsia; *Neoricketsia helminthoeca* is the causative agent of a virulent disease in dogs (Milleman and Knapp, 1970). Two subspecies are reported to infect humans: *Nanophyetus salmincola schikhobalowi*, found in eastern Siberia (Skrjabin and Podjapolskaja, 1931) and *Nanophyetus salmincola salmincola* located in Oregon

(Eastburn et al., 1987). Human infection is asymptomatic or results in diarrhea and other gastrointestinal problems.

10.3.2.3 Family Echinostomatidae: Echinochasmus japonicus

Several species of fish-transmitted echinostomes are classified in the subfamily Echinochasminae—one of the common species is *E. japonicus*. The adult is 7–12 mm long and 3–4 mm wide. The anterior is covered with 24 collar spines, interrupted ventrally and dorsally. Testes are large, round, and tandem, found in the median line of the posterior half of the body. The ovary is small and round, located between the ventral sucker and anterior testis. The uterus is short, filled with 6–8 eggs. Vitelline follicles are large and distributed in the lateral sides of the body from the genital pore to the posterior extremity. Eggs are 84–102 μm × 56–69 μm (Chai, 2009).

10.3.2.4 Family Clinostomatidae: Clinostoma complanatum

Clinostoma metacercariae have been reported in freshwater fish worldwide. The larvae are enclosed by a very thin cyst wall that can be distinguished with the naked eyes; either encysted in the muscle of the fish or moving freely without the cyst wall inside the body cavity of the fish. The metacercariae are stout and whitish yellow, referred to as "yellow grub." After ingestion, metacercariae excysts and either attachs to the esophagus or moves to the trachea. These metacercariae have been known to cause highly irritated allergic infections of the upper digestive/respiratory tract, along with pharyngitis, laryngitis, or laryngo-pharyngitis, a disease commonly known as halzoun syndrome or marrara syndrome (Witenberg, 1944). Rarely, *Clinostoma* can infect the eyes, causing pain and irritation (Tiewchaloern et al., 1999). Human *Clinostoma* infection was first reported in Japan (Yamashita, 1938) and has also appeared in Israel, India, Korea, and Thailand (Witenberg, 1944; Cameron, 1945; Chung et al., 1995; Tiewchaloern et al., 1999; Kim et al., 2009; Park et al., 2009).

10.4 Crustacean borne trematodes

10.4.1 Lung flukes

Paragonimosis typically occurs on the African, American, and Asian continents, but most cases appear in the mountain ranges of Asian and American countries. Several species of *Paragonimus* worms have been reported to infect humans (Table 10.2). The adult worm has an oval, beanlike body, about 1 cm long, 5 mm wide, and 3 mm thick. It is reddish brown in color, and the body is covered with spines arranged either in groups or singly depending on species. The oral and ventral suckers are small, as is the pharynx. The esophagus is short, and the ceca are long and winding, ending at the posterior tip of the body. The paired testes are branched and are positioned opposite each other in the posterior half of the body. The ovary is six lobes or highly branched and lies between the testes and the ventral sucker. The uterus is short, coiled between the ovary and the ventral sucker, and opens at the genital

Table 10.2 Distribution of human *Paragonimus* lung flukes and their crustacean second intermediate hosts

Lung flukes	Second intermediate host	Country
P. africanus	*Sudanonautes africanus*	Nigeria (Voelker and Sachs, 1977)
	S. aubryi	Cameroon (Voelker and Sachs, 1977)
	S. floweri	Cameroon (Voelker and Sachs, 1977)
P. heterotremus	*Larnaudia beusekomae*	Thailand (Hinz, 1992)
	Maydelliathelphusa lugubris	India (Takeda et al., 2012)
	Potamiscus manipurensis	India (Singh et al., 2009)
	Potamon lipkei	Lao PDR (Odermatt et al., 2007)
P. mexicanus	*Eudaniela garmani*	Venezuala (Alarcón de Noya et al., 1985)
	Hypolobocera aequatorialis	Ecuador (Voelker and Arzube, 1979)
	Potamocarcinus magnus	Costa Rica (Miyazaki, 1974)
	Pseudothelphusa chilensis	Peru, Ecuador (Vieira et al., 1992)
	P. cobanensis	Guatemala (Miyazaki et al., 1980)
	P. dilatata	Mexico (Lamothe-Argumedo et al., 1977)
	P. nayaritae	Mexico (Lamothe-Argumedo, 1995)
	P. terrestris	Mexico (Lamothe-Argumedo, 1995)
	Ptychophallus tristani	Costa Rica (Monge et al., 1985)
	Raddaus tuberculatus	Mexico (Lamothe-Argumedo, 1984)
	Tehuana guerreroensis	Mexico (Vargas-Arzola et al., 2014)
	Zilchiopsis ecuadoriensis	Ecuador (Amunárriz, 1991)
P. miyazakii	*Geothelphusa dehaani*	Japan (Lou et al., 1992)
P. psuedoheterotremus	*Larnaudia larnaudii*	Thailand (Waikagul, 2007)
P. uterobilateralis	*Liberonautes chaperi*	Liberia (Sachs and Cumberlidge, 1991)
	L. latidactylus	Liberia, Guinea (Sachs and Voelker, 1982)
	Sudanonautes pelii	Cameroon (Voelker and Sachs, 1977)

Table 10.2 Continued

Lung flukes	Second intermediate host	Country
P. westermani	*Barythelphusa lugubris*	India (Devi et al., 2010)
	Cambaroides similis	Korea (Kim, 1984)
	Ceylonthelphusa rugosa	Sri Lanka (Kannangara and Karunaratne, 1969)
	Chulathelphusa brandti	Lao PDR (Odermatt et al., 2007)
	Eriocheir sinensis	China (Li, 1989)
	E. sinensis	Korea (Kim, 1984)
	E. japonicas	Korea (Kim, 1984) Taiwan (Fan and Khaw, 1965)
	Irmengardia pilosimana	Malaysia (Habe et al., 1993)
	Johora tahanensis	Malaysia (Habe et al., 1993)
	Parathelphusa maculata	Malaysia (Miyazaki et al., 1968)
	P. malaysiana	Malaysia (Habe et al., 1993)
	Parlemon nipponensis	Korea (Soh et al., 1964)
	Phricotelphusa aedes	Thailand (Rangsiruji et al., 2006)
	Potamiscus cognatus	Malaysia (Miyazaki, 1969)
	P. johorensis	Malaysia (Liat and Betterton, 1977)

pore, which lies close to the posterior border of the ventral sucker. Vitelline follicles are small and profusely scattered in the lateral fields of the body from the anterior to the posterior ends. The eggs are 80–118 μm × 48–60 μm, golden brown in color, with flat opercula, and shells of irregular thickness (Yokogawa, 1965; Waikagul and Yoonuan, 2004).

The human-infective stage is either the metacercaria, which encysts in crab or crayfish, or the migrating juveniles in the paratenic/definite hosts, such as wild boar, chickens, and rats. The metacercarial cyst is oval to round, with double-layered cyst walls, approximately 250–500 μm depending on the species. In the infective metacercaria, the oral and ventral suckers, esophagus and ceca, and the excretory bladder are fully developed.

The crustaceans reported as the second intermediate hosts of trematodes include crabs and crayfish, which harbor metacercariae of the *Paragonimus* lung fluke. Metacercariae of the *Paragonimus* species that infect humans are usually found in streams and waterfalls containing crabs and prawns, in mountainous areas where trees are dense and abundant with wildlife. Metacercariae are found all over the body of the crab: gills, liver, and in the muscles of the body and legs. After the metacercariae are digested by the definitive host, they excyst in the duodenum and penetrate the intestinal wall into the body cavity, invade the abdominal wall and wander around for a week before reentering the body cavity and moving upward through the diaphragm and into the pleural cavity. From there, they invade the lungs, wander into the pleura, and finally reside in a cyst which contains a pair of worms or more; a single-worm cyst is quite rare. The eggs are then passed into the respiratory tract and excreted with sputum (Yokogawa et al., 1962; Blair et al., 1999; Waikagul et al., 1986).

During migration in the host muscle or pleura, the *Paragonimus* worms leave the hemorrhage tract along their route filled with red blood cells and polymorphonuclear leukocytes, eosinophils, histiocytes, monocytes, and epithelioid cells. After the migration, the worms are surrounded by fibrous connective tissue and form a worm cyst, which is completely developed within 100 days. The worm cyst contains passages connected to bronchioles in which eggs of the worm are passed into the respiratory tree. A granulomatous reaction is formed around the eggs in the bronchioles. The chief complaint of paragonimosis patient is cough with bloody sputum, particularly in the morning. Other symptoms are bronchiectasis, pneumonitis, and pneumothorax (Harinasuta et al., 1957).

10.4.2 Other crustacean borne flukes

10.4.2.1 Achillurbainia nouvelli

Three species of trematodes in the Family Achillurbainiidae are known to infect humans. Both adults and eggs of the species *A. nouvelli* were found in an abscess behind the earlobe in the mastoid bone area of a man from China (Chen, 1965) and Thailand (Bhanthumkosol and Chinawongse, 1986; Tesjaroen et al., 1989). Eggs from the species *Achillurbainia recondita* were found in a granuloma in the omentum of a man from Honduras (Beaver et al., 1977). Adults and eggs of *Poikilorchis congolensis* were also found in an abscess in the mastoid bone of men from Nigeria, Cameroon (Fain and Vandepitte, 1957; Oyediran et al., 1975), and Malaysia (Lie et al., 1962; Wong and Lie, 1965).

The achillurbainid adult fluke is oval and flattened, 8–11 mm long and 4–5 mm wide, with a subterminal oral sucker, 364 μm in diameter. It has a small pharynx, short esophagus, and narrow ceca and is long and winding. Its ventral sucker is 572 μm in mid body. Testes are numerous, small, and scattered throughout the body from the posterior to the oral sucker to the posterior end of the body. The ovary is oval, small, and located just posterior to ventral sucker. Its uterus is short and coils around the ventral sucker area. Numerous vitelline follicles are scattered throughout the body and overlapping the testes. A genital pore is located between the oral and ventral suckers. Eggs are golden brown with irregular shell thickness, have a wide operculum, and measure 51–74(65) μm × 30–38(34) μm (average). Achillurbainid eggs are morphologically similar to those of *Paragonimus* lung flukes, and it is usually known as the *Paragonimus*-like fluke (Tesjaroen et al., 1989).

Metacercariae of achillurbainids are not encysted and move freely in the liver of the crab host, about 2–3 mm long, 1–2 mm wide. Their oral and ventral suckers are large. Testes are numerous and are scattered all over the body. The ovary is small, located posterior to the ventral sucker. Its excretory bladder is tubular and lies in the middle axis of the body from the posterior end to the ventral sucker (Waikagul and Yaemput, 1999).

Adults are usually found in the sinus or trachea of opossums or rats. Its second intermediate host is mountain crabs, *Parathelphusa rugosa* from Sri Lanka (Miyazaki and Kanagara, 1970) and *Larnaudia beusekomae* from Thailand (Waikagul and Yaemput, 1999).

10.4.2.2 Carneophallus brevicaeca

Another family of trematode that uses shrimp and crab as its second intermediate host is the microphallid. The species was first reported in humans as *Heterophyes breviceca* in the Philippines—its adults were found in the intestines, while its eggs were found in the hearts, brains, and spinal cords of autopsied cases (Africa et al., 1940). The species' name was changed several times, to *Spelotrema breviceca*, *Microphallus breviceca*, and finally to *Carneophallus breviceca*. Metacercariae of this species were first found in freshwater shrimp, *Macrobrachium* sp., by Velasquez (1975). Infection with this species has not been reported outside the Philippines, though many species of the genus *Carneophallus* are distributed in many regions.

The adult body is oval, 360–500 μm long, and 270–330 μm wide, covered with spines. It has a subterminal oral sucker, slightly smaller than the ventral sucker, and a short prepharynx and ceca. Its testes are globular, opposite, and posterior to the ventral sucker, the seminal vesicle thin wall lies between ceca bifurcation and ventral sucker, and a genital pore is on the right side of the ventral sucker, associated with trilobed male papillae. The ovary is globular, larger than the testes, and seven big vitelline follicles are overlapping the testes. The excretory bladder is V-shaped (Velasquez, 1975).

Mature metacercariae resemble the adult stage, covered by a single layer of cyst wall, around 500 μm in diameter. The cysts are attached to the abdominal muscles of the shrimp (second intermediate host) by strands of connective tissue (Velasquez, 1975).

10.5 Other animal borne trematodes

10.5.1 Insect borne

10.5.1.1 Dicrocoelium dendriticum

Adult worms are common parasites in the biliary passages of herbivorous, reptiles, and mammals in all continents. Human cases have been diagnosed in Europe, Asia, and Africa. Adult worms are medium sized, 5–15 mm long, and 1.5–2.5 mm wide. They are thin, transparent, and lancet-shaped; the oral sucker is located at the anterior end, and no prepharynx exist. The pharynx is globular and well developed, the esophagus is relatively long, and the ceca extend nearly to the posterior tip. A ventral sucker is located at the center of the anterior half of the body. Two large testes lie closely together and posterior to the ventral sucker, while the ovary is posterior to the testes. Vitellaria occupy the lateral fields along the middle portion of the body, and the uterus fills the posterior half of the body. The genital pore opens ventrally immediately after the bifurcation of the ceca.

The infective stage of *D. dendriticum* is the encysted metacercaria, which attach to the body walls of ants that serve as the second intermediate hosts. If an infected ant is ingested, such as when vegetables are consumed, the metacercaria excysts in the duodenum of the definitive host and enters the bile or pancreatic ducts, where it develops into the adult form (Krull and Mapes, 1953). Human infections are sporadic, mostly asymptomatic and in many cases are considered spurious (Price and Childs, 1971).

Eurytrema pancreaticum is another liver fluke, transmitted by grasshoppers (Basch, 1965).

10.5.1.2 Plagiorchis *spp.*

At least four species of *Plagiorchis* have been found to infect humans in Asia: *Plagiorchis muris*, *Plagiorchis philippinensis*, *Plagiorchis javensis*, and *Plagiorchis harinasutai*. The genus consists of a large number of species, and differentiation between some of these appears to be based on the minor morphological characteristics, which make the identification of *Plagiorchis* species very difficult (Lie, 1951). The adult worm is medium-sized and pyriform in shape, with no prepharynx, a short esophagus, and long ceca that extend beyond the posterior testes. The ventral sucker is located in the middle of the body. Two oval testes lie obliquely in the posterior half of the body. The ovary is oval and lies immediately posterior to the ventral sucker. Vitelline follicles are scattered in the lateral fields of the body from behind the cecal bifurcation to the posterior end. The excretory bladder is Y-shaped. Its eggs are small, measuring 33–34 μm × 17–18 μm, smooth and thin-shelled, pale yellow, and fully embryonated when laid (Radomyos et al., 1989; Sandground, 1940; Africa and Garcia, 1935; Lie, 1951; McMullen, 1937).

The adult worms live in the small intestine of the definitive vertebrate hosts. Embryonated eggs are excreted with the host's feces, ingested by the lymnaeid snails *Stagnicola angulate*, where the stylet cercaria of the armatae group develops in daughter sporocysts. Some cercariae encyst in the sporocyst and develop into infective metacercariae, but most cercariae leave the snail and encyst in insect larvae, such as nymphs of the stone fly. The natural definitive hosts are rats, dogs, birds, and humans (McMullen, 1937).

10.5.1.3 Phaneropsolus *spp.*

Phaneropsolus bonnei has been reported to infect humans in Indonesia, Laos, and Thailand. The worms in this family are minute, less than 1 mm long. The body is ovoid in shape and covered with spines. The oral sucker and pharynx are well developed, and the ceca wide and short. The ventral sucker is located in the middle of the anterior half of the body. The testes are oval and situated one on each side of the ventral sucker. The ovary is oval and located dorsal to the right testis; the vitelline follicles are large, arranged in two groups, and located postero-laterally to the oral sucker; the uterus is long and winding and occupies the entire posterior half of the body. The cirrus sac is sigmoid in shape and located anterior to the ventral sucker. The genital pore is open to either the left or right side of the oral sucker.

The adult worms live in the small intestine where they lay eggs, which are similar to the eggs of the heterophyid flukes and are embryonated when laid. The first intermediate hosts are the snails in the family Bithyniidae or Thiariidae. The cercaria of this family is the xiphidia or stylet-bearing type. The second intermediate hosts are aquatic larvae (naiads) of dragonflies (Order Odonata). The definitive hosts are insectivores (i.e., bats) and monkeys. Humans acquire the infection by ingesting raw naiads containing the metacercariae. Pathogenesis resulting from the infection has not been reported, even when thousands of worms are present (Lie, 1951; Radomyos et al., 1984).

Phaneropsolus spinicirrus has been reported in humans in northeast Thailand and has the specific characteristic of having tiny spines on the cirrus. The genital pore opens anteriorly close to the ventral border of its oral sucker (Kaewkes et al., 1991).

Prosthodendrium molenkampi has also been reported in Indonesia, Thailand, and Laos. The adult worm differs from *P. bonnie* in the shape of its ovary and the location of the genital pore. The ovary is lobed and located dorsally to the right testis. The cirrus pouch is ovoidal and antero-sinistral to the ventral sucker; the genital pore is also antero-sinistral to the ventral sucker and is surrounded by a pseudo-sucker (Radomyos et al., 1984; 1989).

10.5.2 Snail borne

Transmission of echinostomes to humans occurs through eating raw or undercooked snails, fish, or amphibians. Most human cases have been reported in Asia. Echinostomes are morphologically distinct from other trematodes due to the presence of spines around the oral sucker, known as collar spines. The number and arrangement of these collar spines form the basis of genus identification. Duodenum mucosal bleeding and ulceration are the main pathological findings from mechanical damage caused by the worms. Symptoms include abdominal pain and diarrhea, followed by weakness and weight loss (Chai, 2009).

10.5.2.1 *Echinostoma malayanum*

This species was first found in humans in Malaysia by Lieper (1911), but since then there have been several more reported cases from other countries in Southeast Asia: Indonesia, Singapore, the Philippines, and Thailand. This worm is elongated in shape, reddish in color and measures 7.2–12.4 mm long and 1.7–3.5 mm wide. The body is covered with scalelike spines. There is a collarlike expansion around the oral sucker that is armed with spines interrupted ventrally; the collar or circumoral spines number 43–45. The oral sucker is smaller than the ventral sucker. Testes are branched and lie in tandem in the anterior half of the hind body. The ovary is small, oval, and lies anterior to the testes. The uterus is relatively short and occupies the posterior half of the forebody. Vitellaria are medium-sized follicles and situated along the lateral fields from the posterior of the ventral sucker to the posterior tip of the body. The cirrus pouch is long and prominently situated dorso-lateral to the ventral sucker. The genital pore is immediately anterior to the ventral sucker. Eggs are 120–130 μm × 80–90 μm, thin-shelled, yellowish brown in color, and unsegmented when laid. Relatively few eggs are kept in the uterus at a time (Hadidjaja and Oemijati, 1969).

Echinostoma ilocanum has been found in the Philippines, Thailand, and China. The adult worm measures 2.5–6.5 mm long and 1–1.5 mm wide, has 49–51 circumoral spines, and lobed testes. The eggs are 83–116 μm × 58–69 μm (Chai, 2009).

Echinostoma revolutum is a parasite of waterfowl, but human cases have been reported. Adults measure 7.2–11.4 mm long and 1.6–2.7 mm wide. There are 37–38 circumoral spines; the eggs measure 90–126 μm × 59–71 μm (Chai, 2009).

10.5.2.2 Gymnophalloides seoi

This fluke is minute, 0.3–0.5 mm long, and 0.2–0.3 mm wide and characterized by a ventral pit. The metacercaria are found in oysters, and humans and palearctic oystercatcher *Haematopus ostralegus* are the natural definitive hosts. Korea is an endemic area for human infection, in particular, the western coastal region and islands on the South Sea. The chief complaints of infected persons are indigestion and gastrointestinal problems (Lee et al., 1993; Lee and Chai, 2001).

10.5.3 Amphibian/reptile borne

The body of the worms from the family Diplostomatidae is divided into a flat forebody, which contains suckers and the tribocytic organ, and a cylindrical hind body containing the reproductive organs. They are intestinal parasites of birds and mammals. Their life cycle is different from other trematodes due to having a mesocercarial stage in amphibian second intermediate hosts. In the definitive host, mesocercaria migrates to the lung and transforms to metacercaria (diplostomulum type), which later migrates to the trachea and to the intestine where it develops into an adult. The mesocercariae can also accumulate in the tissue of the paratenic hosts such as snakes or mice, which later become the source of infection to the definitive host (Schell, 1970). Two species have been reported in humans. The first was a fatal case of *Alaria americana*, reported in North America, where it is believed that infection occurred after the consumption of an improperly cooked frog during a hiking expedition. Autopsy revealed that thousands of mesocercariae had migrated throughout all the internal organs (Freeman et al., 1976). The second species is *Neodiplostomum soulense*, an intestinal trematode, which has been reported in humans and animals in Korea. The first intermediate hosts are snails—*Hippeutis cantori*, *Segmentina hemisphaerula*, and *Austrapeplea ollula* (Chung et al., 2002); the mesocercaria is found in frog tadpoles (Hong et al., 1983) and grass snakes (Seo et al., 1988).

10.6 Diagnosis, treatment, and control

10.6.1 Diagnosis

Most particularly light trematode infections are asymptomatic, except those that are acute or chronic. Diagnosis cannot be confirmed from symptoms alone but requires additional information, such as a history of specific consumption of source of infections, presence of parasite eggs, or antibodies/DNA in feces, blood, or other samples, and imaging techniques. In endemic areas, even a nonspecific symptom can prompt patients to seek care, allowing health care workers to identify individuals in need of treatment (Sithiathaworn et al., 2007; Mas-Coma et al., 2009; Keiser and Utzinger, 2009). Conversely, in many nonendemic regions, symptoms from foodborne trematode infection are rarely recognized.

10.6.1.1 Parasitological tools

Various traditional methods are able to detect parasite eggs in fecal samples; however, these have limited sensitivity, since they are unable to detect infections caused by worms that do not achieve sexual maturity in the human host, or those associated with ectopic parasite location (Sithithaworn et al., 2009; Keiser and Utzinger, 2009). The most commonly used method at present is the modified cellophane thick smear, commonly known as the Kato-Katz method. It is inexpensive, rapid, and simple to perform, and practical for simple laboratories as well as in field conditions. FLOTAC is a technique based on flotation and centrifugation. It is more sensitive than the Kato-Katz and McMaster techniques but is more complex to perform and requires some specific laboratory equipment (Cringoli, 2006; Keiser and Utzinger, 2009).

Because sensitivity of fecal examination is much lower than sputum examination for diagnosing Paragonimosis, the normal practice for detecting the infection is to examine the sputum by mixing the sample with 0.3 N NaOH and examining it under a microscope for the characteristic *Paragonimus* egg. Fecal examination is also possible, as the eggs are swallowed and passed out together with the host's feces. Parasitological diagnosis is typically achieved by identifying eggs in feces. However, in cases of opisthorchiosis or clonorchiosis with biliary obstruction, eggs are not released into the intestine and can only be recovered in the bile by needle aspiration, or during surgery or autopsy (Sithithaworn et al., 1991). In such cases, other diagnostic tests are necessary to confirm infection. An additional diagnostic method can be carried out by correlating symptoms and conducting coprological tests, by finding eggs and/or occasionally by identifying expelled adult worms (Weng et al., 1989; Le et al., 2006).

10.6.1.2 Molecular tools

Eggs of parasites of related families are similar in shape and overlap in size. To identify the species, recovered eggs can be tested through molecular methods. DNA from eggs or other biological components or products of the worms can be extracted from stool samples and amplified by polymerase chain reaction (PCR) using nucleotide primers that can be highly sensitive and specific (McGarry et al., 2007; Sithiathaworn et al., 2007). PCR is a good alternative to confirm the diagnosis, but the costs and quality assurance can be obstacles when applying the technology, especially on a large scale. Nevertheless, partial sequences of ITS2 and COI confirmed the first detection of human infection with *P. pseudoheterotremus*, the species previously reported only in experimental animals (Intapan et al., 2012; Waikagul, 2007).

Examining eggs and metacercariae in both human fecal samples and intermediate hosts by PCR can be used for diagnosing *O. viverrini* with a high sensitivity and specificity (Maleewong et al., 2003; Wongratanacheewin et al., 2001, 2002). However, fecal samples generate lower sensitivity, from 40% to 50% in samples with less than 200 eggs per gram of feces (Wongratanacheewin et al., 2002; Stensvold et al., 2006). This test is useful in areas where *O. viverrini* and *C. sinensis* infections overlap geographically (Le et al., 2006) and to discriminate *O. viverrini* from *H. taichui* (Thaenkham et al., 2007).

10.6.1.3 Immunodiagnostic tools

Detecting antibodies against trematodosis is possible in acute and chronic infections and in ectopic cases. Despite a high sensitivity, specific antibody detection cannot differentiate between present and past infections. Also, cross-reactivity with other helminth infections can occur in some tests, reducing the specificity of the diagnosis. Several methods of serodiagnosis can be performed, but enzyme-linked immunoassay (ELISA) or immunoblot techniques are most frequently used. By immunoblot, three polypeptides (32.5, 33, and 35 kDa) of *Paragonimus heterotremus* antigens were specifically reacted with *P. heterotremus* antibody and used for diagnosing paragonimosis heterotremus (Dekumyoy et al., 1998). Detection of antigens is highly specific but less sensitive than detection of antibodies. Detection of antigen indicates current infection, and tests can be performed on serum and fecal samples. Fecal tests are easier to perform and reportedly better accepted by individuals in endemic areas (Sithiathaworn et al., 2007; Keiser and Utzinger, 2009; Adela Valero et al., 2012; Gonzales et al., 2013).

An ELISA for *O. viverrini* is available in a few laboratories and may assist in establishing diagnosis (Wongratanacheewin et al., 1988; Elkins et al., 1991). An alternative antigen, the 53 kDa eluted from the snail *Bithynia goniomphalos*, is useful for antibody detection of *Opisthorchis* cases by indirect-ELISA (Waikagul et al., 2002). Antigen detection by monoclonal-antibody-ELISA is used for the evaluation of opisthorchiosis. This method is based on detecting *O. viverrini* antigen in feces (copro-antigen). The sensitivity of the copro-antigen test is slightly higher compared to microscopic examination, but with lower specificity (Sirisinha et al., 1995).

10.6.1.4 Imaging

X-ray images of the lungs of paragonimosis patients can be divided into five categories: (1) Ring shadow-image of worm cyst is the most common, found in 80% of patients. (2) Opacities with poorly defined borders are found in 45% of X-ray images, similar to Loeffler's syndrome caused by migration of gnathostome or ascarid larvae. (3) Linear infiltration, found in about 20% of patients, in the form of a line shadow associated with fibrosis. (4) Pleural thickening is found in about 20% of patients, mostly in lateral lungs, in particular in the interlobular fissure. (5) Pleural effusion is found in about 10% of patients, 200–300 ml of fluid in both lungs (Suwanik and Harinasuta, 1959).

To detect acute fasciolosis, ultrasound scans (widely used as a complementary diagnostic tool in clinical practice) can identify worms migrating through the liver. In the chronic phase, they can easily detect the typical dilatation and thickening of the bile ducts and gallbladder. Ultrasonography is used for monitoring fasciolosis. Computerized tomography (CT) scans are most useful during the acute phase of fasciolosis, detecting hepatic lesions and "tunnel-like" migration paths, but it is often unavailable in most health care facilities. Endoscopic retrograde cholangiopancreatography (ERCP) is also an alternative as it can show extrahepatic biliary dilatation, caused by the worm attachment (Moghadami and Mardani, 2008; Lim et al., 2008; Mas-Coma et al., 2009; Ezzat et al., 2010; WHO, 1995).

10.6.2 Treatment

The preferred treatment for intestinal fluke infections is praziquantel, taken in a single oral dose of 10–20 mg/kg (Bunnag et al., 1983; Harinasuta et al., 1987; Chai, 2007), a single dose at 40 mg/kg, or 25 mg/kg for 3 consecutive days for small liver flukes. This treatment gives a cure rate of 91–100% (Bunnag and Harinasuta, 1980). Current drug treatment for paragonimosis, with 100% efficacy, is praziquantel at 25 mg/kg body weight, taken three times after meals for 2 consecutive days both for adults and children. After treatment, adult worms are sometimes expectorated during cough, and no eggs are found 1 month after treatment (Vanijanonta et al., 1981). Albendazole can be considered the second-line drug; a single dose gives approximately a 48% cure rate for haplorchiosis (Waikagul et al., 2005), for liver-fluke infection, 400 mg given in two divided doses for 7 days give a cure rate of 63% (Pungpak et al., 1984). Mebendazole in a single dose of 500 mg is also reported to be efficient for the treatment of *G. hominis* (Dada-Adegbola et al., 2004). The efficacy of triclabendazole, oxyclozanide, and rafoxanide has been evaluated in pigs, presenting high efficacy against fasciolopsiosis and with no side effects (Datta et al., 2004). Subacute and chronic infections of fasciolosis may be treated with triclabendazole or praziquantel, which presents high efficacy to trematodes with few collateral effects. Recently, tribendimidine was reported as a promising drug as it gave cure rates similar to praziquantel on opisthorchiosis treatment trials (Soukhathammavong et al., 2011). Alternative drugs, such as artemisinin, and combinations of drugs are proposed in drug-resistant strains (Keiser and Utzinger, 2007, 2009; Chai, 2013). Although the use of drug combinations is an alternative, it is important to exercise caution with regard to the risk of multiple drug resistance (Gaasenbeek et al., 2001; Mas-Coma et al., 2005).

10.6.3 Prevention and control

The main strategies for parasite control programs comprise three interrelated approaches: fecal examination (along with treatment of positive cases for eliminating human reservoir host), health education (which includes promoting well-cooked fish and aquatic vegetables in the endemic areas to prevent infection), and the improvement of hygiene for the interruption of disease transmission. Infection rates have declined dramatically in places where this program was implemented (Jongsuksuntigul and

Imsomboon, 2003). It is important, however, to remember that reinfection can readily occur, so it is crucial to combine treatment with education and transmission-prevention efforts (Upatham et al., 1988). A liver fluke similar to *O. viverrini* was reported in ducks in Vietnam (Dao et al., 2013), and cats and dogs were positive with a high prevalence of opisthorchid eggs in Thailand (Enes et al., 2010). A combination of control measures is required for both domestic animals and humans because human infection is typically related to animal endemicity. It is also important to consider wild animals that are reservoir hosts of infection. Control measures may also include preventing the contamination of water sources by eliminating human excreta as fertilizers, avoiding open-air defecation, and removing and properly disposing of animal excreta.

10.7 Conclusions and future trends

The aforementioned foodborne trematodes have been reported as causative agents of diseases in humans, but there are many more trematodes that infect domestic and wild animals. Many trematodes are zoonotic parasites that are able to infect both animals and humans. Recently there have been a number of reports about domestic animals infected with foodborne trematodes; also poultry and other domestic animals have been found to be reservoir hosts of fish borne zoonotic trematodes in Vietnamese fish farms (Anh et al., 2009, 2011). There is a possibility that these species infect humans in their locality. Further investigations and continued identification of worms recovered after treatment may find new and emerging species in humans.

Investigations on the prevalence and epidemiology of parasitic infections are usually published only in scientific journals and many of them at the international level. Infected people receive treatment and are informed to refrain from eating raw food, which is a source of infection. If salad and raw fish dishes have been part of one's staple diet for a long time, changing these proclivities is difficult. People should receive more specific and practical information and suggestions, such as “don’t eat raw plants from ponds connected to pig farms” or “thoroughly cook fish collected from the rice field ponds especially during October to February” (when metacercarial infection in fish is prevalent). The local environment should also be investigated for parasitic contamination, and health-based parasite control programs could be introduced in schools.

Control programs have been implemented in some countries where foodborne trematodes are endemic. Information about the parasitic infections may raise awareness of populations within and beyond the control programs. Although it is expected that the infection rates and density of foodborne trematodes in endemic areas will decline in the future, the occurrence of these parasite may expand to other areas as a result of globalization of the food supply web. Increasing studies on purged worms after treatment and application of molecular assays to detect eggs of trematodes may lead to the discovery of new emerging species in humans. The zoonotic trematodes that were formerly reported only in animals may find their way to human hosts due to modern agricultural and distribution systems.

Acknowledgments

We would like to thank Tippayarat Yoonuan and Akkarin Poodeepiyasawat for their technical assistance with preparing the figure and tables and Paul Adams and Glad Rotaru for editing the English language of this chapter.

References

Adela Valero, M., Victoria Periago, M., Pérez-Crespo, I., Rodríguez, E., Jesús Perteguer, M., Gárate, T., González-Barberá, E.M., Mas-Coma, S., 2012. Assessing the validity of an ELISA test for the serological diagnosis of human fascioliasis in different epidemiological situations. Trop. Med. Int. Health 17, 630–636. http://dx.doi.org/10.1111/j.1365-3156.2012.02964.x.

Africa, C.M., Garcia, E.Y., 1935. Heterophyid trematodes of man and dog in the Philippines with descriptions of three new species. Philipp. J. Sci. 57, 253–256.

Africa, C.M., de Leon, W., Garcia, E.Y., 1940. Visceral complications in intestinal heterophyidiasis of man. Acta Med. Philipp. 1, 1–132.

Ahluwalia, S.S., 1960. *Gastrodiscoides hominis* (Lewis and McConnell, 1876) Leiper, 1913. The amphistome parasite of man and pigs. Indian J. Med. Res. 48, 315–325.

Alarcón de Noya, B., Noya, O., Torres, J., Botto, C., 1985. A field study of paragonimiasis in Venezuela. Am. J. Trop. Med. Hyg. 34, 766–769.

Amunárriz, M., 1991. Intermediate hosts of *Paragonimus* in the eastern Amazonic region of Ecuador. Trop. Med. Parasitol. 42, 164–166.

Andrews, S.J., 1999. The life cycle of *Fasciola hepatica*. In: Dalton, J.P. (Ed.), Fasciolosis. CAB International, Oxon, pp. 1–29.

Anh, L.T.N., Madsen, H., Dalsgaad, A., Phuong, T.N., Than, H.T.D., Murrell, K.D., 2011. Poultry as reservoir hosts for fishborne zoonotic trematodes in Vietnamese fish farms. Vet. Parasitol. 169, 391–394.

Anh, L.T.N., Phoung, T.N., Murrell, K.D., Johansen, M.V., Dalsgaad, A., Thu, T.L., Chi, K.T.B., Thamsborg, S.M., 2009. Animal reservoir hosts and fish-borne zoonotic trematode infections on fish farms, Vietnam. Emerg. Infect. Dis. 15, 540–546.

Areekul, S., Jaroonvesama, N., Charoenlarp, P., Kasemsuth, R., Cheeramakara, C., 1979. Serum vitamin B12 and folic acid levels in patients with fasciolopsiasis. Southeast Asian J. Trop. Med. Public Health 10, 67–72.

Armignacco, O., Caterini, L., Marucci, G., Ferri, F., Bernardini, G., Raponi, G.N., Ludovisi, A., Bossu, T., Gomez Morales, M.A., Pozio, E., 2008. Human illnesses caused by *Opisthorchis felineus* flukes, Italy. Emerg. Infect. Dis. 14, 1902–1905.

Artigas, P.T., Perez, M.D., 1962. Consideracoes sobre *Opisthorchis pricei* Foster 1939, *O. guayaquilensis* Rodriguez, Gomez e Montalvan 1949 e *O. pseudofelineus* Ward 1901. Descrição de *Amphimerus pseudofelineus minimus* n. sub. sp. Mem. Inst. Butantan 30, 157–166.

Basch, P.F., 1965. Completion of the life cycle of *Eurytrema pancreaticum* (Trematoda: Dicrocoeliidae). J. Parasitol. 51, 350–355.

Beaver, P.C., Duron, R.A., Little, M.D., 1977. Trematodes eggs in the peritoneal cavity of man in Honduras. Am. J. Trop. Med. Hyg. 26, 684–687.

Belding, D.L., 1965. Textbook of Parasitology, third ed. Appleton-Century-Crofts, New York.

Bhanthumkosol, D., Chinawongse, P., 1986. Extrapulmonary paragonimiasis in Chantaburi, report of six cases. J. Prapokklao Hosp. Clin. Med. Educ. Center 3, 85–91.

Blair, D., Xu, Z.B., Agatsuma, T., 1999. Paragonimiasis and the Genus *Paragonimus*. Adv. Parasitol. 42, 113–222.

Boray, J.C., 1969. Experimental fascioliasis in Australia. Adv. Parasitol. 7, 95–210.

Buckley, J.J.C., 1964. The problem of *Gastrodiscoides hominis* (Lewis and McConnell, 1876) Leiper, 1913. J. Helminthol. 38, 1–6.

Bunnag, D., Harinasuta, T., 1980. Studies on the chemotherapy of human opisthorchiasis in Thailand. I. Clinical trial of praziquantel. Southeast Asian J. Trop. Med. Public Health 11, 528–530.

Bunnag, D., Cross, J.H., Bunnag, T., 2000. Liver fluke infection. In: Strickland, G.T. (Ed.), Hunter's Tropical Medicine and Emerging Infectious Diseases, eighth ed. WB Sounders Co., Philadelphia, pp. 840–847.

Bunnag, D., Harinasuta, T., Radomyos, P., 1983. Field trial on the treatment of fasciolopsiasis with praziquantel. Southeast Asian J. Trop. Med. Public Health 14, 216–219.

Calvopina, N., Cevallos, W., Kumazawa, H., Eisenberg, J., 2011. High prevalence of human liver infection by *Amphimerus* spp. Flukes, Ecuador. Emerg. Infect. Dis. 17, 2331–2334.

Cameron, T.W.M., 1945. Fish-carried parasites in Canada. I. Parasites carried by freshwater fish. Can. J. Comp. Med. 9, 245–254.

Chai, J.Y., 2007. Intestinal flukes. In: Murrell, K.D., Fried, B. (Eds.), In: Food-Borne Parasitic Zoonoses: Fish and Plant-Borne Parasites, World Class Parasites, vol. II. Springer, New York, pp. 53–115.

Chai, J.Y., 2013. Praziquantel treatment in trematode and cestode infections: an update. Infect. Chemother. 45, 32–43. http://dx.doi.org/10.3947/ic.2013.45.1.32.

Chai, J.Y., 2009. Echinostomes in humans. In: Fried, B., Toledo, R. (Eds.), The Biology of Echinostomes. Springer, New York, pp. 147–183. http://dx.doi.org/10.1007/978-0-387-09577-6_7.

Chandra, S.S., 1976. A field study on the clinical aspects of *Fasciolopsis buski* in Uttar Pradesh. Med. J. Armed Forces India 32, 181–189.

Chen, H.T., 1965. *Paragonimus*, *Pagumonimus* and a *Paragonimus*-like trematode in man. Chin. Med. J. 84, 781–791.

Chung, D.I., Moon, C.H., Kong, H.H., Choi, D.W., Lim, D.K., 1995. The first human case of *Clinostomum complanatum* (Trematoda: Clinostomatidae) infection in Korea. Korean J. Parasitol. 33, 219–223.

Chung, P.R., Jung, Y., Park, Y.K., Hwang, M.G., 2002. Host specificity of *Austropeplea ollula* (Gastropoda: Lymnaeidae) to miracidial infection with a human intestinal fluke *Neodiplostomum seoulensis* (Trematoda: Diplostomatidae) in Korea. J. Parasitol. 88, 630–631.

Cringoli, G., 2006. FLOTAC, a novel apparatus for a multivalent faecal egg count technique. Parassitologia 48, 381–384.

Dada-Adegbola, H.O., Falade, C.O., Oluwatoba, O.A., Abiadun, O.O., 2004. *Gastrodiscoides hominis* infection in a Nigerian—case report. West Afr. J. Med. 23, 185–186.

Dao, T.H., Nguyen, T.G., Victor, B., Gabriel, S., Dorny, P., 2013. *Opisthorchis viverrini*-like liver fluke in birds from Vietnam: morphological variability and rDNA/mtDNA sequence confirmation. J. Helminthol. 31, 1–6, PubMed PMID: 23721954.

Datta, S., Mukerjee, G.S., Ghosh, J.D., 2004. Comparative efficacy of triclabendazole, oxyclozanide and rafoxanide against *Fasciolopsis buski* in naturally infected pigs. Indian J. Anim. Health 43, 53–56.

De Liberato, C., Scaramozzino, P., Brozzi, A., Lirenzetti, R., Di Cave, D., Martini, E., Lucangeli, C., Pozio, E., Bossu, T., 2011. Investigation on *Opisthorchis felineus* occurrence and life cycle in Italy. Vet. Parasitol. 177, 67–71.

De, N.V., Murrell, K.D., Cong, L.D., Cam, P.D., Chau, L.V., Toan, N.D., Dalsgaard, A., 2003. The food-borne trematode zoonoses of Vietnam. Southeast Asian J. Trop. Med. Public Health 34 (Suppl. 1), 12–34.

Dekumyoy, P., Waikagul, J., Eom, K.S., 1998. Human lung fluke (*Paragonimus heterotremus*): differential diagnosis between *P. heterotremus* and *P. westermani* infections by EITB. Trop. Med. Int. Health 3, 52–56.

Devi, K.R., Narain, K., Agatsuma, T., Blair, D., Nagataki, M., Wickramasinghe, S., Yatawara, L., Mahanta, J., 2010. Morphological and molecular characterization of *Paragonimus westermani* in northeastern India. Acta Trop. 116, 31–38.

Dixon, K.E., 1965. The structure and histochemistry of the cyst wall of the metacercaria of *Fasciola hepatica* L. Parasitology 55, 215–226. http://dx.doi.org/10.1017/S0031182000068712.

Dutt, S.C., Srivastava, H.D., 1966. The intermediate host and cercaria of *Gastrodicoides hominis* (Trematoda: Gastrodiscidae). Preliminary report. J. Helminthol. 40, 45–52.

Dutt, S.C., Srivastava, H.D., 1972. The life history of *Gastrodiscoides hominis* (Lewis and McConnell, 1876) Leiper, 1913. The amphistome parasite of man and pig. J. Helminthol. 46, 35–46.

Eastburn, R.L., Fritsche, T.R., Terhune, C.A., 1987. Human intestinal infection with *Nanophyetus salmincola* from salmonid fishes. Am. J. Trop. Med. Hyg. 36, 586–591.

Elkins, D.B., Sithithaworn, P., Haswell-Elkins, M., Kaewkes, S., Awacharagan, P., Wongratanacheewin, S., 1991. *Opisthorchis viverrini*: relationship between egg counts, worms recovered and antibody levels within an endemic community in northeast Thailand. Parasitology 102, 283–288.

Enes, J.E., Wages, A.J., Malone, J.B., Tesana, S., 2010. Prevalence of *Opisthorchis viverrini* infection in the canine and feline host in three villages, Khon Kaen Province, Northeastern Thailand. Southeast Asian J. Trop. Med. Public Health 41, 36–42.

Esteban, J.G., Flores, A., Angles, R., Strauss, W., Aguirre, C., Mas-Coma, S., 1997. A population-based coprological study of human fascioliasis in a hyperendemic area of the Bolivian Altiplano. Trop. Med. Int. Health 2, 695–699.

Esteban, J.G., Gonzalez, C., Bargues, M.D., Angles, R., Sanchez, C., Naquira, C., Mas-Coma, S., 2002. High fascioliasis infection in children linked to a man-made irrigation zone in Peru. Trop. Med. Int. Health 7, 339–348.

Ezzat, R.F., Karboli, T.A., Kasnazani, K.A., Hamawandi, A.M., 2010. Endoscopic management of biliary fascioliasis: a case report. J. Med. Case Rep. 4, 83. http://dx.doi.org/10.1186/1752-1947-4-83.

Fain, A., Vandepitte, J., 1957. A new trematode, *Poikilorchis congolensis* n.g., n.sp. living in subcutaneous retroauricular cysts in man from Belgian Congo. Nature 179, 740.

Fan, P.C., Khaw, O.K., 1965. *Paragonimus westermani* infection in crustacean host, *Eriocheir japonicus*, in Shen-keng District, Taipei County, Northern Taiwan. Chin. Med. J. 12, 381–396.

Figurnov, V.A., Chertov, A.D., Romanenko, N.A., Grigorenko, A.A., Gavrilov, V.A., Soldatkin, P.K., Prokhorov, P.P., Solozhenkin, V.G., Kalinina, V.V., Katin, I.S., Gavrilov, A.V., Mosolova, N.P., Figurnova, E.V., 2002. Clonorchiasis in the Upper Amur region: biology, epidemiology, clinical presentation. Med. Parazitol. (Mosk) 4, 20–23.

Fox, J.G., Hall, W.C., 1970. Fluke (*Gastrodiscoides hominis*) infection in a rhesus monkey with related intussusception of the colon. J. Am. Vet. Med. Assoc. 157, 714–716.

Freeman, R.S., Stuart, P.F., Cullen, J.B., Ritchie, A.C., Mildon, A., Fernandes, B.J., Bonin, R., 1976. Fatal human infection with mesocercariae of the trematode *Alaria americana*. Am. J. Trop. Med. Hyg. 25, 803–807.

Fried, B., Graczyk, T.K., Tamang, L., 2004. Food-borne intestinal trematodiases in humans. Parasitol. Res. 93, 159–170.

Gaasenbeek, C.P.H., Moll, L., Cornelissen, J.B.W.J., Vellema, P., Borgsteede, F.H.M., 2001. An experimental study on triclabendazole resistance of *Fasciola hepatica* in sheep. Vet. Parasitol. 95, 37–43.

Gonzales, S.B., Dalton, J.P., Vasquez Camargo, F., Parkinson, M., Ndao, M., 2013. The diagnosis of human fascioliasis by enzyme-linked immunosorbent assay (ELISA) using recombinant cathepsin L protease. PLoS Negl. Trop. Dis. 7 (9), e2414. http://dx.doi.org/10.1371/journal.pntd.0002414.

Graczyk, T.K., Gilman, R.H., Fried, B., 2001. Fasciolopsiasis: is it a controllable food-borne disease? Parasitol. Res. 87, 80–83.

Habe, S., Lai, K.P.F., Agatsuma, T., Ow-Yang, C.K., Kawashima, K., 1993. Crab hosts for *Paragonimus westermani* (kerbert, 1878) in Malaysia. Jpn. J. Trop. Med. Hyg. 21, 137–142.

Hadidjaja, P., Oemijati, S., 1969. *Echinostoma* infection in Indonesia with a special study on *Echinostoma malayanum*. In: Proceedings of the Fourth Southeast Asian Seminar on Parasitology and Tropical Medicine. Schistosomes and Other Snail-Transmitted Helminthiasis, Manila, pp. 167–170.

Harinasuta, T., Bunnag, D., Radomyos, P., 1987. Intestinal fluke infections. Baillieres Clin. Trop. Med. Commun. Dis. 2, 695–721.

Harinasuta, T., Kruatrachue, M., Tandhanond, S., 1957. A case of paragonimiasis in Thailand. J. Med. Assoc. Thai. 40, 227–234.

Hartman, H.A., 1961. The intestinal fluke (*Fasciolopsis buski*) in a monkey. Am. J. Vet. Res. 22, 1123–1126.

Haswell-Elkins, M.R., Elkins, D.B., 1998. Lung and liver flukes. In: Cox, F.E.G., Kreir, J.P., Wakelin, D. (Eds.), Topley and Wilson's Microbiology and Microbial Infections: Parasitology, ninth ed., vol. 5. Arnold, London, pp. 507–520.

Herman, L.H., 1967. *Gastrodiscoides hominis* infestation in two monkeys. Vet. Med. 62, 355–356.

Hsieh, H.C., 1960. Studies on the epidemiology of *Fasciolopsis buski* in South Taiwan. Formosan Sci. 14, 95–120.

Hinz, E., 1992. Paragonimiasis in Thailand. Mitt. Österr. Ges. Tropenmed. Parasitol. 14, 79–87.

Hong, T.S., Fang, Y., 2012. *Clonorchis sinensis* and clonorchiasis, an update. Parasitol. Int. 61, 17–24.

Hong, S.J., Lee, S.H., Seo, B.S., Hong, S.T., Chai, J.Y., 1983. Studies on intestinal trematodes in Korea IX. Recovery rate and development of *Fibricola seoulensis* in experimental animals. Korean J. Parasitol. 21, 224–233.

Hussein, A.-N.A., Hassan, I.M., Khalifa, R.M.A., 2010. Description of eggs and larval stages of *Fasciola*, light and scanning electron microscopic studies. Res. J. Parasitol. 5, 1–12. http://dx.doi.org/10.3923/jp.2010.1.12. http://scialert.net/abstract/?doi=jp.2010.1.12.

Ivanov, V.M., Semenova, N.N., 2000. Parasitological consequences of animal introduction. Russ. J. Ecol. 31, 281–283.

Intapan, P.M., Sanpool, O., Thanchomnang, T., Imtawil, K., Pongchaiyakul, C., Nawa, Y., Maleewong, W., 2012. Short report: molecular identification of a case of *Paragonimus pseudoheterotremus* infection in Thailand. Am. J. Trop. Med. Hyg. 87, 706–709.

Jaroonvesama, N., Charoenlarp, K., Areekul, S., 1986. Intestinal absorption studies in *Fasciolopsis buski* infection. Southeast Asian J. Trop. Med. Public Health 17, 582–586.

Jongsuksuntigul, P., Imsomboon, T., 2003. Opisthorchiasis control in Thailand. Acta Trop. 88, 229–232.

Kaewkes, S., Elkins, D.B., Sithithaworn, P., Haswell Elkins, M.R., 1991. Comparative studies on the morphology of the eggs of *Opisthorchis viverrini* and lecithodendriid trematodes. Southeast Asian J. Trop. Med. Public Health 22, 623–630.

Kannangara, D.W.W., Karunaratne, G.N.S., 1969. *Paratelphusa ceylonensis* and *Paratelphusa rugosa* as crab hosts of the human lung fluke *Paragonimus westermani* (Kerbert, 1878) in Ceylon. Ceylon J. Med. Sci. 18, 31–32.

Keiser, J., Utzinger, J., 2007. Food-borne trematodiasis: current chemotherapy and advances with artemisinins and synthetic trioxolanes. Trends Parasitol. 23, 555–562.

Keiser, J., Utzinger, J., 2009. Food-borne trematodiases. Clin. Microbiol. Rev. 22, 466–483. http://dx.doi.org/10.1128/CMR. 00012-09.

Kim, D.C., 1984. *Paragonimus westermani*: life cycle, intermediate hosts, transmission to man and geographical distribution in Korea. Arzneimittelforschung 34, 1180–1183.

Kim, T.S., Cho, S.H., Huh, S., Kong, Y., Sohn, W.M., Hwang, S.S., Chai, J.Y., Lee, S.H., Park, Y.K., Oh, D.K., Lee, J.K., 2009. A nationwide survey on the prevalence of intestinal parasitic infections in the Republic of Korea, 2004. Korean J. Parasitol. 47, 37–47.

Koompirochana, C., Sonakul, D., Chinda, K., Stitnimankarn, T., 1978. Opisthorchiasis: a clinicopathologic study of 154 autopsy cases. Southeast Asian J. Trop. Med. Public Health 9, 60–64.

Krull, W.H., Mapes, C.R., 1953. Studies on the biology of *Dicrocoelium dendriticum* (Rudolphi, 1819) Looss, 1899 (Trematoda: Dicrocoeliidae), including its relation to the intermediate host, *Cionella lubrica* (Muller). IX. Notes on the cyst, metacercaria and infection in the ant, *Formica fusca*. Cornell Vet. 43, 389–409.

Kumar, V., 1980. The digenetic trematodes, *Fasciolopsis buski, Gastrodiscoides hominis* and *Artyfechinostomum malayamun*, as zoonotic infections in South Asian Countries. Ann. Soc. Belg. Med. Trop. 60, 331–339.

Kuntz, R.E., Lo, C.T., 1967. Preliminary studies on *Fasciolopsis buski* (Lankester, 1857) (giant Asian intestinal fluke) in the United States. Trans. Am. Microsc. Soc. 86, 163–166.

Lamothe-Argumedo, R., 1984. Nuevos datos sobre la distribución geográfica de *Paragonimus mexicanus*, y tres nuevos hospederos intermediarios en México. An. Inst. Biol. UNAM Zool. 55, 85–89.

Lamothe-Argumedo, R., 1995. On two new hosts of *Paragonimus mexicanus* in Mexico. An. Inst. Biol. UNAM Zool. 66, 147–150.

Lamothe-Argumedo, R., Caballero Deloya, J., Lazaro Chavez, M.E., 1977. *Pseudothelphusa dilatata*, a second intermediate host of *Paragonimus mexicanus*. An. Inst. Biol. UNAM Zool. 48, 295–298.

Le, T.H., De, N.V., Blair, D., Sithithaworn, P., McManus, D.P., 2006. *Clonorchis sinensis* and *Opisthorchis viverrini*: development of a mitochondrial-based multiplex PCR for their identification and discrimination. Exp. Parasitol. 112, 109–114.

Lee, H.H., 1972. *Fasciolopsis buski* infection among children of Liu-Ying Primary School in Tainan Hsien, South Taiwan. Chin. J. Microbiol. 5, 110–114.

Lee, S.H., Chai, J.Y., 2001. A review of *Gymnophalloides seoi* (Digenea: Gymnophallidae) and human infections in the Republic of Korea. Korean J. Parasitol. 39, 85–118.

Lee, S.H., Chai, J.Y., Hong, S.T., 1993. *Gymnophalloides seoi* n. sp. (Digenea: Gymnophallidae), the first report of human infection by a gymnophallid. J. Parasitol. 79, 677–680.

Li, D., 1991. A case of *Fischoederius elongatus* infection in China. Ann. Bull. Soc. Parasitol. 12 (11–13), 155–156.

Li, Y.S., 1989. A survey of freshwater crabs harbouring parasites in Fujian Province. Acta Hydrobiol. Sin. 13, 83–86.

Liat, L.B., Betterton, C., 1977. *Paragonimus westermani* in Malaysian Felidae and Viverridae: probable modes of transmission in relation to host feeding habits. J. Helminthol. 51, 295–299.

Lie, K.J., 1951. Some intestinal flukes from Indonesia. Doc. Neerl. Indon. Morb. Trop. 3, 105–116.

Lie, K.J., Miyazaki, W.I., Wong, S.K., 1962. A subcutaneous retroauricular abscess in a Dyak boy in Sarawak, probably caused by a trematode of the genus *Poikilorchis,* Fain and Vandepitte, 1957. Med. J. Malaya 17, 37–40.

Lieper, R.T., 1911. A new echinostome parasite in man. J. London School Trop. Med. 1, 27–28.

Lim, J.H., Mairiang, E., Ahn, G.H., 2008. Biliary parasitic diseases including clonorchiasis, opisthorchiasis and fascioliasis. Abdom. Imaging 33, 157–165.

Lin, J., Chen, Y., Li, Y., Lin, J., Chen, Y.Z., Li, Y.S., 2001. The discovery of natural infection of human with *Metorchis orientalis* and the investigation of its focus. Chin. J. Zoonoses 17, 19–21.

Lou, Y.S., Fujino, T., Morita, K., Ishii, Y., 1992. A comparative ultrastructural and histochemical study of the metacercarial cyst walls of four species of Paragonimus (Troglotrematidae: Trematoda). Parasitol. Res. 78 (6), 457–462.

MacLean, J.D., Arthur, J.R., Ward, B.J., Gyorkos, T.W., Curtis, M.A., Kokoskin, E., 1996. Common-source outbreak of acute infection due to the North American liver fluke *Metorchis conjunctus*. Lancet 347, 154–158.

Mairiang, E., Mairiang, P., 2003. Clinical manifestation of opisthorchiasis and treatment. Acta Trop. 88, 221–227.

Maleewong, W., Intapan, P.M., Wongkham, C., Wongsaroj, T., Kowsuwan, T., Pumidonming, W., Pongsaskulchoti, P., Kitikoon, V., 2003. Detection of *Opisthorchis viverrini* in experimentally infected bithynid snails and cyprinoid fishes by a PCR-based method. Parasitology 126, 63–67.

Malviya, H.C., 1985. The susceptibility of mammals to *Fasciolopsis buski*. J. Helminthol. 59, 19–22.

Mas-Coma, S., Bargues, M.D., 1997. Human liver flukes: a review. Res. Rev. Parasitol. 57, 145–218.

Mas-Coma, S., Bargues, M.D., Valero, M.A., 2005. Fascioliasis and other plant-borne trematode zoonoses. Int. J. Parasitol. 35, 1255–1278.

Mas-Coma, S., Bargues, M.D., Valero, M.A., 2007. Plant-borne trematode zoonoses: fascioliasis and fasciolopsiasis. In: Murrell, K.D., Fried, B. (Eds.), World Class Parasites. In: Food-Borne Parasitic Zoonoses. Fish and Plant-Borne Parasites, vol. 11. Springer, New York, pp. 293–334.

Mas-Coma, S., Valero, M.A., Bargues, M.D., 2009. Fasciola, lymnaeids and human fascioliasis, with a global overview on disease transmission, epidemiology, evolutionary genetics, molecular epidemiology and control. Adv. Parasitol. 69, 41–146. http://dx.doi.org/10.1016/S0065-308X(09)69002-3.

McGarry, J.W., Ortiz, P.L., Hodgkinson, J.E., Goreish, I., Williams, D.J., 2007. PCR-based differentiation of Fasciola species (Trematoda: Fasciolidae), using primers based on RAPD-derived sequences. Ann. Trop. Med. Parasitol. 101, 415–421.

McMullen, D.B., 1937. An experimental infection of *Plagiorchis muris* in man. J. Parasitol. 23, 235–243.

Milleman, R.E., Knapp, S.E., 1970. Biology of *Nanophyetus salmincola* and "salmon poisoning" disease. Adv. Parasitol. 8, 1–41.

Miyazaki, I., 1969. *Potamiscus cognatus* (Roux, 1936), a new crab host for *Paragonimus westermani* in Malaysia. J. Parasitol. 55, 459.

Miyazaki, I., 1974. Occurrence of the lung fluke, *Paragonimus peruvianus* in Costa Rica. Jpn. J. Parasitol. 23, 280–284.

Miyazaki, M.I., Kanagara, D.W.W., 1970. Metacercaria of *Achillurbainia* sp. from mountainous crab *Parathelphusa rugosa* in Ceylon (Trematoda: Achillurbainiidae). Jpn. J. Parasitol. 19, 537–540.

Miyazaki, I., Kawashima, K., Tan, M.H., 1968. *Parathelphusa maculata* de Man, 1879, a new crustacean host record for *Paragonimus westermani* (Kerbert, 1878) in Malaysia. J. Parasitol. 54, 178–179.

Miyazaki, I., Kifune, T., Lamothe-Argumedo, R., 1980. Taxonomical and Biological Studies on the Lung Flukes of Central America, vol. 2. Occasional Publications of the Department of Parasitology, School of Medicine, Fukuoka, Japan, pp. 1–28.

Mordvinov, V.A., Yurlova, N.I., Ogorodova, L.M., Katokhin, A.V., 2012. *Opisthorchis felineus* and *Metorchis bilis* are the main agents of liver fluke infection of humans in Russia. Parasitol. Int. 61, 25–31.

Moghadami, M., Mardani, M., 2008. *Fasciola hepatica*: a cause of obstructive jaundice in an elderly man from Iran. Saudi J. Gastroenterol. 14, 208–210. http://dx.doi.org/10.4103/1319-3767.43279.

Monge, E., Brenes, R., Muñoz, G., 1985. Natural infection of *Ptychophallus tristani* (Crustacea: Decapoda) by metacercariae of *Paragonimus mexicanus* (Trematoda) in Tabarcia de Mora, Costa Rica. Rev. Inst. Med. Trop. Sao Paulo 27, 23–26.

Odermatt, P., Habe, S., Manichanh, S., Tran, D.S., Duong, V., Zhang, W., Phommathet, K., Nakamura, S., Barennes, H., Strobel, M., Dreyfuss, G., 2007. Paragonimiasis and its intermediate hosts in a transmission focus in Lao People's Democratic Republic. Acta Trop. 103, 108–115.

Oyediran, A.B.O.O., et al., 1975. Infection of the mastoid bone with a *Paragonimus*-like trematode. Am. J. Trop. Med. Hyg. 24, 268–273.

Park, C.W., Kim, J.S., Joo, H.S., Kim, J., 2009. A human case of *Clinostoma complanatum* infection in Korea. Korean J. Parasitol. 47, 401–404.

Pester, F.R.N., Keymer, I.F., 1968. *Gastrodiscoides hominis* from an orangutan, *Pongo pygmaeus*, Southeast Asia. Trans. R. Soc. Trop. Med. Hyg. 62, 10.

Pick, F., 1964. Informations nouvelles sur la distomatose a *Watsonius watsoni*. Bull. Soc. Pathol. Exot. 57, 502–510.

Pick, F., 1967. Die todliche terminale *Watsonius*-Ileitis. Wien. Klin. Wochenschr. 79, 666–667.

Price, D.L., Childs, P.L., 1971. Dicrocoeliasis. In: Marcial-Rojas, R. (Ed.), Pathology of Protozoal and Helminthic Diseases. Williams and Wilkins, Baltimore, pp. 498–503.

Pungpak, S., Bunnag, D., Harinasuta, T., 1984. Albendazole in the treatment of opisthorchiasis and concomitant intestinal helminthic infections. Southeast Asian J. Trop. Med. Public Health 15, 44–50.

Radomyos, P., Bunnag, D., Harinasuta, T., 1984. Worms recovered in stools following praziquantel treatment. Arzneim. Forsch. 34, 1215–1217.

Radomyos, P., Bunnag, D., Harinasuta, T., 1989. A new intestinal fluke, *Plagiorchis harinasutai* n. sp. Southeast Asian J. Trop. Med. Public Health 20, 101–107.

Radomyos, P., Sirivichayakul, C., Waikagul, J., Krudsood, S., Takeuchi, T., Kojima, S., Looareesuwan, S., 2004. Atlas of Medical Parasitology, first ed. Medical Media, Bangkok.

Rangsiruji, A., Sugiyama, H., Morishima, Y., Kameoka, Y., Donsakul, T., Binchai, S., Ketudat, P., 2006. A new record of Paragonimus other than *P. westermani* in southern Thailand. Southeast Asian J. Trop. Med. Public Health 37 (Suppl. 3), 57–61.

Reinhard, E.G., 1957. Landmarks of parasitology. I. The discovery of the life cycle of the liver fluke. Exp. Parasitol. 6, 208–232.

Rim, H.J., Chai, J.Y., Min, D.Y., Cho, S.Y., Eom, K.S., Hong, S.J., Sohn, W.M., Yong, T.S., Deodato, G., Standgaard, H., Phommasack, B., Yun, C.H., Hoang, E.H., 2003. Prevalence of intestinal parasite infections on a national scale among primary school children in Laos. Parasitol. Res. 91, 267–272.

Rodriguez, J.D., Gomez-Lince, L.F., El Montalvan, J.A., 1949. *Opisthorchis guayaquilensis*. Rev. Ecuat. Hig. Med. Trop. 6, 11–24.

Sachs, R., Cumberlidge, N., 1991. First record of the spiny river crab, *Liberonautes chaperi* (A. Milne-Edwards 1887), as second intermediate host of *Paragonimus uterobilateralis* in Liberia. Ann. Trop. Med. Parasitol. 85, 471–472.

Sachs, R., Voelker, J., 1982. Human paragonimiasis caused by *Paragonimus uterobilateralis* in Liberia and Guinea, West Africa. Tropenmed. Parasitol. 33, 15–16.

Sadun, E.H., Maiphoom, C., 1953. Study on the epidemiology of the human infection with *Fasciolopsis buski* (Lankester) in central Thailand. Am. J. Trop. Med. Hyg. 2, 1070–1084.

Sandground, J.H., 1940. *Plagiorchis javensis* n.sp., a new trematode parasitic in man. Rev. Med. Trop. Parasitol. (Habana) 6, 207–211.

Schell, S.C., 1970. How to Know the Trematodes. WMC Brown, Iowa.

Seo, B.S., Lee, S.H., Chai, J.Y., Hong, S.J., Hong, S.T., 1988. The life cycle and larval development of *Fibricola seoulensis* (Trematoda: Diplostomatidae). Korean J. Parasitol. 26, 179–188.

Shin, H.R., Oh, J.K., Lim, M.K., Shin, A., Kong, H.J., Jung, K.W., Won, Y.J., Park, S., Park, S.J., Hong, S.T., 2010. Descriptive epidemiology of cholangiocarcinoma and clonorchiasis in Korea. J. Korean Med. Sci. 25, 1011–1016.

Singh, T.S., Sugiyama, H., Umehara, A., Hiese, S., Khalo, K., 2009. *Paragonimus heterotremus* infection in Nagaland: a new focus of Paragonimiasis in India. Indian J. Med. Microbiol. 27, 123–127.

Sirisinha, S., Chawengkirttikul, R., Haswell-Elkins, M.R., Elkins, D.B., Kaewkes, S., Sithithaworn, P., 1995. Evaluation of a monoclonal anti-body-based enzyme-linked immunosorbent assay for the diagnosis of *Opisthorchis viverrini* infection in an endemic area. Am. J. Trop. Med. Hyg. 52, 521–524.

Sithiathaworn, P., Yongvanit, P., Tesana, S., Pairojkul, C., 2007. Liver flukes. In: Murrell, K.D., Fried, B. (Eds.), Food-Borne Parasitic Zoonoses: Fish and Plant-Borne Parasites (World Class Parasites), vol. 11. Springer, New York, pp. 3–52.

Sithithaworn, P., Andrews, R.H., De, N.V., Wongsaroj, T., Odermatt, P., Nawa, Y., Liang, S., Brindley, P.J., Sripa, B., 2012. The current status of opisthorchiasis in the Mekong Basin. Parasitol. Int. 61, 10–16.

Sithithaworn, P., Sripa, B., Kaewkes, S., Haswell-Elkins, M., 2009. Food-borne trematodes. In: Cook, G.C., Zumla, A.I. (Eds.), Manson's Tropical Diseases. W.B. Saunders, London, pp. 1461–1476.

Sithithaworn, P., Tesana, S., Pipitgool, V., Kaewkes, S., Pairojkul, C., Sripa, B., Paupairoj, A., Thaiklar, K., 1991. Relationship between faecal egg count and worm burden of *Opisthorchis viverrini* in human autopsy cases. Parasitology 102, 277–281.

Skrjabin, K.J., Podjapolskaja, W.P., 1931. *Nanophyetus schikhobalowi*, n. sp. Ein neuer Trematode aus Darm des Menschen. Zbl. Bakt. I Abt. Orig. 119, 294–297.

Soh, C.T., Lee, K.T., Ahn, Y.K., Lee, Y.H., 1964. A new second intermediat host of genus *Paragonimus*. Korean J. Parasitol. 2, 35–40.

Sohn, W.M., Shin, E.H., Yong, T.S., Eom, K.S., Jeong, H.G., Sinoun, M., Socheat, D., Chai, J.Y., 2011. Adult *Opisthorchis viverrini* flukes in humans, Takeo, Cambodia. Emerg. Infect. Dis. 17, 1302–1304.

Soukhathammavong, P., Odermatt, P., Sayasone, S., Vonghachack, Y., Vounatsou, P., Hatz, C., et al., 2011. Efficacy and safety of mefloquine, artesunate, mefloquine-artesunate, tribendimidine, and praziquantel in patients with *Opisthorchis viverrini*: a randomised, exploratory, open-label, phase 2 trial. Lancet Infect. Dis. 11, 110–118.

Stensvold, C.R., Saijuntha, W., Sithithaworn, P., Wongratanacheewin, S., Strandgaard, H., Ornbjerg, N., Johanson, M.V., 2006. Evaluation of PCR based coprodiagnosis of human opisthorchiasis. Acta Trop. 97, 26–30.

Surinthrangkul, B., Gonthian, S., Pradatsundarasar, A., 1965. *Gastrodescoides hominis* in Thailand. J. Med. Assoc. Thai. 48, 96–103.

Suwanik, R., Harinasuta, C., 1959. Pulmonary paragonimiasis: an evaluation of roentgen findings in 38 positive sputum patients in an endemic area in Thailand. Am. J. Roentgenol. Radium Ther. Nucl. Med. 81, 236–244.

Takeda, M., Sugiyama, H., Singh, T.S., 2012. Some freshwater crabs from Northeast India bordered on Myanmar. J. Teikyo Heisei. Univ. 23, 199–213.

Tesjaroen, S., Ngaotep, P., Lertlaituan, P., 1989. The first report of *Achillurbiania nouveli* Dollfus, 1938 in Thailand. Siriraj Hosp. Gaz. 41, 500–503.

Thaenkham, U., Visetsuk, K., Dung, D.T., Waikagul, J., 2007. Discrimination of *Opisthorchis viverrini* from *Haplorchis taichui* using COI sequence marker. Acta Trop. 103, 26–32.

Tiewchaloern, S., Udomkijdecha, S., Suvouttho, S., Chunchamsri, K., Waikagul, J., 1999. Clinostomum trematode from human eye. Southeast Asian J. Trop. Med. Public Health 30, 382–384.

Traub, R.J., Macaranas, J., Mungthin, M., Leelayuva, S., Cribb, T., Murrell, K.D., Thompson, R.C.A., 2009. A new PCR-based approach indicates the range of *Clonorchis sinensis* now extends to central Thailand. PLoS Negl. Trop. Dis. 3, e367. http://dx.doi.org/10.1371/journal.pntd.0000367.

Traverso, A., Repetto, E., Magnani, S., Meloni, T., Natrella, M., Marchisio, P., Giacomazzi, C., Bernardi, P., Gatti, S., Gomez Morales, M.A., Pozio, E., 2012. A large outbreak of *Opisthorchis felineus* in Italy suggests that opisthorchiasis develops as a febrile eosinophilic syndrome with cholestasis rather than a hepatitis-like syndrome. Eur. J. Clin. Microbiol. Infect. Dis. 31, 1089–1093.

Upatham, E.S., Viyanant, V., Brockelman, W.Y., Kurathong, S., Lee, P., Eraengraeng, R., 1988. Rate of reinfection by *Opisthorchis viverrini* in an endemic northeast Thai community after chemotherapy. Int. J. Parasitol. 18, 643–649.

Valero, M.A., Varea, M.T., Marin, R., 2000. *Fasciola hepatica*: lithogenic capacity in experimental infested rats and chemical determination of the main stone component. Parasitol. Res. 86, 558–562.

Valero, M.A., Santana, M., Morales, M., Hemandez, J.L., Mas-Coma, S., 2003. Risk of gallstone disease in advanced chronic phase of fascioliasis: an experimental study in a rat model. J. Infect. Dis. 188, 787–793.

Vanijanonta, S., Radomyos, P., Bunnag, D., Harinasuta, T., 1981. Pulmonary paragonimiasis with expectoration of worm: a case report. Southeast Asian J. Trop. Med. Public Health 12, 104–106.

Vargas-Arzola, J., Segura-Salvador, A., Reyes-Velasco, L., Díaz-Chiguer, D.L., Márquez-Navarro, A., León-Avila, G., Ibañez-Cervantes, G., Camacho, A.D., Sánchez-Manzano, R.M., Nogueda-Torres, B., 2014. Detection of *Paragonimus mexicanus* (Trematoda) metacercariae in crabs from Oaxaca, Mexico. Acta Trop. 137, 95–98.

Velasquez, C.C., 1975. Observation on the life cycle of *Carneophallus brevi*caeca (Africa et Garcia, 1935) comb. n. (Digenea: Microphallidae). J. Parasitol. 61, 910–914.

Vieira, J.C., Blankespoor, H.D., Cooper, P.J., Guderian, R.H., 1992. Paragonimiasis in Ecuador: prevalence and geographical distribution of parasitisation of second intermediate hosts with *Paragonimus mexicanus* in Esmeraldas province. Trop. Med. Parasitol. 43, 249–252.

Voelker, J., Arzube, M., 1979. A new lung fluke from the coastal range of ecuador: *Paragonimus ecuadoriensis* n.sp. (Paragonimidae, Trematoda). Tropenmed. Parasitol. 30, 249–263.

Voelker, J., Sachs, R., 1977. On the distribution of the lung flukes, *Paragonimus africanus and P. uterobilateralis*, in the South West Province of Cameroon and in Eastern Nigeria as determined by examination of the intermediate crab hosts for infection with metacercariae. Tropenmed. Parasitol. 28, 120–133.

Waikagul, J., 2007. A new species of *Paragonimus* (Trematoda: Troglotrematidae) from a cat infected with metacercariae from mountain crabs *Larnaudia larnaudii*. J. Parasitol. 93, 1496–1500.

Waikagul, J., Thaenkham, U., 2014. Approaches to Research on the Systematic of Fish-Borne Trematodes. Academic Press, Amsterdam, p. 119.

Waikagul, J., Yaemput, S., 1999. Two *Achillurbainia* metacercariae from mountain crabs in Central Thailand. J. Trop. Med. Parasitol. 22, 1–6.

Waikagul, J., Yoonuan, T., 2004. *Paragonimus* and Paragonimiasis in Thailand. In: Arizono, N., Nawa, Y., Chai, J., Takahashi, Y. (Eds.), Food-Borne Helminthiasis in Asia, vol. 1. FAP Journal Ltd., Chiba, pp. 139–148.

Waikagul, J., Dekumyoy, P., Chaichana, K., Anantaphruti, M.T., Komalamisra, C., Kitikoon, V., 2002. Serodiagnosis of human opisthorchiasis using cocktail and electroeluted *Bithynia* snail antigens. Parasitol. Int. 51, 237–247.

Waikagul, J., Watthanakulpanich, D., Muennoo, C., Maipanich, W., Sa-nguankiat, S., Phubampen, S., 2005. Efficacy of benzimidazole carbamate on an intestinal fluke co-infected with nematodes. J. Med. Assoc. Thai. 88, 233–237.

Waikagul, J., Yaemput, S., Visiassuk, K., 1986. The route of migration of *Paragonimus siamensis* Miyazaki and Wykoff, 1965 in the white rat. Southeast Asian J. Trop. Med. Public Health 17, 587–590.

Wang, P., Zhang, K., Wu, F., Yao, T., 1977. Studies on the life history of *Fasciolopsis buski* (Lankester, 1857) with consideration of its seasonal infection in pigs. Acta Zool. Sin. 23, 88–96.

Watson, T.G., Freeman, R.S., Staszak, M., 1979. Parasites in native people of the Sioux Lookout zone, northwestern Ontario. Can. J. Public Health 70, 170–182.

Weng, Y.L., Zhuang, Z.L., Jiang, H.P., Lin, G.R., Lin, J.J., 1989. Studies on ecology of *Fasciolopsis buski* and control strategy of fasciolopsiasis. Zhongguo Ji Sheng Chong Xue Yu Ji Sheng Chong Bing Za Zhi 7, 108–111.

WHO, 1995. Control of foodborne trematode infections. Report of a WHO study group. World Health Organ. Tech. Rep. Ser. 849, 1–157.

WHO, 2004. Joint WHO/FAO Workshop on Food-Borne Trematode Infections in Asia. WHO Report Series, RS/2002/GE/40(VTN).

Witenberg, G., 1944. What is the cause of the parasitic laryngo-pharyngitis in the Near East "Halzoun"? Acta Med. Orient. 3, 191–192.

Wong, S.K., Lie, K.J., 1965. Another periauricular abscess from Sarawak, probably caused by trematode of genus *Poikilorchis* Fain and Vandepitte, 1957. Med. J. Malaya 19, 229–230.

Wongratanacheewin, S., Bunnag, D., Vaeusorn, N., Sirisinha, S., 1988. Characterization of humoral immune response in the serum and bile of patients with opisthorchiasis and its application in immunodiagnosis. Am. J. Trop. Med. Hyg. 38, 356–362.

Wongratanacheewin, S., Pumidonming, W., Sermswan, R.W., Pipitgool, V., Maleewong, W., 2002. Detection of *Opisthorchis viverrini* in human stool specimens by PCR. J. Clin. Microbiol. 40, 3879–3880.

Wongratanacheewin, S., Pumidonming, W., Sermswan, R.W., Maleewong, W., 2001. Development of a PCR-based method for the detection of *Opisthorchis viverrini* in experimentally infected hamsters. Parasitology 122, 175–180.
Xuan, L.T., Hung, N.T., Waikagul, J., 2005. Cutaneous fascioliasis: a case report in Vietnam. Am. J. Trop. Med. Hyg. 72, 508–509.
Yamashita, J., 1938. *Clinostomum complanatum*, a trematode parasite new to man. Annot. Zool. Jpn. 17, 563–566.
Yokogawa, M., 1965. *Paragonimus* and paragonimiasis. Adv. Parasitol. 3, 99–158.
Yokogawa, M., Yoshimura, H., Sano, M., Okura, T., Tsuji, M., 1962. The route of migration of the larva of *Paragonimus westermani* in the final hosts. J. Parasitol. 48, 525–531.
Yong, T.S., Shin, E.H., Chai, J.Y., Sohn, W.M., Eom, K.S., Lee, D.M., Park, K., Jeoung, H.G., Hoang, E.H., Lee, Y.H., Woo, H.J., Lee, J.H., Kang, S.I., Cha, J.K., Lee, K.H., Yoon, C.H., Sinuan, M., Socheat, D., 2012. High prevalence of *Opisthorchis viverrini* infection in a riparian population in Takeo Province, Cambodia. Korean J. Parasitol. 50, 173–176.
Yu, S.H., Mott, K.E., 1994. Epidemiology and morbidity of food-borne intestinal trematode infections. Trop. Dis. Bull. 91, R125–R152.
Zhou, L.X., Luo, L.L., You, C., Wang, B., Xu, J., Liao, L., Hui, X., Cai, B., 2008. Multiple brain hemorrhages and hematomas associated with ectopic fascioliasis in brain and eye. Surg. Neurol. 69, 516–521.

Part Three

Transmission dynamics in food sources

Transmission dynamics of foodborne parasites in pork (pig and wild boar)

11

H.L. Enemark[1], *M.V. Johansen*[2], *L. Alban*[3]
[1]Technical University of Denmark, Frederiksberg, Denmark; [2]University of Copenhagen, Frederiksberg, Denmark; [3]Danish Agriculture and Food Council, Copenhagen, Denmark

11.1 Introduction

Pork is one of the most frequently consumed meats worldwide (Anon., 2014a). As an example, the consumption of pork per year is 40 kg per capita in the European Union (Anon., 2014a). It is eaten raw, cooked, and processed and is popular not only in the Western world but also in Chinese cuisine. However, consumption of pork in some other parts of the world is less widespread or prohibited, primarily due to religious restrictions. Pigs may harbor several zoonotic parasites, but only a limited number (*Alaria* spp., *Sarcocystis suihominis*, *Toxocara* spp. (larva migrans), *Taenia asiatica*, *Taenia solium*, *Toxoplasma gondii*, and *Trichinella* spp.) are transmitted via meat (reviewed by Djurković-Djaković et al., 2013). Of these, *T. solium*, *T. gondii*, and *Trichinella spiralis* were ranked by importance globally as numbers 1, 4, and 7, respectively, in a recent report on risk management of foodborne parasites requested by the Codex Committee on Food Hygiene (CCFH) and produced by the Food and Agriculture Organization (FAO) and the World Health Organization (WHO) (Anonymous, 2012). If infected pork is consumed raw or undercooked, these parasites can be transmitted to humans. In high-income countries, up to 10% of the human population has been estimated to suffer from foodborne zoonotic infections (Schlundt et al., 2004), some of which are parasitic. A recent qualitative risk assessment by the European Food Safety Authority (EFSA) identified *Salmonella* spp., *Yersinia enterocolitica*, *T. gondii*, and *Trichinella* spp. as the most relevant biological hazards in the context of meat inspection of swine in Europe and stated that "a comprehensive pork carcass safety assurance is the only way to ensure their effective control" (EFSA Panels on BIOHAZ, CONTAM, and AHAW, 2011). Meat inspection offers the opportunity to control only some foodborne hazards, such as *Trichinella*, which is directly targeted in many parts of the world through the current meat inspection procedures for pigs and wild boar. However, the most important pork borne zoonotic diseases in humans, including trichinellosis, cause only subclinical infections in pigs, and no apparent or palpable alterations are normally seen in the pig carcasses. Thus, traditional meat inspection with visual inspection, palpation, and incision cannot control these food safety risks.

Foodborne Parasites in the Food Supply Web. http://dx.doi.org/10.1016/B978-1-78242-332-4.00011-4

In recent decades, the pig production industry in high-income countries has undergone major changes, including a significant or marked reduction in the number of farms and a corresponding increase in individual herd size. Today, pig production largely takes place indoors under controlled-housing conditions. This development is attributable primarily for economic and efficiency reasons, but at the same time these changes have been associated with a substantial reduction in the incidence of the major pork borne parasites *T. gondii*, *Trichinella* spp., and *T. solium* (Davies, 2011). Although important differences exist, several risk factors for infection in both humans and animals are identical for these parasites. Thus, measures that control one of them are likely to also reduce the risk of infection with the other in areas where they occur simultaneously. In low-income countries, these parasites continue to be important public health concerns, while the risk of infection may be considered insignificant in high-income countries, particularly regarding the helminths. Nevertheless, modern trends of organic pig production, consuming locally produced foods and raw or rare meat may favor their reemergence. In this chapter, we briefly review where they occur, entry points, methods currently available for diagnosis and detection, risk factors, and points of control. For additional coverage of the subject, readers are referred to chapters in this book and supplementary sources of information mentioned in Section 11.7.

11.2 *Toxoplasma gondii*

The zoonotic protozoan parasite *T. gondii* belongs to the phylum Apicomplexa and is the causative agent of toxoplasmosis in virtually all warm-blooded animals including humans, domestic animals, and wildlife. *T. gondii* comprises clonal lineages or types and numerous subtypes linked to differences in virulence to various hosts (e.g., Howe and Sibley, 1995; Sobanski et al., 2013). *T. gondii* appears to be one of the most common parasites worldwide, although the infections often remain undetected and thus are underreported (EFSA, 2007).

11.2.1 Occurrence of Toxoplasma gondii

11.2.1.1 Toxoplasma gondii *in pigs and wild boar*

In sows, a primary infection established during pregnancy may cause apparent infertility, stillbirths, or abortion, according to the stage of pregnancy at which infection was established. However, under modern intensive farming conditions, where contamination of feed and the indoor environment by *T. gondii* oocysts is absent or minimal, infections are generally expected to be at a very low incidence, causing only mild or subclinical signs of infection (Lind and Buxton, 2000; van der Giessen et al., 2007). Conversely, when pigs are reared outdoors in extensive systems, they are more likely to be exposed to oocysts in higher numbers, and infection will likely be more common (Alvarado-Esquivel et al., 2011; Kijlstra et al., 2004). Age and geographical region are other factors influencing the prevalence of infection in pigs, and several studies have documented that the prevalence increases with the age of the animals (e.g.,

Berger-Schoch et al., 2011; Lopes et al., 2011). Numerous studies worldwide have shown a general downward tendency in the prevalence of *T. gondii* presumably related to improved biosecurity related to indoor housing systems. As an example, surveys of sow populations in the United States documented a decline in the seroprevalence of toxoplasmosis from 20% in 1990 to 6% in 2000 (Patton et al., 1996, 2002). In fattening pigs, on the other hand, a seroprevalence of around 2% has been found repeatedly in intensive farming systems around the world (Patton et al., 2002; de Buhr et al., 2008; Dubey et al., 2014). In organic and free-range pigs, seroprevalences between 1% and 25% have been reported (Kijlstra et al., 2004; van der Giessen et al., 2007; Dubey et al., 2008), while seroprevalences between 7% and 49% were described in European studies of wild boars (EFSA, 2013b; Dubey et al., 2014).

11.2.1.2 Toxoplasmosis *in humans*

Toxoplasmosis is one of the most common parasitic infections of humans infecting approximately one-third of the world's population (Moncada and Montoya, 2012; Flegr, 2013), and the global seroprevalence in women of childbearing age has been reported to range from 6% to 80% (reviewed by Torgerson and Macpherson, 2011). Worldwide, foci of high prevalence exist in parts of Southeast Asia, Africa, Latin America, the Middle East, as well as in parts of Eastern and Central Europe (Pappas et al., 2009). In general, however, the prevalence has decreased over the past decades in Europe and in the United States (Pappas et al., 2009), as exemplified by France, where seroprevalence among pregnant women decreased from 84% in the 1960s to 44% in 2003 (Villena et al., 2010); and American studies showing a decrease in seroprevalence from 23% in the 1990s to 11% in a more recent study (Jones et al., 2001; Jones et al., 2007).

Vertical transmission during pregnancy, which causes congenital toxoplasmosis, is the major public health concern, due to the serious threat to the unborn child if the mother is infected for the first time during the pregnancy (Montoya and Liesenfeld, 2004). Human vaccines are currently unavailable, and present antiparasitic treatments are unsatisfactory. Nevertheless, clinical disease in humans is relatively uncommon despite the widespread occurrence of *T. gondii* (Dubey, 2010). In addition to pregnant women, those particularly at risk include immunosuppressed individuals. In the latter, the infection may be lethal if left untreated, whereas people with no apparent immune deficiency occasionally may develop general malaise, fever, and lymphadenopathy (Montoya and Liesenfeld, 2004). Nevertheless, new concerns have been raised recently about infection in healthy immunocompetent individuals due to the circulation of particularly virulent *T. gondii* genotypes in South America (Khan et al., 2006; Dardé, 2008), and because of the possible correlation between chronic toxoplasmosis and neurological disorders (Torrey and Yolken, 2003; Alvardo-Esquivel et al., 2006). American scientists have ranked *T. gondii* as among the most important causes of foodborne illness and estimated that this pathogen is one of the leading causes of hospitalization surpassed only by *Salmonella* spp., norovirus, and *Campylobacter* spp. The same study found *T. gondii* to be the second-most common cause of death due to the foodborne pathogens (Scallan et al., 2011).

11.2.2 Entry points

11.2.2.1 Parasite stages in meat or meat products

T. gondii has three stages: tachyzoites, bradyzoites, and sporozoites in blood, fluids, and tissues, in tissue cysts, and in oocysts, respectively. It is an obligate intracellular parasite that has a two-stage asexual cycle in warm-blooded animals including humans and a sexual cycle in Felidae, the definitive hosts of this parasite. The life cycle is complex, and the parasite can propagate even in the absence of its definitive hosts (see Chapter 6 for a full description of the life cycle). Pigs become infected with *T. gondii* by ingesting organic matter containing sporulated oocysts, or ingesting infected animal tissues through carnivorism, cannibalism, or scavenging. As the host develops immunity, the parasites transform into the bradyzoite stage within tissue cysts to establish a persistent infection. The parasite remains dormant within these tissue cysts until reactivation or until it is eaten by another host (Dubey, 2010).

Risk factors associated with *T. gondii* infection in pigs include raising pigs outdoors, operating small farms, and having cats on the premises (Assadi-Rad et al., 1995; Patton et al., 1996). Feeding goat milk whey to pigs has also been identified as a source of *T. gondii* infection in pigs (Meersburg et al., 2006), and in Spain, the presence of antibodies against *T. gondii* in wild boar was correlated with a high density of animals (Gauss et al., 2005). A recent Latvian study showed that animals from free-range farms had a 17.6 times higher odds ratio for the presence of antibodies against *T. gondii* compared to animals from intensive farms, and feral wild boars had a 1.7 times higher risk of toxoplasmosis compared to farmed wild boars (Deksne and Kirjušina, 2013).

11.2.2.2 Persistence and infectivity

In pigs, as well as in other intermediate hosts, tissue cysts develop after infection and may remain for the rest of the life of the individual (Dubey, 2010). *T. gondii* persisted as long as 875 days in 14 of 16 experimentally infected pigs (Dubey, 1988). Thus, infective *T. gondii* can be present in raw pork such as minced meat or fresh raw sausages with very short developmental times although the risk of survival in the product is small (Dias et al., 2005). Infective *T. gondii* has been found in pork after 14–21 days and in ham after 24 days (Sommer et al., 1965; Großklaus and Baumgarten, 1967). However, a nationwide American study of retail meat isolated viable *T. gondii* from only 7 of 2094 pork samples (Dubey et al., 2005); whereas a recent study investigated persistence of *T. gondii* in raw sausages and found that only 4 out of 288 (1.4%) laboratory mice contracted the infection after ingestion of contaminated sausages in different ripening stages. It was concluded that raw sausage products represent a risk for consumers, but the likelihood of an infection seems to be quite small (Abdulmawjood et al., 2014).

11.2.2.3 Distribution in carcass and other tissue

Tissue cysts of *T. gondii* are found primarily in the brain (see Figure 11.1) and heart. Yet, virtually all edible parts of an animal may harbor viable *T. gondii* tissue cysts (Dubey et al., 1986b). A recent study used a magnetic capture method for the isolation

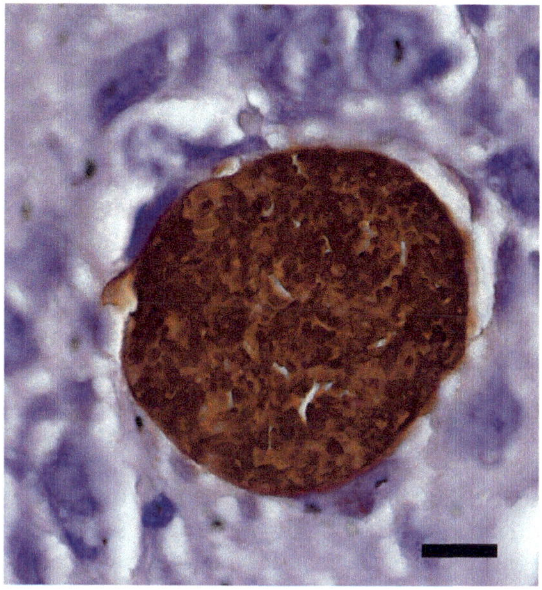

Figure 11.1 *Toxoplasma gondii* tissue cyst in the brain of an experimentally infected mouse. Immunohistochemistry staining (peroxidase–antiperoxidase) using a polyclonal antibody and developed with diaminobenzidine. Scale bar: 10 μm.
Photo by Tim K. Jensen, Technical University of Denmark, National Veterinary Institute.

of *T. gondii* DNA and qualitative real-time polymerase chain reaction (PCR) to estimate the parasite burden in different tissues of experimentally infected pigs. The highest concentration of *T. gondii* DNA was detected in brain tissue, equivalent to 554 tachyzoites per gram, followed by lungs, heart, and dorsal muscles with median values between 0.3 and 2.6 tachyzoites per gram of tissue. The parasite was detected in all tissues except the spleen with parasite burdens equivalent ≤0.2 tachyzoites per gram of tissues in skeletal muscles from fore and hind limb, liver, and kidney (Juránková et al., 2014a).

11.2.2.4 Risk factors and routes of transmission to humans

Infection with *T. gondii* in humans can be congenital, acquired by ingestion of tissue cysts in meat or ingestion of oocysts in food and water (Kapperud et al., 1996; Cook et al., 2000; Dubey, 2004; Bayarri et al., 2012). The most likely sources of human infection are ingestion of raw or undercooked meat containing live *T. gondii* tissue cysts, ingestion of raw or lightly cooked oocyst-contaminated vegetables, or accidental ingestion of oocysts from infected cats (e.g., in children's sand pits or gardens). Cross-contamination during food preparation is another possible mechanism of transmission as suggested by a study that demonstrated increased risk of toxoplasmosis in people who washed kitchen knives infrequently after cutting meat (Kapperud et al., 1996). Until recently, no laboratory tests were available to distinguish a *T. gondii* infection by oocysts from an infection by tissue cysts, and therefore estimates of the relative importance of infection sources have been based on the epidemiological case control studies. Foodborne transmission has been estimated to account for 50% of the human cases in the United States (Scallan et al., 2011).

A sporozoite-specific antigen for determining exposure to oocysts was described in 2011 (Hill et al., 2011), and a subsequent study showed that of 163 patients, 103 (63.2%) had been infected by the ingestion of oocysts (Boyer et al., 2011). Though the relative role of tissue cysts versus oocysts in human toxoplasmosis still remain insufficiently understood and may differ between countries and social habits, the former can be identified and inactivated more efficiently compared to the latter, more complex source of infection (Dubey, 2004; Sroka et al., 2006).

The tasting of raw minced meat or freshly prepared raw sausage in private kitchens is common practice in many regions and is an important risk factor for human toxoplasmosis. This was established in a multicenter study that also identified eating raw or undercooked "other meats" (e.g., wild boar as a significant risk factor) (Cook et al., 2000). Outbreaks linked to eating uncooked pork have been described (e.g., in Korea) (Choi et al., 1997) as well as in a recent Italian study that demonstrated a case of acute toxoplasmosis related to the consumption of homemade fresh sausage made with meat of a backyard-raised pig (Vitale et al., 2014). Eating locally produced smoked, cured, or dried meat sold only in the local area is a well-known risk factor for toxoplasmosis (Jones et al., 2009).

Organic pork products can be expected to be more frequently infected because pigs with outdoor access are more likely to be infected (Kijlstra et al., 2004; Schulzig and Fehlhaber, 2006). However, it is not yet sufficiently evaluated to which extent organic manufactured products entail an increased infection risk for the consumers. Freezing of the raw meat prior to processing might constitute a way of dealing with this putative risk.

11.2.3 Detection of *Toxoplasma gondii* in pigs and pork

11.2.3.1 Diagnosis, including sampling and surveillance

Individual pigs destined for human consumption are usually not tested for *T. gondii* at slaughter anywhere in the world, and no standardized methods for detection and surveillance are currently available, although national and regional regulations may demand collection of *Toxoplasma* data depending on the epidemiological situation. It is not feasible to monitor all pigs used for human consumption for infection with *T. gondii*, and monitoring should focus on free-range pigs, pigs from organic farms, and farmed wild boar, since they are more likely to be exposed to the infection compared to pigs conventionally reared indoors (EFSA, 2007, 2013b). However, focus could also be on the raw material intended for the production of cured products, since these products are often consumed as "ready-to-eat" and therefore potentially contain tissue cysts that are not adequately deactivated.

11.2.3.2 Detection methods

Toxoplasmosis in food animals can be diagnosed by direct as well as indirect methods depending on the purpose and type of matrix. In general, the detection of *T. gondii* infection in animals relies largely on serological assays (Robert-Gangneux and Darde, 2012) where sensitivity and specificity vary according to the specific methods and cut-off values used. Serological tests include the dye test (DT), indirect immunofluorescent antibody test (IFA), direct agglutination test (DAT), indirect haemagglutination test (IHA), latex agglutination test (LAT), and enzyme-linked immunosorbent assay (ELISA). The DT is the "gold standard" for humans and uses live, virulent *Toxoplasma* tachyzoites. IFA (Munday and Corbould, 1971), which is safer and simple, is commonly used in animals. This method uses whole killed tachyzoites that are incubated with diluted test serum and fluorescent antispecies serum and examined with a fluorescence microscope. Alternatively, the DAT (Desmonts and Remington, 1980) or LAT tests can be used. These tests are relatively rapid and do not require sophisticated laboratory facilities. When large numbers of samples needs to be analyzed, the ELISA assay (Voller et al., 1976) is well suited. This test uses a *Toxoplasma* tachyzoite antigen preparation, which is layered into wells in a microtiter plate followed by the addition of test sera and antispecies enzyme-labeled conjugate. The process can be fully automated and has been validated for the detection of *Toxoplasma*-specific antibodies in meat juice (e.g., Meemken and Blaha, 2011), which, used in a multi serology test, can be used to categorize pig herds for risk-based meat inspection (Meemken et al., 2014). In addition, nonspecies-specific detection of toxoplasmosis is possible by a newly developed multihost species-indirect ELISA using protein A/G conjugate for the detection of anti-*T. gondii* IgG antibodies (Al-Adhami and Gajadhar, 2014).

T. gondii can be demonstrated in tissue sections by microscopy and immunohistochemistry (Figure 11.1), although the parasite is often difficult to find. Viability of the organisms may be evaluated by bioassays in mice or cats inoculated with tissue homogenate derived from infected animals. Bioassays in cats increase the sensitivity because larger volumes of tissue can be analyzed compared to mice, but the method is slow and expensive (OIE, 2008; Dubey, 2009) and cannot be used to test large numbers of samples. Brain tissue is particularly well suited for nonserological surveys in pigs and should be used for bioassays, histopathological, immunohistochemical, or molecular studies due to its high concentration of parasites (Juránková et al., 2014a).

Numerous PCR methods have been developed to detect *T. gondii* DNA in blood, fluid, and tissues. Optimal sensitivity is linked to type of matrix, sampling site, sample weight, and choice of method. The specificity of these methods is close to 100%, but the sensitivity is limited partly due to problems with DNA extraction and concentration of large sample quantities (Cenci-Goga et al., 2011), partly because the concentration of *T. gondii* in pigs in most tissues is typically low (one tissue cyst in 25–100g), and the PCR methods detect parasite DNA in only a very small amount of tissue (reviewed by Dubey, 2009). Improved sensitivity can be obtained by magnetic capture concentration of parasite DNA followed by PCR (Opsteegh et al., 2010; Juránková et al., 2014b), but these methods require specialized laboratory facilities and have not yet been evaluated for routine testing of individual carcasses in abattoirs. Multiplex genotyping strategies based on the PCR-restriction fragment length analysis of several loci (Su et al., 2006) or fingerprinting techniques using highly polymorphic microsatellite markers (e.g., Ajzenberg et al., 2005; Demar et al., 2007) should be used to identify atypical genotypes or to trace outbreaks.

11.2.4 Points of control

11.2.4.1 Points of control in animal production

Reduction of environmental oocyst contamination is considered the most effective way to reduce *T. gondii* infections in livestock. At present, the tissue cyst stages of *T. gondii* cannot be killed pharmacologically in the live animals (Kijlstra and Jongert, 2008), and no commercial vaccines are available to prevent oocyst excretion by cats or infection in pigs. The most feasible preventive measures include keeping sties, pastures, feed, and water free from feline feces, combined with rodent control, proper dealing with offal, focus on hygiene, and securing a minimal interface with wildlife (Tenter et al., 2000; Lehmann et al., 2003; Dubey, 2009). Accordingly, production practices that eliminate sources of exposure to *Toxoplasma* decrease the risk of infection in pigs.

Harmonized epidemiological indicators for toxoplasmosis in farmed wild boar have recently been proposed by EFSA (2013b). The proposed scheme includes serological testing of meat juice samples from all wild boars at slaughter. Alternatively, when *T. gondii* prevalence is expected to be low, the serological testing should focus on older animals.

Some may speculate that the concept of controlled housing applied to pig herds with high biosecurity might be used to separate pig herds into herds with a low risk of *T. gondii* (controlled-housing herds) and herds with a high risk (noncontrolled herds). This concept has recently been introduced for *Trichinella* spp. in pigs in the European Union (see Section 11.3.4.1). The usefulness of this approach deserves to be investigated further for *T. gondii*. One suggestion is to freeze raw meat originating from noncontrolled housing if it is destined for the processing of risky products such as sausage that is to be consumed raw.

11.2.4.2 Points of control in food production

Adequate cooking and prevention of cross-contamination are the primary control factors for the prevention of *T. gondii* infection via meat consumption (McCurdy et al., 2006). Heat treatment is the most reliable method to inactivate *T. gondii* tissue cysts. Immediate destruction takes place when the internal temperature of the meat reaches 67 °C (Dubey et al., 1990), or 71.1 °C for ground meat and wild boar (Jones and Dubey, 2012). Cooking in a microwave does not guarantee killing of *T. gondii*, probably due to uneven heating (Lunden and Uggla, 1992).

Likewise, freezing inactivates *T. gondii* tissue cysts, but proper timing and temperature are crucial for a 100% killing efficiency. Freezing at −20 °C for 2 days has been shown to kill the parasite (Sommer et al., 1965), but other studies showed that at least 3 days at −20 °C was necessary to kill tissue cysts from infected mouse brain (Djurković-Djaković and Milenkovic, 2000). Yet, some experiments demonstrated that *T. gondii* could not survive 4 days at −7 to −12 °C (Kuticic and Wikerhauser, 1996), or an internal temperature of −12 °C for more than 2 days (Kotula et al., 1991).

The infectivity of *T. gondii* cysts in meat products depends, among other factors, on pH and salt concentration. Brain tissue cysts from mice can survive for long periods when they are exposed to salt concentrations that are normally used for short-term-fermented sausages (Dubey, 1997). This was further investigated in a study by Pott et al. (2013) showing that *T. gondii* cysts have a high pH tolerance and remained infective for up to 26 days at pH=5. In contrast, muscle cysts survived at a NaCl concentration of up to 2.0% for no longer than 8 days. Following an addition of 2.0% nitrite, the infectivity lasted only 4 days.

Gamma irradiation and high-pressure treatment can kill *T. gondii* tissue cysts at doses between 0.4 and 0.7 kGy (Dubey et al., 1986a; Kuticic and Wikerhauser, 1996) or 300 MPa (Lindsay et al., 2006), but these techniques have adverse effects on meat color and texture. In contrast, a recent study of vacuum-packed *Toxoplasma*-positive goat meat concluded that vacuum packaging increases the survival of *T. gondii* cysts as the parasites were still alive after 6 weeks at 4 °C (Neumayerová et al., 2014).

Despite the various available procedures to kill *T. gondii* muscle cysts, it is difficult to make safety recommendations due to the large variability, and heat treatment or freezing remain the most effective control measures. It should be noted that the effect of strain differences with regard to viability following various eliminating processing steps has not yet been fully investigated. The effect of pH, salting, freezing, and heating on viability of *T. gondii* cysts in pork meat is presented in Table 11.1.

11.3 *Trichinella* spp.

Nematodes of the genus *Trichinella* are the causative agents of *Trichinella* infection in carnivores and omnivores including people and can be found globally in all terrestrial systems and some marine environments (Pozio and Murrell, 2006).

11.3.1 *Occurrence of* Trichinella *spp.*

11.3.1.1 Trichinella *in pigs and wild boar*

In domestic pigs, *T. spiralis* is the predominant species and the etiological agent of most *Trichinella* infections in humans around the world (Pozio, 2007). Nevertheless, a number of other species and genotypes exist of which, for example, *Trichinella britovi*, the main species of wildlife in temperate areas in Europe, has been detected in naturally infected pigs and in particular wild boars; and *Trichinella pseudospiralis*, the only species that is able to infect birds, has been found in wild boar (Nöckler et al., 2006). Both of these species may cause clinical infection in humans (Pozio, 2007). For a more thorough description of *Trichinella* species and its life cycle, see Chapter 8.

In the European Union and in the United States, *Trichinella* is sporadically present in wild boar, free-ranging pigs, and backyard pigs (EFSA, 2011a; CDC, 2014). In addition, available data demonstrate that the risk of *Trichinella* infection in pigs that are raised indoor under high biosecurity levels (i.e., controlled-housing conditions) can be negligible (EFSA, 2011a; Alban et al., 2011; CDC, 2014). The type of production system is therefore the single main risk factor for *Trichinella* infections in domestic pigs.

Table 11.1 Effect of pH, salting, freezing, and heating on viability of *Toxoplasma gondii* tissue cysts in pork meat

Sample	pH	Salt	Temperature (°C)	Time	Efficacy[a]	References
Meat from experimentally infected pigs			−25	6–35 days	+[b]	Groβklaus and Baumgarten (1968)
			−12	3 days	+	Dubey (1988)
			−7 to −12	4 days	+	Kuticic and Wikerhauser (1996)
		Different enhancing solutions	4	8 h	+	Hill et al. (2006)
Pork spiked with *Toxoplasma* cysts			−20	2 days	+	Sommer et al. (1965)
			67	Immediate	+	Dubey et al. (1990)
			>56	10 min		
		2% NaCl	4	7 days	+	Hill et al. (2004)
		1% NaCl	4	45 days	−	
		Up to 2.0% NaCl	4	8 days	−	Pott et al. (2013)
		2.5–3.0% NaCl	4	>1 days	+	
		2.0% NCS[c]	4	>4 days	+	
	5		4	26 days	−	
		15% $NaNO_3$/NaCl	5	4–21 days	+[d]	Scupin (1968)
		Different enhancing solutions	4	8 h	+	Hill et al. (2006)

[a]Unless stated otherwise, the efficacy was scored as "+" (indicating a 100% killing effect of the procedure) or "−" (indicating that the procedure did not kill all parasites). The viability was evaluated by mice or cat bioassay.
[b]After storage at −25 °C for 35 days 1 of 54 samples was still positive in a mouse bioassay.
[c]NaCl plus 0.5% nitrite.
[d]After preparation of smoked hams *T. gondii* cysts could be isolated for up to 13 days.

11.3.1.2 Trichinellosis in humans

Humans are considered to be highly susceptible to infection with *Trichinella* spp., although clinical disease might be mild or absent if the number of ingested infective larvae is low (Malakauskas et al., 2007; Széll et al., 2008; Pozio et al., 2009). The minimal infective dose is estimated to be below 50 larvae (Teunis et al., 2012). It is believed that immunity and individual susceptibility in the human host also play a role in the progression of the disease (Dupouy-Camet and Bruschi, 2007). Therefore, the clinical symptoms range from asymptomatic to fatal and vary over the course of disease (Capó and Despommier, 1996). Fatalities are rare and are mostly associated with complications (Bruschi et al., 2002). Symptoms appear about 8–15 days after the consumption of the contaminated meat (EFSA, 2011a). Further information about symptoms, diagnostics, and treatment can be found in Chapter 8.

In 2011, a total of 363 human cases of trichinellosis were reported in the European Union, of which 268 cases (73.8%) were laboratory confirmed. Cases were only reported by 14 of the 26 EU member states. In 2011, the highest notification rates in the European Union were seen in Latvia (2.24 cases per 100,000), followed by Lithuania, Romania, Bulgaria, and Slovakia (0.89, 0.50, 0.36, and 0.24 cases per 100,000, respectively). These five countries accounted for 84.3% of all confirmed cases reported in 2011 in the European Union. On average, 74% of the confirmed trichinellosis cases were hospitalized. One death due to trichinellosis was reported in Spain in 2011, which gives an EU case fatality rate of 0.49% (EFSA, 2013a).

In the United States, the number of human trichinellosis cases has declined during the last decades. Around 400 cases per year were reported in the late 1940s, when the Public Health Service began tracking cases, and between 2008 and 2010, only 20 cases per year were reported. According to the US CDC, this decline was caused by improved pig-raising practices in the pork industry, extended use of commercial and home freezing of pork, and public awareness of the danger of eating raw or undercooked meat products (CDC, 2014).

In China, 15 outbreaks of human trichinellosis, including 1387 cases and four deaths (corresponding to a case fatality risk of 0.29%), were reported in three southwestern provinces/autonomous regions in China between 2004 and 2009. Of these, 12 outbreaks were caused by eating raw or undercooked pork, and two resulted from the consumption of raw wild boar meat (Cui et al., 2011). In Thailand, 135 outbreaks involving 7340 patients and 97 deaths (corresponding to a case fatality risk of 1.3%) were reported between 1962 and 2006 (Kaewpitoon et al., 2008). Cases of human trichinellosis are also found in many other parts of the world such as Mexico, Central and South America (Ortega-Pierres et al., 2000), Korea (Kim et al., 2011), and sub-Saharan Africa (reviewed by Mukaratirwa et al., 2013).

11.3.2 Entry points

11.3.2.1 Parasite stages in meat or meat products

Trichinella infection in pigs and wild boar is a result of ingestion of the first-stage larvae (see Figure 11.2) in the musculature of an infected animal. The larvae penetrate

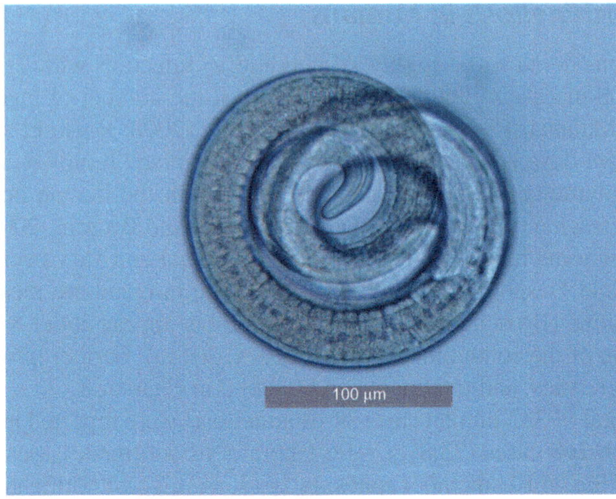

Figure 11.2 *Trichinella spiralis* first-stage muscle larva released from encapsulated tissue cysts by artificial pepsin–HCl digestion. The stichocytes are clearly visible as dark, angular cells in the anterior part of the larva (1000 μm long).
Photo by Heidi L. Enemark, Technical University of Denmark, National Veterinary Institute.

the striated muscles of the host and encapsulate in the tissue, forming a so-called nurse cell (Pozio, 2007). Once encapsulated, they become dormant without any capability to amplify (Pozio and Murrell, 2006).

11.3.2.2 Persistence and infectivity

Trichinella larvae are well protected by the modified muscle fiber ("nurse cell"). Encapsulated larvae can therefore survive and remain infective for years. Certain *Trichinella* species can survive freezing. For example, *T. britovi* and especially *Trichinella nativa* will need to be exposed to −18 °C for prolonged periods of time before they die (Pozio et al., 2006). In general, the parasite's capacity to survive freezing is months to years in muscles of carnivores and horses but only days or weeks in swine (Table 11.2). Most species can survive for at least some time in putrefying flesh (Pozio, 2007; von Köller et al., 2001). The infectivity of *Trichinella* in pork depends on processing prior to consumption. If pork is heat-treated sufficiently, the risk of *Trichinella* infection is absent. However, if the pork is consumed without any eliminating processing steps—such as freezing and heat treatment—then the infectivity remains. For pork, this makes ready-to-eat products risky—in particular dry-cured sausages, bacon, and freshly made sausages intended to be consumed without cooking.

11.3.2.3 Distribution in carcass

In the domestic pig, the three main predilection sites for *T. spiralis*, *T. britovi*, and *T. pseudospiralis* are the diaphragm, the tongue, and the masseter muscle, respectively (Forbes and Gajadhar, 1999), but *Trichinella* larvae may also be present in other

Table 11.2 Required combinations of time and temperature to ensure inactivation of *Trichinella* larvae present in domestic pork

Temperature °F (°C)	Time required to inactivate *Trichinella* larvae: Products in separate pieces not exceeding 6 in. (≈15 cm) (days)	Products in separate pieces exceeding 6 in. (≈15 cm) but not 27 in. (≈69 cm[a]) (days)	References
5 (−15.0)	20	30	EU Comission Regulation No. 2075/2005 (Anon., 2005)
−10 (−23.3)	10	20	
−20 (−28.9)	6	12	Recommendations on methods for the control of *Trichinella* in domestic and wild animals intended for human consumption (ICT, 2006)
120 (49.0)	21 h		United States Department of Agriculture's Code of Federal Regulations; 9CFR318.10 (Anon., 2014c)
122 (50.0)	9.5 h		
124 (51.1)	4.5 h		
126 (52.2)	2 h		
128 (53.4)	1 h		
130 (54.5)	30 min		
132 (55.6)	15 min		
134 (56.7)	6 min		
136 (57.8)	3 min		
138 (58.9)	2 min		
140 (60.0)	1 min		
142 (61.1)	1 min		
144 (62.2)	Instant		

[a] According to the EU Regulation 2075/2005, pieces must be up to 50 cm only.

striated muscles (Ribicich et al., 2001). In wild boars, the main predilection sites are the diaphragm, the forearm muscle, and the tongue (Kapel, 2001).

11.3.2.4 Risk factors and routes of transmission to humans

Consumption of raw, cured, fermented, or undercooked meat containing infective larvae can cause infection in humans. Infection via wild boar is often associated with the consumption of game meat that has not been tested for *Trichinella* spp. Infection via meat from domestic pigs is most commonly related to the consumption of meat from outdoor-reared pigs or backyard pigs. The main risk of infection for these groups of pigs is posed by the feeding of food waste containing pork scraps (Gamble et al., 2000). The presence of *Trichinella* in domestic pigs or wild boar is a risk factor for transmission to humans, with raw home-butchered pork that has not been subject to testing being the major risk factor, in accordance with observations by Petri et al. (1988). However, in a number of countries, *T. spiralis* is also frequently found in wildlife, and in some countries the parasite can occur in the domestic cycle without any documented infection in the human population. This is probably due to the practice of eating only well-cooked pork as well as the execution of *Trichinella* testing as a part of the meat inspection.

11.3.3 Detection of Trichinella in pigs and pork

11.3.3.1 Diagnosis, including sampling and surveillance

Laboratory testing of muscle samples from domestic pigs after slaughter, as a part of routine postmortem inspection, is the only way of reliably diagnosing *Trichinella* spp. in carcasses for food safety purposes. Likewise, meat samples from wild boar should be analyzed for *Trichinella* spp.

For domestic finisher pigs, a sample of a minimum of 1 g of muscle tissue should be taken from the diaphragm musculature after slaughter. For sows and boars, a minimum of 2 g should be taken from the same muscle group. If the main muscles of diaphragm are not available, then a sample twice as large (2 or 4 g) should be taken from the diaphragm's costae musculature or sternal musculature, or the masseter muscles, the tongue, or the abdominal wall musculature (ICT, 2006; Dupouy-Camet and Murrell, 2007).

Surveillance in the large pig abattoirs is more cost-effective, because pooling of up to 100 samples can be used. This means that the price of testing an individual pig is very low on these abattoirs. Contrary, the price of testing pigs delivered to small abattoirs is high, because the possibility of pooling cannot be fully exploited due to the low number of pigs slaughtered in a day. Testing of wild boars shot by hunters is even more expensive; again because pooling cannot be used.

There are special sampling requirements for testing game meats such as wild boar. The guidelines provided by the International Commission of Trichinellosis (ICT) and FAO/WHO/OIE contain detailed instructions on which muscle groups should be tested for a specific kind of animal. According to the guidelines, for wild boar the forearm or the diaphragm musculature should be used. Moreover, a sample size of a minimum of 10 g is recommended, of which a minimum of 5 g should be examined (ICT, 2006; Dupouy-Camet and Murrell, 2007).

Traditionally, the testing of all animals that might harbor *Trichinella* spp. has been recommended. In the European Union, it is mandatory to test all pigs, horses, and relevant wildlife. This has resulted in the testing of hundreds of millions of pig carcasses and revealing only few positives, primarily from outdoor or backyard production systems. As the number of test positives decreased, discussion about risk-based testing began. It was suggested that this could entail testing only of high-risk animals such as sows and boars (because they live longer), as well as all pigs from farms not applying strict biosecurity measures (Alban et al., 2008, 2011; EFSA, 2011b).

For some years the concept of negligible risk status for *Trichinella* spp. in domestic pigs for a country or region was in place in the European Union. Only Denmark (Alban et al., 2008) and Belgium (Anon., 2014b) acquired this status. This status is no longer recognized in an international context by the World Organization for Animal Health (OIE). Instead, such recognition is now linked to compartments of one or more holdings (farms) applying specific controlled-housing conditions.

11.3.3.2 Detection methods

The artificial digestion of meat to reveal *Trichinella* larvae is the only method that is accepted worldwide. The method used should be fit for the purpose and in accordance with required standards. For the European Union, the Commission Regulation 2075/2005, requirements include the preparation of muscle specimens according to Annex 1 in the same regulation. Internationally, the OIE and ICT provide prescribed and recommended methods for this testing, respectively. More information about the artificial digestion methods can be found in Chapter 8 of this book. Furthermore, it can be found in the OIE Diagnostic Manual and in Diagnostic Tests and Vaccines for Terrestrial in Chapter 2.1.16 as well as in the guidelines from the ICT.

Indirect testing methods such as serology are not recommended as a substitute for direct testing of individual carcasses at slaughter by the use of pooled sample digestion, but they may be useful for epidemiological purposes (OIE, 2013; EFSA, 2011b; ICT, 2006).

Trichinoscopic examination, the microscopic examination of small pieces of meat compressed between two glass plates, is time consuming and less sensitive than the digestion assay, particularly for the detection of nonencapsulated *Trichinella* species infecting domestic and wild animals. Therefore, trichinoscopy and similar compression methods are not recommended for the routine examination of food animals and game meats intended for human consumption (ICT, 2006).

11.3.4 Points of control

11.3.4.1 Points of control in animal production

Animal level

Animals do not show any clinical signs of the infection, so a visual inspection cannot be relied on to prevent infection from entering a herd. Experiments have been undertaken to study the protective impact of newborn larval antigens in pigs—see, for example, Marti et al. (1987). However, so far no vaccine is commercially available. Therefore, the focus of control should be on the risk factors for *Trichinella* infection in domestic pigs. These include (1) feeding raw or undercooked food waste containing meat; (2) exposure to infected rodents; and (3) exposure to infected wildlife or infected pig carcasses.

Guidelines have been set up, based on these risk factors, by several bodies such as the European Union (Anon., 2005), the ICT (2006), and the OIE (2013). These guidelines include requirements for the housing facilities, environment, feed and feed storage, rodent control, farm hygiene, introduction of new animals, and animal identification.

Population level

Basically, there are two different overall approaches to ensure the absence of *Trichinella* in pork: (1) by the use of farm audit of the housing and biosecurity practices of the holding or (2) slaughterhouse testing by use of the artificial digestion method of all pigs from the holding as well as for wild boar (EFSA, 2011b).

In the European Union, the concept of controlled housing is used. Controlled housing conditions mean a type of animal husbandry, where pigs are kept at all times under conditions controlled by the food business operator with regard to feeding and housing (Anon., 2014b). This concept is similar to the definition of compartments with negligible risk used by OIE in the Terrestrial Animal Health Code as well as in the coming Codex guidelines for the control of *Trichinella* spp. in meat of suidae (Codex, 2014). All carcasses from holdings that are not part of a negligible risk compartment (which is similar to not being officially recognized as applying controlled-housing conditions) shall be systematically examined for *Trichinella*. Specifically for the European Union, at least 10% of slaughtered carcasses from each holding, officially recognized as applying controlled-housing conditions, should also be examined for *Trichinella*. This provision should remain until the country has demonstrated that accrued data on continuous testing carried out on the slaughtered swine population provide at least 95% confidence that the prevalence of *Trichinella* does not exceed 1 per million in that population. This new approach would ultimately result in a substantial reduction in the number of pigs tested for *Trichinella*—although international acceptance from important pork-importing countries will be required before all countries will apply this risk-based testing approach.

In pigs raised indoors, the risk of infection is primarily related to the lack of compliance with rules on biosecurity, including the treatment of animal waste (EFSA, 2013a). Therefore, auditing of herds applying controlled housing should be undertaken in line with OIE specifications. The frequency of auditing should preferably be risk-based taking into account historical information, slaughterhouse-monitoring results, knowledge of established farm management practices, and the presence of susceptible wildlife. Moreover, a substantial proportion of the audits should be unannounced. The coming Codex guidelines will contain specifications concerning how to establish and maintain a compartment with negligible risk. Consult the home page of Codex for the most updated version of these guidelines.

11.3.4.2 Points of control in food production

Food production often involves some kind of processing such as cooking, freezing, and curing. Such processing steps might have an impact on the viability of infective *Trichinella* larvae. Cooking to a core temperature of 60–70 °C is considered to be sufficient to kill *T. spiralis* (ICT, 2006). For home cooking, the ICT advises cooking to an internal temperature of 71 °C (Gamble et al., 2000). The heating time is also of interest, because *T. spiralis* can survive a core temperature of 77 °C if meat products are rapidly heated up and cooled down (Kotula et al., 1982). Hence, it is the time and temperature combination that determines the survival of *Trichinella* spp. Different combinations of temperature and time are given in Table 11.2 (Anon., 2014c). They apply only when the product reaches and maintains temperatures evenly distributed throughout the meat.

Freezing is also an acceptable way of treating meat to prevent human trichinellosis due to freeze-sensitive *Trichinella* spp. This requires that proper equipment is available for accurately achieving and monitoring time and temperature combinations.

Here, the guidelines set forth for commercial freezing methods in the US Department of Agriculture's Code of Federal Regulations (9CFR318.10) (Anon., 2014c) may be used, as well as the EU Commission Regulation No. 2075/2005 (Anon., 2005) and the ICT guidelines (Table 11.2). Freezing may not eliminate the risk of *Trichinella* in pork unless freezing is properly monitored, particularly in areas where pigs may be exposed to sylvatic species such as *T. britovi* (Pozio et al., 2006; ICT, 2006; Gottstein et al., 2009) that are known to be cold tolerant.

Some specific combinations of salt, temperature, fermentation, and drying time can inactivate *Trichinella* larvae, as shown by Porto-Fett et al. (2010). Still, curing and smoking processes are not recommended for the control of *Trichinella* in meats, because these methods are difficult to control reliably, for example, in artisanal production. Instead, *Trichinella*-free meats should be used in the preparation of cured or smoked products (ICT, 2006; Gottstein et al., 2009). High-pressure processing (HPP) is a relatively new method. It has been evaluated as a way of inactivating *T. spiralis* in (1) pork used for processing of so-called Genoa salami and (2) infected pig masseter muscle. Pressurization at 600 or at 483 MPa for 0.5–12 min was applied in the experimental setup. All HHP treatments inactivated the present larvae as confirmed by both microscopy and mouse bioassays (Porto-Fett et al., 2010). Thus, HPP of contaminated Genoa salami or pork in general appears to effectively inactivate *T. spiralis* larvae. Likewise, irradiation can be an acceptable method for rendering meat safe for human consumption in those countries where irradiation of food is permitted. According to the ICT, levels proven to inactivate *Trichinella* larvae are 0.3 kGy.

11.4 *Taenia solium*

11.4.1 Occurrence of Taenia solium

The human pork tapeworm *T. solium*, for which humans are the only definitive host, is a cosmopolitan parasite transmitted between humans and pigs. The parasite causes taeniosis (infection with the adult tapeworm) in the human host and cysticercosis (infection with the larval tapeworm) in both humans and pigs. Based primarily on the public health concerns, FAO and WHO have ranked *T. solium* as the most important foodborne parasite, and worldwide, 50 million people are estimated to be affected by cysticercosis (WHO, 2011; Anon., 2012).

11.4.1.1 Taenia solium *in pigs and wild boar*

T. solium is primarily found in areas with free-roaming pigs, inadequate meat inspection, and low levels of personal hygiene and sanitation. Despite heavy infections clinical signs in pigs are rarely mentioned in the literature. Mkupasi et al. (2014) observed dullness, sluggishness, somnolence, apathy, and loss of consciousness in naturally infected pigs; Prasad et al. (2006) reported lacrimation, excessive salivation, and excessive blinking to be associated with porcine cysticercosis. However, considerable economic losses are the consequences of infected pigs (Pawlowski et al., 2005).

In Europe and North America, *T. solium* has essentially been eliminated from most countries. This has mainly been achieved through industrialization, including pig confinement and improved hygiene and sanitation. In sub-Saharan Africa, the parasite is emerging and is currently found in 29 countries from Senegal in the west, to Kenya and Tanzania in the east, and Mozambique and South Africa in the south. In Latin America, the parasite is still endemic in most countries despite ongoing efforts to control it. Porcine cysticercosis is frequently detected at meat inspection in abattoirs in these parts of the world. The situation in Asia is more diverse and is not fully understood, but recent data suggest that the parasite is more widespread than previously thought (WHO/FAO/OIE, 2005).

11.4.1.2 Taenia solium *in humans*

Infection with the tapeworm larvae, or cysticerci ("cysts"), affects millions of people in endemic areas and leads to human suffering, including neurologic disorders that can lead to public stigmatization and even death. People become infected with the adult tapeworm by eating raw or undercooked infected pork and become infected with the larval form of the parasite by ingesting *T. solium* eggs either from direct contact with a human tapeworm carrier or from contaminated food or water. Whereas taeniosis typically causes no or minimal clinical symptoms, human cysticercosis can cause severe neurological diseases. Cysts may localize in muscle tissue, in the eye or in the brain. In the brain, the cysts cause neurocysticercosis (NCC), a condition characterized by epileptic seizures, severe headaches, and even death. In endemic areas, NCC has been estimated to be responsible for 30% of cases of acquired epilepsy (Ndimubanzi et al., 2010).

11.4.2 Entry points

11.4.2.1 Parasite stages in meat or meat products

Pigs get infected by ingesting the tapeworm eggs that hatch in the small intestine, and the larvae (oncospheres) penetrate the intestinal mucosa and the vessels in the submucosa (Pal et, al., 2000). After penetration, the oncospheres migrate throughout the body via the bloodstream. Once embedded, the oncospheres enlarge and mature into cysticerci over a period of 3–8 weeks (Flisser, 1994). The cysts appear in the muscles (Figure 11.3) and brain (Figure 11.4) as translucent, thin-walled, whitish structures with an eccentric white nodule containing the invaginated scolex. They measure between 0.2 cm when immature and 2 cm at full growth, and thus are fully macroscopically visible (Pal et al., 2000). The scolex, similar to that of the adult tapeworm, possesses four suckers and a double crown of 22–32 hooks (WHO/FAO/OIE, 2005).

11.4.2.2 Persistence and infectivity

Several studies have determined that at high humidity and low temperatures the eggs of *T. saginata* can stay viable for almost 1 year in the soil (WHO/FAO/OIE, 2005).

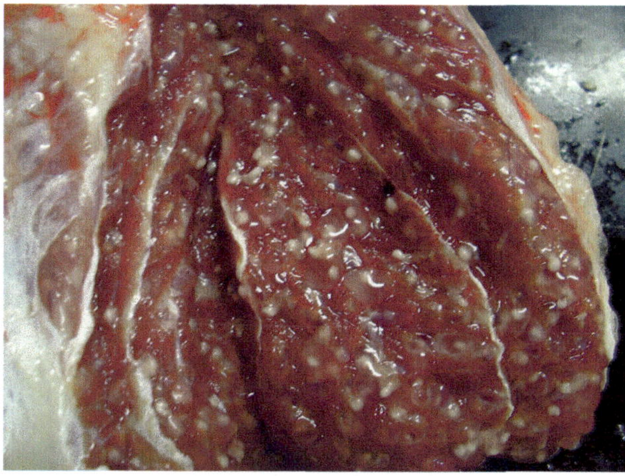

Figure 11.3 Posterior thigh muscles (*semitendinosus*, *semimembranosus*, and *biceps femoris*) from Zambian pig heavily infected with *Taenia solium* cysts.
Photo by Dr. Sikasunge, Lusaka, Zambia.

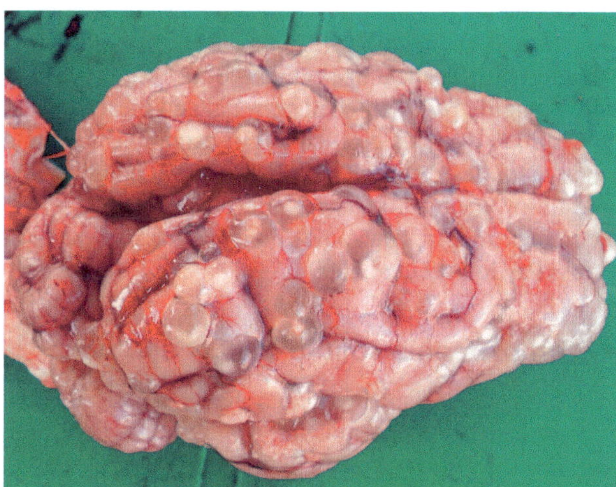

Figure 11.4 Brain from Tanzanian pig heavily infected with live *Taenia solium* cysts.
Photo by Dr. Mkupasi, Morogoro, Tanzania.

Due to morphological similarities, the eggs of *T. solium* are expected to have similar longevity in the environment, but this remains to be assessed. Within the porcine host, cysticerci are infective after about 9–10 weeks. Although the potential longevity of cysticerci is thought to be years, the early age (usually less than 1 year) at which pigs are slaughtered means that the majority of cysts in pork would be viable (Soulsby, 1982). However, most pigs do harbor both live and dead cysts as a result of differences in the age of the cysts and development of host immunity.

11.4.2.3 Distribution in carcass

Predilection sites for cysticerci include the masseter, heart, tongue, neck, shoulder, fore and hind limbs, diaphragm, intercostal and psoas muscles, but cysts can be disseminated throughout the body including the brain (Boa et al., 2002; Mkupasi et al., 2014). In a study from Tanzania, Boa et al. (2002) found by examining 24 naturally infected pigs, the psoas muscles to be the most heavily infected muscles. They also found that all examined pigs had cysts in the brain, none of the pigs had cysts in liver, lung, or kidneys, and the most heavily infected pig harbored more than 80,000 cysts in total. Generally, the total number of cysts per pig varies tremendously even in pigs from endemic areas exposed to similar conditions (Dorny et al., 2004).

11.4.2.4 Risk factors and routes of transmission to humans

As raw or undercooked infected pork is the source of *T. solium*, any insufficient heat treatment of the meat is a risk factor for taeniosis. Roasted pork, as a street food or bar snack, is gaining increased popularity especially in sub-Saharan Africa and as a courtesy to Muslims, pork is called "European goat" in Eastern Africa allowing for consumption across religious borders (Doherty and Johansen, 2013). In the same region, *T. solium* cysticercosis is emerging because of several factors: the demand for pork is increasing, knowledge regarding *T. solium* cysticercosis is almost nonexistent, free-roaming pigs are the norm, meat inspection is either nonexistent or inappropriate, open-air defecation is highly prevalent, and personal and meat hygiene are poor.

Prevalence of *T. solium* depends on the level of economic development as well as hygienic conditions (Morales et al., 2008). However, although the infection is traditionally endemic in low-income countries, tourism as well as economic migration from areas of endemicity into high-income countries is a risk factor for spreading to nonendemic regions (Pawlowski et al., 2005).

11.4.3 Detection of *Taenia solium* in pigs and pork

The most common method for the antemortem diagnosis of porcine cysticercosis in endemic regions is by examining the tongue, using both visual inspection and cyst palpation. Postmortem meat inspection is the routine technique used for the detection of cysticercosis-infected carcasses. Serological tests have been developed for the detection of specific cysticercosis antibodies or antigens but remain primarily as research tools. Likewise have DNA-based PCR methods been described, which are not yet commercially available.

11.4.3.1 Diagnosis including sampling and surveillance

For the detection of *T. solium* in humans, a number of specific serum-IgG antibody ELISA assays are now commercially available. However, simple bedside tests to detect *T. solium*, in particular, live cysts in the brain are not available although urgently needed. For the detection of porcine cysticercosis, a commersial Ag-ELISA test is available, but again, a simple pen-side test not requiring a well-equipped laboratory would be preferred for better surveillance.

11.4.3.2 Detection methods

If tongue inspection is carried out by experienced personnel, the specificity can approach 100% (Dorny et al., 2004). The sensitivity of tongue inspection depends on the level of infection, but even in pigs with more than 100 cysts, the sensitivity is below 50% (Phiri et al., 2002).

Postmortem meat inspection has a low sensitivity (20–25%) in mild infections, whereas heavily infected pigs are easily detected at slaughter (Dorny et al., 2004). In any case, the postmortem examination for porcine cysticercosis should focus on the inspection of muscular surfaces and, in particular, the pillars of the diaphragm, the intercostal muscles, the heart, the tongue, masseters, and possibly the psoas muscles. In addition, the brain should be visually inspected. Incisions should as a minimum be made in the external masseter, the diaphragmatic muscles, and the tongue according to the FAO's *Manual on Meat Inspection for Developing Countries*. However, national rules may prescribe additional procedures (Herenda, 2000).

Cysts found during a meat inspection can be species confirmed (*T. solium*, *T. asiatica*, or *Taenia hydatigena*) by several methods. If cysts are stored in 70% ethanol, DNA can be extracted followed by either PCR (cox-1 gene, HDP2, mitochondrial 12S rDNA fragment), multiplex-PCR, or PCR-RFLP according to Rodriguez-Hidalgo et al. (2002), Yamasaki et al. (2004), and González et al. (2010).

11.4.4 Points of control

Internationally, five strategies have been suggested for the elimination of *T. solium*, such as (1) treatment of humans and pigs, (2) vaccination of pigs, (3) improved pig management and pork production, (4) improved sanitation, and (5) improved knowledge through health education (WHO, 2010). As *T. solium* infects both humans and pigs, control requires an integrated approach. For national control, intersectorial collaboration between the government and the public is vital. Health and veterinary professionals need to collaborate to combine key solutions. Treatment and vaccination against *T. solium* in pigs are not yet commercially available or feasible in most endemic countries; hence, control strategies must include health education, treatment of human taeniosis, pig confinement, and proper pork inspection.

11.4.4.1 Points of control in animal production

T. solium is considered eradicable because of its simple life cycle, with humans as the only tapeworm carrier. Elimination of the parasite in Europe and North America was facilitated through industrialization, including pig confinement and improved public hygiene and sanitation. Whereas porcine cysticercosis is a notifiable disease in most countries, human taeniosis and cysticercosis have not been declared internationally notifiable diseases by WHO. Doing so would be a first real "One Health" approach in the joint fight against this parasite.

If pigs are treated antemortem with oxfendazole (30 mg/kg), muscle cysts will die within 4 weeks posttreatment, but a fair proportion of the cysts in the brain will remain viable, which warrants caution if drug treatment becomes a routine control intervention. Also, although cysts die within 4 weeks posttreatment, visible dead cysts persist for as long as 6 months (Sikasunge et al., 2008).

11.4.4.2 Points of control in food production

If pork is found to be heavily infected, the whole carcass should be condemned and properly disposed of (Herenda, 2000). However, although most meat regulations require total condemnation, for more lightly infected cases there are ways to deal with contaminated carcasses. Cysts will die if the temperature throughout the meat reaches 80 °C (WHO/FAO/OIE, 2005). Freezing is also an option. Sotelo et al. (1986) found that *T. solium* cysts were killed if frozen for 4 days at −5 °C, 3 days at −15 °C, or 1 day at −24 °C. More studies are warranted to confirm optimal temperatures also in relation to age of the cysts and to explore other means of killing the cysts.

11.5 Discussion and future trends

Prevention of parasitic pork borne diseases can be achieved by interventions at the animal and farm level, during slaughter and postslaughter processing, and at the consumer level. Today the combat of these diseases is partly driven by international recommendations, for example, for the surveillance, prevention, and control of *T. solium* (Murrell, 2005). In the case of *Trichinella*, consumer protection is largely directed by international regulations and guidelines (e.g., Gamble et al., 2000; Dupouy-Camet and Murrell, 2007) including the ongoing work by the Codex Alimentarius Commission. Yet, in low-income countries, *Trichinella* control is not always carried out either because pigs are not brought to the abattoirs, inspection is not required or enforced, or there is insufficient education of inspectors (Djordjevic et al., 2005).

International organizations are presently working together to produce guidelines for more general and risk-based control options, such as for *Trichinella*. Current control of *Trichinella* by checking individual slaughtered pigs is very costly and of limited value. Risk-based surveillance may offer an alternative. This type of surveillance focuses on the hazards that make people ill and on high-risk subpopulations; for all three parasites described here, this implies the pigs that are reared outdoors. Hence, surveillance and control should be targeted to wild boar, outdoor-reared pigs, and the products thereof. For low-risk subpopulations, auditing of the biosecurity should be sufficient to ensure that the low-risk herds are, in fact, low risk. This approach will be more cost-effective than the surveillance and control that is currently in place in many regions of the world.

Increasing globalization facilitates the spread of infectious diseases and calls for the integration of veterinary and public health efforts to control infections. This is widely recognized (Newell et al., 2010; Murrell, 2013) and has gained an increased awareness since the avian influenza epidemic in 1997. Nonetheless, although tourists and emigrants may present a source of *T. solium* eggs in nonendemic countries, human taeniosis and cysticercosis are not notifiable internationally. Changing this would facilitate efficient communication between veterinary and public health authorities and would be an important step toward controlling devastating cases of NCC.

Today's global pig production is characterized by two major and opposite trends: expanding highly specialized industrial indoor farming under controlled-housing conditions versus traditional small-scale production and increasing numbers of organic farms with outdoor rearing of pigs. These opposing trends have a major impact on the transmission of pork borne parasites. In addition, the transmission of foodborne parasites is strongly influenced by globalization, which on one hand facilitates the spread of infectious diseases and on the other hand facilitates international collaboration and implementation of measures by regulatory authorities to support the control of these parasites (reviewed by Robertson et al., 2014).

Despite significant differences in modern pig production systems, the majority of commercial pork is produced in confinement in production systems that have practically eliminated the risk of *Trichinella* and *T. solium* infections and reduced the prevalence of *Toxoplasma*. This trend is also seen in low-income countries where increased herd sizes and modernized production systems are changing the way pigs are raised for pork production.

Nevertheless, several trends may cause a reemergence of pork as an infectious meat source in developed countries. In recent years, sociological, ethical, and environmental considerations have led to an increased consumer demand for organically raised and free-range pork products in the Western world, subsequently resulting in an increasing number of pigs being raised in nonconfinement systems (Kijlstra et al., 2004; Davies, 2011; Jones and Dubey, 2012). Due to exposure to wildlife, these systems will inevitably entail an elevated risk of *Trichinella* infections in pigs (Burke et al., 2008; Ribicich et al., 2009), and outdoor access is also well-known as a risk factor for porcine infection with *T. gondii* (e.g., Gamble et al., 1999; van der Giessen et al., 2007; Garcia-Bocanegra et al., 2010).

At the consumer level, the risk associated with pork varies between countries according to local eating habits and prevalence of foodborne parasitic infections in pigs and wild boar. Cooking practices are changing, with an increase in barbecue cooking, whereby the meat is not necessarily fully cooked (Richomme et al., 2010). In many regions, there is a growing interest in traditional local food specialties and small-scale food production (Lücke and Zangerl, 2014). According to Davies (2011), the consumption of such niche market products versus commercial pork products confers an 80-fold greater risk of infection with *Trichinella* in the United States.

11.6 Conclusions

The pork borne parasites *T. gondii*, *Trichinella* spp., and *T. solium* are widespread and may lead to severe illness. Outbreaks of disease in humans caused by zoonotic parasitic infections transmitted via pork can be effectively controlled by adequate treatment of the meat. It is, however, critical for the industry to continuously secure the "safety" of the meat, for example, by reducing exposure of live animals to parasitic infections. In addition, preventive educational campaigns remain necessary to reduce the risk of transmission of these diseases particularly in regions where the prevalence is high or proper meat inspection is not feasible or not in place, or where consumption of wild boar or home-slaughtered backyard pigs is common practice.

11.7 Sources of further information

For supplementary information about zoonotic parasitic infections transmitted via pork, the following sources may be consulted:

The EFSA is the keystone of European Union (EU) risk assessment regarding food and feed safety including zoonotic parasites. EFSA provides independent scientific advice on existing and emerging risks which is made available to the public via the *EFSA Journal* and scientific reports that can be downloaded from www.efsa.europa.eu.

The International Commission on Trichinellosis (ICT) (www.trichinellosis.org) is an international organization of scientists who are interested in all aspects of *Trichinella* or trichinellosis and provides guidelines and recommendations for the control of *Trichinella*. The ICT is a member of the World Federation of Parasitologists, through which it is affiliated with the International Union of Biological Sciences. The Commission cooperates with national and international organizations, for example, WHO, OIE, and FAO who are concerned with the control of *Trichinella*.

The *OIE Manual of Diagnostic Tests and Vaccines for Terrestrial Animals* contains specific chapters that provide information on various aspects of parasitic diseases of mammals and birds, including methods recommended for detecting infection. Standards and recommendations for the control of specific parasitic diseases are included in OIE Terrestrial Animal Health Code.

Dupouy-Camet, J., Murrell, K.D. (Eds.), 2007. FAO/WHO/OIE Guidelines for the Surveillance, Management, Prevention, and Control of Trichinellosis, p.108. Comprehensive guidelines written by a number of leading scientists with expertise on trichinellosis.

Toxoplasmosis of Animals and Humans by Dubey (2010): a comprehensive text book on the subject, written by a world leading expert on toxoplasmosis.

Guidelines for the Surveillance, Prevention and Control of Taeniosis/Cysticercosis by WHO/FAO/OIE (2005). Comprehensive guidelines written by a number of leading scientists with expertise on cysticercosis.

T. solium Cysticercosis: From Basic to Clinical Science by Pawlowsky (2000). Comprehensive textbook written by a number of leading scientists with expertise on cysticercosis.

References

Abdulmawjood, A., Rosa, S., Taubert, A., Bauer, C., Failing, K., Zahner, H., Bülte, M., 2014. Investigation of persistence of infectious *Toxoplasma gondii* in raw sausages using in-house developed and validated real time-PCR. Meat Sci. 97, 542–547. http://dx.doi.org/10.1016/j.meatsci.2014.03.008.

Ajzenberg, D., Dumètre, A., Dardé, M.L., 2005. Multiplex PCR for typing strains of *Toxoplasma gondii*. J. Clin. Microbiol. 43 (4), 1940–1943.

Al-Adhami, B.H., Gajadhar, A.A., 2014. A new multi-host species indirect ELISA using protein A/G conjugate for detection of anti-*Toxoplasma gondii* IgG antibodies with comparison to ELISA-IgG, agglutination assay and Western blot. Vet. Parasitol. 200 (1–2), 66–73. http://dx.doi.org/10.1016/j.vetpar.2013.11.004.

Alban, L., Boes, J., Kreiner, H., Petersen, J.V., Willeberg, P., 2008. Towards a risk-based surveillance for *Trichinella* spp. in Danish pig production. Prev. Vet. Med. 87, 340–357. http://dx.doi.org/10.1016/j.prevetmed.2008.05.008.

Alban, L., Pozio, E., Boes, B., Boireau, P., Boué, F., Claes, M., Cook, A.J.C., Dorny, P., Enemark, H.L., van der Giessen, J., Hunt, K.R., Howell, M., Kirjusina, M., Nöckler, K., Rossi, P., Smith, G.C., Snow, L., Taylor, M.A., Theodoropoulos, G., Vallée, I., Viera-Pinto, M.M., Zimmer, I.A., 2011. Towards a standardised surveillance for *Trichinella* in the European Union. Prev. Vet. Med. 99, 148–160. http://dx.doi.org/10.1016/j.prevetmed.2011.02.008.

Alvarado-Esquivel, C., García-Machado, C., Alvarado-Esquivel, D., González-Salazar, A.M., Griones-Fraire, C., Vitela-Corrales, J., Villena, I., Dubey, J.P., 2011. Seroprevalence of *Toxoplasma gondii* infection in domestic pigs in Durango State, Mexico. J. Parasitol. 97, 616–619.

Alvardo-Esquivel, C., Alanis-Quiñones, O.P., Arreola-Valenzuela, M.A., Rodríguwz-Briones, A., Piedra-Navarez, L.J., Duran-Morales, E., Estrada-Martínez, S., Mariínez-García, S.A., Liesenfeld, O., 2006. Seroepidemiology of *Toxoplasma gondii* infection in psychiatric inpatients in a northern Mexican city. BMC Infect. Dis. 6, 178. http://dx.doi.org/10.1186/1471-2334.

Anonymous, 2005. Commission regulation (EU) No 2075/2005 laying down specific rules on official controls for *Trichinella* in meat. The EU Commission.

Anonymous, 2012. Multicriteria-based ranking for risk management of foodborne parasites. In: Report of a Joint FAO/WHO Expert Meeting, 3–7 September. FAO Headquarters, Rome, Italy. http://www.fao.org/fileadmin/user_upload/agns/news_events/Parasite%20report%20final%20draft-25October2012.pdf.

Anonymous, 2014a. Livestock and Poultry: World Markets and Trade. Circular Series DL&P, Foreign Agricultural Service, United States Department of Agriculture, April. http://apps.fas.usda.gov/psdonline/circulars/livestock_poultry.pdf.

Anonymous, 2014b. Commission regulation (EU) No216/2014 amending Regulation (EC) No 2075/2005 laying down specific rules on official controls for *Trichinella* in meat.

Anonymous, 2014c. Prescribed Treatment of Pork and Pork Products Containing Pork to Destroy Trichinae. Food Safety and Inspection Service, The United States Department of Agriculture's Code of Federal Regulations (9CFR318.10). http://www.gpo.gov./fdsys/pkg/CFR-2001-title9-vol2/pdf/CFR-2001-title9-vol2-sec318-10.pdf.

Assadi-Rad, A.M., New, J.C., Patton, S., 1995. Risk factors associated with transmission of *Toxoplasma gondii* to sows kept in different management systems in Tennessee. Vet. Parasitol. 57, 289–297.

Bayarri, S., Gracia, M.J., Perez-Arquillue, C., Lazaro, R., Herrera, A., 2012. *Toxoplasma gondii* in commercially available pork meat and cured ham: a contribution to risk assessment for consumers. J. Food Prot. 75, 597–600.

Berger-Schoch, A.E., Bernet, D., Doherr, M.G., Gottstein, B., Frey, C.F., 2011. *Toxoplasma gondii* in Switzerland: a serosurvey based on meat juice analysis of slaughtered pigs, wild boar, sheep and cattle. Zoonoses Public Health 58, 472–478.

Boa, M.E., Kassuku, A.A., Willingham III, A.L., Keyyu, J.D., Phiri, I.K., Nansen, P., 2002. Distribution and density of cysticerci of *Taenia solium* by muscle groups and organs in naturally infected local finished pigs in Tanzania. Vet. Parasitol. 106, 155–164.

Boyer, K., Hill, D., Mui, E., Wroblewski, K., Karrison, T., Dubey, J.P., Sautter, M., Noble, A.G., Withers, S., Swisher, C., Heydemann, P., Hosten, T., Babiarz, J., Lee, D., Meier, P., McLeod, R., Toxoplasmosis Study Group, 2011. Unrecognized ingestion of *Toxoplasma gondii* oocysts leads to congenital toxoplasmosis and causes epidemics in North America. Clin. Infect. Dis. 53, 1081–1089. http://dx.doi.org/10.1093/cid/cir667.

Bruschi, F., Dupouy-Camet, J., Kociecka, W., Pozio, E., Bolas-Fernandez, F., 2002. Opinion on the diagnosis and treatment of human trichinellosis. Expert Opin. Pharmacother. 3, 1117–1130. http://dx.doi.org/10.1517/14656566.3.8.1117.

Burke, R., Masuoka, P., Murell, K.D., 2008. Swine *Trichinella* infection and geographic information system tools. Emerg. Infect. Dis. 14, 1109–1111. http://dx.doi.org/10.3201/eid1407.071538, http://dx.doi.org/10.3201%2Feid1407.071538#pmc_ext.

Capó, V., Despommier, D.D., 1996. Clinical aspects of infection with *Trichinella* spp. Clin. Microbiol. Rev. 9, 47–54.

CDC, 2014. Trichinellosis—Epidemiology and Risk Factors. CDC, Atlanta, GA. http://www.cdc.gov/parasites/trichinellosis/epi.html.

Cenci-Goga, B.T., Rossitto, P.V., Sechi, P., McCrindle, C.M., Cullor, J.S., 2011. *Toxoplasma* in animals, food, and humans: an old parasite of new concern. Foodborne Pathog. Dis. 8, 751–762.

Choi, W.Y., Nam, H.W., Kwak, N.H., Huh, W., Kim, Y.R., Kang, M.W., Cho, S.Y., Dubey, J.P., 1997. Foodborne outbreaks of human toxoplasmosis. J. Infect. Dis. 175, 1280–1282.

Codex, 2014. Proposed Draft Guidelines for the Control of *Trichinella* spp. in Meat of Suidae (At step 5/8). ftp://ftp.fao.org/codex/reports/reports_2014/REP14_FHe.pdf.

Cook, A.J., Gilbert, R.E., Buffolano, W., Zufferey, J., Petersen, E., Jenum, P.A., Foulon, W., Semprini, A.E., Dunn, D.T., 2000. Sources of *Toxoplasma* infection in pregnant women: European multicentre case–control study. European Research Network on Congenital Toxoplasmosis. Br. Med. J. 321 (7254), 142–147.

Cui, J., Wang, Z.Q., Xu, B.L., 2011. The epidemiology of human trichinellosis in China during 2004–2009. Acta Trop. 118 (1), 1–5. http://dx.doi.org/10.1016/j.actatropica.2011.02.005.

Dardé, M.L., 2008. *Toxoplasma gondii*, "new" genotypes and virulence. Parasite 15, 366–371.

Davies, P.R., 2011. Intensive swine production and pork safety. Foodborne Pathog. Dis. 8, 189–201.

de Buhr, K., Ludewig, M., Fehlhaber, K., 2008. *Toxoplasma gondii*-seroprevalence—current results in German swine herds. Arch. Lebensmittelhyg. 59, 5–8.

Deksne, G., Kirjušina, M., 2013. Seroprevalence of *Toxoplasma gondii* in domestic pigs (*Sus scrofa domestica*) and wild boars (*Sus scrofa*) in Latvia. J. Parasitol. 99 (1), 44–47.

Demar, M., Ajzenberg, D., Maubon, D., Djossou, F., Panchoe, F., Punwasi, W., Valery, N., Peneau, C., Daigre, J.L., Aznar, C., Cottrelle, B., Terzan, L., Dardé, M.L., Carme, B., 2007. Fatal outbreak of human toxoplasmosis along Maroni River: epidemiological, clinical and parasitological aspects. Clin. Infect. Dis. 45, e88–e95.

Desmonts, G., Remington, J.S., 1980. Direct agglutination test for diagnosis of *Toxoplasma* infection: method for increasing sensitivity and specificity. J. Clin. Microbiol. 11, 562–568.

Dias, R.A.F., Navarro, I.T., Ruffolo, B.B., Bugni, F.M., de Castro, M.V., Freire, R.L., 2005. *Toxoplasma gondii* in fresh pork sausage and seroprevalence in butchers from factories in Londrina, Parana State Brazil. Rev. Inst. Med. Trop. Sao Paulo 47, 185–189.

Djordjevic, M., Cuperlovic, K., Savic, M., Pavlovic, S., 2005. The need for implementation of International Commission on Trichinellosis recommendations, quality assurance standards, and proficiency sample programs in meat inspection for trichinellosis in Serbia. Vet. Parasitol. 132, 185–188.

Djurković-Djaković, O., Milenkovic, V., 2000. Effect of refrigeration and freezing on survival of *Toxoplasma gondii* tissue cysts. Acta Vet. (Beograd) 50, 375–380.

Djurković-Djaković, O., Bobić, B., Nikolić, A., Klun, I., Dupouy-Camet, J., 2013. Pork as a source of human parasitic infection. Clin. Microbiol. Infect. 19, 586–594. http://dx.doi.org/10.1111/1469.12162.

Doherty, T., Johansen, M.V., 2013. Cysticercosis. In: Mabey, D., Gill, G., Parry, E., Weber, M.W., Whitty, C.J.M. (Eds.), Principles of Medicine in Africa. Cambridge University Press, Cambridge, pp. 466–467.

Dorny, P., Phiri, I.K., Vercruysse, J., Gabriel, S., Willingham III, A.L., Brandt, J., Victor, B., Speybroeck, N., Berkvens, D., 2004. A Bayesian approach for estimating values for prevalence and diagnostic test characteristics of porcine cysticercosis. Int. J. Parasitol. 34, 569–576. http://dx.doi.org/10.1016/j.ijpara.2003.11.014.

Dubey, J.P., 1988. Long-term persistence of *Toxoplasma gondii* in tissues of pigs inoculated with *T. gondii* oocysts and effect of freezing on viability of tissue cysts in pork. Am. J. Vet. Res. 49, 910–913.

Dubey, J.P., 1997. Survival of *Toxoplasma gondii* tissue cysts in 0.85%–6% NaCl solutions at 4–20°C. J. Parasitol. 83, 946–949.

Dubey, J.P., 2004. Toxoplasmosis—a waterborne zoonosis. Vet. Parasitol. 126, 57–72.

Dubey, J.P., 2009. Toxoplasmosis in pigs—the last 20 years. Vet. Parasitol. 164 (2–4), 89–103.

Dubey, J.P., 2010. Toxoplasmosis of Animals and Humans. CRC Press, Boca Raton, FL, p. 313.

Dubey, J.P., Brake, R.J., Murell, K.D., Fayer, R., 1986a. Effect of irradiation on the viability of *Toxoplasma gondii* in tissues of mice and pigs. Am. J. Vet. Res. 47, 518–522.

Dubey, J.P., Murrell, K.D., Fayer, R., Schad, G.A., 1986b. Distribution of *Toxoplasma gondii* tissue cysts in commercial cuts of pork. J. Am. Vet. Med. Assoc. 188, 1035–1037.

Dubey, J.P., Kotula, A.W., Sharar, A., Andrews, C.D., Lindsay, D.S., 1990. Effect of high-temperature on infectivity of *Toxoplasma gondii* tissue cysts in pork. J. Parasitol. 76, 201–204. http://dx.doi.org/10.2307/3283016.

Dubey, J.P., Hill, D.E., Jones, J.L., Hightower, A.W., Kirkland, E., Roberts, J.M., Marcet, P.L., Lehmann, T., Vianna, M.C., Miska, K., Sreekumar, C., Kwok, O.C., Shen, S.K., Gamble, H.R., 2005. Prevalence of *Toxoplasma gondii* in beef, chicken, and pork from retail meat stores in the United States: risk assessment to consumers. J. Parasitol. 91, 1082–1093.

Dubey, J.P., Hill, D.E., Sundar, N., Velmurugan, G.V., Bandini, L.A., Kwok, O.C.H., Pierce, V., Kelly, K., Dulin, M., Thulliez, P., Iwueke, C., Su, C., 2008. Endemic toxoplasmosis in pigs on a farm in Maryland: isolation and genetic characterization on *Toxoplasma gondii*. J. Parasitol. 94, 36–41.

Dubey, J.P., Hotea, I., Olariu, T.R., Jones, J.L., Dărăbuş, G., 2014. Epidemiological review of toxoplasmosis in humans and animals in Romania. Parasitology 141, 311–325.

Dupouy-Camet, J., Bruschi, B., 2007. Management and diagnosis of human trichinellosis. In: Dupouy-Camet, J., Murrell, K.D. (Eds.), FAO/WHO/OIE Guidelines for the Surveillance, Management, Prevention and Control of Trichinellosis. Office International des Epizooties, Paris 108 978-92-9044-704-7.

Dupouy-Camet, J., Murrell, K.D., 2007. FAO/WHO/OIE Guidelines for the Surveillance, Management, Prevention and Control of Trichinellosis. Office International des Epizooties, Paris, 108 pp.

EFSA Panels on Biological Hazards (BIOHAZ), on Contaminants in the Food Chain (CONTAM), and on Animal Health and Welfare (AHAW), 2011. Scientific opinion on the public health hazards to be covered by inspection of meat (swine). EFSA J. 9 (10), 2351. http://dx.doi.org/10.2903/j.efsa.2011.2351, 198 pp.

EFSA, European Food Safety Authority, 2007. Scientific opinion of the panel on biological hazards on a request from EFSA on surveillance and monitoring of *Toxoplasma* in humans, food and animals. EFSA J. 583, 1–64. http://dx.doi.org/10.2903/j.efsa.2007.583.

EFSA, European Food Safety Authority, 2011a. Scientific opinion on the public health hazards to be covered by inspection of meat (swine). EFSA J. 9 (10), 2351. http://www.efsa.europa.eu/en/efsajournal/doc/2351.pdf.

EFSA, European Food Safety Authority, 2011b. Technical specifications on harmonised epidemiological indicators for public health hazards to be covered by meat inspection of swine. EFSA J. 9 (10), 2371. http://www.efsa.europa.eu/en/efsajournal/doc/2371.pdf.

EFSA, European Food Safety Authority, 2013a. The European Union summary report on trends and sources of zoonoses, zoonotic agents and food-borne outbreaks in 2011. EFSA J. 11 (4), 3129. http://www.efsa.europa.eu/en/efsajournal/doc/3129.pdf.

EFSA, European Food Safety Authority, 2013b. Technical specifications on harmonised epidemiological indicators for biological hazards to be covered by meat inspection of farmed game. EFSA J. 11 (6), 3267. http://dx.doi.org/10.2903/j.efsa.2013.3267, 60pp.

Flegr, J., 2013. Influence of latent *Toxoplasma* infection on human personality, physiology and morphology: pros and cons of the *Toxoplasma*-human model in studying the manipulation hypothesis. J. Exp. Biol. 216 (Pt 1), 127–133.

Flisser, A., 1994. Taeniasis and cysticercosis due to *T. solium*. In: Sun, T. (Ed.), Progress in Clinical Parasitology. CRC Press Inc., Florida, pp. 77–116. http://dx.doi.org/10.1242/jeb.073635.

Forbes, L.B., Gajadhar, A.A., 1999. A validated *Trichinella* digestion assay and an associated sampling and quality assurance system for use in testing pork and horse meat. J. Food Prot. 62 (11), 1308–1313.

Gamble, H.R., Brady, R.C., Dubey, J.P., 1999. Prevalence of *Toxoplasma gondii* infection in domestic pigs in the New England states. Vet. Parasitol. 82, 129–136.

Gamble, H.R., Bessonov, A.S., Cuperlovic, K., Gajadhar, A.A., van Knapen, F., Noeckler, K., Schenone, H., Zhu, X., 2000. International Commission on Trichinellosis: recommendations on methods for the control of *Trichinella* in domestic and wild animals intended for human consumption. Vet. Parasitol. 93, 393–408.

Garcia-Bocanegra, I., Dubey, J.P., Simon-Grife, M., Cabezon, O., Casal, J., Allepuz, A., Napp, S., Almeria, S., 2010. Seroprevalence and risk factors associated with *Toxoplasma gondii* infection in pig farms from Catalonia, north-eastern Spain. Res. Vet. Sci. 89, 85–87.

Gauss, C.B., Dubey, J.P., Vidal, D., Ruiz, F., Vicente, J., Marco, I., Lavin, S., Gortazar, C., Almeria, S., 2005. Seroprevalence of *Toxoplasma gondii* in wild pigs (*Sus scrofa*) from Spain. Vet. Parasitol. 131, 151–156.

González, L.M., Bailo, B., Ferrer, E., Fernandez, G., Harrison, L.J.S., Parkhouse, M.R.E., McManus, D.P., Gárate, T., 2010. Characterization of the *Taenia* spp. HDP2 sequence and development of a novel PCR-based assay for discrimination of *Taenia saginata* from *Taenia asiatica*. Parasit. Vectors 3, 51.

Gottstein, B., Pozio, E., Nöckler, K., 2009. Epidemiology, diagnosis, treatment and control of trichinellosis. Clin. Microbiol. Rev. 22 (1), 127–145. http://dx.doi.org/10.1128/CMR.00026-08.

Groβklaus, D., Baumgarten, H.J., 1967. Die Überlebensdauer von *Toxoplasma*-Cysten in Schweinfleisch. Fleischwirtschaft 47, 1372–1374.

Groβklaus, D., Baumgarten, H.J., 1968. Die Überlebensdauer von *Toxoplasma*-Cysten in Schweinfleisch. Fleischwirtschaft 48, 930–932.

Herenda, D., 2000. Manual on Meat Inspection for Developing Countries. Food and Agriculture Organization of the United Nations, Rome. http://www.fao.org/docrep/003/t0756e/t0756e00.HTM.

Hill, D.E., Sreekumar, C., Gamble, H.R., Dubey, J.P., 2004. Effect of commonly used enhancement solutions on the viability of *Toxoplasma gondii* tissue cysts in pork loin. J. Food Prot. 67, 2230–2233.

Hill, A.E., Benedetto, S.M.C., Coss, C., McCrary, J.L., Fournet, V.M., Dubey, J.P., 2006. Effects of time and temperature on the viability of *Toxoplasma gondii* tissue cysts in enhanced pork loin. J. Food Prot. 69, 1961–1965.

Hill, D., Coss, C., Dubey, J.P., Wroblewski, K., Sautter, M., Hosten, T., Muñoz-Zanzi, C., Mui, E., Withers, S., Boyer, K., Hermes, G., Coyne, J., Jagdis, F., Burnett, A., McLeod, P., Morton, H., Robinson, D., McLeod, R., 2011. Identification of a sporozoite-specific antigen from *Toxoplasma gondii*. J. Parasitol. 97, 328–337. http://dx.doi.org/10.1645/GE-2782.1.

Howe, D.K., Sibley, L.D., 1995. *Toxoplasma gondii* comprises three clonal lineages: correlation of parasite genotype with human disease. J. Infect. Dis. 172, 1561–1566.

ICT, International Commission on Trichinellosis, 2006. Recommendations on Methods for the Control of *Trichinella* in Domestic and Wild Animals Intended for Human Consumption. International Commission on Trichinellosis. 22 pp. http://www.trichinellosis.org/uploads/ICT_Recommendations_for_Control_English.pdf.

Jones, J.L., Dubey, J.P., 2012. Foodborne toxoplasmosis. Clin. Infect. Dis. 55 (6), 845–851.

Jones, J.L., Kruszon-Moran, D., Wilson, M., McQuillan, G., Navin, T., McAuley, J.B., 2001. *Toxoplasma gondii* infection in the United States: seroprevalence and risk factors. Am. J. Epidemiol. 154, 357–365.

Jones, J.L., Kruszon-Moran, D., Sanders-Lewis, K., Wilson, M., 2007. *Toxoplasma gondii* infection in the United States, 1999–2004, decline from the prior decade. Am. J. Trop. Med. Hyg. 77 (3), 405–410.

Jones, J.L., Dargelas, V., Roberts, J., Press, C., Remington, J.S., Montoya, J.G., 2009. Risk factors for *Toxoplasma gondii* infection in the United States. Clin. Infect. Dis. 49, 878–884.

Juránková, J., Basso, W., Neumayerová, H., Baláž, V., Jánová, E., Sidler, X., Deplazes, P., Koudela, B., 2014a. Brain is the predilection site of *Toxoplasma gondii* in experimentally inoculated pigs as revealed by magnetic capture and real-time PCR. Food Microbiol. 38, 167–170.

Juránková, J., Hurková-Hofmannová, L., Volf, J., Piálek, J., 2014b. Efficacy of magnetic capture in comparison with conventional DNA isolation in a survey of *Toxoplasma gondii* in wild house mice. Eur. J. Protistol. 50 (1), 11–15. http://dx.doi.org/10.1016/j.ejop.2013.08.002.

Kaewpitoon, N., Kaewpitoon, S.J., Pengsaa, P., 2008. Food-borne parasitic zoonosis: distribution of trichinosis in Thailand. World J. Gastroenterol. 14 (22), 3471–3475. http://dx.doi.org/10.3748/wjg.14.3471, http://dx.doi.org/10.3748%2Fwjg.14.3471#pmc_ext.

Kapel, C.M.O., 2001. Sylvatic and domestic *Trichinella* spp. in wild boars: infectivity, muscle larvae distribution, and antibody response. J. Parasitol. 87 (2), 309–314. http://dx.doi.org/10.1645/0022-3395(2001)087[0309:SADTSI]2.0.CO;2, http://dx.doi.org/10.1645/0022-3395(2001)087%5b0309:SADTSI%5d2.0.CO;2.

Kapperud, G., Jenum, P.A., Stray-Pedersen, B., Melby, K.K., Eskild, A., Eng, J., 1996. Risk factors for *Toxoplasma gondii* infection in pregnancy. Results of a prospective case-control study in Norway. Am. J. Epidemiol. 144, 405–412.

Khan, A., Jordan, C., Muccioli, C., Vallochi, A.L., Rizzo, L.V., Belfort, R., Vitor Jr., R.W., Sibley, L.D., 2006. Genetic divergence of *Toxoplasma gondii* strains associated with ocular toxoplasmosis, Brazil. Emerg. Infect. Dis. 12, 942–949.

Kijlstra, A., Jongert, E., 2008. Control of the risk of human toxoplasmosis transmitted by meat. Int. J. Parasitol. 38, 1359–1370. http://dx.doi.org/10.1016/j.ijpara.2008.06.002.

Kijlstra, A., Eissen, O.A., Cornelissen, J., Munniksma, K., Eijck, I., Kortbeek, T., 2004. *Toxoplasma gondii* infection in animal-friendly pig production systems. Invest. Ophthalmol. Vis. Sci. 45, 3165–3169.

Kim, G., Choi, M.-H., Kim, J.-H., Kang, Y.M., Jeon, H.J., Jung, Y., Lee, M.J., Oh, M.-D., 2011. An outbreak of trichinellosis with detection of *Trichinella* larvae in leftover wild boar meat. J. Korean Med. Sci. 26 (12), 1630–1633. http://dx.doi.org/10.3346/jkms.2011.26.12.1630, http://dx.doi.org/10.3346%2Fjkms.2011.26.12.1630#pmc_ext.

Kotula, A.W., Murrell, K.D., Acosta-Stein, L., Tennent, I., 1982. Influence of rapid cooking methods on the survival of *Trichinella spiralis* in pork chops from experimentally infected pigs. J. Food Sci. 47, 1006–1007. http://dx.doi.org/10.1111/j.1365-2621.1982.tb12765.x.

Kotula, A.W., Dubey, J.P., Sharar, A.K., Andrews, C.D., Shen, S.K., Lindsay, D.S., 1991. Effect of freezing on infectivity of *Toxoplasma gondii* tissue cysts in pork. J. Food Prot. 54, 587–690.

Kuticic, V., Wikerhauser, T., 1996. Studies of the effect of various treatments on the viability of *Toxoplasma gondii* tissue cysts and oocysts. Curr. Top. Microbiol. Immunol. 219, 261–265.

Lehmann, T., Graham, D.H., Dahl, E., Sreekumar, C., Launer, F., Corn, J.L., Gamble, H.R., Dubey, J.P., 2003. Transmission dynamics of *Toxoplasma gondii* on a pig farm. Infect. Genet. Evol. 3 (2), 135–141.

Lind, P., Buxton, D., 2000. Veterinary aspects of *Toxoplasma* infection. In: Ambroise-Thomas, P., Petersen, E. (Eds.), Congenital Toxoplasmosis; Scientific Background, Clinical Management and Control. Springer, Paris, France, pp. 261–269.

Lindsay, D.S., Collins, M.V., Holliman, D., Dubey, J.P., 2006. Effects of high-pressure processing on *Toxoplasma gondii* tissue cysts in ground pork. J. Parasitol. 92, 195–196.

Lopes, A.P., Sargo, R., Rodrigues, M., Cardoso, L., 2011. High seroprevalence of antibodies to *Toxoplasma gondii* in wild animals from Portugal. Parasitol. Res. 108, 1163–1169.

Lücke, F., Zangerl, P., 2014. Food safety challenges associated with traditional foods in German-speaking regions. Food Control 42, 217–230. http://dx.doi.org/10.1016/j.foodcont.2014.03.014.

Lunden, A., Uggla, A., 1992. Infectivity of *Toxoplasma gondii* in mutton following curing, smoking, freezing or microwave cooking. Int. J. Food Microbiol. 15, 357–363.

Malakauskas, A., Paulauskas, V., Järvis, T., Keidans, P., Eddi, C., Kapel, C.M.O., 2007. Molecular epidemiology of *Trichinella* spp. in three Baltic countries: Lithuania, Latvia, and Estonia. Parasitol. Res. 100, 687–693. http://dx.doi.org/10.1016/j.ijpara.2008.06.006.

Marti, H.P., Murrell, K.D., Gamble, H.R., 1987. *Trichinella spiralis*: immunization of pigs with newborn larval antigens. Exp. Parasitol. 63, 68–73.

McCurdy, S.M., Takeuchi, M.T., Edwards, Z.M., Edlefsen, M., Kang, D.H., Mayes, V.E., Hillers, V.N., 2006. Food safety education initiative to increase consumer use of food thermometers in the United States. Br. Food J. 108, 775–794.

Meemken, D., Blaha, T., 2011. "Meat juice multi-serology" – a tool for the continuous improvement of herd health and food safety in the framework of the risk based meat inspection of slaughter pigs. J. Food Saf. Food Qual. 62, 192–199.

Meemken, D., Tangeman, A.H., Meermeier, D., Gundlach, S., Mischok, D., Geriner, M., Blaha, T., 2014. Establishment of serological herd profiles for zoonoses and production diseases in pigs by "meat juice multi-serology". Prev. Vet. Med. 113 (4), 589–598. http://dx.doi.org/10.1016/j.prevetmed.2013.12.006.

Meersburg, B.G., van Riel, J.W., Cornelissen, J.B., Kijlstra, A., Mul, M.F., 2006. Cats and goat whey associated with *Toxoplasma gondii* infection in pigs. Vector Borne Zoonotic Dis. 6, 266–274.

Mkupasi, E.M., Ngowi, H.A., Sikasunge, C.S., Leifsson, P.S., Johansen, M.V., 2014. Distribution and histopathological changes induced bv cysts of *Taenia solium* the brain of pigs from Tanzania. J. Helminthol. 6, 1–6. http://dx.doi.org/10.1017/S0022149X1400042X.

Moncada, P.A., Montoya, J.G., 2012. Toxoplasmosis in the fetus and newborn: an update on prevalence, diagnosis and treatment. Expert Rev. Anti Infect. Ther. 10 (7), 815–828.

Montoya, J.G., Liesenfeld, O., 2004. Toxoplasmosis. Lancet 363, 1965–1976.

Morales, J., Martínez, J.J., Rosetti, M., Fleury, A., Maza, V., Hernandez, M., Villalobos, N., Fragoso, G., de Aluja, A.S., Larralde, C., Sciutto, E., 2008. Spatial distribution of *Taenia solium* porcine cysticercosis within a rural area of Mexico. PLoS Negl. Trop. Dis. 2, e284. http://dx.doi.org/10.1371/journal.pntd. 0000284.

Mukaratirwa, S., La Grange, L., Pfukenyi, D.M., 2013. *Trichinella* infections in animals and humans in sub-Saharan Africa: a review. Acta Trop. 125, 82–89. http://dx.doi.org/10.1016/j.actatropica.2012.09.005.

Munday, B.L., Corbould, A., 1971. The application of the *Toxoplasma* indirect fluorescent-antibody test to sheep sera. Aust. J. Med. Technol. 2, 3–6.

Murrell, K.D., 2005. Epidemiology of taeniosis and cysticercosis. In: Murell, K.D. (Ed.), FAO/WHO/OIE Guidelines for the Surveillance, Prevention and Control of Taeniosis/Cysticercosis. OIE, Paris, pp. 27–34.

Murrell, K.D., 2013. Zoonotic foodborne parasites and their surveillance. Rev. Sci. Tech. 32, 559–569.

Ndimubanzi, P.C., Carabin, H., Budke, C.M., Nguyen, H., Qian, Y.J., Rainwater, E., Dickey, M., Reynolds, S., Stoner, J.A., 2010. A systematic review of the frequency of neurocysticercosis with a focus on people with epilepsy. PLoS Negl. Trop. Dis. 4 (11), e870. http://dx.doi.org/10.1371/journal.pntd.0000870.

Neumayerová, H., Juránková, J., Saláková, A., Gallas, L., Kovařčík, K., Koudela, B., 2014. Survival of experimentally induced *Toxoplasma gondii* tissue cysts in vacuum packed goat meat and dry fermented goat meat sausages. Food Microbiol. 39, 47–52. http://dx.doi.org/10.1016/j.fm.2013.11.001.

Newell, D.G., Koopmans, M., Verhoef, L., Duizer, E., Aidara-Kane, A., Sprong, H., Opsteegh, M., Langelaar, M., Threfall, J., Scheutz, F., van der Giessen, J., Kruse, H., 2010. Food-borne diseases – the challenges of 20 years ago still persist while now ones continue to emerge. Int. J. Food Microbiol. 139, S3–S15. http://dx.doi.org/10.1016/j.ijfoodmicro.2010.01.021.

Nöckler, K., Reckinger, S., Pozio, E., 2006. *Trichinella spiralis* and *Trichinella pseudospiralis* mixed infection in a wild boar (*Sus scrofa*) of Germany. Vet. Parasitol. 137, 364–368. http://dx.doi.org/10.1016/j.vetpar.2006.01.031.

OIE, World Organization for Animal Health, 2008. Toxoplasmosis. In: Manual of Diagnostic Tests and Vaccines for Terrestrial Animals 2013, eighth ed., pp. 1284–1293 (Chapter 2.9.10).

OIE, World Organization for Animal Health, 2013. Infection with *Trichinella* species. In: Terrestrial Animal Health Code (Chapter 8.14). http://www.oie.int/index.php?id=169&L=0&htmfile=chapitre_1.8.14.htm.

Opsteegh, M., Langelaar, M., Spong, H., den Hartog, L., De Craeye, S., Bokken, G., Ajzenberg, D., Kijlstra, A., van der Giessen, J., 2010. Direct detection and genotyping of *Toxoplasma gondii* in meat samples using magnetic capture and PCR. Int. J. Food Microbiol. 139, 193–201.

Ortega-Pierres, M.G., Arriaga, C., Yépez-Mulia, L., 2000. Epidemiology of trichinellosis in Mexico, Central and South America. Vet. Parasitol. 93 (3–4), 201–225.

Pal, D.K., Carpio, A., Sander, J.W.A.S., 2000. Neurocysticercosis and epilepsy in developing countries. J. Neurol. Neurosurg. Psychiatry 68, 137–143. http://dx.doi.org/10.1136/jnnp.68.2.137.

Pappas, G., Roussos, N., Falagas, M.E., 2009. Toxoplasmosis snapshot: global status of *Toxoplasma gondii* seroprevalence and implications for pregnancy and congenital toxoplasmosis. Int. J. Parasitol. 39 (12), 1385–1394.

Patton, S., Zimmerman, J., Roberts, T., Faulkner, C., Diderrich, V., Assadi-Rad, A., Davies, P., Kliebenstein, J., 1996. Seroprevalence of *Toxoplasma gondii* in hogs in the National Animal Health Monitoring System (NAHMS). J. Eukaryot. Microbiol. 43, 121S.

Patton, S., Faulkner, C., Anderson, A., Smedley, K., Bush, E., 2002. *Toxoplasma gondii* infection in sows and market weight pigs in the United States and its potential impact on consumer demand for pork. National Pork Board report. http://www.pork.org/PorkScience/Documents/00-130%20-Patton-UofTenn.pdf.

Pawlowski, Z., Allan, J., Sarti, E., 2005. Control of *Taenia solium* taeniasis/cysticercosis: from research towards implementation. Int. J. Parasitol. 35, 1221–1232. http://dx.doi.org/10.1016/j.ijpara.2005.07.015.

Pawlowsky, Z.S., 2000. Basic biology and transmission. In: Singh, G., Prabhakar, S. (Eds.), *Taenia solium* Cysticercosis: From Basic to Clinical Science. CABI, Wallingford, UK, pp. 1–13. http://dx.doi.org/10.1079/9780851996288.0000, http://dx.doi.org/10.1079/9780851996288.0000#_blank.

Petri, W.A., Holsinger, J.R., Pearson, R.D., 1988. Common-source outbreak of trichinosis associated with eating raw home-butchered pork. South. Med. J. 81 (8), 1056–1058. http://dx.doi.org/10.1097/00007611-198808000-00029.

Phiri, I.K., Dorny, P., Gabriel, S., Willingham III, A.L., Speybroeck, N., Vercruysse, J., 2002. The prevalence of porcine cysticercosis in Eastern and Southern provinces of Zambia. Vet. Parasitol. 108, 31–39.

Porto-Fett, A.C., Call, J.E., Shoyer, B.E., Hill, D.E., Pshebniski, C., Cocoma, G.J., Luchansky, J.B., 2010. Evaluation of fermentation, drying, and/or high pressure processing on viability of *Listeria monocytogenes*, *Escherichia coli* O157:H7, *Salmonella* spp., and *Trichinella spiralis* in raw pork and Genoa salami. Int. J. Food Microbiol. 140 (1), 61–75. http://dx.doi.org/10.1016/j.ijfoodmicro.2010.02.008.

Pott, S., Koethe, M., Bangoura, B., Zöller, B., Daugschies, A., Straubinger, R.K., Fehlhaber, K., Ludewig, M., 2013. Effects of pH, sodium chloride, and curing salt on the infectivity of *Toxoplasma gondii* tissue cysts. J. Food Prot. 76 (6), 1056–1061.

Pozio, E., 2007. Taxonomy, biology and epidemiology of *Trichinella* parasites. In: Dupouy-Camet, J., Murrell, K.D. (Eds.), FAO/WHO/OIE Guidelines for the Surveillance, Management. Prevention and Control of Trichinellosis. OIE, Paris, France, pp. 1–32.

Pozio, E., Murrell, K.D., 2006. Systematics and epidemiology of *Trichinella*. Adv. Parasitol. 63, 367–439. http://dx.doi.org/10.1016/S0065-308X(06)63005-4.

Pozio, E., Kapel, C.M.O., Gajadhar, A.A., Boireau, P., Dupouy-Camet, J., Gamble, H.R., 2006. *Trichinella* in pork: current knowledge on the suitability of freezing as a public health measure. Euro Surveill. 11, E061116.1.

Pozio, E., Rinaldi, L., Marucci, G., Musella, V., Galati, F., Cringoli, G., Boireau, P., La Rosa, G., 2009. Hosts and habitat of *Trichinella spiralis* and *Trichinella britovi* in Europe. Int. J. Parasitol. 39, 71–79. http://dx.doi.org/10.1016/j.ijpara.2008.06.006.

Prasad, K., Chawla, S., Prasad, A., Tripathi, M., Husain, N., Gunta, R., 2006. Clinical signs for identification of neurocysticercosis in swine naturally infected with *Taenia solium*. Parasitol. Int. 55, 151–154.

Ribicich, M., Miguez, M., Argibay, T., Basso, N., Franco, A., 2001. Localization of *Trichinella spiralis* in muscles of commercial and parasitologic interest in pig meat. Parasite 8, 246–248.

Ribicich, M., Gamble, H.R., Bolpe, J., Sommerfelt, I., Cardillo, N., Scialfa, E., Gimenez, R., Pasqualetti, M., Pascual, G., Franco, A., Rosa, A., 2009. Evaluation of the risk of transmission of *Trichinella* in pork production systems in Argentina. Vet. Parasitol. 159, 350–353.

Richomme, C., Lacour, S.A., Ducrot, C., Gilot-Fromont, E., Casabianca, F., Maestrini, O., Vallée, I., Grasset, A., van der Giessen, J., Boireau, P., 2010. Epidemiological survey of trichinellosis in wild boar (*Sus scrofa*) and fox (*Vulpes vulpes*) in a French insular region, Corsica. Vet. Parasitol. 172, 150–154. http://dx.doi.org/10.1016/j.vetpar.2010.04.026.

Robert-Gangneux, F., Darde, M.L., 2012. Epidemiology of and diagnostic strategies for toxoplasmosis. Clin. Microbiol. Rev. 25, 264–296.

Robertson, L.J., Sprong, H., Ortega, Y.R., van der Giessen, J.W.B., Fayer, R., 2014. Impacts of globalization on foodborne parasites. Trends Parasitol. 30, 37–52. http://dx.doi.org/10.1016/j.pt.2013.09.005.

Rodriguez-Hidalgo, R., Geysen, D., Benítez-Ortiz, W., Geerts, S., Brandt, J., 2002. Comparison of conventional techniques to differentiate between *Taenia solium* and *Taenia saginata* and an improved polymerase chain reaction-restriction fragment length polymorphism assay using a mitochondrial 12s rDNA fragment. J. Parasitol. 88, 1007–1011. http://dx.doi.org/10.1645/0022-3395(2002)088[1007:COCTTD]2.0.CO;2.

Scallan, E., Hoekstra, R.M., Angulo, F.J., Tauxe, R.V., Widdowson, M.A., Roy, S.L., Jones, J.L., Griffin, P.M., 2011. Foodborne illness acquired in the United States. Major pathogens. Emerg. Infect. Dis. 17, 7–15. http://dx.doi.org/10.3201/eid1701.P11101.

Schlundt, J., Toyofoku, H., Jansen, J., Herbst, S.A., 2004. Emerging food-borne zoonoses. Rev. Sci. Tech. 23, 513–533.

Schulzig, H.S., Fehlhaber, K., 2006. Seroprevalence of *Toxoplasma gondii* in conventionally and organically produced pork and pork-products. Fleischwirtschaft 86 (12), 106–108.

Scupin, E., 1968. Weitere Untersuchungen der überlebensmöglichkeiten von *Toxoplasma* in Schinken. Arch. Lebensmittelhyg. 12, 11–13.

Sikasunge, C.S., Johansen, M.V., Willingham III, A.L., Leifsson, P.S., Phiri, I.K., 2008. *Taenia solium* cysticercosis in pigs: viability of cysticerci and persistency of antibodies and cysticercal antigens after treatment with Oxfendazole. Vet. Parasitol. 158, 57–66. http://dx.doi.org/10.1016/j.vetpar.2008.08.014.

Sobanski, V., Ajzenberg, D., Delhaes, L., Bautin, N., Just, N., 2013. Severe toxoplasmosis in immunocompetent hosts: be aware of atypical strains. Am. J. Respir. Crit. Care Med. 187 (10), 1143–1145.

Sommer, R., Rommel, M., Levetzow, R., 1965. Die Überlebensdauer von Toxoplasmazysten in fleisch und Fleischzubereitungen. Fleischwirtschaft 45, 454–457.

Sotelo, J., Rosas, N., Palencia, G., 1986. Freezing of infested pork muscle kills cysticerci. JAMA 256, 893–894. http://dx.doi.org/10.1001/jama.1986.03380070099027.

Soulsby, E.J.L., 1982. Helminths, Arthropods and Protozoa of Domesticated Animals. Bailliere Tindall, London, pp. 50–59.

Sroka, J., Wojcik-Fatla, A., Dutkiewicz, J., 2006. Occurrence of *Toxoplasma gondii* in water from wells located on farms. Ann. Agric. Environ. Med. 13, 169–175.

Su, C., Zang, X., Dubey, J.P., 2006. Genotyping of *Toxoplasma gondii* by multilocus PCR-RFLP markers: a high resolution and simple method for identification of parasites. Int. J. Parasitol. 36, 841–848.

Széll, Z., Marucci, G., Bajmóczy, E., Cséplo, A., Pozio, E., Sréter, T., 2008. Spatial distribution of *Trichinella britovi*, *T. pseudospiralis* and *T. spiralis* in red foxes (*Vulpes vulpes*) in Hungary. Vet. Parasitol. 156, 210–215. http://dx.doi.org/10.1016/j.vetpar.2008.06.014.

Tenter, A.M., Heckeroth, A.R., Weiss, L.M., 2000. *Toxoplasma gondii*: from animals to humans. Int. J. Parasitol. 30, 1217–1258.

Teunis, P.F., Koningstein, M., Takumi, K., van der Giessen, J.W., 2012. Human beings are highly susceptible to low doses of *Trichinella* spp. Epidemiol. Infect. 140, 201–218. http://dx.doi.org/10.1017/S0950268811000380, http://dx.doi.org/10.1017/S0950268811000380#_blank.

Torgerson, P.R., Macpherson, C.N.L., 2011. The socioeconomic burden of parasitic zoonoses: global trends. Vet. Parasitol. 182, 79–95.

Torrey, E.F., Yolken, R.H., 2003. *Toxoplasma gondii* and schizophrenia. Emerg. Infect. Dis. 9, 1375–1380.

van der Giessen, J., Fonville, M., Bouwknegt, M., Langelaar, M., Vollema, A., 2007. Seroprevalence of *Trichinella spiralis* and *Toxoplasma gondii* in pigs from different housing systems in The Netherlands. Vet. Parasitol. 148, 371–374. http://dx.doi.org/10.1016/j.vetpar.2007.06.009.

Villena, I., Ancelle, T., Delmas, C., Garcia, P., Brezin, A.P., Thulliez, P., Wallon, M., King, L., Goulet, V., 2010. Toxosurv network and National Reference Centre for Toxoplasmosis, Congenital toxoplasmosis in France in 2007: first results from a national surveillance system. Euro Surveill. 15 (25), 19600.

Vitale, M., Tumino, G., Partanna, S., La Chiusa, S., Mancuso, G., La Giglia, M., Presti, V.D., 2014. Impact of traditional practices on food safety: a case of acute toxoplasmosis related to the consumption of contaminated raw pork sausage in Italy. J. Food Prot. 77 (4), 643–646. http://dx.doi.org/10.4315/0362-028X.JFP-13-285.

Voller, A., Bidwell, D.E., Bartlett, A., Fleck, D.G., Perkins, M., Oladehin, B., 1976. A microplate enzyme-immunoassay for toxoplasma antibody. J. Clin. Pathol. 29, 150–153.

von Köller, J., Kapel, C.M.O., Enemark, H.L., Hindsbo, O., 2001. Infectivity of *Trichinella* spp. recovered from decaying mouse and fox muscle tissue. Parasite 8, S209–S2012.

WHO, 2010. Working to overcome the global impact of neglected tropical diseases. First WHO report on neglected tropical diseases. France. http://whqlibdoc.who.int/publications/2010/9789241564090_eng.pdf?ua=1.

WHO, 2011. Neglected zoonotic diseases: an open-ended list. In: The Control of Neglected Zoonotic Diseases: Community Based Interventions for NZDs Prevention and Control. Report of the Third Conference Organized with ICONZ, DFID-RiU, SOS, EU, TDR and FAO with the Participation of ILRI and OIE, 23–24 November 2010. WHO Headquarters, Geneva, Switzerland, pp. 5–10.

WHO/FAO/OIE, 2005. Guidelines for the Surveillance, Prevention and Control of Taeniosis/Cysticercosis. World Organisation for Animal Health, Paris. http://www.oie.int/doc/ged/d11245.pdf.

Yamasaki, H., Allan, J.C., Sato, M.O., Nakao, M., Sako, Y., Nakaya, K., Qiu, D., Mamuti, W., Craig, P.S., Ito, A., 2004. DNA differential diagnosis of taeniasis and cysticercosis by multiplex PCR. J. Clin. Microbiol. 42, 548–553.

Transmission dynamics of foodborne parasites in fish and shellfish

12

S.R.M. Jones
Pacific Biological Station, Nanaimo, BC, Canada

12.1 Introduction

Finfish, crustaceans, and molluscs (i.e., seafood) belonging to freshwater or marine species are known to host parasites with zoonotic potential (Butt et al., 2004; Dorny et al., 2009). There is evidence that some of these infections have been endemic for millennia (Wu et al., 1996), and, based on contemporary accounts, the same or related parasite species are still involved, with similar life cycles and definitive and intermediate hosts. The longevity of these host–parasite associations reflects one of the greatest challenges in the development of control strategies; that is, many have survived because of cultural practices combined with poverty and ignorance that are entrenched in endemic regions, often despite the availability of contemporary parasitological and epidemiological knowledge. This cultural inertia combined with limited awareness and funding hampers the implementation of mitigation and risk-avoidance strategies. Given that we have known about these infections and the associated risks for a long time, a thoughtful reader might enquire as to the rationale for another review of this subject. The timeliness of this chapter reflects a number of recent trends that influence the risk of parasite transmission and exposure and which support a growing consensus of foodborne parasites in seafood as a reemerging global health risk. More generally, Broglia and Kapel (2011) cite changing eating habits, including an increased preference for exotic, fresh, or raw foods; population growth and movement; increased global trade in food; improved awareness of food safety and disease surveillance; and incipient patterns of changing climate as contributors to the reemergence of foodborne parasitoses. More specifically, seafood is becoming increasingly important globally as a source of nutrition. In 2012, the fisheries' production were approximately 158 million tons, of which 48% derived from aquaculture and the remainder from capture fisheries (FAO, 2014). Between 2006 and 2012, capture fisheries production was relatively stable around 90 million tons, whereas production from aquaculture increased by more than 40% (Figure 12.1). Risk to consumers caused by the presence of parasites is relatively well understood and stems from the consumption of raw or inadequately processed seafood. The parasites of the greatest concern are the larval stages of species belonging to the digenetic trematodes (flukes), cestodes (tapeworms), or nematodes (roundworms), which occur in seafood and normally mature in other mammals or birds. Regulatory oversight in several regions or countries seeks to minimize risk from potentially harmful parasites consumed with

Foodborne Parasites in the Food Supply Web. http://dx.doi.org/10.1016/B978-1-78242-332-4.00012-6

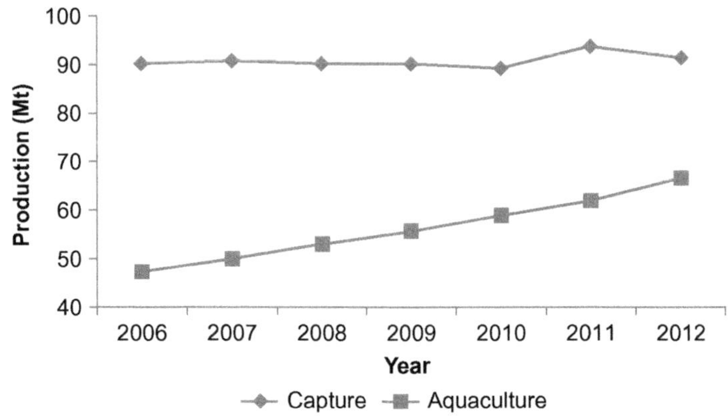

Figure 12.1 Global production of aquatic animals (finfish, crustaceans, mollusks, etc.) in capture and culture fisheries (FAO, 2014). Mt, metric tons.

seafood including, for example, in the European Union, Council Directive 91/493/EEC, and in the United States, the Food and Drug Administration Fish and Fishery Products Hazards and Control Guide. In areas subject to such oversight, it is unlikely that increased seafood consumption will translate into a greater risk of infection with foodborne parasites; however, in all jurisdictions, there remains an ongoing risk of exposure from seafood obtained in recreational or subsistence fisheries. In the absence of strict control measures, the growth of freshwater aquaculture is expected to increase the risk of exposure to foodborne parasites (WHO, 2004).

The purpose of this chapter is to review the transmission dynamics of medically, culturally, or economically important aquatic foodborne parasites by a major taxonomic group. Sampling and diagnostic methods are described and compared. In addition, control points in aquatic animal and food production will be reviewed with special emphasis on opportunities for the identification, removal, or inactivation of zoonotic parasites in the seafood chain. The chapter will conclude with a summary and discussion of future trends.

12.2 Life history of parasites and transmission

12.2.1 Trematodes

12.2.1.1 Background

The scientific literature on foodborne trematodoses has been summarized in several reviews (Keiser and Utzinger, 2009; Fried and Abruzzi, 2010; Sripa et al., 2010; Conlan et al., 2011; Hong and Fang, 2012; Toledo et al., 2012; Fürst et al., 2012). With the exception of members of the family Fasciolidae, which are acquired by the consumption of contaminated vegetation, most infections are acquired through the consumption of seafood infected with viable metacercariae. The life cycles of these parasites include a gastropod as the first intermediate host, and several freshwater or brackish water snails are important hosts that acquire infections either by ingesting embryonated eggs or by exposure to miracidia hatched from eggs shed in the feces of infected definitive hosts. Thus, inadequate sewage treatment is also an important risk factor for trematodosis, and this has been linked with poverty, lack of education, malnutrition, and the absence of food inspection (Gracyk and Fried, 2007). Including cases acquired from the consumption of contaminated aquatic vegetables, the World Health Organization (WHO) estimated that there are more than 56 million cases of foodborne trematodes (WHO, 1995, 2004) with, in 2005, an estimated 7000 associated mortalities worldwide (WHO, 2014). Both wild and cultured fish can be sources of infections. In Vietnam, fish are cultured in ponds containing untreated urban wastewater as well as untreated animal and human feces (De et al., 2012). Elevated nutrient loadings resulting from these practices increase the growth of algae upon which the fish feed. However, the presence of suitable snail species also provides the opportunity for the propagation of trematode life cycles, some of which have zoonotic potential. The prevalence of metacercariae of liver and intestinal flukes in urban fish farms ranged from 2% to 10% and in rural farms from 3% to 33% (De et al., 2012). However, despite this evidence of significant impact to public health, the general absence of well-defined symptoms, along with a strong association with poverty, means that the real impacts of trematodoses are likely to be underestimated, and these infections have been described as the most neglected of the neglected tropical diseases (Sripa, 2008; Keiser and Utzinger, 2009).

Of the more than 56 million people worldwide estimated to be infected with food borne trematodes, more than 95% of these are acquired through the consumption of raw or inadequately prepared seafood (Fürst et al., 2012). Paragonimoses represent 43% of the infections followed by clonorchioses (29%), opisthorchioses (16%), and intestinal flukes (12%). Although the proportions of heavy infections are 21.9%, 7.4%, 3.9%, and 13.8%, respectively, deaths have only been attributed to clonorchiosis (0.5% of heavy infections), opisthorchiosis (0.4%), and paragonimoses (0.005%). There is a tendency for infections with higher prevalence and intensity in males. The more significant socioeconomic impacts are those of years lived with disability and years of lost life, which for all fish borne trematodoses were 315,820 and 314,326 (data from Fürst et al., 2012). The overly simple control recommendation is to cook your fish well and avoid contaminating the groundwater with feces. The reality is that poverty and tradition, combined with a rapidly growing freshwater aquaculture sector, provide the socioeconomic context for these statistics to worsen.

12.2.1.2 Liver flukes

Zoonotic fish borne liver flukes belonging to the family Opisthorchiidae are morphologically alike, and the similarities among life cycles reinforce common epidemiologies. There is a widespread distribution of opisthorchiid liver fluke infections in Europe, Asia, North America, and Greenland. *Opisthorchis felineus* occurs throughout Russia, central, eastern, and southern Europe. *Opisthorchis viverrini* occurs in Cambodia, Laos, Thailand, and Vietnam (Table 12.1). The range of the Chinese or Oriental liver fluke, *Clonorchis sinensis*, includes China, the Korean peninsula, Taiwan, Vietnam, and far eastern Russia (Chai et al., 2005a; WHO, 2008; Sripa et al., 2010) and that of *Metorchis conjunctus* includes eastern North America and Greenland (EFSA, 2010).

Table 12.1 Prevalence of opisthorchid liver flukes by country

Species	Country	Prevalence
Clonorchis sinensis	Republic of Korea	1.4–45.5%
	China	0.4–57%
	Vietnam	13.7–73%
Opisthorchis viverrini	Thailand	9.4–97%
	Laos	70.3%
	Vietnam	15.2–36.9%
Opisthorchis felineus	Russia	45%
	Ukraine	5–40%

From Chai et al. (2005a).

The ranges of these parasites are sympatric with those of the gastropod host, the most important species of which are listed in Table 12.2. Freshwater cyprinid fish are common second intermediate hosts and harbor the infective metacercariae in skin or skeletal muscle (see Table 12.2). Definitive hosts include a broad range of feral and domestic mammals as well as humans (see Table 12.2). Following consumption of metacercariae, adult flukes migrate to and inhabit the hepatic bile ducts and the prepatent period ranges from 2 weeks (*O. felineus*) to 1 month (*C. sinensis*). In humans, many infections are asymptomatic; however, a wide range of gastrointestinal and abdominal symptoms are reported, particularly in heavy infections (WHO, 2008; Hong and Fang, 2012). An important consequence of infection with *C. sinensis* and *O. viverrini* is an increased risk of cholangiocarcinoma. *C. sinensis* is classified as a group 1 carcinogen.

The potential health impact of liver flukes is reflected in the more than 200 million people at risk of infection (Hong and Fang, 2012). As many as 35 million people are infected with *C. sinensis* including 15 million in China (Keiser and Utzinger, 2005), although Chai et al. (2005a) estimated 6 million are infected; the declining trends, they say, are due to control measures in place in larger centers (Chen et al., 1994). In Thailand and Laos, 8–10 million people are infected with *O. viverrini* (WHO, 1995; Jongsuksuntigul and Imsomboon, 2003; Andrews et al., 2008). Overall, Yossepowitch et al. (2004) have estimated that 1.6 million people are infected with *O. felineus*. There is considerable variation in prevalence among sites or communities within endemic regions. This variation may relate to local demographic or gender effects, local eating habits, or the presence of certain fish species among which the prevalence and intensity of infections can vary (De et al., 2012).

12.2.1.3 Intestinal flukes

Zoonotic trematodes parasitic in the intestine and acquired from the ingestion of viable metacercariae in seafood belong to the families Heterophyidae, Lecithodendriidae, Echinostomatidae, Diplostomidae, and Gymnophallidae. The heterophyids are small (<2.5 mm in length) and often occur as mixed infections along with members of the

Table 12.2 **Molluscan and fish hosts of the zoonotic liver flukes *Clonorchis sinensis*, *Opisthorchis viverrini*, *O. felineus*, and *Metorchis conjunctus***

Species	Intermediate hosts		Definitive hosts
	First (snail)	**Second (fish)**	
C. sinensis	*Parafossarulus manchouricus*, *P. anomalospiralis*, *Alocinma longicornis*, *Bithynia fuchsiana*, *B. misella*, *Melanoides tuberculata*, *Semisulcospira libertine*, *Assiminea lutea*, *Thiagra granifera*	*Pseudorasbora parva*, *Abbottina rivularis*, *Ctenopharyngodon idellus*, *Carassius carassius*, *C. auratus*, *Hemiculter* spp., *Cyprinus carpio*, *Opsariichthys* spp., *Rhodeus* spp., *Sarcocheilichthys* spp., *Zacco platypus*, *Z. temminckii*, *Hypomesus olidus*	Dogs, cats, rats, pigs, badgers, weasels, camels, buffalo
O. viverrini	*Bithynia (siamensis) goniomphalus*, *B. (siamensis) funiculate*, *B. (siamensis) siamensis*	*Cyclocheillichthys siaja*, *Hampala dispar*, *Puntius orphoides*, *P. gonionotus*, *P. proctozysron*, *P. viehoever*, *Labiobarbus lineatus*, *Esomus metallicus*, *Osteochilus* sp.	Dogs, cats, rats, pigs
O. felineus	*Bithynia leachii*, *B. inflate*, *B. tentaculata*	*Idus melanotus*, *Tinca tinca*, *T. vulgaris*, *Abramis brama*, *A. sapa*, *Barbus barbus*, *C. carpio*, *Blicca bjorkna*, *Leuciscus idus*, *Alburnus lucidus*, *Aspius aspius*, *Scardinius erythophthalmus*	Dogs, foxes, cats, rats, pigs, rabbits, seals, lions, wolverines, martens, polecats
M. conjunctus	*Amnicola limosa limosa*	*Catostomus catostomus*, *Salvelinus fontinalis*, *Perca flavescens*	Dogs, cats, wolves, foxes, coyotes, raccoons, muskrats, minks, fisher

From Chai et al. (2005a).

Lecithodendriidae, the so-called minute intestinal flukes. The eggs of worms in the Opisthorchiidae and Lecithodendriidae are small, operculated, and morphologically similar, rendering species-specific diagnosis a challenge. *Metagonimus yokogawai* is most frequently reported in China, Japan, the Republic of Korea, and Taiwan, and primarily in Russia (Chai et al., 2005a; Keiser and Utzinger, 2009). Chai et al. (2005a) reported that prevalence (percent of egg-positive stool samples) ranged from 10% to 70% in the Republic of Korea. Other species of zoonotic significance are *Heterophyes heterophyes*, *Heterophyes nocens*, and *Haplorchis* spp. The infections can have highly variable levels of prevalence and intensity throughout the range (Chai et al., 2005a); however, there are few data on numbers at risk and prevalence (Keiser and Utzinger, 2009). The echinostomatids *Echinostoma hortense* and *Echinochasmus japonicus* occur widely throughout Korea, Japan, and China and the range of other *Echinochasmus* spp. (e.g., *Echinochasmus perfoliatus*, *Echinochasmus liliputanus*) also includes the Middle East and Southeastern Europe (Chai et al., 2005a). As with the heterophyids, infections are distributed focally, with highly variable prevalence and intensity.

In the definitive host, zoonotic heterophyids occur closely associated with villi of the intestinal mucosa. Embryonated eggs shed with the feces are ingested by the gastropod host (Table 12.3) leading to the development of cercariae, which escape into the water, ultimately encysting as metacercariae in the muscle of fresh- or brackish water fish or crustaceans. When conditions are favorable, large numbers of metacercariae

Table 12.3 Molluscan and fish hosts of certain zoonotic heterophyid and echinostomatid intestinal flukes

Species	Intermediate hosts		Definitive hosts
	First (snail)	**Second (fish)**	
Metagonimus yokogawai	*Semisulcospira libertine*, *S. coreana*	*Plecoglossus altivelis*, *Tribolodon taczanowskii*, *Lateolabrax japonicus*	Dogs, cats, rats
Heterophyes heterophyes	*Pirenella conica*	*Mugil cephalus*, *Tilapia nilotica*, *Aphanius fasciatus*, *Acanthogobius* sp.	Dogs, cats, foxes, wolves, pelicans
Echinostoma hortense	*Limnaea pervia*, *Radix auricularia coreana*	*Misgurnus anguillicaudatus*, *M. mizolepis*, *Odontobutis obscura interrupta*, *Moroco oxycephalus*, *Coreoperca kawamebari*, *Squalidus coreanus*	Dog, cats, rats, mice, chickens, ducks
Echinochasmus japonicus	*Parafossarulus manchouricus*	*Pseudorasbora parva*, *Hypomesus olidus*, *Gnathopogon strigatus*	Chickens, ducks

From Chai et al. (2005a).

can occur, greatly increasing the risk of harmful infection (Cho et al., 1984). The resulting metacercariae develop into adults within 5–10 days following ingestion (Sripa et al., 2010). Echinostomatids have low host specificity, and infections may be acquired by the consumption of viable metacercariae in snails, bivalves, amphibians, and fish (Sripa et al., 2010). Most infections with intestinal flukes are asymptomatic. However, with increased intensity, infections are accompanied by an eosinophilic gastroenteritis, ulceration, and bleeding of the intestinal mucosa. Mortality associated with heterophyid infection is rare and caused by lesions in cardiac muscle or the central nervous system following the dissemination of fluke eggs in the lymph or circulatory system.

12.2.1.4 Lung flukes

Zoonotic trematodes of the genus *Paragonimus* (Troglotrematidae) are parasitic in the lungs of mammals. *Paragonimus westermani*, one of the 17 species of lung flukes, is most commonly reported in humans and occurs in three broadly defined regions: eastern and southern Asia, equatorial West Africa, and equatorial South America and Central America. *Paragonimus africanus* and *Paragonimus mexicana* cause zoonoses in West Africa and Central and South America, respectively, as does *Paragonimus kellicotti* in North America (Akuthota and Weller, 2012). About 13 other species are known to occur in tropical and temperate regions, and all are transmissible via the consumption of viable metacercariae which occur in freshwater crab, crayfish, or shrimp. Wild boars may also serve as paratenic hosts (Toledo et al., 2012). An estimated 293 million people are at risk of infection, and between 20 and 23 million people are infected (WHO, 1995; Keiser and Utzinger, 2005; Fürst et al., 2012). The prevalence of paragonimoses based on the national surveys or expert opinion ranges from 0.002% to 4.568% (Fürst et al., 2012).

Adult flukes are robust (7.5–12 mm long × 4–6 mm wide × 3.5–5 mm thick), and comparable in size, shape, and color to coffee beans. Unembryonated, operculated eggs are transported to the pharynx by bronchial cilia and either expectorated or swallowed and passed in the feces. Following embryonation and hatching, miracidia invade snails belonging to the genera *Brotia*, *Melanoides*, *Semisulcospira*, *Tarebia*, and *Thiara*, in which they develop through sporocysts and rediae to cercariae. The released cercariae crawl on the substrate and infect susceptible crustaceans by penetrating skin that is not protected by the carapace or by ingestion of infected snails. Freshwater crabs of the genera *Eriocheir*, *Potamon*, and *Potamiscus* are preferred second intermediate hosts and metacercariae encyst in skeletal muscle, viscera, or gills (Diaz, 2013). Following ingestion of metacercariae by the human definitive host, migration of excysted larvae from the upper gastrointestinal tract, temporary encystment on the diaphragm followed by migration to the lungs requires 2–15 days and can be associated with abdominal pain and diarrhea. Migration through the diaphragm to the lungs leads to an eosinophilic pulmonary effusion (Akuthota and Weller, 2012). Fibrous capsules (often containing a pair of worms) and associated inflammatory lesions can be mistaken for tuberculosis (Lall et al., 2013). In humans, a small percentage of infections (0.7%) occur ectopically, caused by migration of larvae to the brain (Fürst et al., 2012).

12.2.2 Cestodes

12.2.2.1 Background

Fish borne zoonotic tapeworms have multihost life cycles consisting of the first and the second intermediates, and definitive host, stages. Those for which fish serve as the second intermediate host use piscivorous fish, birds, or mammals as definitive hosts. The body of most mature cestodes consists of three morphologically distinct regions: a small and slender attachment organ or scolex, a proliferative neck region, and a strobila, which is a series of anatomically identical, reproductively active segments (or proglottids) each containing male and female reproductive organs. Human infections are generally asymptomatic, and although the passage of eggs in the feces goes unnoticed, the shedding of large worm fragments or detached proglottids can be conspicuous. The cestode family Diphyllobothriidae includes several genera with species known to infect humans, including *Diplogonoporus* (marine parasites of baleen whales and otarid seals), *Pyramicocephalus* (marine parasites of phocid seals), *Schistocephalus* (freshwater parasites of birds and mammals), and *Diphyllobothrium* (Jenkins et al., 2013). Because of their widespread distribution and number of human infections, this section will focus on fish borne infections with cestodes belonging to the genus *Diphyllobothrium*.

12.2.2.2 Diphyllobothrium *spp.*

Diphyllobothrium is a speciose genus including 50 accepted species, 14 of which are known to infect humans. Also called broad fish tapeworms, these are among the largest parasites that infect humans, with some species reaching lengths of 15–25 m and including as many as 4000 proglottids (Scholtz et al., 2009; Jenkins et al., 2013). The life cycles are similar, with unembryonated operculated eggs shed into freshwater and, after 8 or more days, depending on the water temperature, the emergence of a ciliated first stage larvae or coracidium. The swimming behavior of the coracidium attracts copepods that serve as the first intermediate host. Approximately 40 species of copepods within the genera *Acanthodiaptomus*, *Arctodiaptomus*, *Diaptomus*, *Eudiaptomus*, *Eurytemora*, *Boeckella*, *Cyclops*, and *Mesocyclops* serve as the first intermediate hosts among the species of *Diphyllobothrium*. Soon after ingestion by the copepod, the coracidium sheds its cilia and migrates through the gut wall to the haemocoel, where it elongates over approximately 3 weeks to become a procercoid. No further growth or development of the procercoid occurs until the infected copepod is eaten by a suitable species of fish which serves as the second intermediate host. In the fish, the larval cestode migrates through the gut wall and develops into a plerocercoid larva at a site that depends on the parasite species (Table 12.4). Plerocercoids may occur freely within the peritoneum or skeletal muscle or be encapsulated by a host response (Table 12.4; Dezfuli et al., 2007). The plerocercoid may transfer to a paratenic fish host, such as a pike (*Esox lucius*) or salmonid following ingestion of the second intermediate host. In all cases, the definitive host becomes infected by the consumption of a viable plerocercoid contained within raw or inadequately processed fish. Infections in the definitive host usually become patent within 2 weeks.

Table 12.4 Range of hosts and geographic distributions among *Diphyllobothrium* spp. occurring in freshwater and anadromous fish and known to infect humans

Species	Host		Site of infection[a]	Distribution
	Definitive	Second intermediate		
D. alascense	Dogs	*Lota lota*, *Osmerus mordax*	Stomach lumen (no)	NA (Alaska)
D. dalliae	Dogs, Arctic foxes	*Dallia pectoralis*, *Salvelinus malma*	Peritoneum (no)	NA (Alaska)
D. dendriticum	Gulls, piscivorous birds, and mammals	Salmonids, coregonids	Peritoneum (no)	CP-B
D. latum	Piscivorous mammals	*Esox lucius*, *Perca fluviatilis*, *L. lota*, *Sander vitreum*, *Gymnocephalus cernuus*, *P. flavescens*	Skeletal muscle (no)	CP-T
D. nihonkaiense	Brown bear	*Oncorhynchus* spp., *Hucho perryi*	Skeletal muscle (yes/no)	NPO
D. ursi	Bear	Unknown	Gastric serosa (yes)	NA (Alaska)

NA, North America; CP-B, circumpolar boreal; CP-T, circumpolar temperate; NPO, North Pacific Ocean.
a In the second intermediate (or paratenic: see text) host: encapsulated (yes or no).
From Scholtz et al. (2009).

Diphyllobothriosis is an ancient parasitosis, with evidence of the infection found in 6000-year-old mummified human remains found in the Attacama region of Peru and Chile (Arriaza et al., 2010). Today, human infections have a global distribution, but overall the number of infected people appears to be declining from the high of 20 million estimated near the end of the twentieth century (Chai et al., 2005a; Scholtz et al., 2009; Torgerson and Macpherson, 2011). However, there is uncertainty in estimates of the number of infections or prevalence rates because most infections go unreported and because the symptoms tend to be nonspecific leading to misdiagnosis. Risk of exposure, exemplified by the consumption of raw or inadequately processed fish, reflects both well-established cultural practices, which often have strong regional and demographic characteristics, and more recently, increasing demands for raw fish products facilitated by the global transport of food commodities.

The regional declines in the number of human cases in areas with historically high rates of infection (e.g., Alaska, Finland) and generally in North America and most of Europe and Asia is in contrast to increases in Russia, South Korea, Japan, and in parts of South America (see Scholtz et al., 2009). Diphyllobothrioses persist locally in Switzerland and northern Italy (Vaiani et al., 2006). Of the 14 *Diphyllobothrium* spp. responsible for infections in humans, *Diphyllobothrium latum* and *Diphyllobothrium nihonkaiense* are considered most pathogenic (Scholtz et al., 2009). However, a third species, *Diphyllobothrium dendriticum*, is an emerging human pathogen with a widespread distribution (Kutchta et al., 2013). Historically, the geographic ranges of infections with each *Diphyllobothrium* spp. are reasonably well defined. The high Arctic remains a region in which ancestral hosts and life histories of several *Diphyllobothrium* spp. may still be observed (Hoberg et al., 2012; Jenkins et al., 2011; Schurer et al., 2013). Surveys conducted in the latter half of the twentieth century revealed that the prevalence of human diphyllobothrioses (various species) ranged from 6% to 53% in Alaska and from 1.7% to 77% in Northern Canada (Jenkins et al., 2013). However, global distribution of highly valued fish has increased the range of infections with those species (e.g., *D. nihonkaiense*) using salmon as a paratenic or the second intermediate host (Yéra et al., 2006; Wicht et al., 2007). The possible long-distance transport of diphyllobothriids by piscivorous birds or human immigration may explain the occurrence of northerly species such as *D. latum* and *D. dendriticum* appearing in Chile (Scholtz et al., 2009). Six of the 14 species infecting humans are acquired from exclusively freshwater and anadromous fish (see Table 12.4). The remaining eight *Diphyllobothrium* spp. are strictly marine and use pinnipeds and cetaceans as definitive hosts. Second intermediate hosts are unknown for most marine species, and reports of human infections are rare (Scholtz et al., 2009).

Salmon aquaculture includes freshwater and marine phases in which fish are typically reared in carefully controlled environments and fed manufactured diets that exclude the presence of viable parasites. However, salmon smolts are occasionally reared in cages in freshwater lakes prior to the marine grow-out phase. Larval *Diphyllobothrium* spp. have been found in cultured Atlantic salmon, rainbow trout, and other trouts in the United States, Scotland, Ireland, Finland, Russia, and Chile (Cabello, 2007; Lima dos Santos and Howgate, 2011). These findings confirm that despite being fed a commercial diet free of viable larval cestodes, cultured salmonids are exposed to and will ingest procercoid-infected zooplankton that occur naturally in lakes. It is important to emphasize that the likelihood of larval cestode infection in farmed salmon is low.

12.2.3 Nematodes

12.2.3.1 Background

Anisakidosis is a disease afflicting humans caused by infection with larval nematodes belonging to the family Anisakidae. Most frequently, these infections are caused by *Anisakis simplex* (anisakiosis) and *Pseudoterranova decipiens* (Kuhn et al., 2011), but human infections with *Anisakis physeteris*, *Anisakis pegreffii*, *Contracecum* spp., and *Thynnascaris* spp. have also been reported. The definitive hosts of anisakid nematodes are marine mammals and occasionally birds, in which the nematodes reside in the gastrointestinal tract. Analysis of the ranges of anisakid species identified by using molecular methods suggests the occurrence of species-specific distribution patterns that map to the distribution of definitive host species (Kuhn et al., 2011). Unembryonated eggs are shed into the marine environment with the feces. The developing embryo molts before hatching as a second- or third-stage larva, depending on species. The life cycles of anisakids have become integrated into numerous marine food webs and can include several intermediate, paratenic, and definitive hosts. The paratenic host serves as an ecological bridge for the parasite to move through the food web, but within which it does not undergo further development. The larvae are ingested by copepod, decapod, or amphipod crustaceans and migrate to the haemocoel and develop to the infective third stage. Larger crustaceans can serve as paratenic hosts by ingesting smaller copepods. Similarly, larval *Anisakis* spp. appear not to undergo further development while encysted in tissues of fish and cephalopods (ICES, 2012), which therefore serve as paratenic hosts bridging the trophic gap between the crustacean and definitive hosts. In the definitive host, the nematode matures to the adult stage in the gastrointestinal tract. Following ingestion of the infective third-stage larvae by humans, no further development occurs. However, the larva remains viable, and clinical signs of anisakidosis are related to the severity of the localized irritation to the esophageal, gastric, or intestinal mucosa caused by larval movement and tissue migrations.

12.2.3.2 Anisakis *and* Pseudoterranova

Parasites belonging to the *A. simplex* complex (*A. simplex sensu stricto*, *A. simplex* C, *A. pegreffii*, *A. physeteris*) are widely distributed in the North Atlantic and Pacific Ocean basins, congruent with the ranges of their most frequent definitive hosts, which are pinnipeds and cetaceans belonging to several odontocete species (Hochberg and Hamer, 2010; Kuhn et al., 2011; Jenkins et al., 2013). *P. decipiens* types A, B, and C occupy somewhat distinct marine food webs (Jenkins et al., 2013). Fish hosts believed to harbor the third-stage larvae of *A. simplex* complex include Pacific salmon (*Oncorhynchus* spp.), herring (*Clupea harengus*), and hake (*Merluccius merluccius*). Those harboring infective *P. decipiens* larvae include mackerel (*Scomber japonicus*), Atlantic cod (*Gadus morhua*), Pacific cod (*Gadus macrocephalus*), and Pacific halibut

Hippoglossus stenolepis (Hochberg and Hamer, 2010). These lists of host species are much abbreviated, and throughout the ranges of these parasites the European Food Safety Authority concluded that virtually all edible marine fish should be considered potentially infected (EFSA, 2010). Alternatively farmed salmon, because they are fed a processed commercial diet, had been considered to present a low risk of harboring larval anisakids (EFSA, 2010), in agreement with Angot and Brasseur (1993). However, Marty (2008) described a larval anisakid from the viscera of one of the 894 farmed Atlantic salmon and (Mo et al., 2014) reported 59 *A. simplex* larvae in the muscle or viscera from 9 of 50 salmon discarded at harvest because they were runts of small size (mean weight of 1.1 kg). In the latter study, no larvae were observed in 50 harvest-quality salmon (mean weight of 5.4 kg). The authors suggested the risk of infection in subsize fish reflected their basal status in the feeding hierarchy in the net pen, and the consequent dependence on natural food rather than the high-quality processed diet. Overall, the evidence suggests that harvest-weight salmon are unlikely to serve as a source of anisakiosis.

Similar to infections caused by trematodes and cestodes, there are no systematic efforts to document anisakidoses, suggesting that reported figures underestimate the true prevalence (or incidence) of infections. Nevertheless, anisakidoses have been reported from several countries, and there is evidence that the number of reports has increased more recently, possibly because of regulations limiting the harvest of marine mammals (Hochberg and Hamer, 2010). Although it may be tempting to suggest that increases in anisakidosis reporting rates are related to increased abundances of cetaceans, this relationship is difficult to measure. In contrast, there are good statistics demonstrating increases in seafood consumption (EFSA, 2010). Hochberg and Hamer (2010) estimated that prior to the 1990s, 20,000 cases of anisakidosis had been diagnosed, with more than 90% of these from Japan and the remainder from coastal areas of the Netherlands, Germany, France, and Spain. The recent increase represents reports from Brazil, Canada, Chile, Egypt, and New Zealand. Similar to diphyllobothriosis, the geographic range of anisakidosis is no longer restricted to coastal regions and has expanded with global transportation of fresh seafood (Couture et al., 2003).

Despite the uncertainty surrounding true incidence, the epidemiology of anisakidosis is well-established and results from the ingestion of raw or inadequately processed marine seafood that is infected with the third-stage larvae. Typically, the first symptoms of anisakidosis are experienced less than a day after infection, and collectively three sequential syndromes are related to the presence and migratory behavior of viable third-stage larvae: gastric, intestinal, and ectopic. Gastric pain and nausea accompanied by vomiting and fever are early symptoms of infection, and there is evidence that the gastric syndrome is more frequent in Japan, whereas in Europe the intestinal syndrome predominates (Hochberg and Hamer, 2010). The intestinal symptoms occur 5–7 days later, resulting from inflammation associated with larvae, which cause abdominal pain and ascites. Rarely, migration of larvae into the peritoneum results in chronic ectopic infections with complications. Exposure to parasite antigens present in fresh or processed seafood of some individuals previously sensitized to *Anisakis* spp. causes allergic reactions, ranging from mild hypersensitivity reactions to life-threatening anaphylactic shock (Audicana and Kennedy, 2008;

Hochberg and Hamer, 2010). The epidemiology and characteristics of gastro-allergic anisakiasis (GAA) in Spain has been well described (see EFSA, 2010). Infections with *P. decipiens* larvae are primarily confined to the stomach and can be accompanied by coughing and expectoration or vomiting of larvae.

12.3 Sampling and detection methods

12.3.1 Introduction

Over the last three decades, advances in molecular biology have made available a number of assays with characteristics that make them suitable tests for parasite detection, screening, and surveillance. For example, conventional or quantitative polymerase chain reactions (PCRs) are highly sensitive, and specific assays can quickly amplify a defined segment of parasite nucleic acid. A positive result confirms the presence of parasite nucleic acid in the sample, often at extremely low concentrations. However, PCRs are relatively costly and require specialized instruments and trained technologists. Existing field-based programs often use traditional methods such as microscopic examination of fecal samples, which can have low sensitivity and specificity. Therefore, care must be taken when integrating newer methods with inherently high sensitivity, which can show an apparent low specificity (high rate of false positives) when compared with accepted standard methods (Johansen et al., 2010). This section will review sampling and detection methods for foodborne trematodes, cestodes, and nematodes derived from seafood.

12.3.2 Trematodes

The extensive body of knowledge on the diagnosis of foodborne trematodoses derived from seafood has been recently reviewed (Johansen et al., 2010; Keiser et al., 2010; Sripa et al., 2010; Toledo et al., 2012). The "gold standard" diagnostic assay for the presence of biliary or liver infections (i.e., *O. viverrini* or *O. sinensis*) is microscopic detection of eggs in fecal samples. This method will also detect infections with intestinal or lung flukes—also in sputum samples in the case of *Paragonimus* spp. There are several variations in this method that involve a variety of flotation, concentration, and staining techniques, and overall the parasitological methods remain widely used because they are simple, relatively quick, and inexpensive (Lovis et al., 2009; Keiser et al., 2010). Among these methods, there is indication that the formalin-ether concentration technique is more sensitive than the Kato-Katz thick smear method and has been recommended for the detection of low-intensity infections (Hong and Fang, 2012). Long-term fecal egg data sets provide a reference against which the effectiveness of treatment or other mitigation strategies may be gaged. The limitations of parasitological detection methods include reduced sensitivity during infections of low intensity and an inability to accurately identify parasites to species because of morphological similarities of eggs among flukes belonging to the Opisthorchiidae, Heterophyidae, and Lecithodendriidae. Periodicity in the passage of eggs in feces contributed to reduced sensitivity of these and other screening tools (Keiser et al., 2010). In endemic regions, infections with *O. viverrini* occur together with the less harmful minute intestinal flukes (Chai et al., 2005b; Lovis et al., 2009; Traub et al., 2009; Keiser et al., 2010) leading to an increased likelihood of incorrect parasitological estimates of the distribution, prevalence, and intensity of the more pathogenic infections. In contrast, the specific amplification of minute quantities of parasite ribosomal genomic or mitochondrial DNA from fecal or sputum samples has provided the means to confirm infection and identify the parasites involved (Lovis et al., 2009; Sato et al., 2010). The amount of *C. sinensis* DNA in fecal samples, determined by quantitative PCR, was shown to correlate significantly with egg counts (Kim et al., 2009), supporting a quantitative capacity for this approach, in addition to its increased sensitivity.

Protein or carbohydrate parasite antigens may be detected by using enzyme-linked immunosorbent assays (ELISA), which have proven to be more sensitive than microscopic examination of fecal preparations. Monoclonal antibodies that recognize potentially valuable diagnostic antigens of *O. viverrini* form the basis of such antigen-capture ELISAs (Chaicumpa et al., 1991; Sirisinha et al., 1995; Wongratanacheewin et al., 2003). The ELISA is also used to screen for host antibodies present in the plasma in response to trematode infections. The performance of the assay reflects the quality and composition of parasite antigens used in the ELISA (Ruangsittichai et al., 2006; Hu et al., 2007; Ma et al., 2007). A key drawback to serological screening is that it reflects the host response to an infection that may no longer persist. Also, some antibodies show a tendency to cross-react with different antigens or with homologous antigens from different parasite species (Johansen et al., 2010) and therefore may not be a specific indicator of the infection under study.

Johansen et al. (2010) discuss the need to carefully match the diagnostic method with the stated objectives of the work, for example, the reduction of morbidity versus transmission control. These authors also conclude that diagnostic oversimplification and economic constraints have contributed to increased ignorance of the biology and epidemiology of fish borne trematodes. However, given that the risk factors associated with acquisition of infections with these parasites are well-known, it is important to emphasize that adequate diagnosis is one of the three pillars of disease mitigation: public awareness through education, implementation of risk-avoidance strategies (adequate food preparation, hygienic defecation practices), and systematic surveillance. The introduction of a nationwide liver fluke control program in Thailand provides an example of this principle. The overall prevalence of opisthorchiid infections fell from 63.6% between 1984 and 1987 to less than 10% between 1997 and 2001, following implementation of the program (Jongsuksuntigul and Imsomboon, 2003). In the case from Thailand, diagnosis was achieved by using trained teams of technicians conducting parasitological examinations of fecal preparations. Thus, integrated programs that involve carefully planned systematic surveillance can be effective even when simple diagnostic methods are used. Alth`ough demonstrating the potential for a reduced level of infection, the program in Thailand was not equally effective in all parts of the country and illustrated the need for ongoing political commitment (Ziegler et al., 2011). In addition, effective control at the community level will require that reservoir hosts, including cats, dogs, and swine, are included to the extent possible in the three-pillared mitigation effort (Anh et al., 2009).

The detection of zoonotic trematode larvae in seafood remains dependent on simple traditional methods of squashing skeletal muscle or skin, artificial digestion, and visual or microscopic assessment, and species identification is based on the recognition of diagnostic anatomical features (Sohn, 2009; Toledo et al., 2012). The increasing availability of PCR-based technologies as described will also be useful in confirming the identity of larval parasites in the mollusc or fish intermediate hosts (e.g., Parvathi et al., 2008).

12.3.3 Cestodes

The detection and diagnosis of diphyllobothriosis is most frequently achieved through the identification of characteristic proglottids and eggs in fecal samples. From a strictly clinical perspective, confirmation of the infection as a diphyllobothriosis is sufficient, regardless of the species involved (Scholtz et al., 2009). However, when necessary for epidemiology or other research purposes, amplification of parasite-specific genomic or mitochondrial DNA from fecal samples provides the opportunity to confirm the identity of the parasite. Diagnosis is rarely attempted, however, because of the high incidence of asymptomatic infections.

Identification of plerocercoid larvae of diphyllobothriids in fish is hampered by morphological similarity among species, although the site of encystment may be informative (see Table 12.4). Until recently, the use of molecular methods to confirm the identification of cestode larvae in fish capable of infecting humans has been limited by the few available sequences. However, the molecular taxonomy of cestodes is an active field of research, and a number of novel approaches show promise (Yéra et al., 2008; Arizono et al., 2009; Wicht et al., 2010). Despite this, the cryptic occurrence of *D. latum* and *D. nihonkaiense* plerocercoids in skeletal muscle suggests a high rate of undetected infections in food fish. As discussed in Section 12.5, efforts to increase consumer awareness regarding food safety are strongly encouraged.

12.3.4 Nematodes

Unlike for fluke and tapeworm infections, fecal examinations are inappropriate for the detection and diagnosis of anisakidoses. In rare cases, larvae expelled by coughing or spitting may be identified based on the morphological features or by using PCR to determine the presence of parasite-specific DNA. However, symptoms tend to be nonspecific, and a correct diagnosis is unlikely in most cases. Evidence of ongoing or historical exposure can be obtained from allergen sensitivity skin tests.

Anisakid infections in seafood on the processing line are detected by candling (see Section 12.5). Alternative approaches include fluorescent imaging (Yang et al., 2013), amplification of parasite DNA by quantitative PCR (Lopez and Pardo, 2010; Herrero et al., 2011; Mossali et al., 2010), and serological methods (Xu et al., 2010). Although these methods are sensitive, they are not necessarily reliable estimators of parasite viability. However, some serological methods may permit the quantification of parasite-allergen levels in seafood (Rodriguez-Mahillo et al., 2010).

12.4 Points of control in the food chain

12.4.1 Traditional and thermal processing

Light salting, marinating, or cold-smoking of seafood harboring zoonotic trematode, cestode, or nematode larvae are insufficient to affect parasite viability as suggested by the list of traditional dishes associated with heightened risk of infection: ceviche (fish and spices marinated in lime juice), lomi lomi (salmon marinated in lemon juice, onion, and tomato), poisson cru (fish marinated in citrus juice, onion, tomato, and coconut milk), herring roe, sashimi (sliced raw fish), sushi (raw fish with rice and other ingredients), green herring (lightly brined herring), drunken crabs (crab marinated in wine and pepper), cold-smoked fish (lox), and undercooked grilled fish (Kuipers et al., 1960; Karl et al., 1995; FDA, 2011; ESFA, 2010). The importance of aquacultured fish as sources of infection is increasing, for example, due to metacercariae in pond-cultured fish in Southeast Asia, but mitigation of this risk may be feasible by interventions made during production practices (Figure 12.2; Hung et al., 2013).

However, occurrence of fish borne parasites in the food chain occurs primarily from wild-caught fishery products, and intervention and control is feasible only during processing following capture. Automated, semi-automated, or manual finfish processing is unlikely to reduce the risk of parasites completely within the filet (skeletal muscle), although manual intervention (e.g., candling) can enable recognition and manual removal of some larvae (e.g., *P. decipiens* or *Diphyllobothrium* spp.). Visual inspection of fresh fish filets for parasites by candling is required in Canada, the United States, and the EC (Murrell and Dalsgaard, 2014). Sample units can be rejected if they contain two or more parasites per kg (FAO, 2001).

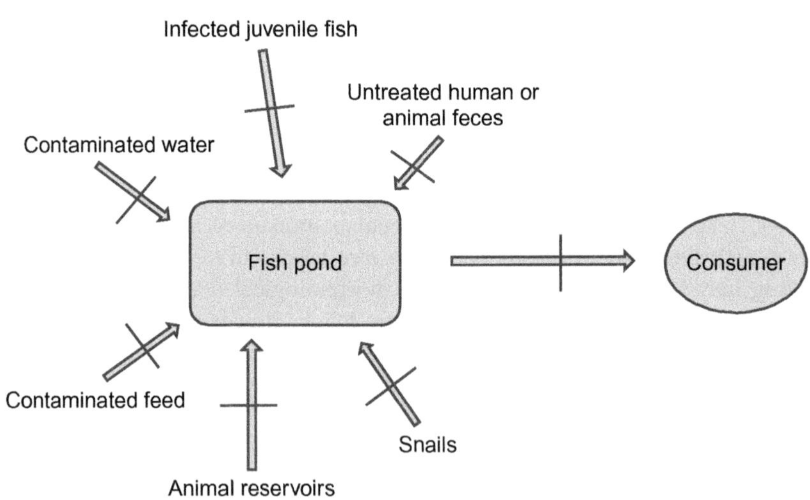

Figure 12.2 Risk factors facilitating the life cycle and transmission of foodborne trematodes in an aquaculture facility. Bars across arrows identify pathways of risk for which intervention is possible.
From WHO (1995).

With essentially a global distribution and a wide host range, *Anisakis* spp. have been the subject of numerous studies focusing on the larvicidal effects of various treatments (Table 12.5). Freezing remains the most widely accepted method for killing parasite larvae in seafood while retaining the appearance, texture, and flavor of the product and has been adopted by regulatory bodies in the United States and the European Union. The practice of freezing had initially been adopted by the Netherlands in 1968 as a method of inactivating *Anisakis* larvae in herring. The original Dutch regulations required that within 12 h of capture, the product be frozen to −20 °C (or below) and stored at this temperature for at least 24 h. Current EC regulation requires freezing to a core temperature −20 °C (or below) for at least 24 h for seafood products to be consumed raw or almost raw, for those from high-risk species (herring, mackerel, sprat, wild salmon) destined for cold-smoking in which the core temperature does not exceed 60 °C, and for traditionally marinated or salted seafood products. Similarly, the US Food and Drug Administration (USFDA) requires that for any seafood product destined for consumption raw or in a semiraw state, it must be frozen to a core temperature of −20 °C (or below) for at least 7 days, to a core temperature of −35 °C (or below) for at least 15 h, or to a core temperature of −35 °C or below with storage at −20 °C (or

Table 12.5 Conditions reported to kill larval *Anisakis* spp. in products from fisheries

Product	Treatment	Parameters
Herring	Salting	5% NaCl, >17 weeks
		6–7% NaCl, 10–12 weeks
		8–9% NaCl, 6 weeks
	Dry salting	20 days
Anchovy	Marinating	10% acetic acid, 12% NaCl, >5 days
		2.4% acetic acid, 6% NaCl, 35 days
Sardine	Marinating	6% acetic acid, 10% NaCl, 4 °C, 24 h to 13 days
Herring	Marinating	3.7% acetic acid, 6.3% NaCl, 28 days
Salmon, rockfish	Freezing	−35 °C, 15 h; −18 °C, 24 h
Flounder	Freezing	−15 °C, 96 h; −20 °C, 60 h; −30 °C, 20 h; −40 °C, 9 h
Salmon, flounder	High pressure	414 MPa, 30–60 s; 276 MPa, 90–180 s; 207 MPa, 180 s
Herring	Irradiation	6–10 kGy
Eel	Irradiation	>1 kGy
In vitro larvae	Freezing	−15 °C, <1 h
	Heating	60 °C, >15 min
		>60 °C, 1 min
		60 °C, 10 min (3 cm thick filet)
	Plant extract	[6]Shogaol (62.5 µg/ml), [6]gingerol (62.5 µg/ml)

From EFSA (2010).

below) for at least 24 h. It is important to note that the larvicidal heating or freezing regimes do not abrogate the allergenic potential of *Anisakis* spp., so treated fish may still pose a risk of GAA (Baird et al., 2014). These regulations provide the framework and rationale for the development of hazard analysis critical control point (HACCP) plans by seafood producers to systematically identify hazards (e.g., *Anisakis* larvae), determine their significance (e.g., consumption of raw seafood), identify critical control points (e.g., freezing), and define control strategies (Butt et al., 2004; FDA, 2011).

Conditions outlined by US and EC regulations for *Anisakis* are also likely to be effective against *Diphyllobothrium* plerocercoids, which are inactivated by freezing to −18 °C for at least 24 h (Salminen, 1970) (inactivation of *Diphyllobothrium* plerocercoids at −23 °C for 7 days or −35 °C for 15 h was also reported by Murrell and Dalsgaard, 2014). Heating to a temperature of 60 °C or greater for at least 1 min will kill *Anisakis* and *Diphyllobothrium* larvae (ESFA, 2010; Murrell and Dalsgaard, 2014). Therefore, whereas hot smoking, in which the core temperature of the filet reaches or exceeds 60 °C, is larvicidal, cold-smoking is not. Although the freezing and heating conditions confirmed to be effective for *Anisakis* and *Diphyllobothrium* will likely be effective in killing metacercariae belonging to zoonotic trematodes (Fan, 1998), more research in this area will be beneficial.

12.4.2 Chemical inactivation, irradiation

Salting and marinating have traditionally been used to preserve seafood. When the concentrations of the preservative are sufficient, these processes are also known to kill larval parasites (see Table 12.5). Although it is advantageous in circumstances where electrical power (for freezing or cooking) is not available, salting and marinating lose their larvicidal properties if NaCl and/or acetic acid concentrations are insufficient or when contact times are too short (Fan, 1998). The larvicidal effects of certain plant extracts, high hydrostatic pressure, and irradiation have been explored experimentally (see Table 12.5); however, more research is required to determine efficacy, safety, and consumer acceptance.

12.5 Conclusions

The natural occurrence of parasites in seafood can pose a risk of serious infection or allergic reactions to consumers in many parts of the world. There are two principal at-risk groups: (1) those living in endemic regions and practicing traditional food preparation and eating habits (e.g., liver, lung, and intestinal flukes in several tropical and temperate regions and diphyllobothrioses in Arctic communities) and (2) those within the general population exposed because of the increased popularity of exotic or ethnic foods, both in endemic and nonendemic regions, which can be facilitated by tourism and the global transport of fresh seafood. The biology of these parasites is well understood, as are the risk factors associated with infection. Infections with *Diphyllobothrium* spp. and *Anisakis* spp. are acquired primarily from wild sources, whereas liver and intestinal flukes are increasingly associated with the rapid growth of extensive freshwater aquaculture, particularly in developing countries. In all cases, the risk of infection persists because of the presence of viable larvae in inadequately processed seafood. Regulatory agencies in some regions require that seafood be processed in the food chain to minimize risk of infection. Such oversight is often lacking or poorly developed in regions endemic for liver and intestinal trematodes. However, in these regions, the integration of education, strategic control, and systematic surveillance programs implemented at the community level have shown local benefits. The greatest opportunity for reducing the prevalence and impacts of fish borne trematodes is in aquaculture, which is increasingly being used in endemic regions. Specifically, the risk of exposure to metacercariae-infected fish will be lessened through the implementation of quality-assured farm practices that interrupt the cycle of transmission. Examples include snail control, use of commercial diets rather than the traditional feces-based pond enrichment methods, and livestock exclusion from fish ponds (see Li et al., 2013). In addition, regardless of the population at-risk, elevated awareness through consumer education will lessen the risk of infection.

References

Akuthota, P., Weller, P.F., 2012. Eosinophilic pneumonias. Clin. Microbiol. Rev. 25, 649–660.

Andrews, R.H., Sithithaworn, P., Petney, T.N., 2008. *Opisthorchis viverrini*: an under-estimated parasite in world health. Trends Parasitol. 24, 497–501.

Angot, V., Brasseur, P., 1993. European farmed Atlantic salmon (*Salmo salar* L.) are safe from anisakid larvae. Aquaculture 118, 339–344.

Anh, N.T.L., Phuong, N.T., Murrell, K.D., Johansen, M.V., Dalsgaard, A., Thu, L.T., Chi, T.T.K., Thamsborg, S.M., 2009. Animal reservoir hosts and fish-borne zoonotic trematode infection on fish farms, Vietnam. Emerg. Infect. Dis. 15, 540–546.

Arizono, N., Shedko, M., Yamada, M., Uchikawa, R., Tegoshi, T., Takeda, K., Hashimoto, K., 2009. Mitochondrial DNA divergence in populations of the tapeworm *Diphyllobothrium nihonkaiense* and its phylogenetic relationship with *Diphyllobothrium klebanovskii*. Parasitol. Int. 58, 22–28.

Arriaza, B.T., Reinhard, K.J., Araújo, A.G., Orellana, N.C., Standen, V.G., 2010. Possible influence of the ENSO phenomenon on the pathoecology of diphyllobothriasis and anisakiasis in ancient Chinchorro populations. Mem. Inst. Oswaldo Cruz 105, 66–72.

Audicana, M.T., Kennedy, M.W., 2008. *Anisakis simplex*: from obscure infectious worm to inducer of immune hypersensitivity. Clin. Microbiol. Rev. 21, 360–379.

Baird, F.J., Gasser, R.B., Jabbar, A., Lopata, A.L., 2014. Foodborne anisakiasis and allergy. Mol. Cell. Probes 28, 167–174.

Broglia, A., Kapel, C., 2011. Changing dietary habits in a changing world: emerging drivers for the transmission of foodborne parasitic zoonoses. Vet. Parasitol. 182, 2–13.

Butt, A.A., Aldridge, K.E., Sanders, C.V., 2004. Infections related to the ingestion of seafood. Part II: parasitic infections and food safety. Lancet Infect. Dis. 4, 294–300.

Cabello, F.C., 2007. Acuicultura y salud pública. 'La expansión de la difilobotriasis en Chile y el mundo'. Rev. Med. Chil. 135, 1064–1071.

Chai, J.-Y., Murrell, K.D., Lymbery, A.J., 2005a. Fish-borne parasitic zoonoses: status and issues. Int. J. Parasitol. 35, 1233–1254.

Chai, J.-Y., Park, J.-H., Han, E.-T., Guk, S.-M., Shin, E.-H., Lin, A., Kim,, E.-H., Phommmasack, B., Insigiengmay, B., Rim, H.-J., 2005b. Mixed infections with *Opisthorchis viverrini* and intestinal flukes in residents of Vientiane Municipality and Saravane Province in Laos. J. Helminthol. 79, 283–289.

Chaicumpa, W., Ruangkunaporn, Y., Kalambaheti, T., Limavongpranee, S., Kitikoon, V., Khusmith, S., Pungpak, S., Chongsa-Nguan, M., Sornmani, S., 1991. Specific monoclonal antibodies to *Opisthorchis viverrini*. Int. J. Parasitol. 21, 969–974.

Chen, M.G., Lu, Y., Hua, X., Mott, K.E., 1994. Progress in assessment of morbidity due to *Clonorchis sinensis* infection: a review of recent literature. Trop. Dis. Bull. 91, R7–R65.

Cho, S.Y., Kang, S.Y., Lee, J.B., 1984. Metagonimiasis in Korea. Arzneimittelforschung 34, 1211–1213.

Conlan, J.V., Sripa, B., Attwood, S., Newton, P.N., 2011. A review of parasitic zoonoses in a changing Southeast Asia. Vet. Parasitol. 182, 22–40.

Couture, C., Measures, L., Gagnon, J., 2003. Human intestinal anisakiosis due to consumption of raw salmon. Am. J. Surg. Pathol. 27, 1167–1172.

De, N.V., Le, T.H., Murrell, K.D., 2012. Prevalence and intensity of fish-borne zoonotic trematodes in cultured freshwater fish from rural and urban areas of Northern Vietnam. J. Parasitol. 98, 1023–1025.

Dezfuli, B.S., Pironi, F., Simoni, E., Shinn, A.P., Giari, L., 2007. Selected pathological, immunohistochemical and ultrastructural changes associated with an infection by *Diphyllobothrium dendriticum* (Nitzsch, 1824) (Cestoda) plerocercoids in *Coregonus lavaretus* (L.) (Coregonidae). J. Fish Dis. 30, 471–482.

Diaz, J.H., 2013. Paragonimiasis acquired in the United States: native and non-native species. Clin. Microbiol. Rev. 26, 493–504.

Dorny, P., Praet, N., Deckers, N., Gabriel, S., 2009. Emerging food-borne parasites. Vet. Parasitol. 163, 196–206.

EFSA Panel on Biological Hazards (BIOHAZ), 2010. Scientific opinion on risk assessment of parasites in fishery products. EFSA J. 8 (4), 91 pp. Article 1543.

Fan, P.C., 1998. Viability of metacercariae of *Clonorchis sinensis* in frozen or salted freshwater fish. Int. J. Parasitol. 28, 603–605.

FAO, 2001. Codex Alimentarius. Fish and Fishery Products, vol. 9A, Food and Agriculture Organization of the United Nations, Rome. Available from: http://www.codexalimentarius.net.

FAO, 2014. FAO Yearbook, Fishery and Aquaculture Statistics, 2012. Available from: http://www.fao.org/3/a-i3740t/index.html.

FDA, 2011. Fish and Fishery Products Hazards and Controls Guidance. Available from: http://www.fda.gov/FoodGuidances.

Fried, B., Abruzzi, A., 2010. Food-borne trematode infections of humans in the United States of America. Parasitol. Res. 106, 1263–1280.

Fürst, T., Keiser, J., Utzinger, J., 2012. Global burden of human food-borne trematodiasis: a systematic review and meta-analysis. Lancet Infect. Dis. 12, 201–221.

Gracyk, T.K., Fried, B., 2007. Human waterborne trematode and protozoan infections. Adv. Parasitol. 64, 111–160.

Herrero, B., Vieites, J.M., Espiñeira, M., 2011. Detection of anisakids in fish and seafood products by real-time PCR. Food Control 22, 933–939.

Hoberg, E.P., Galbreath, K.E., Cook, J.A., Kutz, S.J., Polley, L., 2012. Northern host-parasite assemblages: history and biogeography on the borderlands of episodic climate and environmental transition. Adv. Parasitol. 79, 3–97.

Hochberg, N.S., Hamer, D.H., 2010. Anisakidosis: perils of the deep. Emerg. Infect. Dis. 51, 806–812.

Hong, S.-T., Fang, Y., 2012. *Clonorchis sinensis* and clonorchiasis, an update. Parasitol. Int. 61, 17–24.
Hu, F.Y., Yu, X.B., Ma, C.L., Zhou, H.J., Li, Y.W., Lu, F., Xu, J., Wu, Z., Hu, H., 2007. *Clonorchis sinensis*: expression, characterization, immunolocalization and serological reactivity of one excretory/secretory antigen-LPAP homologue. Exp. Parasitol. 117, 157–164.
Hung, N.M., Duc, N.V., Stauffer, J.R., Madsen, H., 2013. Use of black carp (*Mylopharyngodon piceus*) in biological control of intermediate host snails of fish-borne zoonotic trematodes in nursery ponds in the Red River delta, Vietnam. Parasit. Vectors 6, 142.
ICES, 2012. *Anisakis* larvae ("herringworm"; Nematoda) in fish. Revised and updated by Matt Longshaw. ICES Identification Leaflets for Diseases and Parasites of Fish and Shellfish, Leaflet No. 8, 5 pp.
Jenkins, E.J., Schurer, J.M., Gesy, K.M., 2011. Old problems on a new playing field: helminth zoonoses transmitted among dogs, wildlife, and people in a changing northern climate. Vet. Parasitol. 182, 54–69.
Jenkins, E.J., Castrodale, L.J., de Rosemond, S.J.C., Dixon, B.R., Elmore, S.A., Gesy, K.M., Hoberg, E.P., Polley, L., Schurer, J.M., Simard, M., Thompson, R.C.A., 2013. Tradition and transition: parasitic zoonoses of people and animals in Alaska, Northern Canada, and Greenland. Adv. Parasitol. 82, 33–204.
Johansen, M.V., Sithithaworn, P., Berquist, R., Utzinger, J., 2010. Towards improved diagnosis of zoonotic trematode infections in Southeast Asia. Adv. Parasitol. 73, 171–195.
Jongsuksuntigul, P., Imsomboon, T., 2003. Opisthorchiasis control in Thailand. Acta Trop. 88, 229–232.
Karl, H., Roepstorff, A., Huss, H.H., Bloemsa, B., 1995. Survival of *Anisakis* larvae in marinated herring fillets. Int. J. Food Sci. Technol. 29, 661–670.
Keiser, S., Utzinger, J., 2005. Emerging food-borne trematodiasis. Emerg. Infect. Dis. 11, 1507–1514.
Keiser, J., Utzinger, J., 2009. Food-borne trematodiases. Clin. Microbiol. Rev. 22, 466–483.
Keiser, J., Duthaler, U., Utzinger, J., 2010. Update on the diagnosis and treatment of food-borne trematode infections. Curr. Opin. Infect. Dis. 23, 513–520.
Kim, E.M., Verweij, J.J., Jalili, A., van Lieshout, L., Choi, M.-H., Bae, Y.M., Lim, M.K., Hong, S.-T., 2009. Detection of *Clonorchis sinensis* in stool samples using real-time PCR. Ann. Trop. Med. Parasitol. 103, 513–518.
Kuhn, T., García-Màrquez, J., Klimpel, S., 2011. Adaptive radiation within marine anisakid nematodes: a zoogeographical modeling of cosmopolitan, zoonotic parasites. PLoS One 6 (12), e28642.
Kuipers, F.C., Rodenburg, W., Wielinga, W.J., Roskam, R.T., 1960. Eosinophilic phlegmon of the alimentary canal caused by a worm. Lancet 2, 1171–1173.
Kutchta, R., Brabec, J., Kubáčková, P., Scholz, T., 2013. Tapeworm *Diphyllobothrium dendriticum* (Cestoda) – neglected or emerging human parasite? PLoS Negl. Trop. Dis. 7 (12), e2535.
Lall, M., Sahni, A.K., Rajput, A.K., 2013. Pleuropulmonary paragonimiasis: mimicker of tuberculosis. Pathog. Glob. Health 107, 40–42.
Li, K., Clausen, J.H., Murrell, K.D., Liu, L., 2013. Risks for fishborne zoonotic trematodes in tilapia production systems in Guangdong province, China. Vet. Parasitol. 198, 223–229.
Lima dos Santos, C.A.M., Howgate, P., 2011. Fishborne zoonotic parasites and aquaculture: a review. Aquaculture 318, 253–261.
Lopez, I., Pardo, M.A., 2010. Evaluation of a real-time polymerase chain reaction (PCR) assay for the detection of *Anisakis simplex* parasite as a food-borne allergen source in seafood products. J. Agric. Food Chem. 58, 1469–1477.

Lovis, L., Mak, T.K., Phongluxa, K., Soukhathammavong, P., Sayasone, S., Akkhavong, K., Odermatt, P., Keiser, J., Felger, I., 2009. PCR diagnosis of *Opisthorchis viverrini* and *Haplorchis taichui* infections in a Lao community in an area of endemicity and comparison of diagnostic methods for parasitological field surveys. J. Clin. Microbiol. 47, 1517–1523.

Ma, C.L., Hu, X.C., Hu, F.Y., Li, Y.W., Chen, X.X., Zhou, Z.W., Lu, F.L., Xu, J., Wu, Z.D., Yu, X.B., 2007. Molecular characterization and serodiagnosis analysis of a novel lysophospholipase from *Clonorchis sinensis*. Parasitol. Res. 101, 419–425.

Marty, G.D., 2008. Anisakid larvae in the viscera of a farmed Atlantic salmon (*Salmo salar*). Aquaculture 279, 209–210.

Mo, T.A., Gahr, A., Hansen, H., Hoel, E., Oaland, Ø., Poppe, T.T., 2014. Presence of *Anisakis simplex* (Rudolphi, 1809 det. Krabbe, 1878) and *Hysterothylacium aduncum* (Rudolphi, 1802) (Nematoda; Anisakidae) in runts of farmed Atlantic salmon, *Salmo salar* L. J. Fish Dis. 37, 135–140.

Mossali, C., Palermo, S., Capra, E., Piccolo, G., Botti, S., Bandi, C., D'Amelio, S., Giuffra, E., 2010. Sensitive detection and quantification of anisakid parasite residues in food products. Foodborne Pathog. Dis. 7, 391–397.

Murrell, K.D., Dalsgaard, A., 2014. Parasites. In: Ryder, J., Karunasagar, I., Ababouch, L. (Eds.), Assessment and Management of Seafood Safety and Quality: Current Practices and Emerging Issues. FAO Fisheries and Aquaculture Technical Paper No. 574. Rome, pp. 93–105.

Parvathi, A., Umesha, K.R., Kumar, S., Sithithaworn, P., Karunasagar, I., Karunasagar, I., 2008. Development and evaluation of a polymerase chain reaction (PCR) assay for the detection of *Opisthorchis viverrini* in fish. Acta Trop. 107, 13–16.

Rodriguez-Mahillo, A.I., Gonzalez-Munoz, M., de las Heras, C., Tejada, M., Moneo, I., 2010. Quantification of *Anisakis simplex* allergens in fresh, long-term frozen, and cooked fish muscle. Foodborne Pathog. Dis. 7, 967–973.

Ruangsittichai, J., Viyanant, V., Vichasri-Grams, S., Sobhon, P., Tesana, S., Upatham, E.S., Hofmann, A., Korge, G., Grams, R., 2006. *Opisthorchis viverrini*: identification of a glycine-tyrosine rich eggshell protein and its potential as a diagnostic tool for human opisthorchiasis. Int. J. Parasitol. 36, 1329–1339.

Salminen, K., 1970. The infestiveness of heat and cold exposed *Diphyllobothrium latum* plerocercoids on golden hamster. Acta Vet. Scand. 11, 247–253.

Sato, M., Thaenkham, U., Dekumyoy, P., Waikagul, J., 2010. Discrimination of *O. viverrini, C. sinensis, H. pumilio* and *H. taichui* using nuclear DNA-based PCR targeting ribosomal DNA ITS regions. Acta Trop. 109, 81–83.

Scholtz, T., Garcia, H.H., Kuchta, R., Wicht, B., 2009. Update on the human broad tapeworm (Genus *Diphyllobothrium*), including clinical relevance. Clin. Microbiol. Rev. 22, 146–160.

Schurer, J.M., Ndao, M., Skinner, S., Irvine, J., Elmore, S.A., Epp, T., 2013. Parasitic zoonoses: one health surveillance in Northern Saskatchewan. PLoS Negl. Trop. Dis. 7 (3), e2141.

Sirisinha, S., Chawengkirttikul, R., Haswell-Elkins, M.R., Elkins, D.B., Kaewkes, S., Sithithaworn, P., 1995. Evaluation of a monoclonal antibody-based enzyme linked immunosorbent assay for the diagnosis of *Opisthorchis viverrini* infection in an endemic area. Am. J. Trop. Med. Hyg. 52, 521–524.

Sohn, W.M., 2009. Fish-borne zoonotic trematode metacercariae in the Republic of Korea. Korean J. Parasitol. 47, S103–S113.

Sripa, B., 2008. Concerted action is needed to tackle liver fluke infections in Asia. PLoS Negl. Trop. Dis. 2 (5), e232.

Sripa, B., Kaewkes, S., Intapan, P.M., Maleewong, W., Brindley, P.J., 2010. Food-borne trematodiases in Southeast Asia: epidemiology, pathology, clinical manifestation and control. Adv. Parasitol. 72, 305–350.

Toledo, R., Esteban, J.G., Fried, B., 2012. Current status of food-borne trematode infections. Eur. J. Clin. Microbiol. Infect. Dis. 31, 1705–1718.

Torgerson, P.R., Macpherson, C.N.L., 2011. The socioeconomic burden of parasitic zoonoses: global trends. Vet. Parasitol. 182, 79–95.

Traub, R.J., Macarana, J., Mungthin, M., Leelayoova, S., Cribb, T., Murrell, K.D., Thompson, R.C.A., 2009. A new PCR-based approach indicates the range of *Clonorchis sinensis* now extends to central Thailand. PLoS Negl. Trop. Dis. 3, e367.

Vaiani, R., Terramocci, R., Crotti, D., Gustinelli, A., Invernizzi, S., Fioravanti, M.L., Pampiglione, S., 2006. Diphyllobothriasis in Como Lake, northern Italy: an update. Parassitologia 48, 297.

WHO, 1995. Control of foodborne trematode infections. WHO Tech. Rep. Ser. 849, 1–157.

WHO, 2004. Report of joint WHO/FAO workshop on food-borne trematode infections in Asia, Hanoi, 58 pp.

WHO, 2008. Foodborne Disease Outbreaks: Guidelines for Investigation and Control. World Health Organization, Geneva, 146 pp.

WHO, 2014. Multicriteria-Based Ranking for Risk Management of Food-Borne Parasites. Available from: http://www.fao.org/food/food-safety-quality.

Wicht, B., de Marval, F., Peduzzi, R., 2007. *Diphyllobothrium nihonkaiense* (Yamane et al., 1986) in Switzerland: first molecular evidence and case reports. Parasitol. Int. 56, 195–199.

Wicht, B., Ruggeri-Bernardi, N., Yanagida, T., Nakao, M., Peduzzi, R., Ito, A., 2010. Inter- and intra-specific characterization of tapeworms of the genus *Diphyllobothrium* (Cestoda: Diphyllobothriidae) from Switzerland, using nuclear and mitochrondrial DNA targets. Parasitol. Int. 59, 35–39.

Wongratanacheewin, S., Sermswan, R.W., Sirisinha, S., 2003. Immunology and molecular biology of *Opisthorchis viverrini* infection. Acta Trop. 88, 195–207.

Wu, Z., Guan, Y., Zhou, Z., 1996. Study of an ancient corpse of the Warring States period unearthed from Tomb No. 1 at Guo-Jia Gang in Jingmen City (A Comprehensive Study). J. Tongji Med. Univ. 16, 10.

Xu, X., Sui, J., Cao, L., Lin, H., 2010. Direct competitive enzyme-linked immunosorbent assay (ELISA) for rapid screening of anisakid larvae in seafood. J. Sci. Food Agric. 90, 877–881.

Yang, X., Nian, R., Lin, H., Duan, C., Sui, J., Cao, L., 2013. Detection of anisakid larvae in cod fillets by UV fluorescent imaging based on principal component analysis and gray value analysis. J. Food Prot. 76, 1288–1292.

Yéra, H., Nicoulaud, J., Dupouy-Camet, J., 2008. Use of nuclear and mitochondrial DNA PCR and sequencing for molecular identification of *Diphyllobothrium* isolates potentially infective for humans. Parasite 15, 402–407.

Yéra, H., Estran, C., Delaunay, P., Gari-Toussaint, M., Dupouy-Camet, J., Marty, P., 2006. Putative *Diphyllobothrium nihonkaiense* acquired from a Pacific salmon (*Oncorhynchus keta*) eaten in France; genomic identification and case report. Parasitol. Int. 55, 45–49.

Yossepowitch, O., Gotesman, T., Assous, M., Marva, E., Zimlichman, R., Dan, M., 2004. Opisthorchiasis from imported raw fish. Emerg. Infect. Dis. 10, 2122–2126.

Ziegler, A.D., Andrews, R.H., Grundy-Warr, C., Sithithaworn, P., Petney, T.N., 2011. Fighting liverflukes with food safety education. Science 331, 282–283.

Transmission dynamics of foodborne parasites on fresh produce

13

B.R. Dixon
Health Canada, Ottawa, ON, Canada

13.1 Introduction

Fresh produce contaminated with the infectious stages of parasites is an important source of infection in humans worldwide. For example, cysts and oocysts of protozoa such as *Giardia duodenalis*, *Cryptosporidium* spp., and *Cyclospora cayetanensis* have been reported on a wide variety of fresh produce worldwide and have resulted in numerous illness outbreaks and cases. In recent years, outbreaks of orally acquired Chagas' disease have been associated with the contamination of juices with the infectious stage of *Trypanosoma cruzi*. The eggs of helminth parasites, such as the nematode *Ascaris* spp. and the cestodes *Taenia solium* and *Echinococcus* spp., have also frequently been reported on fresh fruits and vegetables, and the infectious larval stage of the trematode *Fasciola* spp. has been reported on a variety of edible aquatic plants.

Contamination of fresh produce with parasites may occur through a number of different routes. Contamination of food or equipment during harvesting, packaging, transport, or food preparation may occur directly from the hands of food handlers who are infected, or who have family members that are infected, and is often associated with poor personal hygiene. The irrigation of crops with contaminated water and the use of contaminated water to mix pesticides or wash produce or equipment are other possible sources of contamination, particularly in regions where water treatment and sanitation systems are poor. Contamination of fresh produce with parasites such as *Cryptosporidium* and *Giardia* by livestock, either through direct access or through the application of manure to croplands, is also likely a factor, as is the use of human feces (night soil) as fertilizer. Domestic and wild animals are also responsible for the transmission of other produce-borne parasites. For example, cats and other felines shed infectious *Toxoplasma gondii* oocysts into the environment, likely resulting in the direct or indirect contamination of fresh produce. Dogs and other canines are solely responsible for the spread of *Echinococcus* spp. eggs into the environment and for the contamination of fresh produce and other foods. Freshwater snails serve as intermediate hosts of *Fasciola* spp., with the resulting cercariae exiting the snail before encysting on aquatic vegetation as infectious metacercariae. Also, unpasteurized tropical juices have been associated with outbreaks of Chagas' disease in South America, likely resulting from the contamination of the juice with infected triatomine bugs, or their feces, during preparation.

Foodborne Parasites in the Food Supply Web. http://dx.doi.org/10.1016/B978-1-78242-332-4.00013-8

Foodborne transmission of parasites by means of contaminated fresh produce is of growing importance, and numerous foodborne cases and outbreaks of illness due to infections with these parasites have been reported in recent years. Surveillance studies of foodborne parasites on a wide variety of fresh produce have also been conducted in many countries around the world, with a wide range of prevalences reported, likely due to different levels of sanitation and hygiene, agricultural practices, and methods used for detection. Many factors are involved in this emerging issue, including the globalization of the food trade, international travel, the increased number of immunocompromised and other susceptible individuals, and changes in consumer habits, particularly the increasing consumption of raw foods. There are, unfortunately, very few barriers to the transmission of parasitic infections associated with the consumption of fresh produce. For example, the infectious stages of most of these parasites have protective surfaces, are environmentally resistant, and can survive for long periods on moist and sheltered surfaces of many fresh fruits and vegetables (Gajadhar and Allen, 2004). Even vigorous washing of the surface of produce is not fully effective in removing the infectious stages, which are often sticky and/or are protected by crevasses or other surface structures on the produce; nor is it even feasible in the case of more delicate fruits such as raspberries. Furthermore, many of these parasites are highly resistant to chemical disinfectants used in the food industry and in water treatment. Finally, fresh produce is very often consumed raw, with no further treatments such as freezing or cooking that would otherwise readily kill most contaminating parasites.

This chapter provides an overview of the parasites of high public health significance that may be transmitted to humans via fresh produce and highlights the food surveillance studies performed worldwide, as well as the associated illness outbreaks reported. Possible sources of contamination of fresh produce are also discussed, along with potential control measures. The parasites highlighted in this chapter were selected based on their association with fresh produce with respect to surveillance studies and outbreak investigations and the availability of epidemiological data. The selection of parasites was also based on the findings of a report by the Food and Agriculture Organization of the United Nations (FAO) and the World Health Organization (WHO) on multicriteria-based ranking for risk management of foodborne parasites (FAO/WHO, 2012).

13.2 Protozoan parasites on fresh produce

13.2.1 Cyclospora cayetanensis

13.2.1.1 Overview

Cyclospora cayetanensis is a recently identified protozoan parasite of the human small intestine (Ortega et al., 1993). The life cycle of *C. cayetanensis* is similar to other coccidia and has been described in detail elsewhere (Mansfield and Gajadhar, 2004; Ortega and Sanchez, 2010). The transmission stage of *C. cayetanensis*, known as an oocyst, is spherical and is 8–10 μm in diameter. Unsporulated (immature) oocysts are shed into the environment with the feces of infected individuals. Although the oocysts do not multiply outside the host, they do undergo sporulation, depending on conditions such as temperature and humidity, becoming mature and infective within 7–15 days (Ortega and Sanchez, 2010). Details on the biology and life cycle of *C. cayetanensis* are provided in Chapter 6.

13.2.1.2 Prevalence in humans

C. cayetanensis has been identified as a cause of diarrheal illness in natives and travelers to North, Central, and South America, the Caribbean, Southeast Asia, Eastern Europe, the United Kingdom, India, and Africa (Ortega and Sanchez, 2010). Most of the prevalence data, however, come from studies conducted in endemic countries such as Nepal, Haiti, Peru, and Guatemala (Cama, 2006; Ortega and Sanchez, 2010).

13.2.1.3 Transmission

Although some earlier outbreaks of cyclosporosis (syn. cyclosporiasis) were thought to have resulted from the consumption of fecally contaminated tap water, waterborne outbreaks appear to be less common than the foodborne route (Ortega and Sanchez, 2010). Person-to-person transmission (fecal–oral route) is considered to be unlikely due to the relatively long sporulation period required before oocysts become infective. Zoonotic transmission has also been suggested, but not substantiated, and *Cyclospora*-like organisms, and/or positive polymerase chain reactions (PCRs) for *Cyclospora*, have been observed in the feces of chickens, ducks, dogs, monkeys, chimpanzees, and baboons (Ortega and Sanchez, 2010). However, to date, there is only anecdotal evidence for this method of transmission to humans.

Since 1995, numerous foodborne outbreaks and cases of cyclosporosis have been reported in North America (Ortega and Sanchez, 2010; Dixon et al., 2011). It has been estimated that 90–99% of cyclosporosis cases in the United States are foodborne (Mead et al., 1999; Scallan et al., 2011).

13.2.1.4 Surveillance studies and outbreaks associated with fresh produce

A number of surveillance studies worldwide have reported the presence of *Cyclospora* oocysts on a variety of fresh fruits and vegetables (Table 13.1). Although two small outbreaks associated with fresh produce occurred in the United States during the spring and summer of 1995, the first large outbreak of cyclosporosis in North America occurred in 1996. As summarized by Herwaldt et al. (1997), a total of 1465 cases of diarrheal illness due to *Cyclospora* infection were reported in the United States and Canada during May and June 1996. The only exposure that was consistently linked epidemiologically to *Cyclospora* infection was the consumption of imported fresh raspberries. In the spring of 1997, 1012 cases of diarrheal illness due to cyclosporosis were reported in the United States and Canada (Herwaldt et al., 1999). Fresh imported raspberries were again the only food common to all events, although one Canadian cluster suggested a possible link to fresh blackberries. In subsequent years, fresh berries and

Table 13.1 Surveillance studies reporting the presence of *Cyclospora*, *Cryptosporidium*, *Giardia*, or *Entamoeba* on fresh produce worldwide

Parasite	Country	Produce testing positive	Prevalence	Reference
Cyclospora	Cambodia	Water spinach	8%	Anh et al. (2007)
	Canada	Packaged leafy greens	1.7%[a]	Dixon et al. (2013)
	Costa Rica	Lettuce	8%	Calvo et al. (2004)
	Egypt	Lettuce	–[b]	Abou el Naga (1999)
	Egypt	Rocket, lettuce, parsley, leek, green onions	21.3%[a]	El Said Said (2012)
	Nepal	Cabbage, lettuce, mustard leaves	–[b]	Sherchand et al. (1999)
	Nepal	Lettuce, spinach, mustard leaves, basil	–[b]	Sherchan et al. (2010)
	Nepal	Radishes, cauliflower, cabbage, mustard leaves	3.3–10.0%	Ghimire et al. (2005)
	Peru	Yerba buena, huacatay, lettuce	1.8% and 1.6%[a] (two collections)	Ortega et al. (1997)
	Vietnam	Basil, coriander, mint, marjoram, persicaria, lettuce	3.75–11.6%	Tram et al. (2008)
Cryptosporidium	Cambodia	Water spinach	17%	Anh et al. (2007)
	Canada	Unpasteurized apple cider, washed apples	1–5%	Garcia et al. (2006)
	Canada	Spinach	0.6%[a]	Bohaychuk et al. (2009)
	Canada	Packaged leafy greens	5.9%[a]	Dixon et al. (2013)
	Costa Rica	Cilantro leaves, cilantro roots, lettuce, carrots, cucumbers, radishes, tomatoes	1.2–8.7%	Monge and Chinchilla (1996)
	Costa Rica	Lettuce, parsley, cilantro, blackberries	4–24%	Calvo et al. (2004)
	Egypt	Rocket, lettuce, parsley, leek, green onions	29.3%[a]	El Said Said (2012)
	Iran	Mint, leek, cress, green onions, coriander, basil	1.1–14.8%	Ranjbar-Bahadori et al. (2013)
	Nepal	Radishes, cabbage, mustard leaves	3.3–16.7%	Ghimire et al. (2005)
	Norway	Lettuce, mung bean sprouts	4%[a]	Robertson and Gjerde (2001)
	Norway	Mung bean sprouts	8% of all sprouted seed products tested	Robertson et al. (2002)
	Peru	Cabbage, celery, cilantro, green onions, green chili, leek, lettuce, parsley, yerba buena, basil	14.5% and 19.35%[a] (two collections)	Ortega et al. (1997)

	Poland	Leek, celery, white cabbage, red cabbage, Peking cabbage	4.7%[a] (all fruit samples negative)	Rzeżutka et al. (2010)
	Saudi Arabia	Watercress, leek	2.2%[a]	Al-Binali et al. (2006)
	Saudi Arabia	Onions, radishes, parsley	13%[a]	Ammar and Omar (2013)
	Spain	Lollo rosso lettuce, Romaine lettuce, Chinese cabbage	63.1%[a]	Amorós et al. (2010)
Giardia	Brazil	Lettuce (oily leaves and crisphead varieties), endive, watercress	4.0–24.0%	de Oliveira and Germano (1992b)
	Brazil	Vegetables	4.1%[a]	da Silva et al. (1995)
	Brazil	Lettuce	–[b]	Takayanagui et al. (2000)
	Brazil	Vegetables	–[b]	Coelho et al. (2001)
	Cambodia	Water spinach	56%	Anh et al. (2007)
	Canada	Packaged leafy greens	1.8%[a]	Dixon et al. (2013)
	Costa Rica	Cilantro leaves, cilantro roots	2.5–5.2%	Monge and Arias (1996)
	Egypt	Carrots, coriander, cucumbers, peppers parsley, radishes, tomatoes	8.2%[a]	Hassan et al. (2012)
	Egypt	Rocket, lettuce, parsley, leek	6.7%[a]	El Said Said (2012)
	Egypt	Lettuce, watercress, parsley, green onions, leek	8.8%[a]	Eraky et al. (2014)
	Eritrea	Cabbage, lettuce, green vegetables, tomatoes	22–50%	Srikanth and Naik (2004)
	Iran	Vegetables	6.5% of farm samples tested; 9.0% of market samples tested	Gharavi et al. (2002)
	Iran	Vegetables	7% of all market vegetables tested; 9% of all garden vegetables tested	Daryani et al. (2008)
	Iran	Leek, basil	1.83%[a]	Shahnazi and Jafari-Sabet (2010)
	Iran	Vegetables	10% of all market vegetables tested; 4% of all garden vegetables tested	Garedaghi et al. (2011)
	Iran	Spearmint, scallions, basil, cress, leek, radishes, purslane	8.2%[a]	Fallah et al. (2012)

Continued

Table 13.1 **Surveillance studies reporting the presence of *Cyclospora*, *Cryptosporidium*, *Giardia*, or *Entamoeba* on fresh produce worldwide—Cont'd**

Parasite	Country	Produce testing positive	Prevalence	Reference
	Iran	Chamomile, coriander, herb king, basil, savory, parsley, mint	17.4%[a]	Nazemi et al. (2012)
	Iran	Vegetables	8.1%[a]	Ebrahimzadeh et al. (2013)
	Iran	Vegetables	4.8%[a]	Olyaei and Hajivandi (2013)
	Iran	Vegetables	13.3%[a]	Saki et al. (2013)
	Iran	Leek, radishes, garden cress, mint	5.8% (spring) and 1.1% (winter)[a]	Ezatpour et al. (2013)
	Iran	Basil, scallions, spinach, coriander, green onions, green mint, parsley, garden cress, lettuce	10.5%[a]	Siyadatpanah et al. (2013)
	Iraq	Lettuce, celery, cress, parsley, tomatoes, radishes, cucumbers	17.28%[a]	Al-Kassar (2012)
	Iraq	Leek, celery, cress, green onion, lettuce	6.7%[a]	Ali and Ameen (2013)
	Kenya	Vegetables	–[b]	Nyarango et al. (2008)
	Libya	Tomatoes, cucumbers, lettuce, cress	10%[a]	Abougrain et al. (2010)
	Morocco	Mint, coriander, potatoes, carrots, radishes	25–83.3%	Amahmid et al. (1999)
	Norway	Dill, lettuce, mung bean sprouts, radish sprouts, strawberries	2%[a]	Robertson and Gjerde (2001)
	Norway	Mung bean sprouts, radish sprouts	2% of all sprouted seed products tested	Robertson et al. (2002)
	Palestine	Dill, rocket, cucumbers, cabbage, purslane	10.7%[a]	Al-Shawa and Mwafy (2007)
	Philippines	Vegetables	1%	de Leon et al. (1992)
	Philippines	Pechay	1.25%[a]	Sia Su et al. (2012)
	Poland	Strawberries	–[b]	Kasprzak et al. (1981)
	Saudi Arabia	Leafy vegetables	5.1%[a]	Al-Megrin (2010)
	Saudi Arabia	Lettuce, leek	1.1%[a]	Al-Binali et al. (2006)
	Saudi Arabia	Onions, radishes, rocket, lettuce, parsley	20.7%[a]	Ammar and Omar (2013)

	Spain	Iollo rosso lettuce, Romaine lettuce, Chinese cabbage	52.6%[a]	Amorós et al. (2010)
	Turkey	Lettuce, strawberries	20.0%[a]	Erdoğrul and Şener (2005)
Entamoeba histolytica	Brazil	Lettuce (oily leaves and crisphead varieties), endive, watercress	8.0–26.0% (*Entamoeba* sp. 4N)	de Oliveira and Germano (1992b)
	Brazil	Lettuce, endive	–[b]	Takayanagui et al. (2000)
	Costa Rica	Cilantro leaves, cilantro roots, lettuce, radishes, carrots, cucumbers, cabbage, tomatoes	2.0–6.2%	Monge and Arias (1996)
	Egypt	Coriander, cucumbers, peppers, radishes	7.1%[a]	Hassan et al. (2012)
	Egypt	Lettuce, watercress, parsley, green onions, leek	6.8%[a] (*Entamoeba* spp.)	Eraky et al. (2014)
	Iran	Leek, spearmint	1.37%[a]	Shahnazi and Jafari-Sabet (2010)
	Iran	Leek	1.1%[a]	Nazemi et al. (2012)
	Iran	Vegetables	5.0%[a]	Ebrahimzadeh et al. (2013)
	Iran	Vegetables	2.9%[a] (*E. histolytica/dispar*)	Saki et al. (2013)
	Iran	Scallions, spinach, parsley	1.5%[a] (*E. histolytica/dispar*)	Siyadatpanah et al. (2013)
	Iraq	Lettuce, celery, cress, parsley, tomatoes, radishes, cucumbers, peppers	25.30%[a] (*Entamoeba* spp.)	Al-Kassar (2012)
	Iraq	Leek, celery, cress, green onion, lettuce	13.8%[a]	Ali and Ameen (2013)
	Kenya	Vegetables	–[b]	Nyarango et al. (2008)
	Mexico	Carrots	0.9%	Vázquez Tsuji et al. (1997)
	Nigeria	Market vegetables	5.0%[a]	Damen et al. (2007)
	Nigeria	Cabbage, lettuce, garden egg, tomatoes	2.5%[a]	Idahosa (2011)
	Palestine	Parsley, dill, rocket, cucumbers, cabbage, purslane	13.9%[a]	Al-Shawa and Mwafy (2007)
	Philippines	Pechay	2.50%[a]	Sia Su et al. (2012)
	Saudi Arabia	Radishes, green onions	1.1%[a]	Al-Binali et al. (2006)
	Saudi Arabia	Onions, rocket, lettuce, parsley	10.7%[a] (*Entamoeba* spp.)	Ammar and Omar (2013)
	Turkey	Lettuce, parsley, strawberries	27.6%[a]	Erdoğrul and Şener (2005)

[a] Percent positive in all fresh produce samples tested.
[b] Produce tested positive but the actual prevalence was not reported.

a variety of other fresh produce items (e.g., mesclun, cilantro, snow peas, and basil) were epidemiologically linked to cyclosporosis outbreaks in North America (Ortega and Sanchez, 2010; Dixon et al., 2011). Most recently, there were large multistate outbreaks in the United States in the late spring and summer of 2013, which were associated with the consumption of imported salad mix and fresh cilantro (CDC, 2013). There has been a distinct seasonality in the foodborne outbreaks of cyclosporosis in North America, with most being reported in the spring to early summer. The first European foodborne cyclosporosis outbreak occurred in Germany in 2000 and was associated with salad consumption (Döller et al., 2002). A second European outbreak occurred in Sweden in 2009 and was associated with the consumption of imported sugar snap peas (Insulander et al., 2010). In Australia, an outbreak of cyclosporosis occurred in 2010 among passengers and crew members of two successive voyages of a cruise ship (Gibbs et al., 2013). Illnesses were thought to have been associated with the consumption of fresh produce onboard the ship, but specific foods were not identified. A few outbreaks associated with fresh produce, including watercress, salads, and raspberry juice, have also been reported in developing countries (Chacín-Bonilla, 2010).

13.2.2 Cryptosporidium *spp.*

13.2.2.1 Overview

Cryptosporidium spp. is a protozoa in the phylum Apicomplexa. It is found worldwide in a large number of different hosts, including humans. There are currently more than 20 valid species of *Cryptosporidium* and greater than 40 distinct genotypes (see list of species in Chapter 6). Some species, such as *C. hominis*, have very narrow host ranges, whereas others, such as *C. parvum*, have a wide range of hosts. A growing number of *Cryptosporidium* species have been reported to infect humans, and several genotypes have also been identified. However, approximately 90% of reported human infections involve *C. hominis*, which is found primarily in humans, and *C. parvum*, which is an important zoonotic species. *Cryptosporidium* oocysts are shed with the feces of a host and are immediately infective to subsequent hosts. Oocysts are, however, environmentally resistant and can survive for many weeks under cool and moist conditions. *C. parvum* oocysts are round, thick-walled structures of about 4–5 μm in diameter and contain four sporozoites. Further details of the biology and other characteristics of *Cryptosporidium* spp. are available in Chapter 6.

13.2.2.2 Prevalence in humans

In recent years, human infection with *Cryptosporidium* has emerged as a global public health problem and this parasite is now considered to be a common cause of gastroenteritis in immunocompetent individuals and of severe illness in immunocompromised individuals. Prevalence rates based on oocyst excretion vary from approximately 1–3% in industrialized countries, up to 10% or higher in developing countries. The higher prevalence in developing countries is likely due to a lack of clean water, poor sanitation, crowded housing conditions, and closer contact with domestic animals.

Those people at greatest risk of infection include young children, people in contact with young animals or children, international travelers, recreational water users, and consumers of poor-quality drinking water. *Cryptosporidium* oocysts are found in the stools of 10–20% of patients with AIDS-associated diarrhea, and chronic intestinal cryptosporidiosis is currently listed as an AIDS-defining disease. The prevalence of *Cryptosporidium* spp. in some animals can be very high. A 100% cumulative prevalence has been reported numerous times in young cattle and pigs, suggesting that they are important reservoir hosts (Dixon, 2009).

13.2.2.3 Transmission

Routes of transmission of cryptosporidiosis include waterborne, person-to-person (i.e., the fecal–oral route), zoonotic, and foodborne. Although there is considerable overlap among these routes of transmission, water is numerically the most important mode of transmission, with numerous outbreaks having occurred worldwide as a result of oocyst contamination of drinking water and recreational water. Direct person-to-person transmission may occur following the ingestion of oocysts in fecal matter and may be associated with poor hygiene. In the case of zoonotic species of *Cryptosporidium*, such as *C. parvum*, calves, rodents, puppies, kittens, and many other animals serve as important reservoir hosts in zoonotic transmission.

Approximately 8% of domestically acquired cases of cryptosporidiosis in the United States are foodborne (Scallan et al., 2011). The contamination of fresh produce during harvest, packaging, transport, or food preparation can occur directly from the hands of food handlers who are infected, or have family members who are infected, and is largely associated with poor personal hygiene, namely insufficient hand washing. The irrigation of crops with contaminated water and the use of contaminated water to mix pesticides or wash produce are other possible sources. The contamination of produce by livestock, either through direct access or through the application of manure to croplands, has also been proposed (Dixon, 2009).

13.2.2.4 Surveillance studies and outbreaks associated with fresh produce

Although foods are not as important in the transmission of cryptosporidiosis as water or person-to-person contact in terms of the numbers of cases or outbreaks reported, numerous surveillance studies worldwide have reported the presence of *Cryptosporidium* oocysts on fresh produce (Table 13.1).

A number of foodborne outbreaks of cryptosporidiosis associated with the consumption of fresh produce have been reported (Dixon et al., 2011). Uncooked green onions were epidemiologically associated with one such outbreak following a catered dinner in Washington State, in 1997. In another outbreak in 1998, a large number of cases were associated with eating at a university cafeteria in Washington, DC. Although no specific food item was implicated in this outbreak, an ill food handler with laboratory-confirmed cryptosporidiosis prepared raw produce used in meals served during the expected exposure period. This outbreak illustrates the need for good hygienic practices by food handlers, and a restriction from working during periods of diarrheal illness. More recently, an outbreak at a summer camp in North Carolina in 2009 was associated with sandwich-bar ingredients, including ham and lettuce, and possibly tomatoes and onions. There have also been at least four cryptosporidiosis outbreaks associated with drinking unpasteurized apple cider, all in the United States.

Fresh produce has also been implicated in a number of recent cryptosporidiosis outbreaks reported in Northern Europe (Robertson and Chalmers, 2013). An outbreak in Sweden following a wedding reception resulted in gastroenteritis in both guests and restaurant employees. Fresh parsley was determined to be the most likely source of these illnesses. Another outbreak was associated with the consumption of peeled whole carrots, grated carrots, or red peppers at a company cafeteria in Denmark. Again, the vegetables in this case were thought to have been contaminated by an infected food handler. A large outbreak in Finland was thought to have been associated with the consumption of contaminated lettuce mixture.

13.2.3 Toxoplasma gondii

13.2.3.1 Overview

Toxoplasma gondii is an obligate intracellular protozoa found worldwide in virtually all warm-blooded animals, including humans, livestock, marine mammals, and birds (Hill et al., 2005; Dubey, 2009). *T. gondii* oocysts are produced following the sexual phase of the life cycle and are shed with the feces of cats and other felids, which represent the only definitive hosts. These unsporulated oocysts require 1–5 days under favorable environmental conditions to sporulate and become infectious (Pereira et al., 2010). Intermediate hosts can also become infected through the ingestion of *T. gondii* tissue cysts from infected animals. See Chapter 6 for more details on the life cycle and biology of *T. gondii*.

13.2.3.2 Prevalence in humans

Toxoplasmosis in humans occurs worldwide. Although the prevalence varies widely among different regions, the overall prevalence of infection is thought to be extremely high, estimated at one-third of the world's population (Pereira et al., 2010). The seroprevalence of toxoplasmosis is much higher in countries and regions in which more meat is consumed raw or undercooked. For example, a prevalence of anti-*Toxoplasma* antibodies of over 90% was reported in France and South America (McCabe and Remington, 1988; Remington, 1990).

13.2.3.3 Transmission

Transmission of toxoplasmosis is primarily foodborne, and Scallan et al. (2011) estimated that 50% of domestically acquired cases of toxoplasmosis in the United States are foodborne. Foodborne transmission is thought to occur primarily through the consumption of raw or poorly cooked meats or organ tissues containing tissue cysts or through the consumption of unpasteurized milk containing tachyzoites (Pereira et al., 2010). Very little information is available regarding the potential for transmission through the ingestion of oocysts on contaminated fresh produce.

13.2.3.4 Surveillance studies and outbreaks associated with fresh produce

There are few methods for the detection of *T. gondii* oocysts on produce, and as a result, very little information is available regarding their prevalence. Al-Megrin (2010) reported a 1.1% prevalence of *T. gondii* oocysts on leafy vegetables in Saudi Arabia. Another study reported the detection of *Toxoplasma* DNA by real-time PCR in 9.7% of fruit and vegetable samples collected in Poland (Lass et al., 2012). Direct contact with cat feces (i.e., cats actively shedding oocysts) or oocyst-contaminated water may represent important sources of food contamination. There have been very few reported outbreaks of toxoplasmosis associated with fresh produce. Ekman et al. (2012) described an outbreak of acute toxoplasmosis in Brazil, which was associated with the consumption of green vegetables.

13.2.4 Entamoeba histolytica

13.2.4.1 Overview

Entamoeba histolytica is a parasitic amoeba belonging to the phylum Sarcomastigophora, which has an environmentally resistant infectious stage, known as a cyst. In the intestine, cysts undergo excystation, and the intestinal stage, known as a trophozoite, is released and begins to multiply asexually. *E. histolytica* has been reported in humans worldwide but is more prevalent in the tropics and subtropics than in cooler regions (Ortega, 2006). *E. histolytica* trophozoites are between 12 and 60 μm in diameter, and cysts are typically 10–20 μm (Ortega, 2006). Mature cysts have four characteristic nuclei. *E. histolytica* is morphologically very similar to the nonpathogenic species, *E. dispar*.

13.2.4.2 Prevalence in humans

Although humans are thought to be the primary reservoirs for *E. histolytica,* this parasite also infects nonhuman primates (Ortega, 2006). The WHO has estimated that there are 50 million infections per year, and up to 50% of the population in endemic regions can be infected (Ortega, 2006).

13.2.4.3 Transmission

Transmission of *E. histolytica* occurs through the ingestion of cysts by means of the direct person-to-person route, including sexual transmission, or indirectly through cyst-contaminated water or food. Because *E. histolytica* is found primarily in humans and nonhuman primates, zoonotic transmission does not play as important a role as it does for some other parasites. Fresh produce and other foods can become contaminated with cysts of *E. histolytica* through the use of sewage-contaminated water for irrigation, washing, or processing, and poor hygiene among farm workers or food handlers.

13.2.4.4 Surveillance studies and outbreaks associated with fresh produce

Several surveillance studies have reported the presence of *E. histolytica* cysts on fresh produce (Table 13.1). Foodborne illness due to infection with *E. histolytica* is largely sporadic and few large outbreaks have been documented (de Lalla et al., 1992).

13.2.5 Giardia duodenalis

13.2.5.1 Overview

Giardia duodenalis (syn. *G. lamblia, G. intestinalis*) is a flagellate protozoa infecting humans and a wide variety of other mammals worldwide. *G. duodenalis* has a direct life cycle consisting of an environmentally resistant transmission stage known as a cyst, which is oval in shape, 8–12 μm in length, and contains four nuclei. Cysts are shed with the feces of the host and are transmitted to new hosts primarily through contaminated water or by direct contact with feces containing cysts, as well as through contaminated foods. Despite their morphological similarity, isolates of *G. duodenalis* show considerable genetic heterogeneity. It is generally believed that humans are only infected with two lineages: Assemblages A and B. In addition to humans, these two assemblages are also infective to hosts such as livestock, dogs, and beavers (Feng and Xiao, 2011). Other assemblages of less zoonotic significance have also been identified by DNA analysis. Further details on the taxonomy and biology of *Giardia* spp. are available in Chapter 7.

13.2.5.2 Prevalence in humans

G. duodenalis is one of the most common intestinal parasites in humans throughout the world. Prevalence rates for giardiosis (syn. giardiasis) generally range from 2% to 7% in developed countries, and, according to most studies, from 20% to 30% in developing countries (Dixon et al., 2011). Giardiosis is more prevalent in children than in adults, possibly because many individuals seem to have a lasting immunity after infection. Age-specific prevalence rises through infancy and childhood and declines in adolescence. High-risk groups include infants and young children, travelers, and immunocompromised individuals.

13.2.5.3 Transmission

The transmission of giardiosis is dependent on the ingestion of viable cysts. Transmission of giardiosis occurs predominantly by means of fecal–oral contamination, and this route is responsible for many outbreaks, particularly in institutional settings where personal hygiene may be poor. Waterborne transmission is probably the most widely recognized means of transmission, with numerous outbreaks associated with cyst-contaminated drinking water or recreational water. Although humans probably represent the most important reservoir for *G. duodenalis*, a large number of mammals, including most domestic animals and pets, also serve as hosts, and there is considerable evidence supporting zoonotic transmission (Feng and Xiao, 2011). Considerably less common than other routes, foodborne transmission of giardiosis nevertheless has become more widely recognized in recent years. Scallan et al. (2011) estimated that 7% of domestically acquired cases of giardiosis in the United States are foodborne.

13.2.5.4 Surveillance studies and outbreaks associated with fresh produce

In surveillance studies, *Giardia* cysts have been detected on fresh produce in many countries, particularly in the Middle East (Table 13.1). Foodborne outbreaks of giardiosis have been reported worldwide. An outbreak was reported following a party in New Jersey (Porter et al., 1990). The implicated food in this outbreak was fruit salad, which had been prepared by a woman who became ill 9 days after the party. She had a young child in diapers who attended a day care and was subsequently found to be infected. Another outbreak was reported following a dinner for members of a church youth group in New Mexico (Grabowski et al., 1989). The most likely vehicles of transmission in this outbreak were taco ingredients including lettuce, tomatoes, and onions. In yet another outbreak originating in the cafeteria of a corporate office in Connecticut, the probable vehicle was raw sliced vegetables served in the cafeteria and prepared by an infected, asymptomatic food handler (Mintz et al., 1993).

13.2.6 Trypanosoma cruzi

13.2.6.1 Overview

T. cruzi is a flagellate protozoa responsible for Chagas' disease or South American trypanosomosis (syn. trypanosomiasis). *T. cruzi* multiplies in the gut of triatomine bugs, which serve as intermediate hosts. A variety of mammals serve as definitive hosts, including humans. The infectious form of *T. cruzi* is shed with the insect's feces, which may be deposited on the lips or near mucous membranes, and subsequent scratching in the area of irritation after the deposition of the feces or bite of the insect allows the parasite to enter the body. The parasite then circulates in the blood, eventually reaching skeletal muscle or heart tissues (Pereira et al., 2009). The life cycle is completed when trypomastigote stages circulating in the blood are ingested by triatomine bugs during feeding on definitive hosts.

13.2.6.2 Prevalence in humans

Approximately 8 million people are currently infected with Chagas' disease in North, Central, and South America (Bern et al., 2011).

13.2.6.3 Transmission

Although transmission of *T. cruzi* is primarily vector-borne, other mechanisms include blood transfusions, organ transplants, congenital transmission, and oral transmission. Orally acquired Chagas' disease may result from the ingestion of contaminated mother's milk, raw or poorly cooked meat from infected animals, foods contaminated with infected triatomine bugs or their feces, or foods contaminated with anal gland secretions of marsupials (Pereira et al., 2009). It has also been associated with the consumption of a variety of unpasteurized juices in South America (e.g., açaí juice, sugarcane juice, guava juice) contaminated with trypanosomes (Pereira et al., 2009). The contamination of juice is thought to occur in a number of different ways depending on the type of juice. For example, sugarcane juice may become contaminated when the cane is ground up along with infected triatomine bugs. When açaí juice is prepared at night it is thought that light inside the grinding machine attracts triatomine bugs, which then fall into the juice being prepared. Alternatively, the fruit may be stored and transported together with infected insects and/or their feces.

13.2.6.4 Surveillance studies and outbreaks associated with fresh produce

No surveillance studies have been reported on *T. cruzi* in fresh produce or juices. A number of outbreaks of orally acquired Chagas' disease associated with the consumption of unpasteurized juices have been reported, particularly in the Amazon Basin of Brazil and in Venezuela (Pereira et al., 2009; Bern et al., 2011). A variety of juices have been implicated in these outbreaks (see Section 13.2.6.3). Severe infections have been reported in many of these outbreaks, with several cases resulting in death.

13.2.7 Other protozoan parasites

A few other protozoa of concern to public health have occasionally been reported on fresh produce. *Cystoisospora belli* (formerly *Isospora belli*) oocysts were reported on 2% of raw vegetables tested in Iran (Ebrahimzadeh et al., 2013). The ciliate *Balantidium coli* was reported on 2.2% of vegetables collected from farms in Iran (Nazemi et al., 2012) and 0.8% of market vegetables in Nigeria (Ogbolu et al., 2009). *B. coli* was also reported on vegetables in Kenya, but no prevalence was given (Nyarango et al., 2008). Similarly, a recent study in Saudi Arabia reported this parasite at a prevalence of 2.3% on vegetables (Ammar and Omar, 2013). *Blastocystis hominis* cysts have been reported on leafy vegetables in Saudi Arabia by Al-Binali et al. (2006) (4.4% prevalence) and Al-Megrin (2010) (2.8% prevalence). The microsporidia are an emerging concern in fresh produce. Thurston-Enriquez et al. (2002) reported the presence of human pathogenic microsporidia in 28% of irrigation water samples collected in the United States, Costa Rica, Mexico, and Panama, and a recent study done in Egypt reported *Microsporidium* spp. spores on raw vegetables at a prevalence of 25.3% (El Said Said, 2012). The first reported foodborne outbreak associated with microsporidia (*Enterocytozoon bieneusi*) occurred in Sweden in 2009 and was associated with the consumption of contaminated cucumber slices (Decraene et al., 2012).

13.3 Helminth parasites on fresh produce

13.3.1 *Ascaris* spp.

13.3.1.1 Overview

The nematode *Ascaris lumbricoides* is a common intestinal parasite of humans. It is one of a group of so-called soil-transmitted helminths that are responsible for a large number of human infections worldwide. In addition to *A. lumbricoides* (roundworms), this group includes whipworms (*Trichuris trichiura*) and hookworms (*Ancylostoma duodenale* and *Necator americanus*), and it is common for individuals, especially children, in developing countries to be infected with all three types of parasites (Bethony et al., 2006). Upon ingestion, *Ascaris* eggs hatch and larvae penetrate the intestine and migrate to the liver and lungs, where they are coughed up and swallowed. The larvae then develop into mature adult male and female worms in the intestine. *A. lumbricoides* are very large parasites, measuring 15–45 cm in length as adults (Ojha et al., 2014). Eggs are shed with the feces of the host. Further details on the biology and life cycle of *Ascaris* spp. and other foodborne nematodes are available in Chapter 8.

13.3.1.2 Prevalence in humans

Ascaris lumbricoides is a very common intestinal nematode, which is estimated to infect 1.4 billion people, particularly in the tropics and subtropics (Scott, 2008).

13.3.1.3 Transmission

Ascaris are generally known as soil-transmitted parasites as their eggs are often ingested through either accidental or intentional ingestion of soil. However, the consumption of fresh produce contaminated with *Ascaris* eggs is another important mechanism of transmission. The latter mechanism is thought to be increasing due to a trend toward the use of organic fertilizers, and the reuse of wastewater to fertilize and irrigate crops (Scott, 2008).

13.3.1.4 Surveillance studies and outbreaks associated with fresh produce

Ascaris lumbricoides eggs have been detected in numerous surveillance studies on fresh produce worldwide (Table 13.2). Amahmid et al. (1999) demonstrated that irrigating crops with raw wastewater led to the contamination of the vegetables with *Ascaris* eggs and *Giardia* cysts.

Table 13.2 Surveillance studies reporting the presence of *Ascaris* spp. eggs on fresh produce worldwide

Country	Produce testing positive	Prevalence	Reference
Brazil	Lettuce (oily leaves and crisphead varieties), endive, watercress	8.0–32.0%	de Oliveira and Germano (1992a)
Brazil	Vegetables	7.3%[a]	da Silva et al. (1995)
Brazil	Lettuce	–[b]	Takayanagui et al. (2000)
Brazil	Vegetables	–[b]	Coelho et al. (2001)
Egypt	Rocket, lettuce, parsley, leek, green onions	20.3%[a]	El Said Said (2012)
Egypt	Lettuce, watercress	0.6%[a]	Eraky et al. (2014)
Ghana	Lettuce, cabbage, spring onion	55–65%	Amoah et al. (2006)
India	Vegetables	36%[a]	Gupta et al. (2009)
Iran	Vegetables	1.1% of all farm samples tested; 6.6% of all market samples tested	Gharavi et al. (2002)
Iran	Vegetables	2%[a]	Daryani et al. (2008)
Iran	Leek, spring onion	2.29%[a]	Shahnazi and Jafari-Sabet (2010)
Iran	Vegetables	2%[a]	Garedaghi et al. (2011)
Iran	Spearmint, scallions, basil, cress, leek, radishes, purslane	14.1%[a]	Fallah et al. (2012)
Iran	Chamomile, herb king, basil, mint	5.4%[a]	Nazemi et al. (2012)
Iran	Vegetables	3.3%[a]	Olyaei and Hajivandi (2013)
Iran	Leek, green onions, garden cress, mint	4.7% (spring) and 1.1% (winter)[a]	Ezatpour et al. (2013)
Iran	Vegetables	6.1%[a]	Ebrahimzadeh et al. (2013)
Iraq	Lettuce, celery, cress, parsley, tomatoes, radishes, cucumbers	20.37%[a]	Al-Kassar (2012)
Iraq	Leek, celery, cress	11.3%[a]	Ali and Ameen (2013)
Kenya	Vegetables	–[b]	Nyarango et al. (2008)
Libya	Tomatoes, cucumbers, lettuce, cress	68%[a]	Abougrain et al. (2010)
Mexico	Carrots, potatoes, mushrooms, coriander, sweet potatoes, spinach	1.9–20.0%	Vázquez Tsuji et al. (1997)

Table 13.2 **Continued**

Country	Produce testing positive	Prevalence	Reference
Morocco	Potatoes, turnips, squash, marrow, coriander, carrots, mint, radishes	25–50%	Amahmid et al. (1999)
Morocco	Mint, parsley/coriander, cabbage, lettuce, radishes	10.2%[a]	Hajjami et al. (2013)
Nigeria	Green vegetable, fluted pumpkin, water leaf, cabbage, carrots, guava, oranges, pineapples	–[b]	Uneke (2007)
Nigeria	Market vegetables	6.2%[a]	Damen et al. (2007)
Nigeria	Market vegetables	16.7%[a]	Ogbolu et al. (2009)
Nigeria	Lettuce, spinach, pumpkin	1.5%[a]	Idahosa (2011)
Nigeria	Lettuce, garden egg	0.5%[a]	Adamu et al. (2012)
Nigeria	Fruits and vegetables	0.78%[a]	Omowaye and Odikamnoro (2013)
Palestine	Parsley, rocket, cucumber, cabbage, purslane	7.4%[a]	Al-Shawa and Mwafy (2007)
Philippines	Pechay, lettuce	45.00%[a]	Sia Su et al. (2012)
Poland	Leek, onions, rhubarb, beetroot	5.4%[a] (organic farms); 7.7%[a] (conventional farms)	Kłapeć and Borecka (2012)
Saudi Arabia	Lettuce, watercress, radishes, leek	5.6%[a]	Al-Binali et al. (2006)
Saudi Arabia	Leafy vegetables	4.3%[a]	Al-Megrin (2010)
Turkey	Lettuce, parsley, spinach, strawberries	31.4%[a]	Erdoğrul and Şener (2005)
Turkey	Lettuce	0.98%[a]	Kozan et al. (2005)
Turkey	Lettuce, parsley	1.8%[a]	Adanir and Tasci (2013)
Vietnam	Pumpkin leaves, water morning glory, coriander, sawtooth coriander, basil, *Houttuynia*, *Centella*, lettuce, King-guy-soy, taro, jicama, carrots, tomato	21%[a]	Uga et al. (2009)

[a] Percent positive in all fresh produce samples tested.
[b] Produce tested positive but the actual prevalence was not reported.

Very few foodborne outbreaks of ascariosis (syn. ascariasis) have been reported. Räisänen et al. (1985) described a local epidemic of ascariosis in Finland that was associated with imported vegetables. The intentional contamination of food with *A. suum* eggs caused illness in several people in Quebec, Canada, in 1970.

13.3.2 *Fasciola spp. and Fasciolopsis buski*

13.3.2.1 Overview

The liver flukes, *Fasciola* spp., are digenetic trematodes, which are common parasites of sheep and cattle worldwide. Both *F. hepatica* and *F. gigantica* have also been reported in humans. *Fasciolopsis buski* is a large intestinal fluke infecting humans and pigs primarily in India and in other areas of South and Southeast Asia. The life cycle of both *Fasciola* spp. and *Fasciolopsis buski* is similar. Eggs are shed with the feces of the livestock or human hosts and require a source of freshwater for further development to take place. Upon hatching, the miracidium larvae penetrate freshwater snails and undergo further development through a sporocyst stage to a redia, and finally a cercaria, which then exits the snail host and becomes free-swimming. The cercariae larvae then encyst on aquatic vegetation, and the resulting metacercariae await ingestion by suitable final hosts. Cercariae can also encyst without attaching to vegetation and can be transmitted through contaminated drinking water. Upon ingestion, the larvae excyst in the small intestine and, in the case of *Fasciola* spp., travel to the liver and eventually the bile ducts where they mature and produce eggs (Fried and Abruzzi, 2010). Conversely, *F. buski* develop into mature adults within the small intestine. Further details on the biology and life cycle of foodborne trematodes are provided in Chapter 10.

13.3.2.2 Prevalence in humans

F. hepatica is found in humans and livestock worldwide, whereas *F. gigantica* is reported mainly in Asia and Africa (Adams, 2006; Mas-Coma et al., 2007). Although *F. hepatica* is reported much more commonly in humans than *F. gigantica*, estimates of the total combined human infections range from 2.4 to 17 million or more (Mas-Coma et al., 2007). The prevalence of fasciolopsiosis (syn. fasciolopsiasis) has been reported to be 50% or greater of the population in some endemic regions (Mas-Coma et al., 2007).

13.3.2.3 Transmission

Transmission of both *Fasciola* spp. and *F. buski* in humans occurs by means of the consumption of raw aquatic plants contaminated with encysted metacercariae. Watercress is most commonly associated with *Fasciola* spp. infections in humans, although mint, lettuce, parsley, and wild watercress may also be contaminated with these parasites (Adams, 2006). In the case of *F. buski*, the most commonly implicated aquatic plants are water chestnut, water caltrop, lotus, bamboo, water hyacinth, water mimosa, and water spinach (Adams, 2006). The contamination of aquatic plants with *Fasciola* spp. and *F. buski* is often associated with agricultural practices, particularly the application of livestock manure or human feces, which may contain eggs, to fields as fertilizer.

13.3.2.4 Surveillance studies and outbreaks associated with fresh produce

There are very little data available on the prevalence of metacercariae on natural watercress or other aquatic plants. Dreyfuss et al. (2005) reported the presence of low numbers of *F. hepatica* metacercariae in watercress beds (2.6–6.3 per bed) in central France over a 15-year surveillance study. Numerous studies, however, have reported the presence of *Fasciola* spp. eggs on fresh produce (de Oliveira and Germano, 1992a; Daryani et al., 2008; Al-Megrin, 2010; Garedaghi et al., 2011; Al-Kassar, 2012; Nazemi et al., 2012; Olyaei and Hajivandi, 2013; Omowaye and Odikamnoro, 2013; Ezatpour et al., 2013; Ebrahimzadeh et al., 2013; Ali and Ameen, 2013; Siyadatpanah et al., 2013). Although these eggs are not directly infectious to humans, their presence is indicative of fecal contamination of the produce by infected humans or livestock.

Mas-Coma et al. (2007) provided an overview of the cases and outbreaks of fasciolosis (syn. fascioliasis) reported in endemic regions. Fried and Abruzzi (2010) listed case reports of fasciolosis in the United States, almost all of which were acquired outside the continental United States. Only a few outbreaks of fasciolosis have been reported. Bjorland et al. (1995) reported an outbreak among Aymara Indians in Bolivia in 1991, which was associated with the consumption of an aquatic plant called kjosco. Espino et al. (1998) described an outbreak in Cuba in 1995, which was linked to the consumption of lettuce contaminated with metacercariae. Mailles et al. (2006) reported the first outbreak associated with commercialized cultivated watercress in France. Eighteen confirmed cases were identified in this outbreak. Weisenberg and Perlada (2013) reported on two related domestically acquired cases of fasciolosis in California, which were associated with the consumption of watercress.

13.3.3 Taenia solium

13.3.3.1 Overview

Humans can serve as both intermediate and definitive hosts for *Taenia solium*. The adult stage of this tapeworm is parasitic only in human hosts, where it inhabits the small intestine. Pigs serve as intermediate hosts in the life cycle and become infected by ingesting *T. solium* eggs in human feces. Infection with adult tapeworms in humans, known as taeniosis (syn. taeniasis), results from the ingestion of cysticerci larvae in raw or undercooked pork. Taeniosis is generally characterized by mild symptoms or may be asymptomatic. Of much greater public health concern is human infection with the cysticercus larval stage, which results from ingestion of *T. solium* eggs produced by adult tapeworms in infected persons. Invasive oncospheres within the eggs are released in the intestine of the host, enter the bloodstream, and are carried to the muscles and other tissues where they encyst as cysticerci larvae. Cysticerci eventually reach a size of 1–2 cm. Although the cysticerci larvae may be present throughout the body, cysts that establish outside the central nervous system do not generally cause significant symptoms (Garcia et al., 2003). However, cysts commonly become established in the central nervous system and may result in severe or fatal neurological disease (neurocysticercosis). For example, neurocysticercosis is the most common cause of acquired epilepsy worldwide (Garcia et al., 2003). Details on the life cycle and biology of foodborne cestodes are provided in Chapter 9.

13.3.3.2 Prevalence in humans

Human infections with adult *T. solium* are endemic in developing countries worldwide, especially in rural areas where people live in close contact with pigs, and consume raw or undercooked pork. Neurocysticercosis is prevalent in humans in Latin America, as well as in much of Asia, sub-Saharan Africa, and parts of Oceania (Garcia et al., 2003). Bern et al. (1999) estimated that 20 million people worldwide are infected with *T. gondii* cysticerci, and 400,000 people have symptomatic neurocysticercosis in Latin America alone. Neurocysticercosis has also been reported in many developed countries as a result of increased immigration, international travel, and improved diagnostic methods (Pawlowski et al., 2005; Bowman et al., 2006).

13.3.3.3 Transmission

Transmission of *T. solium* taeniosis occurs through the ingestion of cysticerci in raw or undercooked pork. Cysticercosis is transmitted to humans, and to pigs, through the ingestion of *T. solium* eggs shed with the feces of humans infected with the adult tapeworms. In humans, the ingestion of eggs often occurs within households where persons with asymptomatic taeniosis are present. Autoinfection can also play a role in neurocysticercosis, as the intestinal form of the infection is often reported in patients diagnosed with neurocysticercosis (Garcia et al., 2003; Bowman et al., 2006). *T. solium* eggs may also be ingested along with fecally contaminated water or food, particularly fresh fruit and vegetables.

13.3.3.4 Surveillance studies and outbreaks associated with fresh produce

Numerous studies have reported the presence of *Taenia* spp. eggs on fresh produce. None of these studies, however, identified the species of *Taenia* present. In Brazil, de Oliveira and Germano (1992a) reported a *Taenia* sp. prevalence of 2.5% on a variety of leafy greens, and da Silva et al. (1995) reported a prevalence of 0.5% on all vegetables tested. In Nigeria, Ogbolu et al. (2009) reported these eggs on 4.2% of market vegetables, while Omowaye and Odikamnoro (2013) reported only a 0.04% prevalence on fruits and vegetables. Kozan et al. (2005) reported *Taenia* spp. eggs on 3.45% of unwashed vegetables in Turkey, whereas Adanir and Tasci (2013) reported a 2.7% prevalence in the same country. *Taenia* spp. eggs were also reported on 3.2% of leafy vegetables in Saudi Arabia (Al-Megrin, 2010). In Iraq, Al-Kassar (2012) reported the presence of *Taenia* spp. eggs on 4.32% of all vegetables tested. In another study done in Iraq, Ali and Ameen (2013) reported the presence of these eggs on 10.0% of all vegetables tested. Several surveillance studies in different regions of Iran have also reported *Taenia* spp. eggs on fresh produce. Gharavi et al. (2002) reported a relatively low prevalence of *Taenia* spp. eggs on vegetables from farms (0.8%) and markets (0.6%) in Tehran, Iran. Fallah et al. (2012) reported that 9.2% of unwashed vegetable samples were contaminated with taeniid eggs in Shahrekord, Iran. Shahnazi and Jafari-Sabet (2010) reported a prevalence of 1.83% on vegetables (parsley and lettuce) in villages of Qazvin Province, Iran. Olyaei and Hajivandi (2013) reported that 20%

of all vegetables tested in southern Iran contained *Taenia* spp. eggs. Ebrahimzadeh et al. (2013) reported a 13.1% prevalence in Zahedan, Iran. Similarly, Daryani et al. (2008) reported a 14% prevalence on market vegetables and a 16% prevalence on garden vegetables collected in Ardabil, Iran. Garedaghi et al. (2011) reported a 22% prevalence on market vegetables and a 10% prevalence on garden vegetables collected in Tabriz, Iran. Siyadatpanah et al. (2013) reported a 1.5% prevalence on vegetables in Amol, Iran. In Vietnam, Uga et al. (2009) reported a 1% prevalence of *Taenia* sp. eggs on vegetables (water morning glory). A few additional published studies reported the presence of eggs on vegetables, but did not differentiate between *Taenia* spp. and *Echinococcus* spp.

Schantz et al. (1992) reported on a now widely cited outbreak of neurocysticercosis in an Orthodox Jewish community in New York City. Although the infected individuals did not eat pork, they appear to have acquired the infections from *T. solium*-infected housekeepers who had recently emigrated from Latin America. At least one of these employees was actively shedding *T. solium* eggs and may have contaminated prepared foods.

13.3.4 Echinococcus *spp.*

13.3.4.1 Overview

In humans, the tapeworms *Echinococcus granulosus* and *E. multilocularis* are the two most important species within this genus from a public health perspective (Bowman et al., 2006). The adult stage of *E. granulosus* is only 3–6 mm long and inhabits the small intestine of dogs, which serve as definitive hosts. Eggs are shed with the dogs' feces and must be ingested by an appropriate intermediate host for the completion of the life cycle. Sheep serve as the most important intermediate hosts, although cattle, goats, pigs, and other livestock are also potential hosts. Adults of *E. multilocularis* are 1.2–4.5 mm long and exist in the small intestine of foxes, coyotes, and other wild canids and, increasingly, in dogs. The intermediate hosts of *E. multilocularis* include a variety of rodents. Humans can serve as accidental, or dead-end, intermediate hosts in the life cycle of *Echinococcus* spp. through the ingestion of eggs shed in definitive host feces. This disease in humans is known as echinococcosis and may be either cystic echinococcosis (CE), also known as hydatid disease, caused by infection with the larval stage of *E. granulosus*, or alveolar echinococcosis (AE), caused by infection with the larval stage of *E. multilocularis*. CE is generally asymptomatic in humans, although gradually enlarging cysts in the liver and lungs can cause problems years later. AE is rarer in humans but may result in much more severe symptoms, including liver dysfunction or failure. Eggs are shed with the feces of the definitive hosts, and when ingested with food or water by intermediate hosts, including humans, oncospheres are released and penetrate the intestinal wall before entering the bloodstream and traveling to various organs, most importantly, the liver and lungs. Oncospheres then develop into cysts that continue to slowly enlarge. The life cycle is completed when the infected intermediate host is eaten by a suitable definitive host.

13.3.4.2 Prevalence in humans

CE is the most common form of echinococcosis in humans worldwide. The highest prevalence of CE in humans and animals is found in temperate regions, including the Mediterranean region, central and southern Russia, China, Australia, South America, northern and eastern Africa (Bowman et al., 2006). Human AE occurs widely in the northern hemisphere, where there are a number of endemic foci with particularly high prevalences (Torgerson et al., 2010). Overall, however, AE is relatively rare in humans, despite a high prevalence of infection in wild canids in some regions.

13.3.4.3 Transmission

Human infection (echinococcosis) may occur through direct contact with infected canids or indirectly through the ingestion of eggs in contaminated water or food.

13.3.4.4 Surveillance studies and outbreaks associated with fresh produce

There is very little data available on the prevalence of *Echinococcus* spp. eggs on fresh produce or other foods. As noted previously, a number of published studies have reported the presence of taeniid eggs on fresh vegetables, but did not differentiate between *Taenia* spp. and *Echinococcus* spp. Outbreaks of echinococcosis associated with consumption of contaminated fresh produce have not been reported.

13.3.5 Other helminth parasites

In addition to ascarids, the eggs of a number of other important soil-transmitted helminths have been reported worldwide on fresh produce and also pose a risk to consumers. For example, pinworm eggs, *Enterobius vermicularis*, have been reported on a variety of fresh produce items in Brazil (de Oliveira and Germano, 1992a; da Silva et al., 1995), Egypt (Eraky et al., 2014), Iran (Gharavi et al., 2002; Ebrahimzadeh et al., 2013; Olyaei and Hajivandi, 2013; Ezatpour et al., 2013), Iraq (Ali and Ameen, 2013), Nigeria (Maikai et al., 2012; Omowaye and Odikamnoro, 2013), Palestine (Al-Shawa and Mwafy, 2007), the Philippines (Sia Su et al., 2012), Saudi Arabia (Al-Binali et al., 2006; Ammar and Omar, 2013), and Turkey (Erdoğrul and Şener, 2005; Adanir and Tasci, 2013). Eggs of *Toxocara* spp. have been reported on fruits and vegetables in Brazil (de Oliveira and Germano, 1992a), Egypt (El Said Said, 2012), Iran (Gharavi et al., 2002; Fallah et al., 2012; Olyaei and Hajivandi, 2013; Ebrahimzadeh et al., 2013; Siyadatpanah et al., 2013), Iraq (Al-Kassar, 2012), Libya (Abougrain et al., 2010), Mexico (Vázquez Tsuji et al., 1997), Morocco (Hajjami et al., 2013), Nigeria (Maikai et al., 2012), Poland (Kłapeć and Borecka, 2012), Saudi Arabia (Al-Binali et al., 2006; Ammar and Omar, 2013), Turkey (Kozan et al., 2005; Adanir and Tasci, 2013), and Vietnam (Uga et al., 2009). *Trichuris* spp. eggs have been reported on fresh produce in Brazil (da Silva et al., 1995), Ghana (Amoah et al., 2006), India (Gupta et al., 2009), Iran (Gharavi et al., 2002; Shahnazi and Jafari-Sabet, 2010; Olyaei and Hajivandi, 2013; Ebrahimzadeh et al., 2013), Iraq (Al-Kassar, 2012),

Kenya (Nyarango et al., 2008), Nigeria (Damen et al., 2007; Uneke, 2007; Adamu et al., 2012; Idahosa, 2011; Maikai et al., 2012; Omowaye and Odikamnoro, 2013), Palestine (Al-Shawa and Mwafy, 2007), the Philippines (Sia Su et al., 2012), Poland (Kłapeć and Borecka, 2012), Saudi Arabia (Ammar and Omar, 2013), and Vietnam (Uga et al., 2009).

The eggs and larval stages of *Ancylostoma* spp. and *Strongyloides stercoralis* have also been reported on fresh produce in many studies, but the risk of infection to humans is less clear as these parasites are generally transmitted by means of skin-penetration by the filariform larvae. Zeehaida et al. (2011), however, reported the presence of *S. stercoralis* rhabditiform larvae in the water used to elute parasites from fresh vegetables and herbs in Malaysia and suggested that vegetable sellers and food handlers are the groups at highest risk of infection.

The infectious stages of a few other helminth parasites have also been widely reported on fresh produce. For example, eggs of the cestode, *Hymenolepis nana*, have been reported on produce in Brazil (Takayanagui et al., 2000), Egypt (El Said Said, 2012; Eraky et al., 2014), Iran (Daryani et al., 2008; Shahnazi and Jafari-Sabet, 2010; Garedaghi et al., 2011; Olyaei and Hajivandi, 2013; Ebrahimzadeh et al., 2013; Siyadatpanah et al., 2013), Iraq (Al-Kassar, 2012), Nigeria (Damen et al., 2007; Idahosa, 2011), and Palestine (Al-Shawa and Mwafy, 2007). In Saudi Arabia, Al-Megrin (2010) reported the presence of *Hymenolepis* sp. eggs in leafy vegetables. Eggs and larvae of the nematode, *Trichostrongylus* spp. have also been frequently reported in surveillance studies on fresh vegetables, including studies in Brazil (de Oliveira and Germano, 1992a), Iran (Gharavi et al., 2002; Daryani et al., 2008; Shahnazi and Jafari-Sabet, 2010; Garedaghi et al., 2011; Fallah et al., 2012; Ebrahimzadeh et al., 2013; Olyaei and Hajivandi, 2013; Siyadatpanah et al., 2013), the Philippines (Sia Su et al., 2012), and Saudi Arabia (Al-Binali et al., 2006; Al-Megrin, 2010).

13.4 Sources of contamination and methods for control

13.4.1 Sources of contamination of fresh produce

Fresh produce may become contaminated with parasites at any one of a number of points from farm level to the consumer level. Indirect contamination of produce with protozoan cysts or oocysts, or helminth eggs or larvae may occur through the use of fecally contaminated water for irrigation, mixing of pesticides, or washing of produce, hands or equipment. Many parasites, such as *Giardia duodenalis*, *Cryptosporidium* spp., *Cyclospora cayetanensis*, *Entamoeba histolytica*, *Ascaris lumbricoides*, and *Taenia* spp. are commonly found in raw water sources that have been contaminated with human sewage. Although some of these parasites (e.g., *G. duodenalis*, *Cryptosporidium* spp.) may also originate from the feces of wild and domestic animals, others such as the oocysts of *Toxoplasma gondii* (cats/felines) and the eggs of *Echinococcus* spp. (dogs/canids) are shed exclusively in the feces of animals, and may indirectly contaminate fresh produce by means of water used on the farm, or even during postharvest processing or washing. In the case of *Fasciola* spp., a water source is, in fact, required for the completion of the life cycle.

Direct contamination of fresh produce with the infectious stages of parasites may occur at the farm level through the application of animal or human feces to croplands. Although manure as fertilizer is applied widely in agriculture, the use of human feces is also commonly used in some regions. These practices are important risk factors in the contamination of produce due to the high prevalence of enteric parasites such as *Cryptosporidium* and *Giardia* in livestock, as well as in humans in some regions. For the same reasons, the direct access to croplands by livestock or wildlife represents another risk of fecal contamination. Surface contamination of fresh produce may also occur by means of transport hosts such as birds and flies (Slifko et al., 2000b). Finally, contamination of produce can also occur through direct contact with parasite-infected or contaminated persons or equipment during harvesting, packaging, transport, food handling, or preparation. Direct contact with infected farm workers or food handlers is considered to be a very important source of contamination of fruits and vegetables, and has been identified as the direct cause of a number of illness outbreaks (Dixon et al., 2011).

Because fresh produce is often consumed raw, effective control measures to minimize the risk of parasite contamination of the foods in the first place, to destroy the parasites or their viability, or to physically remove the parasites, are imperative to reduce the risk of illness in consumers. Numerous control measures applicable to the farm level (i.e., preharvest and postharvest), or to the consumer and food-industry level, may be implemented to achieve this.

13.4.2 Preharvest control measures

Control measures to reduce the likelihood of contamination of produce with parasites at the preharvest stage include the use of treated water and improved sanitation, restricted access of livestock and other animals to croplands and surface waters, and addressing the health and hygiene of farm workers.

Surface water used in the production of produce can become contaminated with the infectious stages of parasites through a number of means, including agricultural runoff, sewage discharge, storm water discharge, and direct access to water sources by domestic and wild animals. Parasites have been detected in irrigation water in numerous studies (Robertson and Gjerde, 2001; Robertson et al., 2002; Thurston-Enriquez et al., 2002; Tram et al., 2008; Andoh et al., 2009; Mota et al., 2009; Sherchan et al., 2010; Amorós et al., 2010). Wastewater irrigation, in particular, has been cited as an important source of parasite contamination of vegetables in several surveillance studies (Amahmid et al., 1999; Srikanth and Naik, 2004; Gupta et al., 2009; El Said Said, 2012). Water treated with chlorine still poses a risk as the infectious stages of many parasites are much more resistant to chlorine than are bacterial pathogens. However, many filtration methods routinely used in water treatment are effective in removing parasites such as *Cryptosporidium* and *Giardia*. Although other technologies used in the water industry, such as ultraviolet light, ozone, and irradiation, can be effective in inactivating parasites, these technologies are expensive and are not generally available in many smaller communities or in developing regions. Effective sanitation systems for the safe disposal of human wastes is another important control measure. Sanitation is particularly important in minimizing the transmission of parasites, such as the tapeworm *Taenia solium*, whose life cycles depend on the direct exposure of animals to human feces.

The proximity and access of domestic and wild animals to croplands, and to surface water, is another important concern in terms of potential contamination of fresh produce. Some of these animals have a high prevalence of infection with parasites, and may serve as important reservoir hosts for human infections (e.g., *Cryptosporidium* spp. in cattle, *Fasciola* spp. in sheep and cattle). Produce may become contaminated with parasites through direct contact with the feces of these animals, or indirectly through agricultural runoff. As such, it is very important that these animals be kept away from croplands or any surface waters used for drinking or agricultural purposes. In the case of *Toxoplasma gondii*, it is imperative that farm cats be kept away from growing areas to prevent the contamination of fresh produce with oocysts. Similarly, as dogs and wild canids are responsible for the dispersion of *Echinococcus* spp. eggs into the environment, these animals must be kept away from field crops and vegetable gardens. Dogs should also be regularly dewormed and should not be fed the offal of sheep or other livestock.

The intentional application of animal manure or human feces (night soil) to croplands as fertilizer is widely practiced and represents another potential source of contamination of fresh produce. The effectiveness of composting in destroying any parasites that may be present in manure is not entirely clear. Olson et al. (1999) concluded that the application of cattle manure contaminated with *Giardia* and *Cryptosporidium* should be done in warmer weather, as degradation of cysts and oocysts was accelerated at 25 °C, and following at least 12 weeks of storage to inactivate the cysts and oocysts. However, in another study, composting manure was demonstrated to be effective in inactivating both *Giardia* cysts and *Cryptosporidium* oocysts when temperatures exceeded 55 °C for just 15 days (Van Herk et al., 2004).

The risk of transmission of parasites through the consumption of fresh produce may be greatly reduced by means of good hygienic practices by any farm workers directly or indirectly involved in the cultivation, harvesting, or processing of fresh fruits and vegetables. This control measure is particularly important in endemic and developing regions of the world where the prevalence of parasitic infections is greater. The availability of suitable toilets and hand-washing facilities for farm workers is of greatest concern in this regard. To ensure that hygienic practices are strictly followed, both educational and health-monitoring programs should be established for these individuals.

The environmental resistance of infectious stages should also be taken into consideration with respect to the control of parasites on fresh produce. For example, *C. parvum* oocysts were found to survive for considerable periods of time in water which was frozen at −10, −15, or −20 °C, or for up to 2 weeks at temperatures as high as 30 °C (Fayer et al., 1996; Fayer and Nerad, 1996). Similarly, *Toxoplasma gondii* oocysts stored in water at 35 °C were infective for 32 days, and there was no loss of infectivity after 106 days at either −5 or −10 °C (Dubey, 1998). *Entamoeba histolytica* cysts remain viable and infective in feces for several days, or in soil for at least 8 days at 28–34 °C. *Cyclospora cayetanensis* appears to be slightly more susceptible to adverse environmental conditions, as sporulation was found to be delayed in oocysts stored at either 4 or 37 °C for 14 days (Smith et al., 1997). However, Sathyanarayanan and Ortega (2006) reported that, on basil, sporulation of *Cyclospora cayetanensis* oocysts still occurred after incubation for up to 2 days at −20 °C and up to 4 days at 37 °C. Very little information is available on the temperature resistance of helminth eggs or larval stages in the environment, although most are thought to survive for long periods under suitable conditions. Desiccation is another important factor limiting the survival time of parasites in the environment. Studies have reported very low viability rates of *C. parvum* oocysts after only 2 h of air drying on glass slides at room temperature, or after 4 h of air drying at room temperature on stainless-steel surfaces (Robertson et al., 1992; Deng and Cliver, 1999). Although there are little supporting data, desiccation may be responsible for significant inactivation of parasite stages on fresh produce in the field or during storage and on surfaces and equipment. However, some fruits and vegetables have moist, irregular surfaces, and it has been suggested that this may protect contaminating parasites from desiccation (Warnes and Keevil, 2003).

Several studies have noted seasonal differences in the prevalences of parasites on fresh produce. It is not clear whether these differences are the result of environmental influences (e.g., temperature, desiccation) or are associated with seasonal differences in parasite prevalences in humans and animals. Studies in Egypt, Iran, and Saudi Arabia, for example, all reported the highest prevalences in the spring (Al-Megrin, 2010; El Said Said, 2012; Fallah et al., 2012; Ezatpour et al., 2013; Olyaei and Hajivandi, 2013). One study in Egypt reported the highest rate of contamination of vegetables in the summer (Eraky et al., 2014). Conversely, Al-Kassar (2012) reported a significantly higher frequency of parasites on winter vegetables than summer vegetables in Iraq. In Costa Rica, a greater percentage of *Cryptosporidium*-positive vegetable samples were reported during the rainy season (Monge and Chinchilla, 1996), whereas a study in Vietnam reported higher parasite prevalences on produce in the dry season than in the rainy season (Uga et al., 2009) and suggested that this may have been a result of the lack of rain to wash the parasites off the produce.

13.4.3 Postharvest control measures

Similar to the preharvest considerations described above, postharvest control measures include primarily the use of treated water for washing and processing produce, and for cleaning equipment, as well as the monitoring and enforcement of good personal hygiene in food handlers. Ensink et al. (2007) reported higher concentrations of helminth eggs and the fecal indicator *Escherichia coli* on vegetables collected from markets in Pakistan than on those collected from agricultural fields and suggested that food handling was an even more important factor in contamination than was irrigation water quality.

The use of chemical and physical disinfectants, either directly on foods or on surfaces and equipment, represents other potential barriers to the foodborne transmission of parasites (Erickson and Ortega, 2006). It is, however, well known that the infectious stages of waterborne parasites are highly resistant to many chemical and physical disinfectants (Gajadhar and Allen, 2004). Much of the information available on the effectiveness of chemical disinfectants on parasites stems from work on the inactivation of *Cryptosporidium* spp. oocysts and *Giardia* spp. cysts in drinking water and wastewater. Much work has been done, for example, on the effectiveness of chlorine, chlorine dioxide, and ozone as disinfectants (Erickson and Ortega, 2006). In general, ozone has been found to be a more effective disinfectant than either chlorine or chlorine dioxide against protozoan parasites in water. Many other chemical disinfectants commonly used for sanitizing surfaces and equipment have also been evaluated on *C. parvum* oocysts. Some chemical agents, including ammonia, formaldehyde, and hydrogen peroxide, can be effective as aqueous solutions, while others are more effective as fumigants (Erickson and Ortega, 2006). The effectiveness of commercial sanitizing agents against *C. parvum* oocysts has been variable. As with other protozoan parasites, *Cyclospora cayetanensis* oocysts are thought to be resistant to the chemical disinfectants commonly used in the food industry, as well as in water treatment (Ortega and Sanchez, 2010). *Giardia* cysts were found to be considerably more susceptible to commercially available disinfectants, during a 1-min contact time, than *Cryptosporidium* oocysts (Lee, 1992).

In terms of physical disinfection, a variety of technologies have been shown to be effective, or to have great promise, in the destruction of parasites on fresh produce. Pasteurization has been demonstrated to be effective in inactivating *Cryptosporidium* oocysts in apple cider (Deng and Cliver, 2001). There was a 3.0 log inactivation at 70 °C for 5 s and a 4.8 log inactivation at 71.7 °C. Gamma irradiation of protozoa has also been shown to be an effective means of decontaminating fresh fruits and vegetables. For example, Dubey et al. (1998) reported that sporulated *T. gondii* oocysts inoculated onto raspberries were inactivated at 0.4 kGy and concluded that 0.5 kGy would be effective in killing coccidian oocysts on fruits and vegetables. High hydrostatic pressure (or high pressure processing (HPP)) has also shown some promise in the inactivation of protozoa on fresh produce and in juices. For example, this technology was found to be effective in inactivating *Cryptosporidium* oocysts in fruit juices (Slifko et al., 2000a). Lindsay et al. (2008) reported that *Toxoplasma* oocysts inoculated onto raspberries were rendered noninfectious to mice when the berries were exposed to 340 MPa for 60 s in a commercial HPP unit. However, HPP was not found to be fully effective at 550 MPa for 2 min in inactivating *Eimeria acervulina* oocysts, which were used as a surrogate for *Cyclospora cayetanensis* (Kniel et al., 2007). Further studies are needed to evaluate these technologies on other parasites contaminating fresh produce. With respect to irradiation, in particular, public perception and acceptance remain major hurdles in its widespread use.

13.4.4 Consumer and food-industry level control measures

There are also some important control points at the consumer and food-industry level. Good personal hygiene, particularly hand washing, is of considerable importance in reducing the risk of transmission. The use of disposable gloves is also recommended for food handlers employed in the food industry. Food handlers either at home or in food service operations, who are experiencing symptoms such as diarrhea, or who have a confirmed infection, should not handle any food until after they have fully recovered. It is important that these control measures become common practice and are regularly monitored in commercial settings. Personal hygiene, however, has less to do with the contamination of foods with parasites such as *Toxoplasma*, *Trypanosoma*, and *Fasciola*, because humans do not shed the infectious stage in feces; it is nevertheless an extremely important component of good food hygiene.

Although rinsing fresh fruits and vegetables with water is recommended for reducing the risk of transmission of pathogens in general, it is unlikely that this practice will remove all parasites from these foods. Many fruits and vegetables have crevices and surface structures that act to retain the infectious stages of parasites. Several studies have, however, demonstrated a higher prevalence of parasites in unwashed vegetables than in washed vegetables (Kozan et al., 2005; Shahnazi and Jafari-Sabet, 2010; Avcioglu et al., 2011; Fallah et al., 2012). As with preharvest and postharvest activities, the quality of the water used for washing fresh produce before consumption is a major consideration, and only treated, potable water should be used for this purpose. In the case of *Fasciola* spp., the metacercarial stage strongly adheres to aquatic vegetation and cannot easily be washed off with water alone. The addition of vinegar, lemon juice, or salt to the wash water, however, has been shown to have a detaching effect on these metacercariae (Fawzi et al., 2004). As with other foods, the adherence to safe food-handling practices, such as using separate cutting boards and knives, proper storage, and hand washing will help to reduce the likelihood of cross-contamination of fresh produce with parasites or other foodborne pathogens.

Treatments such as cooking and freezing may be used as final barriers against transmission, although fresh produce is very often consumed raw, rendering such measures irrelevant. As discussed previously in this chapter, protozoan parasites have been shown to be resistant to temperature extremes in the environment, but relatively little information is available on the resistance of parasites on fresh produce to household freezing or cooking. Based on temperature tolerance studies done with *C. parvum* and other parasites suspended in water, it is likely that cooking with sufficiently high temperatures can be effective in inactivating any contaminating parasites. For example, *Cyclospora cayetanensis* oocysts will not sporulate following exposure to high temperatures, including 70 and 100 °C (Ortega and Sanchez, 2010). Household freezing should not be recommended as the sole means of inactivating parasites in foods because *C. parvum* and *T. gondii* oocysts have been shown to tolerate temperatures as low as –20 °C, and evidence from survival studies suggests that helminth eggs are also somewhat resistant to freezing.

13.5 Conclusions

The infectious stages of a large number of different parasites, including both protozoa and helminths, have been reported on a wide variety of fruits and vegetables in surveillance studies done worldwide. The relatively high prevalence of contamination shown in many of these studies, along with the numerous reported cases and outbreaks of illness associated with the consumption of contaminated fresh produce, suggests that parasites on fresh produce represent a global public health concern. Contamination of fresh produce with parasites may occur anywhere from primary production on farms through to the consumer and food service levels. Contamination may occur as a result of direct contact of the produce with animal or human feces, or contaminated hands and equipment, or through indirect means such as fecally contaminated water used in irrigation, washing, or processing. The control of foodborne parasitic diseases associated with fresh produce relies on the prevention of parasite contamination in the first place, or the destruction or removal of the infectious stages. At the farm level, control measures include the use of noncontaminated water and the implementation of other good farm management practices, such as supporting and monitoring the hygiene of workers, taking steps to minimize infections in domestic animals, and restricting animal access to croplands or water sources. A number of control measures can also be taken at the postharvest stage, including good personal hygiene, the use of treated water, and the use of chemical and/or physical disinfection. Control measures at the level of the consumer, or food service workers, represent final barriers to the transmission of foodborne parasites, and include good personal hygiene and safe food-handling practices.

13.6 Future considerations

Further surveillance studies are required on the prevalence of parasites on fresh produce, particularly from developed countries where such data are currently scarce. Optimization and standardization of laboratory methods for the detection, molecular characterization, and viability determination of parasites on fresh produce will also be extremely important in determining the level of risk posed to consumers, as well as the potential sources of contamination. This information will be of significant value in developing health risk assessments, policies, and guidelines with the aim of minimizing the risk of transmission to consumers. The global implementation of control measures such as good agricultural practices, use of good-quality water for irrigation and processing, and education of farm workers and food handlers will also be essential for minimizing the contamination of fresh produce and reducing the numbers of cases of foodborne illness associated with parasites. Further studies will also be required on the susceptibility of these parasites to various environmental conditions, as well as to chemical and physical treatments and disinfectants. As well, sustained efforts should be put into monitoring exercises, and identifying and characterizing emerging foodborne parasites on fresh produce, especially in light of the globalization of the food trade.

References

Abou el Naga, I.F., 1999. Studies on a newly emerging protozoal pathogen: *Cyclospora cayetanensis*. J. Egypt. Soc. Parasitol. 29, 575–586.

Abougrain, A.K., Nahaisi, M.H., Madi, N.S., Saied, M.M., Ghenghesh, K.S., 2010. Parasitological contamination in salad vegetables in Tripoli–Libya. Food Control 21, 760–762.

Adams, A.M., 2006. Foodborne trematodes. In: Ortega, Y.R. (Ed.), Foodborne Parasites. Springer, New York, pp. 161–196.

Adamu, N.B., Adamu, J.Y., Mohammed, D., 2012. Prevalence of helminth parasites found on vegetables sold in Maiduguri, northeastern Nigeria. Food Control 25, 23–26.

Adanir, R., Tasci, F., 2013. Prevalence of helminth eggs in raw vegetables consumed in Burdur, Turkey. Food Control 31, 482–484.

Al-Binali, A.M., Bello, C.S., El-Shewy, K., Abdulla, S.E., 2006. The prevalence of parasites in commonly used leafy vegetables in south western Saudi Arabia. Saudi Med. J. 27, 613–616.

Ali, S.A., Ameen, H.A., 2013. Prevalence of human intestinal parasites in selected vegetables in Sulaimani city. J. Sulaimani Med. Coll. 3, 75–79.

Al-Kassar, N.R., 2012. Prevalence of different parasitic stages in commercial vegetables in Al-Nassiriyah city, Iraq. J. Coll. Educ. Pure Sci. 2, 172–186.

Al-Megrin, W.A.I., 2010. Prevalence intestinal parasites in leafy vegetables in Riyadh, Saudi Arabia. Int. J. Trop. Med. 5, 20–23.

Al-Shawa, R.M., Mwafy, S.N., 2007. The enteroparasitic contamination of commercial vegetables in Gaza Governorates. J. Infect. Dev. Ctries 1, 62–66.

Amahmid, O., Asmama, S., Bouhoum, K., 1999. The effect of waste water reuse in irrigation on the contamination level of crops by *Giardia* cysts and *Ascaris* eggs. Int. J. Food Microbiol. 49, 19–26.

Ammar, A.S., Omar, H.M., 2013. The prevalence of leafy vegetable-borne parasites in Al-Qassim Region, Saudi Arabia. J. Agric. Vet. Sci. 6, 29–40.

Amoah, P., Drechsel, P., Abaidoo, R.C., Ntow, W.J., 2006. Pesticide and pathogen contamination of vegetables in Ghana's urban markets. Arch. Environ. Contam. Tox. 50, 1–6.

Amorós, I., Alonso, J.L., Cuesta, G., 2010. *Cryptosporidium* oocysts and *Giardia* cysts on salad products irrigated with contaminated water. J. Food Prot. 73, 1138–1140.

Andoh, L.A., Abaidoo, R.C., Obiri-Danso, K., Drechsel, P., Kondrasen, F., Klank, L.T., 2009. Helminth contamination of lettuce and associated risk factors at production sites, markets and street food vendor points in urban and peri-urban Kumasi, Ghana. Res. J. Microbiol. 4, 13–22.

Anh, V.T., Tram, N.T., Klank, L.T., Cam, P.D., Dalsgaard, A., 2007. Fecal and protozoan parasite contamination of water spinach (*Ipomoea aquatica*) cultivated in urban wastewater in Phnom Penh, Cambodia. Trop. Med. Int. Health 12 (Suppl. 2), 73–81.

Avcioglu, H., Soykan, E., Tarakci, U., 2011. Control of helminth contamination of raw vegetables by washing. Vector Borne Zoonotic Dis. 11, 189–191.

Bern, C., Garcia, H.H., Evans, C., Gonzalez, A.E., Verastegui, M., Tsang, V.C., Gilman, R.H., 1999. Magnitude of the disease burden from neurocysticercosis in a developing country. Clin. Infect. Dis. 29, 1203–1209.

Bern, C., Kjos, S., Yabsley, M.J., Montgomery, S.P., 2011. *Trypanosoma cruzi* and Chagas' disease in the United States. Clin. Microbiol. Rev. 24, 655–681.

Bethony, J., Brooker, S., Albonica, M., Geiger, S.M., Loukas, A., Diemert, D., Hotez, P.J., 2006. Soil-transmitted helminth infections: ascariosis, trichuriasis, and hookworm. Lancet 367, 1521–1532.

Bjorland, J., Bryan, R.T., Strauss, W., Hillyer, G.V., McAuley, J.B., 1995. An outbreak of acute fasciolosis among Aymara Indians in the Bolivian Altiplano. Clin. Infect. Dis. 21, 1228–1233.

Bohaychuk, V.M., Bradbury, R.W., Dimock, R., Fehr, M., Gensler, G.E., King, R.K., Rieve, R., Romero Barrios, P., 2009. A microbiological survey of selected Alberta-grown fresh produce from farmers' markets in Alberta, Canada. J. Food Prot. 72, 415–420.

Bowman, N., Donroe, J., Gilman, R., 2006. Cestodes. In: Ortega, Y.R. (Ed.), Foodborne Parasites. Springer, New York, pp. 197–229.

Calvo, M., Carazo, M., Arias, M.L., Chaves, C., Monge, R., Chinchilla, M., 2004. Prevalence of *Cyclospora* sp., *Cryptosporidium* sp., microsporidia and fecal coliform determination in fresh fruit and vegetables consumed in Costa Rica. Arch. Latinoam. Nutr. 54, 428–432.

Cama, V., 2006. Coccidian parasites. In: Ortega, Y.R. (Ed.), Foodborne Parasites. Springer, New York, pp. 33–55.

CDC, 2013. Cyclosporosis outbreak investigations—United States, 2013 (final update). Centers for disease control and prevention. Available from: http://www.cdc.gov/parasites/cyclosporiasis/outbreaks/investigation-2013.html (accessed 22 July 2014).

Chacín-Bonilla, L., 2010. Epidemiology of *Cyclospora cayetanensis*: a review focusing in endemic areas. Acta Trop. 115, 181–193.

Coelho, L.M.P.S., de Oliveira, S.M., Milman, M.H.S.A., Karasawa, K.A., Santos, R.P., 2001. [Detection enteroparasites transmissible forms in water and raw vegetables consumed in pre-schools from Sorocaba, São Paulo state, Brazil]. Rev. Soc. Bras. Med. Trop. 34, 479–482.

da Silva, J.P., Marzochi, M.C.A., Camillo-Coura, L., Messias, A.A., Marques, S., 1995. Estudo da contaminação por enteroparasitas em hortaliças comercializadas nos supermercados da cidade do Rio de Janeiro. Rev. Soc. Bras. Med. Trop. 28, 237–241.

Damen, J.G., Banwat, E.B., Egah, D.Z., Allanana, J.A., 2007. Parasitic contamination of vegetables in Jos, Nigeria. Ann. Afr. Med. 6, 115–118.

Daryani, A., Ettehad, G.H., Sharif, M., Ghorbani, L., Ziaei, H., 2008. Prevalence of intestinal parasites in vegetables consumed in Ardabil, Iran. Food Control 19, 790–794.

de Lalla, F., Rinaldi, E., Santoro, D., Nicolin, R., Tramarin, A., 1992. Outbreak of *Entamoeba histolytica* and *Giardia lamblia* infections in travellers returning from the tropics. Infection 20, 78–82.

de Leon, W.U., Monzon, R.B., Aganon, A.A., Arceo, R.E., Ignacio, E.J., Santos, G., 1992. Parasitic contamination of selected vegetables sold in metropolitan Manila, Philippines. Southeast Asian J. Trop. Med. Public Health 23, 162–164.

de Oliveira, C.A., Germano, P.M., 1992a. [Study on the occurrence of intestinal parasites on vegetables commercially traded in the metropolitan area of S.Paulo, SP, Brazil. I – Search for helminths]. Rev. Saúde públ., S.Paulo 26, 283–289.

de Oliveira, C.A., Germano, P.M., 1992b. [Study of the occurrence of intestinal parasites on vegetables commercially traded in the metropolitan area of S.Paulo, SP – Brazil. II – Research into protozoan cysts]. Rev. Saúde públ., S.Paulo 26, 332–335.

Decraene, V., Lebbad, M., Botero-Kleiven, S., Gustavsson, A.-M., Löfdahl, M., 2012. First reported foodborne outbreak associated with microsporidia, Sweden, October 2009. Epidemiol. Infect. 140, 519–527.

Deng, M.Q., Cliver, D.O., 1999. *Cryptosporidium parvum* studies with dairy products. Int. J. Food Microbiol. 46, 113–121.

Deng, M.Q., Cliver, D.O., 2001. Inactivation of *Cryptosporidium parvum* oocysts in cider by flash pasteurization. J. Food Prot. 64, 523–527.

Dixon, B.R., 2009. The role of livestock in the foodborne transmission of *Giardia duodenalis* and *Cryptosporidium* spp. to humans. In: Ortega-Pierres, M.G., Cacciò, S., Fayer, R., Mank, T., Smith, H., Thompson, R.C.A. (Eds.), *Giardia* and *Cryptosporidium:* From Molecules to Disease. CAB International, Wallingford, UK, pp. 107–122.

Dixon, B.R., Fayer, R., Santin, M., Hill, D.E., Dubey, J.P., 2011. Protozoan parasites: *Cryptosporidium*, *Giardia*, *Cyclospora*, and *Toxoplasma*. In: Hoorfar, J. (Ed.), Rapid Detection, Characterization and Enumeration of Food-Borne Pathogens. ASM Press, Washington, USA, pp. 349–370.

Dixon, B., Parrington, L., Cook, A., Pollari, F., Farber, J., 2013. Detection of *Cyclospora, Cryptosporidium* and *Giardia* in ready-to-eat packaged leafy greens in Ontario, Canada. J. Food Prot. 76, 307–313.

Döller, P.C., Dietrich, K., Filipp, N., Brockmann, S., Dreweck, C., Vonthein, R., Wagner-Wiening, C., Wiedenmann, A., 2002. Cyclosporosis outbreak in Germany associated with the consumption of salad. Emerg. Infect. Dis. 8, 992–994.

Dreyfuss, G., Vignoles, P., Rondelaud, D., 2005. *Fasciola hepatica*: epidemiological surveillance of natural watercress beds in central France. Parasitol. Res. 95, 278–282.

Dubey, J.P., 1998. *Toxoplasma gondii* oocyst survival under defined temperatures. J. Parasitol. 84, 862–865.

Dubey, J.P., 2009. Toxoplasmosis of Animals and Humans, second ed. CRC Press, Boca Raton, FL.

Dubey, J.P., Thayer, D.W., Speer, C.A., Shen, S.K., 1998. Effect of gamma irradiation on unsporulated and sporulated *Toxoplasma gondii* oocysts. Int. J. Parasitol. 28, 369–375.

Ebrahimzadeh, A., Jamshidi, A., Mohammadi, S., 2013. The parasitic contamination of raw vegetables consumed in Zahedan, Iran. Health Scope 1, 205–209.

Ekman, C.C.J., Chiossi, M.F.d.V., Meireles, L.R., de Andrade Junior, H.F., Figueiredo, W.M., Marciano, M.A.M., Luna, E.J.d.A., 2012. Case-control study of an outbreak of acute toxoplasmosis in an industrial plant in the state of São Paulo, Brazil. Rev. Inst. Med. Trop. Sao Paulo 54, 239–244.

El Said Said, D., 2012. Detection of parasites in commonly consumed raw vegetables. Alexandria J. Med. 48, 345–352.

Ensink, J.H.J., Mahmood, T., Dalsgaard, A., 2007. Wastewater-irrigated vegetables: market handling versus irrigation water quality. Trop. Med. Int. Health 12, 2–7.

Eraky, M.A., Rashed, S.M., El-Sayed Nasr, M., El-Hamshary, A.M.S., El-Ghannam, A.S., 2014. Parasitic contamination of commonly consumed fresh leafy vegetables in Benha, Egypt. J. Parasitol. Res. 2014, 1–7. http://dx.doi.org/10.1155/2014/613960.

Erdoğrul, Ö., Şener, H., 2005. The contamination of various fruit and vegetable with *Enterobius vermicularis, Ascaris* eggs, *Entamoeba histolytica* and *Giardia* cysts. Food Control 16, 559–562.

Erickson, M.C., Ortega, Y.R., 2006. Inactivation of protozoan parasites in food, water, and environmental systems. J. Food Prot. 69, 2786–2808.

Espino, A.M., Díaz, A., Pérez, A., Finlay, C.M., 1998. Dynamics of antigenemia and coproantigens during a human *Fasciola hepatica* outbreak. J. Clin. Microbiol. 36, 2723–2726.

Ezatpour, B., Chegeni, A.S., Abdollahpour, F., Aazami, M., Alirezaei, M., 2013. Prevalence of parasitic contamination of raw vegetables in Khorramabad, Iran. Food Control 34, 92–95.

Fallah, A.A., Pirali-Kheirabadi, K., Shirvani, F., Saei-Dehkordi, S.S., 2012. Prevalence of parasitic contamination in vegetables used for raw consumption in Shahrekord, Iran: influence of season and washing procedure. Food Control 25, 617–620.

FAO/WHO, 2012. Preliminary report: multicriteria-based ranking for risk management of foodborne parasites. Joint FAO/WHO Expert Meeting on Foodborne Parasites, Rome, Italy, 3–7 September, 2012. Available from: http://www.who.int/foodsafety/micro/jemra/meetings/parasite_report_preliminary_251012.pdf?ua=1 (accessed 22 July 2014).

Fawzi, M., El-Sahn, A.A., Ibrahim, H.F., Shehata, A.I., 2004. Vegetable-transmitted parasites among inhabitants of El-Prince, Alexandria and its relation to housewives' knowledge and practices. J. Egypt. Public Health Assoc. 79, 13–29.

Fayer, R., Nerad, T., 1996. Effects of low temperatures on viability of *Cryptosporidium parvum* oocysts. Appl. Environ. Microbiol. 62, 1431–1433.

Fayer, R., Trout, J.M., Nerad, T., 1996. Effects of a wide range of temperatures on the infectivity of *Cryptosporidium parvum* oocysts. J. Eukaryot. Microbiol. 43, S64.

Feng, Y., Xiao, L., 2011. Zoonotic potential and molecular epidemiology of *Giardia* species and giardiasis. Clin. Microbiol. Rev. 24, 110–140.

Fried, B., Abruzzi, A., 2010. Food-borne trematode infections of humans in the United States of America. Parasitol. Res. 106, 1263–1280.

Gajadhar, A.A., Allen, J.R., 2004. Factors contributing to the public health and economic importance of waterborne zoonotic parasites. Vet. Parasitol. 126, 3–14.

Garcia, H.H., Gonzalez, A.E., Evans, C.A.W., Gilman, R.H., 2003. *Taenia solium* cysticercosis. Lancet 361, 547–556.

Garcia, L., Henderson, J., Fabri, M., Oke, M., 2006. Potential sources of microbial contamination in unpasteurized apple cider. J. Food Prot. 69, 137–144.

Garedaghi, Y., Hashemzade, F.H., Pooryagoobi, S., 2011. Parasitic contamination of fresh vegetables consumed in Tabriz, Iran. Res. J. Biol. Sci. 6, 518–522.

Gharavi, M.J., Jahani, M.R., Rokni, M.B., 2002. Parasitic contamination of vegetables from farms and markets in Tehran. Iran J. Public Health 31, 83–86.

Ghimire, T.R., Mishra, P.N., Sherchand, J.B., 2005. The seasonal outbreaks of *Cyclospora* and *Cryptosporidium* in Kathmandu, Nepal. J. Nepal Health Res. Counc. 3, 39–48.

Gibbs, R.A., Nanyonjo, R., Pingault, N.M., Combs, B.G., Mazzucchelli, T., Armstrong, P., Tarling, G., Dowse, G.K., 2013. An outbreak of *Cyclospora* infection on a cruise ship. Epidemiol. Infect. 141, 508–516.

Grabowski, D.J., Tiggs, K.J., Hall, J.D., Senke, H.W., Salas, A.J., Powers, C.M., Knott, J.A., Nims, L.J., Sewell, C.M., 1989. Epidemiologic notes and reports common-source outbreak of giardiosis. Morb. Mortal. Wkly Rep. 38, 405–407.

Gupta, N., Khan, D.K., Santra, S.C., 2009. Prevalence of intestinal helminth eggs on vegetables grown in wastewater-irrigated areas of Titagarh, West Bengal, India. Food Control 20, 942–945.

Hajjami, K., Ennaji, M.M., Amdiouni, H., Fouad, S., Cohen, N., 2013. Parasitic contamination on fresh vegetable consumed in Casablanca City (Morocco) and risk for consumer. Int. J. Sci. Tech. 2, 543–549.

Hassan, A., Farouk, H., Abdul-Ghani, R., 2012. Parasitological contamination of freshly eaten vegetables collected from local markets in Alexandria, Egypt: a preliminary study. Food Control 26, 500–503.

Herwaldt, B.L., Ackers, M.-L., The Cyclospora Working Group, 1997. An outbreak in 1996 of cyclosporosis associated with imported raspberries. New Engl. J. Med. 336, 1548–1556.

Herwaldt, B.L., Beach, M.J., The Cyclospora Working Group, 1999. The return of *Cyclospora* in 1997: another outbreak of cyclosporosis in North America associated with imported raspberries. Ann. Intern. Med. 130, 210–220.

Hill, D.E., Chirukandoth, S., Dubey, J.P., 2005. Biology and epidemiology of *Toxoplasma gondii* in man and animals. Anim. Health Res. Rev. 6, 41–61.

Idahosa, O.T., 2011. Parasitic contamination of fresh vegetables sold in Jos markets. Global J. Med. Res. 11, 21–25.

Insulander, M., Svenungsson, B., Lebbad, M., Karlsson, L., de Jong, B., 2010. A foodborne outbreak of *Cyclospora* infection in Stockholm, Sweden. Foodborne Pathog. Dis. 7, 1585–1587.

Kasprzak, W., Rauhut, W., Mazur, T., 1981. Transmission of *Giardia* cysts. II. Fruit and vegetables as the source of infection. Wiad. Parazytol. 27, 565–571.

Kłapeć, T., Borecka, A., 2012. Contamination of vegetables, fruits and soil with geohelminths eggs on organic farms in Poland. Ann. Agric. Environ. Med. 19, 421–425.

Kniel, K.E., Shearer, A.E.H., Cascarino, J.L., Wilkins, G.C., Jenkins, M.C., 2007. High hydrostatic pressure and UV light treatment of produce contaminated with *Eimeria acervulina* as a *Cyclospora cayetanensis* surrogate. J. Food Prot. 70, 2837–2842.

Kozan, E., Gonene, B., Sarimehmetoglu, O., Aycicek, H., 2005. Prevalence of helminth eggs on raw vegetables used for salads. Food Control 16, 239–242.

Lass, A., Pietkiewicz, H., Szostakowska, B., Myjak, P., 2012. The first detection of *Toxoplasma gondii* DNA in environmental fruits and vegetables samples. Eur. J. Clin. Microbiol. Infect. Dis. 31, 1101–1108.

Lee, M.B., 1992. The effectiveness of commercially available disinfectants upon *Giardia lamblia* cysts. Can. J. Public Health 83, 171–172.

Lindsay, D.S., Holliman, D., Flick, G.J., Goodwin, D.G., Mitchell, S.M., Dubey, J.P., 2008. Effects of high pressure processing on *Toxoplasma gondii* oocysts on raspberries. J. Parasitol. 94, 757–758.

Maikai, B.V., Elisha, I.A., Baba-Onoja, E.B.T., 2012. Contamination of vegetables sold in markets with helminth eggs in Zaria metropolis, Kaduna state, Nigeria. Food Control 28, 345–348.

Mailles, A., Capek, I., Ajana, F., Schepens, C., Ilef, D., Vaillant, V., 2006. Commercial watercress as an emerging source of fascioliasis in Northern France in 2002: results from an outbreak investigation. Epidemiol. Infect. 134, 942–945.

Mansfield, L.S., Gajadhar, A.A., 2004. *Cyclospora cayetanensis*, a food- and waterborne coccidian parasite. Vet. Parasitol. 126, 73–90.

Mas-Coma, S., Bargues, M.D., Valero, M.A., 2007. Plant-borne trematode zoonoses: fasciolosis and fasciolopsiosis. In: Murrell, K.D., Fried, B. (Eds.), Food-Borne Parasitic Zoonoses: Fish and Plant-Borne Parasites. World Class Parasites, vol. 11. Springer, New York, pp. 293–334.

McCabe, R., Remington, J.S., 1988. Toxoplasmosis: the time has come. New Engl. J. Med. 318, 313–315.

Mead, P.S., Slutsker, L., Dietz, V., McCaig, L.F., Bresee, J.S., Shapiro, C., Griffin, P.M., Tauxe, R.V., 1999. Food-related illness and death in the United States. Emerg. Infect. Dis. 5, 607–625.

Mintz, E.D., Hudson-Wragg, M., Mshar, P., Cartter, M.L., Hadler, J.L., 1993. Foodborne giardiosis in a corporate office setting. J. Infect. Dis. 167, 250–253.

Monge, R., Arias, M.L., 1996. Presence of various pathogenic microorganisms in fresh vegetables in Costa Rica. Arch. Latinoam. Nutr. 46, 292–294.

Monge, R., Chinchilla, M., 1996. Presence of *Cryptosporidium* oocysts in fresh vegetables. J. Food Prot. 59, 202–203.

Mota, A., Mena, K.D., Soto-Beltran, M., Tarwater, P.M., Cháidez, C., 2009. Risk assessment of *Cryptosporidium* and *Giardia* in water irrigating fresh produce in Mexico. J. Food Prot. 72, 2184–2188.

Nazemi, S., Raei, M., Amiri, M., Chaman, R., 2012. Parasitic contamination of raw vegetables in Shahroud, Semnan. Zahedan J. Res. Med. Sci. 14, 84–86.

Nyarango, R.M., Aloo, P.A., Kabiru, E.W., Nyanchongi, B.O., 2008. The risk of pathogenic intestinal parasite infections in Kisii Municipality, Kenya. BMC Public Health 8, 237. http://dx.doi.org/10.1186/1471-2458-8-237.

Ogbolu, D.O., Alli, O.A., Ogunleye, V.F., Olusoga-Ogbolu, F.F., Olaosun, I., 2009. The presence of intestinal parasites in selected vegetables from open markets in south western Nigeria. Afr. J. Med. Med. Sci. 38, 319–324.

Ojha, S.C., Jaide, C., Jinawath, N., Rotjanapan, P., Baral, P., 2014. Geohelminths: public health significance. J. Infect. Dev. Ctries. 8, 5–16.

Olson, M.E., Goh, J., Phillips, M., Guselle, N., McAllister, T.A., 1999. *Giardia* cyst and *Cryptosporidium* oocyst survival in water, soil, and cattle feces. J. Environ. Qual. 28, 1991–1996.
Olyaei, A., Hajivandi, L., 2013. Parasitological contamination of markets and farms in vegetables consumed in southern Iran. Global Vet. 10, 327–331.
Omowaye, O.S., Odikamnoro, O.O., 2013. Examination of food-borne parasites in northern-part of Nigeria. Stand. Sci. Res. Essays 1, 113–115.
Ortega, Y.R., 2006. Amoeba and ciliates. In: Ortega, Y.R. (Ed.), Foodborne Parasites. Springer, New York, pp. 1–14.
Ortega, Y.R., Sanchez, R., 2010. Update on *Cyclospora cayetanensis*, a food-borne and waterborne parasite. Clin. Microbiol. Rev. 23, 218–234.
Ortega, Y.R., Sterling, C.R., Gilman, R.H., Cama, V.A., Diaz, F., 1993. *Cyclospora* species – a new protozoan pathogen of humans. New Engl. J. Med. 328, 1308–1312.
Ortega, Y.R., Roxas, C.R., Gilman, R.H., Miller, N.J., Cabrera, L., Taquiri, C., Sterling, C.R., 1997. Isolation of *Cryptosporidium parvum* and *Cyclospora cayetanensis* from vegetables collected in markets of an endemic region in Peru. Am. J. Trop. Med. Hyg. 57, 683–686.
Pawlowski, Z., Allan, J., Sarti, E., 2005. Control of *Taenia solium* taeniosis/cysticercosis: from research towards implementation. Int. J. Parasitol. 35, 1221–1232.
Pereira, K.S., Schmidt, F.L., Guaraldo, A.M.A., Franco, R.M.B., Dias, V.L., Passos, L.A.C., 2009. Chagas' disease as a foodborne illness. J. Food Prot. 72, 441–446.
Pereira, K.S., Franco, R.M.B., Leal, D.A.G., 2010. Transmission of toxoplasmosis (*Toxoplasma gondii*) by food. Adv. Food Nutr. Res. 60, 1–19.
Porter, J.D.H., Gaffney, C., Heymann, D., Parkin, W., 1990. Food-borne outbreak of *Giardia lamblia*. Am. J. Public Health 80, 1259–1260.
Räisänen, S., Ruuskanen, L., Nyman, S., 1985. Epidemic ascariasis – evidence of transmission by imported vegetables. Scand. J. Prim. Health Care 3, 189–191.
Ranjbar-Bahadori, S., Mostoophi, A., Shemshadi, B., 2013. Study on *Cryptosporidium* contamination in vegetable farms around Tehran. Trop. Biomed. 30, 193–198.
Remington, J.S., 1990. The tragedy of toxoplasmosis. Pediatr. Infect. Dis. J. 9, 762–763.
Robertson, L.J., Chalmers, R.M., 2013. Foodborne cryptosporidiosis: is there really more in Nordic countries? Trends Parasitol. 29, 3–9.
Robertson, L.J., Gjerde, B., 2001. Occurrence of parasites on fruits and vegetables in Norway. J. Food Prot. 64, 1793–1798.
Robertson, L.J., Campbell, A.T., Smith, H.V., 1992. Survival of *Cryptosporidium parvum* oocysts under various environmental pressures. Appl. Environ. Microbiol. 58, 3494–3500.
Robertson, L.J., Johannessen, G.S., Gjerde, B.K., Loncarevic, S., 2002. Microbiological analysis of seed sprouts in Norway. Int. J. Food Microbiol. 75, 119–126.
Rzeżutka, A., Nichols, R.A., Connelly, L., Kaupke, A., Kozyra, I., Cook, N., Birrell, S., Smith, H.V., 2010. *Cryptosporidium* oocysts on fresh produce from areas of high livestock production in Poland. Int. J. Food Microbiol. 139, 96–101.
Saki, J., Asadpoori, R., Khademvatan, S., 2013. Prevalence of intestinal parasites in vegetables consumed in Ahvaz, South West of Iran. J. Med. Sci. 13, 488–492.
Sathyanarayanan, L., Ortega, Y., 2006. Effects of temperature and different food matrices on *Cyclospora cayetanensis* oocyst sporulation. J. Parasitol. 92, 218–222.
Scallan, E., Hoekstra, R.M., Angulo, F.J., Tauxe, R.V., Widdowson, M.A., Roy, S.L., Jones, J.L., Griffin, P.M., 2011. Foodborne illness acquired in the United States – major pathogens. Emerg. Infect. Dis. 17, 7–15.
Schantz, P.M., Moore, A.C., Muñoz, J.L., Hartman, B.J., Schaefer, J.A., Aron, A.M., Persaud, D., Sarti, E., Wilson, M., Flisser, A., 1992. Neurocysticercosis in an Orthodox Jewish community in New York City. New Engl. J. Med. 327, 692–695.

Scott, M.E., 2008. *Ascaris lumbricoides*: a review of its epidemiology and relationship to other infections. Ann. Nestle 66, 7–22.

Shahnazi, M., Jafari-Sabet, M., 2010. Prevalence of parasitic contamination of raw vegetables in villages of Qazvin Province, Iran. Foodborne Pathog. Dis. 7, 1025–1030.

Sherchan, J.B., Sherpa, K., Tandukar, S., Cross, J.H., Gajadhar, A., Sherchand, J.B., 2010. Infection of *Cyclospora cayetanensis* in diarrhoeal children of Nepal. J. Nepal Paediatr. Soc. 30, 23–30.

Sherchand, J.B., Cross, J., Jimba, M., Sherchand, S., Shrestha, M.P., 1999. Study of *Cyclospora cayetanensis* in health care facilities, sewage water and green leafy vegetables in Nepal. Southeast Asian J. Trop. Med. Public Health 30, 58–63.

Sia Su, G.L., Mariano, C.M.R., Matti, N.S.A., Ramos, G.B., 2012. Assessing parasitic infestation of vegetables in selected markets in Metro Manila, Philippines. Asian Pac. J. Trop. Dis. 2012, 51–54.

Siyadatpanah, A., Tabatabaei, F., Emami Zeydi, A., Spotin, A., Fallah-Omrani, V., Assadi, M., Moradi, S., Rostami, A., Memari, F., Hajialiani, F., 2013. Parasitic contamination of raw vegetables in Amol, North of Iran. Arch. Clin. Infect. Dis. 8, e15983.

Slifko, T.R., Raghubeer, E., Rose, J.B., 2000a. Effect of high hydrostatic pressure on *Cryptosporidium parvum* infectivity. J. Food Prot. 63, 1262–1267.

Slifko, T.R., Smith, H.V., Rose, J.B., 2000b. Emerging parasite zoonoses associated with water and food. Int. J. Parasitol. 30, 1379–1393.

Smith, H.V., Paton, C.A., Mtambo, M.A., Girdwood, R.W.A., 1997. Sporulation of *Cyclospora* sp. oocysts. Appl. Environ. Microbiol. 63, 1631–1632.

Srikanth, R., Naik, D., 2004. Prevalence of giardiosis due to wastewater reuse for agriculture in the suburbs of Asmara City, Eritrea. Int. J. Environ. Health Res. 14, 43–52.

Takayanagui, O.M., Febrônio, L.H.P., Bergamini, A.M., Okino, M.H.T., Castro e Silva, A.A.M.C., Santiago, R., Capuano, D.M., Oliveira, M.A., Takayanagui, A.M.M., 2000. [Monitoring of lettuce crops of Ribeirão Preto, SP, Brazil]. Rev. Soc. Bras. Med. Trop. 33, 169–174.

Thurston-Enriquez, J.A., Watt, P., Dowd, S.E., Enriquez, R., Pepper, I.L., Gerba, C.P., 2002. Detection of protozoan parasites and microsporidia in irrigation waters used for crop production. J. Food Prot. 65, 378–382.

Torgerson, P.R., Keller, K., Magnotta, M., Ragland, N., 2010. The global burden of alveolar echinococcosis. PLoS Negl. Trop. Dis. 4, e722. http://dx.doi.org/10.1371/journal.pntd.0000722.

Tram, N.T., Hoang, L.M.N., Cam, P.D., Chung, P.T., Fyfe, M.W., Isaac-Renton, J.L., Ong, C.S.L., 2008. *Cyclospora* spp. in herbs and water samples collected from markets and farms in Hanoi, Vietnam. Trop. Med. Int. Health 13, 1415–1420.

Uga, S., Hoa, N.T.V., Noda, S., Moji, K., Cong, L., Aoki, Y., Rai, R.K., Fujimaki, Y., 2009. Parasite egg contamination of vegetables from a suburban market in Hanoi, Vietnam. Nepal Med. Coll. J. 11, 75–78.

Uneke, C.J., 2007. Potential for geohelminth parasite transmission by raw fruits and vegetables in Nigeria: implication for a risk profile. J. Nutr. Environ. Med. 16, 59–68.

Van Herk, F.H., McAllister, T.A., Cockwill, C.L., Guselle, N., Larney, F.J., Miller, J.J., Olson, M.E., 2004. Inactivation of *Giardia* cysts and *Cryptosporidium* oocysts in beef feedlot manure by thermophilic windrow composting. Compost. Sci. Util. 12, 235–241.

Vázquez Tsuji, O., Martínez Barbabosa, I., Tay Zavala, J., Ruiz Hernández, A., Pérez Torres, A., 1997. [Vegetables for human consumption as probable source of *Toxocara* sp. infection in man]. Bol. Chil. Parasitol. 52, 47–50.

Warnes, S., Keevil, C.W., 2003. Survival of *Cryptosporidium parvum* in faecal wastes and salad crops. Teagasc, Agriculture and food development authority (Ireland). Available from: http://www.teagasc.ie/publications/2003/conferences/cryptosporidiumparvum/paper02.asp (accessed 22 July 2014).

Weisenberg, S.A., Perlada, D.E., 2013. Domestically acquired fasciolosis in northern California. Am. J. Trop. Med. Hyg. 89, 588–591.

Zeehaida, M., Zairi, N.Z., Rahmah, N., Maimunah, A., Madihah, B., 2011. *Strongyloides stercoralis* in common vegetables and herbs in Kota Bharu, Kelantan, Malaysia. Trop. Biomed. 28, 188–193.

Part Four

Prevention and Control

Components of control for foodborne parasites and their application in the food production chain

14

W.B. Scandrett
Canadian Food Inspection Agency, Saskatoon, SK, Canada

14.1 Introduction

Compared to other pathogens, the detection and control of foodborne parasites can be especially challenging due to factors such as long incubation periods and nonspecific clinical manifestations of infection, lack of *in vitro* or *in vivo* propagation methods, and environmental robustness. As well, there has been relatively little awareness of these parasites by regulators, producers, and consumers, particularly in developed countries (Gajadhar et al., 2006). Although regional elimination and global eradication of foodborne parasitic disease is possible for some foodborne parasites, such as *Taenia solium*, there must be the socioeconomic and political justification for the costs and benefits of eradication versus control of a particular parasite, as health resources are limited and may be better directed elsewhere (Dowdle, 1999). Thus, in most cases, control, not eradication, is the only practical approach to mitigating the risks of foodborne parasite transmission.

When developing control programs for foodborne parasites, important aspects of disease control must be considered. These components of control, their effectiveness, and challenges to their implementation, are described in this chapter. For each component this includes examples of related interventions, strategies, or programs implemented in developed and developing regions for the control of select foodborne parasites representative of the diversity of these pathogens and the food matrices they affect: the cestodes *Taenia saginata* and *T. solium*, the nematodes of the genus *Trichinella*, the trematodes *Clonorchis* and *Opisthorchis* of the family Opisthorchiidae, and the coocidian protozoa *Cyclospora*, *Cryptosporidium*, and *Toxoplasma*. The Food and Agricultural Organisation (FAO) and World Health Organisation (WHO) have jointly recognized these among those foodborne parasites deemed most significant from a public health and socioeconomic perspective (FAO/WHO, 2014a). Further details on the risk factors for transmission of these parasites, and their biology, epidemiology, diagnosis, significance, and control are presented in the respective chapters elsewhere in this book.

Foodborne Parasites in the Food Supply Web. http://dx.doi.org/10.1016/B978-1-78242-332-4.00014-X

14.2 Components of control for foodborne parasites

Control measures to mitigate the risk of foodborne parasitic disease can be applied at any stage of the food production chain, to humans, definitive or intermediate animal hosts, foods, water, and/or the environment. One or multiple interventions may be implemented to form the basis of a control program or strategy. Countries may have limited veterinary and public health infrastructure, regulatory oversight, or other capacity to plan and implement control programs for foodborne parasites. However, the most successful outcome will be achieved by incorporating the following components of disease control: regulations and standards, detection and diagnosis, surveillance, incursions and outbreak investigations, treatment and inactivation, prevention of infection and contamination, and education and training.

14.3 Regulations and standards

Developing countries in particular are hampered by weaknesses in veterinary and public health infrastructure, inadequate cooperation between medical and veterinary authorities, and the clandestine slaughter of animals without regulated inspection, which provides a route for even heavily infected carcasses to enter the food chain. To effectively prevent and control foodborne parasitic disease, an established regulatory framework should exist to enable decisions on policy, risk assessment, risk management (i.e., disease eradication vs. control), and risk communication, and to apply practical regulations that are acceptable to the food industry (Hastein, 2000). The goal and objectives of the control program should be clearly defined (OIE, 2014a). Ideally, this framework has a legal basis supported by legislation, with a competent authority empowered accordingly. Because of the zoonotic nature of most foodborne parasites, both the veterinary community and public health authorities should share responsibility for such a framework. The provisions within the framework should include: (i) a list of prioritized or notifiable foodborne parasites foreign to and/or of socioeconomic concern within a country; (ii) procedures for inspection, traceability, health control, and disease prevention; (iii) import/export regulations; (iv) quarantine measures; (v) transport regulations and controls on the movement and sale of susceptible animals and food products; and (vi) sanitation and disinfection procedures (Hastein, 2000).

Whenever possible, these provisions should be based on available international guidelines and standards provided by the World Organisation for Animal Health (OIE) and the Codex Alimentarius Commission (CAC) for preharvest and postharvest control, respectively, and the International Standards Organisation (ISO). Other international guidelines or recommendations, such as those provided by the International Commission on Trichinellosis (ICT) and other scientific bodies, should also be considered, as relevant. Regulated procedures should be standardized and incorporate quality control principles such as those espoused by Good Agricultural Practices (GAPs) and the hazard analysis critical control points (HACCP) system. Chapter 17 provides further details on the roles that regulatory and standards-setting organizations play in foodborne parasite control.

14.3.1 Taenia *spp.*

Successful control for both *T. saginata* and *T. solium* should focus on both taeniosis in human definitive hosts and cysticercosis in cattle and swine intermediate hosts, respectively (FAO, 2013a). However, even in developed countries, although regulations exist for the reporting and control of cysticercosis in livestock, they rarely exist for human taeniosis. Thus, human infections with *T. solium*, as well as *T. saginata*, imported via immigration or travel from endemic regions are an emerging public health problem. Foci of autochthonous transmission of *T. solium* exist in Spain, Portugal, and the United States, where this is now recognized as a neglected parasitic infection (Fabiani and Bruschi, 2013; Cantey et al., 2014). *Taenia saginata* remains endemic even in Western Europe and sporadic cases of human taeniosis and of epizootic outbreaks of bovine cysticercosis occur in nonendemic regions in spite of better public health and veterinary infrastructure, including regulated inspection of cattle carcasses at slaughter and trace back procedures to identify, quarantine, and monitor infected herds (Dorny and Praet, 2007).

Because of the high costs of implementing the insensitive inspection procedure for the screening of cattle for cysticercosis in developed countries with low prevalence, models have been developed to demonstrate the negligible residual risk to the consumer in domestic or export markets if inspection measures were reduced or even eliminated (Van Der Logt et al., 1997; Calvo-Artavia et al., 2013). A similar model has recently been used by FAO/WHO to develop risk-based examples to provide country authorities with a tool to assess the effects of various control measures, including meat inspection, on residual risk (CAC, 2013; FAO/WHO, 2014b).

A collaborative effort by WHO/FAO/OIE has provided guidelines for the prevention and control of taeniosis/cysticercosis, as have other organizations such as the Cysticercosis Working Group in Peru (WHO/FAO/OIE, 2005; Garcia et al., 2007). *Taenia solium* is more amenable to eradication compared to *T. saginata*, due to the reduced potential for widespread contamination of the environment with infective eggs disseminated only via active defecation. Although sustained interventions targeted solely at livestock or at human taeniosis could in theory be effective in reducing the transmission of *T. saginata* and *T. solium*, simultaneous treatment of taeniosis combined with effective interventions in livestock is the ideal approach. Such a program is currently being carried out in Peru for *T. solium*, although the feasibility and sustainability of such a complex and expensive undertaking remains to be seen (Garcia et al., 2010; Lightowlers, 2013).

14.3.2 Trichinella *spp.*

Trichinellosis in humans is a reportable or notifiable disease in most developed countries, as is *Trichinella* infection in domestic livestock. Historically, most outbreaks of human trichinellosis have been associated with *Trichinella spiralis*-infected swine (Dupouy-Camet, 2000). Regulations for control in swine have been applied in many countries for over a century, and typically entail restrictions on access to infected food waste, carcasses, rats, and wild animals, testing to detect positive carcasses and/ or treatment to inactivate any parasites present (FAO, 2013b). Consequently, in these countries, human trichinellosis from commercial meat is rare (Gajadhar et al., 2006). Standard biosecurity measures inherent in modern swine production in industrialized countries facilitate the certification of *Trichinella*-free farms and herds in nonendemic areas (Pyburn et al., 2005). However, even in these countries, human outbreaks linked to imported meat or consumption of wild game continue to occur, and much effort and expense is expended in the monitoring and demonstration of negligible risk of infection for food safety and trade purposes. For example, more than 167 million pigs have been tested annually for *Trichinella* in the European Union (EU) in accordance with their meat hygiene regulations (Alban et al., 2011). This is disproportionate to the relatively low global burden posed by trichinellosis compared to other foodborne parasitic diseases (Devleesschauwer et al., 2014).

The OIE and Codex have responsibilities for establishing guidelines for trade and control to reduce the risk of *Trichinella* in food animals and their products, respectively (CAC, 2013; FAO, 2013b; OIE, 2014c). Additionally, the ICT and the FAO/WHO/OIE have provided guidelines for control (Gamble et al., 2000; FAO/WHO/OIE, 2007). At the national and local levels, veterinary and public health authorities are, in turn, responsible for the control of *Trichinella* at the farm, processing and distribution levels (FAO, 2013b). Chapter 8.15 of the current OIE Terrestrial Animal Health Code and Codex draft guidelines for the control of *Trichinella* meat are designed to achieve a level of negligible risk in a swine herd or compartment, regardless of the status of *Trichinella* spp. in any particular country (CAC, 2013; OIE, 2014c). The OIE provides the conditions and criteria to be met for mitigating the risk of infection to pigs to establish a negligible risk compartment, and Codex provides the recommendations for verifying the maintenance of the compartment or for processing and treatment of carcasses to ensure consumer safety. Testing of pigs and auditing, taking into account historical data such as surveillance of domestic pigs and wildlife, public health records of trichinellosis occurrences, and the like is required to verify the successful establishment and maintenance of a compartment. What constitutes an acceptable negligible risk in terms of the potential number of *Trichinella*-infected pigs in the population in spite of these measures must be determined by the competent authority in each country and will depend on the proportion of the population tested and other mitigating factors such as carcass processing and consumption habits. For the EU, the standard target is one in a million pigs (Alban et al., 2011). To support this decision making by country risk managers, FAO/WHO (2014b) has recently developed a model to provide risk-based examples enabling the determination of residual risk for *Trichinella* based on the pre- and postharvest measures implemented, including the proportion of pigs to be tested in a particular population.

The control of *Trichinella* infection in free-range pasturing and backyard rearing practices, for organic pork and for "traditional" or artisanal ready-to-eat meat products bypassing conventional treatments to inactivate *Trichinella* can be more challenging. In addition to *T. spiralis*, sylvatic species which establish well in pigs include *T. britovi*, *T. pseudospiralis*, *T. papuae*, and *T. zimbabwensis* (Kapel, 2000; OIE, 2014b; FAO, 2013b). Minimum regulations for these commodities should entail individual carcass testing or appropriate treatment to inactivate any parasites present. Because natural infections with *T. spiralis*, *T. britovi*, and *T. murrelli* have occurred in horses, since

1994 there has been mandatory testing of all fresh horsemeat consumed in Europe. However, outbreaks linked to horsemeat still occur, and further requirements in quality assurance to ensure reliability of the testing performed may be necessary (Boireau et al., 2000).

14.3.3 Opisthorchiidae

In general, the risk of infection with the foodborne trematodes (FBTs) *Clonorchis sinensis* and *Opisthorchis* spp. is greatest from the consumption of native wild fish, because most of the susceptible cyprinid host species are of relatively low commercial value and are usually cultured only on a small scale for domestic consumers. However, this is changing, with several species of cyprinid carps being cultured more extensively for international trade. This is contributing to the reemergence of these FBTs globally, including in developed regions, due to the growing propensity to consume local or imported fish from endemic regions uncooked (Fried and Abruzzi, 2010; Pozio et al., 2013). Thus, several factors, such as deeply imbedded cultural habits, poverty, and increasing international markets and demographics make effective control difficult (Toledo et al., 2012). However, if aquaculture is to establish itself as a major sector in worldwide food production, recognition and regulated control of these food safety risks is increasingly important. Although long recognized as an emerging and significant public health issue, international control campaigns previously initiated by FAO and WHO have languished, and only recently have these parasites been included in the priority list of the WHO (Toledo et al., 2012; FAO/WHO, 2014a).

Chapters 10 and 12 provide additional details on these FBTs and their infection in fish. Although there are several stages in the life cycle where control can be applied, it is unlikely that control of any single stage would be effective across the variety of cultural practices employed in the countries endemic for these parasites. Regulations pertaining to the inactivation of these FBTs in fish are prescribed by most developed countries or regions, including the European Community (EC), the United States, and Canada. However, the ideal strategy should integrate multiple interventions and be based on a disciplined systematic appraisal of the entire production system to identify where controls will most effectively mitigate the risk of infection, such as the HACCP system (Lima dos Santos and Howgate, 2011; Hung et al., 2013b). As with any foodborne parasite control program, ongoing success requires a multidisciplinary approach, incorporating all aspects of the food chain, including production, processing, trade, and consumption of fish. This requires an enabling policy from governments and a national and international regulatory environment with defined standards, establishment of appropriate food control systems and programs, including surveillance, at national and local levels, and provision of appropriate training and capacity building (WHO/FAO, 2002). Since 2005, the Denmark-funded FIBOZOPA (Fish-borne Zoonotic Parasites in Vietnam) project has been operating in Vietnam to increase awareness of the occurrence, risks, and preventative measures for fish-borne zoonotic parasitic infections in humans and to acquire knowledge and tools to address the challenges at central government and provincial levels. However, although there are similar initiatives in other endemic countries, in general, wide-scale prevention activities are not currently implemented at the primary fish production level, especially in small-scale operations (Lima dos Santos and Howgate, 2011).

14.3.4 Coccidian protozoa

Cyclospora cayetanensis, *Cryptosporidium* spp., and *Toxoplasma gondii* occur worldwide with the highest prevalence in those regions where poor hygiene, sanitation, animal husbandry, and agricultural practices facilitate contamination of food and water with oocysts. *Toxoplasma* is also most prevalent in regions where raw meat is consumed, as the meat may be infected with the tissue stages of the parasite. Further details on these parasites and the foods they infect or contaminate are found in Chapters 6, 11, and 13.

Recent attention in the EU has focused on the establishment of serological herd profiles and risk categorization for a number of zoonotic and production diseases of livestock, including *Toxoplasma*, to enable risk categorization and risk-based decisions required by European food safety regulations (Meemken et al., 2014). This will hopefully pave the way for other countries to adopt a similar approach. Because practical and reliable treatments for removal or inactivation of oocysts from contaminated fresh produce and other foods are not yet available, developed countries also need to take an active role in assisting endemic countries to minimize risk. In 1999, in response to the growing problem of cyclosporosis attributed to contaminated Guatemalan raspberries, the Model Plan of Excellence (MPE) was developed through cooperation between the US Food and Drug Administration, the Guatemalan government, and the Guatemalan Berry Commission. The MPE is a system based on GAPs and designed to guard against contamination by monitoring important food-safety aspects of berry production, including oversight and surveillance of sanitation practices, water source development, irrigation methods, food handling, and employee hygiene (Orlandi et al., 2002). Even for *Toxoplasma*, which is ubiquitous, there are geographically associated strains with differences in virulence, and the global trade in fresh-chilled meat and produce may result in the spreading of more virulent strains (Robertson et al., 2013). Clinical toxoplasmosis cases in France have been attributed to the consumption of imported raw horsemeat infected with atypical, more virulent strains of the parasite (Pomares et al., 2011). Some of this infected horsemeat was from Brazil, which is known to harbor a diversity of genotypes that tend to be more virulent than those in Europe and North America (Carneiro et al., 2013; Clementino Andrade et al., 2013). Therefore food safety awareness and training, under regulatory oversight, is an absolute necessity if progress is to be made in the provision of safe food internationally (Ortega and Sanchez, 2010).

14.4 Detection and diagnosis

Methods for the detection and diagnosis of foodborne parasites in humans, animals, and their products have evolved from primarily traditional visual inspection and microscopic confirmation to include an array of immunological and molecular techniques, many of which are available as commercial kits. Further information on these diagnostic methods is provided in Chapter 16, and in other chapters as indicated for the parasite-specific examples below. Also, information on the diagnosis of *Taenia*, *Trichinella*, *Cryptosporidium*, and *Toxoplasma*, including any prescribed tests for international trade, is provided in Chapters 2.9.5, 2.1.16, 2.9.4, and 2.9.10, respectively, of the OIE *Manual of Diagnostic Tests and Vaccines for Terrestrial Animals* (OIE, 2014b). Limitations of available assays include inadequate sensitivity and specificity, host species-specific reliability, and ability to determine viability and infectivity of the detected parasite. Unlike bacteria and viruses, most parasites cannot be readily propagated *in vitro* and/or *in vivo* to increase their numbers and resultant sensitivity of detection.

Regardless of the method used, it must fit the intended purpose. Whenever feasible, only reliable methods that are standardized, validated, and performed under appropriate conditions of quality assurance should be used. In additional to the OIE terrestrial animal manual and code, ISO and ICT provide standards and guidelines, respectively, for acceptable methods and quality assurance requirements for the testing of some foodborne parasites. Further information on standard-setting organizations is provided in Chapter 17. International reference laboratories with pathogen-specific expertise such as those designated by OIE and WHO are also important sources for the provision of scientific advice, reference materials, controls, reagents, and confirmatory testing.

14.4.1 Taenia *spp.*

The control measures most commonly implemented for porcine and bovine cysticercosis rely on the organoleptic detection of cysticerci in carcass "predilection" sites during postslaughter inspection, with treatment or disposal of affected carcasses (Saini et al., 1997; CAC, 2013). Identification of suspect cysticerci is based on morphology and host-specificity, with histological, immunohistochemical, or molecular confirmation of degenerating parasite lesions (Scandrett et al., 2012). For pigs, tongue palpation can be a practical means to detect infections in endemic developing regions. However, all these procedures have a low sensitivity of detecting light infections, which is further reduced in nonendemic regions where inspectors are unfamiliar with the appearance and detection of the *in situ* cysticerci (Dewhirst et al., 1967). Serological assays to detect cysticercus antibodies or antigen (Ab- and Ag ELISA, respectively) for the detection of bovine and porcine cysticercosis have the potential to be much more sensitive than meat inspection, but these methods are currently unreliable for determining the status of individual animals, particularly when low numbers of cysts are present. They are nevertheless valuable for surveillance and epidemiological investigations (Dorny et al., 2000; Abuseir et al., 2007). Immunodiagnosis of porcine cysticercosis has benefited from the adaptation of serological tools developed for diagnosis of human neurocysticercosis.

The routine method for diagnosing human taeniosis is coprological examination for *Taenia* eggs. This method, however, has relatively low sensitivity, particularly for single samples, and does not differentiate among *Taenia* species. Coproantigen

ELISAs have been developed; these are purported to be more sensitive, and in some cases species-specific. Molecular assays have also been developed to enable species-specific tapeworm detection in feces. Validation of these newer methods has been limited. Serological diagnosis of *T. solium* taeniosis by methods such as enzyme-linked immune-electrotransfer blot (EITB) and Western blot (WB) have been developed but are currently used only for research purposes (DeGiorgio et al., 2005; Praet et al., 2013). There are no reliable methods for the detection of *Taenia* eggs in feed, water, or the environment (Scandrett and Gajadhar, 2004). This also applies to the detection of *T. solium* eggs contaminating fruits and vegetables for human consumption (Uga et al., 2009). Although eggs of these *Taenia* are morphologically indistinguishable from those of all other taniids, molecular methods are available to differentiate them (Nkouawa et al., 2009). Additional information on the detection and diagnosis of taeniosis and cysticercosis is provided in Chapters 9 and 11.

14.4.2 Trichinella *spp.*

The test method currently recommended by the OIE, Codex, and ICT for trade and food safety purposes is the magnetic stirrer digestion assay, which enables the direct detection of *Trichinella* larvae in meat (Gajadhar et al., 2009; CAC, 2013; OIE, 2014b,c). Although predilection sites vary according to host species, the tongue and the diaphragm are often among the preferred sites. The ICT has recently provided guidelines for essential quality assurance standards for *Trichinella* digestion assays (ICT, 2014). An ISO standard for this method (ISO/DIS 18743) is also currently under development and should be available in the near future. Trichinoscopy, another direct method used historically, is less sensitive than digestion and is not recommended for food safety testing (Forbes et al., 2003; OIE, 2014b). However, in countries where resources are limited and *Trichinella* is endemic or emerging in domestic host species, use of this method may have merit as the only practical tool available to mitigate parasite transmission and disease. Molecular methods are available to determine genotype or species of recovered *Trichinella* larvae for epidemiological purposes and to determine the risk to domestic livestock and options for treatment (e.g., freezing of susceptible species) to inactivate the parasite (Zarlenga et al., 1999).

Serological testing of pre- or postmortem serum or meat juice samples is currently recommended by the OIE and ICT only for the detection and control of *Trichinella* infection at the herd or population level, but not to reliably determine individual animal status for food safety purposes (OIE, 2014b,c). Serological testing typically employs an indirect Ab ELISA using *Trichinella* excretory–secretory (ES) antigen to detect host IgG, with confirmation by WB. It is an important tool for establishing baseline estimates of *Trichinella* prevalence by serosurveillance of human and domestic animal and wildlife populations, and for epidemiological and disease control investigations (Gajadhar and Forbes, 2010; Nga et al., 2013; Meemken et al., 2014). Whenever feasible, corresponding tissue samples or biopsies for digestion assay should also be collected so that seropositive results can be corroborated by the detection of larvae, and genotyping can be performed. Additional information on the detection and diagnosis of *Trichinella* is provided in Chapters 8 and 11.

A quality assurance system for *Trichinella* digestion testing of pork and horsemeat has been implemented in Canada to meet the requirements for the export of fresh pork and horsemeat to the EU (Forbes et al., 1998; Forbes and Gajadhar, 1999). Similar systems have been adopted, in whole or in part, in Europe and elsewhere (Vallee et al., 2007; Larrat et al., 2012). However, in many cases, more stringent adherence to quality assurance is required; a recent study of laboratory performance of *Trichinella* testing in Germany indicated that many labs were performing far below an acceptable standard for food safety (Petroff et al., 2014). The ICT provides recommendations on essential components and minimum requirements for a *Trichinella* testing laboratory certification (or similar qualification) program (ICT, 2014).

14.4.3 Opisthorchiidae

The most common control measures against opisthorchiids entail their detection and inactivation in fish. The identification of fluke larvae in fish remains the best method for detection and relies on morphological characterization by visual inspection, including direct tissue examination and stereoscopic examination of samples processed by muscle compression or pepsin–HCl artificial digestion. Specific identification of metacercariae requires examination of characteristic features and dimensions observed under compound microscopy. Although the application of molecular methods to detect metacercariae is limited, a number of species-specific PCR-based methods have been developed, and some of the molecular tools already applied to the diagnosis of human infection are also available for testing food (Toledo et al., 2012).

Several approaches are available for the diagnosis of human and other definitive host infections, of which direct detection of eggs in feces or bile is the preferred method. However, such egg-based assays have low sensitivity in detecting light infections and low specificity due to the morphological similarities of eggs from a variety of trematodes. This lack of specificity is more of an issue in surveillance activities where the prevalence and response to intervention measures requires accurate identification of the agents. However, this is not as important for decisions regarding the administration of mass or individual chemotherapy as the drugs used are broad spectrum with few side effects. Other assays to detect these infections in feces include detection of fecal antigen by ELISA and molecular methods. Several serological tests have been developed, of which the indirect ELISA is the most common approach. Sensitivity and specificity vary, based on the antigen used. Use of specific recombinant antigens has yielded higher sensitivities and specificities than for native antigens. Regardless of antigen quality, the main limitation of this indirect approach is the inability to determine past from current infection, inasmuch as antibodies in clonorchiasis and opisthorchiasis persist for months to years after curative treatment of infected human hosts (Johansen et al., 2010). For any diagnostic method to be useful, particularly in poor regions where FBTs are endemic, it needs to be accurate, simple, and affordable. This is a challenge, because increasing accuracy usually entails more complexity and costs. Further information on the detection and diagnosis of these FBTs is provided in Chapters 10 and 12.

14.4.4 Coccidian protozoa

Various methods are available for the detection of foodborne coccidia in humans, animals, food, and the environment. These include parasite isolation and identification by traditional parasitological methods, immunoassays, bioassays, and PCR and other molecular assays. Additional information on the detection and diagnosis of these parasites is available in Chapters 6 and 11. The most commonly used methods rely on the detection of oocysts or their antigens in stool or other samples, with some of these assays available as commercial kits. Microscopic examination and identification of oocysts based on morphology can be challenging due to their small size and difficulty in differentiating from artifact (Goodgame, 1996). In the United Kingdom during the period from 1993 to 1998, only 58% of participating laboratories correctly identified *Cyclospora*-positive samples in a wet preparation (Cann et al., 2000). Various staining techniques are available to increase sensitivity and specificity, but require expertise in interpretation. Demonstration of autofluorescence under an epifluorescence microscope can also aid in detection, as do more costly direct and indirect immunofluorescence assays. Sporulation of *Cyclospora* and *Toxoplasma* oocysts will also facilitate sensitivity and specificity of identification; however, sporulation does not necessarily correlate with infectivity, and for *Cyclospora* no animal models exist for bioassay (Ortega and Sanchez, 2010). Samples may be concentrated using standard flotation techniques, but the recovery percentage of oocysts varies by the method and matrix being tested. Detection in large volume samples of water used for irrigation or processing vegetables or other foods requires filtration or other techniques to concentrate any oocysts present (Sturbaum et al., 1998; Bellamy, 2004). General quality assurance recommendations for the detection of these parasites, using *Cryptosporidium* as an example, have been provided by Bellamy (2004). An ISO international standard (ISO/DIS 18744) is also under development for the detection and enumeration of *Cryptosporidium* in fresh, green leafy vegetables and berries.

Serology is the most common method for routine diagnosis and surveillance of human and animal exposure to *Toxoplasma*. A number of commercial serological kits are available, most of which using native antigens prepared from tachyzoites grown in mice and/or tissue culture. However, recent studies have indicated that the use of recombinant antigens may have potential advantages of improved method specificity, standardization, and cost-effectiveness. Also, selected antigens corresponding to acute or chronic infection could enable differentiation between the two stages (Holec-Gasior, 2013). Serology is not routinely used for the diagnosis of *Cryptosporidium*, and efforts to develop such methods for detection of *Cyclospora* in humans have been hindered by the lack of an animal model needed to generate the large numbers of oocysts required (Ortega and Sanchez, 2010).

14.5 Surveillance

Surveillance refers to the ongoing systematic collection of data to determine the prevalence and severity of a disease or pathogen in a population. It should begin with the establishment of baseline data on the epidemiological, economic, and social impact of the pathogen (OIE, 2014a). Surveillance also implies the intent to implement timely corrective actions when there is evidence for increased incidence of disease or infection. For practical reasons, surveillance programs are typically designed to collect data from a convenience sector of the population (with potential sample bias), but can be an effective means to control and limit the impact of foodborne parasites on public health (Orlandi et al., 2002; Collett, 2013). For foodborne parasitic diseases, different surveillance methods are applicable in the veterinary and public health sectors, and a balance between animal health and public health interests must be considered (Berman and Shimshony, 2013). The design of surveillance and control strategies for the various foodborne parasite species and the respective involvement of veterinary and public health agencies vary considerably based on the diverse epidemiological aspects and life cycles of these parasites (Murrell, 2013). Surveillance can be active or passive; because many foodborne parasites cause subclinical infections that can evade diagnosis, passive surveillance only cannot be relied on for effective control (Berman and Shimshony, 2013). Regardless, integrating surveillance programs across animal and public health sectors to harmonize the collection and interpretation of data is essential to rapidly report and respond to any foodborne parasite occurrences (Acar and Moulin, 2013). Surveillance activities can target any stage of the food production chain and should be designed to provide guidance on priorities and targets for the application of interventions and to demonstrate the impact of any such interventions (Carr and Bartram, 2004; OIE, 2014a). The OIE terrestrial code's Chapter 1.4 and WHO provide guidance on the design and assessment of animal health surveillance systems, and on surveillance to detect foodborne disease outbreaks, respectively (WHO, 2008a; OIE, 2014c). For the reasons indicated in the previous section on detection and diagnosis, serology is often the test method of choice when conducting surveillance of human and animal populations, but the method used ultimately will depend on the nature of the sample matrix and fitness for purpose.

14.5.1 Taenia *spp.*

Surveillance for *T. solium* and *T. saginata* in countries with control programs for these parasites mostly entails the mandatory slaughter inspection of pig and cattle carcasses for the presence of cysticercosis. Because the overall sensitivity of this inspection procedure is low, estimates of true overall prevalence must take this into account. With the suboptimal sensitivity and specificity of current serological assays, these indirect methods have yet to be widely adopted for the regulated surveillance of porcine or bovine cysticercosis, especially in nonendemic countries where false-positive results are particularly problematic. However, they can be used for the antemortem screening of suspect herds identified as such via meat inspection, and have proven to be valuable tools in seroprevalence studies to elucidate the epidemiology of these infections in endemic and nonendemic regions (Dorny et al., 2000; de Cassia Paulan et al., 2013).

Because human taeniosis is not notifiable in most countries, relatively little attention has focused on its surveillance for disease control purposes. Prevalence estimates based on surveillance data are further compromised by the fact that taeniosis is frequently underdiagnosed and underreported by physicians, and many patients hesitate to seek medical care due to sociological reasons. Thus, such estimates must often be determined indirectly, for example, by extrapolation from sales figures for specific anthelmintics (Dupuy et al., 2014). In addition to surveillance data accrued via fecal testing, serological tests have been used to conduct seroprevalence studies of *T. solium* taeniosis in populations at risk (DeGiorgio et al., 2005). Surveillance studies of human cysticercosis using assays such as the Ag ELISA and EITB to detect antigen and antibody, respectively, have also been particularly valuable in establishing baseline estimates of incidence or prevalence in endemic regions such as Ecuador, for input into epidemiological models to enable a better understanding of parasite transmission and the effects of control interventions (Coral-Almeida et al., 2014).

14.5.2 Trichinella *spp.*

Although surveillance data for trichinellosis have been accrued in those countries with mandatory reporting of human cases, surveillance for *Trichinella* has consisted mainly of the slaughter testing of domestic swine by digestion assay or serology for food safety and/or trade purposes. Surveillance data for horses are similarly generated from the regulated slaughter testing of horses. Although no longer recognized as such under the new OIE terrestrial code, Belgium and Denmark achieved previous international recognition of countrywide negligible status for *Trichinella* by testing all slaughtered swine by digestion assay. In other low-prevalence countries such as Canada, regulated slaughter testing of a representative subpopulation of the national swine herd using digestion assay or serology has been conducted annually to demonstrate negligible levels of infection. Such subpopulations should include high-risk sows and boars, and pigs not raised under controlled housing conditions (Alban et al., 2011; Vanderstichel et al., 2013). The importance of ongoing surveillance has been recently highlighted by outbreaks of trichinellosis in Italy and Argentina due to *T. britovi* in wild boar and *T. spiralis* in domestic pigs, respectively, in areas thought to be free of these parasites (Calcagno et al., 2014; Fichi et al., 2014).

To meet current OIE requirements for surveillance of domestic pigs and wildlife to establish compartments with negligible risk for *Trichinella*, only the digestion assay is recommended for testing. Although serological testing by ELISA may be acceptable in the future, it is currently recommended only for epidemiological purposes due to the lack of standardization and unreliable sensitivity and specificity. Serology will likely be of limited use in the surveillance of horses for *Trichinella* because antibody levels in this species can drop below detectable levels despite the existence of infective larvae in muscle (Hill et al., 2007).

14.5.3 Opisthorchiidae

Surveillance for these FBTs has focused primarily on humans in endemic regions to establish baseline prevalence estimates and to assess the impact of control measures. However, as a neglected tropical disease (NTD) primarily of poor and marginalized populations, reliable estimates of prevalence have been difficult to obtain. The resulting lack of accurate data about disease burden compromises the effectiveness of any control programs attempted (Whittaker et al., 2013). Although serological and molecular assays are available, even for recent surveillance studies, standard egg-based assays of fecal samples have been the methods most commonly used (Suwannahitatorn et al., 2013). This widespread reliance on relatively insensitive fecal egg detection methods may be sufficient to establish initial baseline estimates of disease burden in regions with little control and high prevalence, but once controls are implemented and prevalence and intensity decline, diagnosis using these methods becomes ambiguous and low-intensity infections may be overlooked. This negative bias can lead to an overestimation of the success of control programs and the subsequent redirection of control efforts to other areas, eventually facilitating the reemergence of the original problem (Whittaker et al., 2013). More sensitive and specific methods such as PCR are available and recommended to overcome the diagnostic limitations of these conventional parasitological methods (Traub et al., 2009).

Comparatively little surveillance of definitive host livestock or wildlife species has been conducted, which also typically relies on the detection of trematode eggs in fecal samples, although prevalence studies based on postmortem examination for adult flukes have also been conducted (Johansen et al., 2010; Lin et al., 2011). Surveys of snail and fish intermediate hosts have been conducted mostly using tissue compression or digestion assay to detect the respective larval stages of the parasite, although molecular methods are increasingly being used (Zhang et al., 2007; Wiriya et al., 2013).

14.5.4 Coccidian protozoa

Numerous serological and epidemiological studies have been conducted, but few countries have implemented comprehensive surveillance programs for these coccidial infections in humans or animals (Gajadhar et al., 2006; Murrell, 2013; Steinparzer et al., 2014). Most of the surveillance so far has focused on *Toxoplasma*. When implemented for humans, surveillance often relies on voluntary reporting and follow-up on presumptive cases only, or targeting high-risk populations rather than the general population at large (Alvarado-Esquivel et al., 2014). Prevalence estimates for human infection with these ubiquitous coccidia are further compromised by underreporting and the benign or nonspecific nature of the clinical manifestations of most infections. Similarly, the numerous surveillance studies of livestock, wildlife, or foods for these parasites typically have been on a relatively small scale. Serological monitoring of food animals is further hindered by a lack of general agreement among the tests to be used, of availability of reference sera and other materials, and of laboratory certification programs (Kijlstra and Jongert, 2008). Methods available for animals have been validated only in a few common domestic species, such as the pig and cat for *T. gondii*, and are limited by a requirement for species-specific secondary conjugated antibody. A recently developed indirect ELISA using a nonspecies-specific protein A/G conjugate has proved effective for the detection of *T. gondii* in a variety of mammalian hosts, including wildlife (Al-Adhami and Gajadhar, 2014). This may help address the many knowledge gaps in the overall epidemiology and significance of this parasite regionally and globally. Establishing serological herd profiles for *Toxoplasma* in swine and other species of concern will also enable the risk categorization and risk-based decisions necessary for targeted interventions to improve food safety (Meemken et al., 2014).

Because transmission of *Toxoplasma* can occur via the consumption of tissue cysts in meat and does not require ingestion of oocysts, the domestic cat definitive host has perhaps been unfairly vilified in the perpetuation of this parasite (Thompson, 2014). However, a large-scale nationwide survey of retail meats in the United States found viable *Toxoplasma* in only a few pork samples, concluding that consumption of retail meats could not account for the level of *Toxoplasma* in the US population (Hill and Dubey, 2013). A recently developed serological assay incorporating a sporozoite-specific antigen to determine oocyst exposure will hopefully help to better elucidate this in the future (Jones and Dubey, 2012). Most surveillance studies to determine the prevalence of *Cyclospora*, *Cryptosporidium*, and *Toxoplasma* oocyst contamination of fresh fruit and vegetables have examined produce at the farm level or at local markets in developing countries. However, similar surveillance is increasingly being conducted in developed countries, on imported and domestic produce, and at the retail level (Lass et al., 2012). For example, the detection of *Cyclospora* and *Cryptosporidium* oocyst contamination of retail leafy greens has been incorporated into the ongoing surveillance by the C-EnterNet Program of the Public Health Agency of Canada (Dixon et al., 2013). Further information on surveillance studies of these parasites on fresh produce is provided in Chapter 13.

14.6 Incursions and outbreak investigations

A systematic procedure to investigate the cause and source of incursions or outbreaks detected via surveillance, or otherwise, is necessary to control and prevent future occurrences of foodborne parasites. Such an outbreak investigation is an important responsibility of the relevant competent authority to ensure that preventative and control measures are applied, to recognize control strategy deficiencies and achievements, to identify changes in the pathogen, environment, or other aspects that may be beyond the scope of the control program, and to help demonstrate the effectiveness of the surveillance program. Important steps in an outbreak investigation include determining the validity of any reports triggering an investigation and confirming the diagnosis. When appropriate, national laboratories can submit samples to international reference laboratories for confirmation of findings and more detailed analysis (WHO, 2008b; OIE, 2014a). Effective systems for identification and traceability of animals, based on the principles in Chapter 4.1 of the OIE terrestrial code, and of food products are also required (Britt et al., 2013; OIE, 2014c). Additional provisions or contingencies include rapid diagnosis and communication of results, quarantine, slaughter and depopulation, sanitation, disinfection, disposal, and food recall, as appropriate (Hastein, 2000).

14.6.1 Taenia *spp.*

When epizootics of porcine or bovine cysticercosis, or of neurocysticercosis, occur in nonendemic countries, there is often little data available on the occurrence of human taeniosis to aid investigators in determining the source of infection. Because of the stigma associated with taeniosis, even when more sensitive diagnostic assays such as the coproantigen ELISA are used to screen suspected tapeworm carriers, results are usually unrewarding due to compliance problems with the provision of reliable fecal samples. Even when a particular contaminated feed or water source is suspected, processing of relatively large sample volumes, usually contaminated at low levels, is problematic. Modified flotation methods have been attempted in such cases, but the high specific gravity of *Taenia* eggs, and confounding artifacts and adherent debris in the assayed matrix negatively impact sensitivity (Scandrett and Gajadhar, 2004). In addition, usually a minimum of several months have elapsed after presumed exposure before the cysticerci can be detected at slaughter, or before clinical neurocysticercosis is evident, and the contaminated source may no longer remain or may have undergone degeneration, further confounding recovery of the agent and interpretation of results. Because taeniid eggs cannot be speciated based on morphology, and there are no baseline data available for levels of environmental contamination with other domestic and wildlife taeniid species, any positive findings not confirmed by molecular methods must be interpreted with caution. Therefore, in most outbreak investigations of cysticercosis, neither the human source of infective eggs, nor the contaminated feed or water matrix is definitively identified (Schantz et al., 1992; Jenkins et al., 2013a). This poses challenges to determining effective preventative measures and can result in prolonged quarantine and/or monitoring of suspect herds until there is no further evidence of ongoing exposure to infective eggs.

14.6.2 Trichinella *spp.*

Trichinella in domestic swine is well controlled in most developed countries; hence outbreaks of pastoral trichinellosis are uncommon in these regions. However, occasional outbreaks associated with free-ranging backyard swine herds, and with feral swine, wild boar, horsemeat, and wild game, persist. Outbreaks of pastoral and sylvatic trichinellosis increasingly are being reported from developing countries, particularly China and Southeast Asia, and trichinellosis has reemerged in Eastern Europe as a result of widespread breakdowns in the veterinary public heath infrastructure due to regional conflicts and economic collapse. The increasing occurrence of trichinellosis outbreaks in China, particularly in urban areas, appears due in part to increasing affluence, which makes pork more accessible to the masses (Bruschi, 2012). Although outbreaks are rare in predominantly Muslim or Jewish countries where consumption of pork is prohibited for religious reasons, outbreaks have occurred due to food adulteration with infected pork (Turk et al., 2006). The adulteration of beef with horsemeat, which has caused a recent scandal in Europe, also constitutes an increased risk for trichinellosis (Boyaci et al., 2014). Although infection of horses is rare, one infected horse can result in an outbreak affecting hundreds of people (Boireau et al., 2000). Because of the typically less rigid animal identification and trace back requirements for horses compared to most other livestock, determining the on-farm source of infection is usually impossible.

As for many parasitic infections, early clinical diagnosis of trichinellosis is difficult because there are no pathognomonic symptoms, and physicians in nonendemic countries are unfamiliar with the disease (Gottstein et al., 2009). In addition, the reliability of testing samples for *Trichinella* in an outbreak investigation can be compromised if the implicated meat has been processed or otherwise treated, since the digestion assay has been extensively validated only on fresh muscle tissue.

14.6.3 Opisthorchiidae

There are relatively few recent reports of outbreaks due to *C. sinensis* and *O. viverrini* in endemic regions in Asia, presumably due to inadequate surveillance and public health infrastructure, and the usually chronic and insidious nature of these infections. However, there are increasing reports of outbreaks due to *O. felineus* from Europe where this parasite is endemic, as well as from other nonendemic regions (Yossepowitch et al., 2004; Pozio et al., 2013). This has been most evident in central Italy where there have been several outbreaks of human opisthorchiasis since it was first reported in 2004. Most of these outbreaks have implicated raw tench (*Tinca tinca*) as the source of infection. The challenges associated with these investigations have included a high percentage of asymptomatic infections, unfamiliarity with the disease by physicians, and poor sensitivity of diagnosis by laboratories performing only microscopic examination for trematode eggs in feces, instead of using serological or molecular detection methods. This has led to delays in diagnoses and recognition of these outbreaks (Armignacco et al., 2013).

A subsequent extensive investigation related to these outbreaks conducted by De Liberato et al. (2011) used standard egg detection assays, muscle compression and digestion assays, and molecular methods to analyze a variety of snails, fish, and definitive host species for this parasite. A high prevalence of infection was found in tench and domestic cat intermediate and definitive hosts, respectively, confirming the endemic presence of the parasite in the region. However, as there is a widespread distribution and variety of competent intermediate and definitive (primary and reservoir) host species for these parasites, further investigation will be required to better elucidate the epidemiology of these outbreaks (Diaz, 2013). In particular, additional species of native cyprinid fish, of which the raw consumption has become increasingly popular in recent years, should be evaluated (De Liberato et al., 2011).

14.6.4 Coccidian protozoa

Foodborne outbreaks caused by zoonotic coccidia are difficult to investigate because their incubation periods are relatively prolonged compared to other common foodborne pathogens, and by the time the outbreak is identified, the implicated food has usually been consumed, discarded, or is no longer suitable for testing. This is particularly true for *Toxoplasma*, where manifestation of infection can take weeks to years. Therefore, outbreak investigations must generally rely on microbiological analysis of clinical samples, retrospective interviews for epidemiological descriptions and analysis, and environmental inspection of suspected food premises (Robertson and Chalmers, 2013). In addition, the nonspecific clinical nature of these infections results in underreporting and presents challenges to establishing case definition criteria. Identification of the original source and mode of contamination is further complicated for implicated foods that have been imported. Because oocysts of many species are ubiquitous in the environment and are often difficult to distinguish morphologically, molecular methods are essential to identify species, genotype, and subtype as relevant, to determine the organism responsible for the outbreak, and the source and routes of transmission. The current limitations of molecular tools available for these purposes can hopefully be addressed in the future using techniques such as next-generation sequencing (Ryan et al., 2014).

An example of an effective outbreak investigation infrastructure possibly leading to an apparent excess of foodborne outbreaks is the relatively high number of cases in Nordic countries linked to contamination of produce with *Cryptosporidium*. This, at first, seems unreconcilable with the fact that Nordic countries are among the most privileged in the world, with relatively low population densities, comprehensive social welfare and health care systems, and a very high global ranking for quality of life. However, this same status may better enable optimization of diagnostic techniques and implementation of effective epidemiological investigation, follow-up, and reporting, compared to other countries (Robertson and Chalmers, 2013). Further information on outbreaks linked to produce contaminated with these parasites is provided in Chapter 13.

14.7 Treatment and inactivation

Infection or contamination of food products by parasites can occur at any stage in the food production chain. Chemotherapeutic, chemical, or physical destruction or inactivation of foodborne parasites in susceptible humans or animals, foods, or contaminated environments are currently the most commonly implemented control measures. Depending on the parasite and the affected matrix, a variety of treatment options exist, and international standards for postharvest treatments of particular parasites and foods are provided by Codex. Of these, cooking is still the most reliable control measure, since most parasites will be killed or inactivated by temperatures as low as 60 °C. However, the heat must uniformly penetrate the entire food matrix to destroy any parasites that may be encysted within (Orlandi et al., 2002). Washing of produce contaminated with protozoan parasites will not reliably remove them, and conventional disinfectants such as chlorine will not inactivate them. For contaminated source water, filtration is an effective means to remove all but the smallest of parasites (Orlandi et al., 2002). Freezing at specified temperature and time combinations can be recommended for the reliable inactivation of many protozoan and helminth foodborne parasites in a variety of food matrices, but some parasites have evolved to survive extremely low temperatures. Freezing, particularly in the short term and at the consumer level, can be unpredictable and may, in fact, preserve rather than inactivate parasites under certain conditions (Orlandi et al., 2002). Increasing consumer preferences for raw or semicooked fish and meat, and the consumption of fresh fruit and vegetables also preclude the use of heat or cold as control measures. Other traditional processes such as smoking, brining, and curing can be effective for inactivation of some foodborne helminth parasites in particular food matrices if specified protocols are followed, but much work remains to develop and validate reliable methods using these processes. Newer technologies such as ozone oxidation, UV and gamma irradiation, and hydrostatic pressure can also inactivate many foodborne parasites, but their effectiveness is dependent on the parasite, the stage of the parasite, and the characteristics of the food matrix (Farkas, 1998). Also, the economic feasibility and consumer concerns regarding some of these technologies may limit their application.

Treatment of infected or susceptible human and animal hosts with effective antiparasitic agents is another intervention measure to reduce the transmission of foodborne parasites. This has been used mainly for the control of foodborne cestodes and trematodes for which humans and domestic animals are definitive hosts, and is most effective for those parasite cycles in which infected wildlife do not play a significant role in transmission. The availability of effective anthelmintics with few side effects such as praziquantel has facilitated this process. The WHO and OIE provide guidelines on chemotherapeutics, dose, and frequency of treatment for humans and animals, respectively.

14.7.1 Taenia *spp.*

For carcasses in which cysticerci have been detected or are suspected, freezing the meat and viscera at a minimum of −10 °C for at least 10 days should render any cysticerci nonviable. Cooking to attain a core temperature of at least 60 °C is also considered sufficient to kill cysticerci, and low dose irradiation of 0.5 kGy will inactivate them (Hilwig et al., 1978; WHO, 1995). Obviously, beef and pork produced in endemic regions and distributed locally is less likely to have received such treatments compared to exported products that often have been frozen to extend shelf life.

Anthelmintics such as praziquantel and oxfendazole are effective in killing bovine and porcine cysticerci *in vivo*. However, because of the relatively high doses and costs required to treat cattle, this is not practical. In pigs, use of oxfendazole has proven more feasible; although cysticeri in the brain are not reliably killed, they presumably do not play a significant role in disease transmission. In all cases, anthelmintic treatment kills only those cysticerci present at the time of treatment. The resultant necrotic lesions, if numerous, can render the meat unpalatable. Because complete dissolution can take months, chronic lesions detected during meat inspection could still result in the carcass being considered infected (Gallie and Sewell, 1983; Lightowlers, 2010).

Because human taeniosis can be safely and effectively treated with a single oral dose of praziquantel or niclosamide, mass taeniacidal campaigns against *T. solium* waged in rural villages and jurisdictions in a variety of endemic regions have proved cost-effective in reducing the local prevalence of this parasite, but their long-term effect as a standalone measure is unclear (Craig and Ito, 2007; Alexander et al., 2011; Lightowlers, 2013).

Taenia eggs contaminating food or the environment can remain infective for months, particularly under cool moist conditions, eventually succumbing to the effects of environmental UV irradiation and dessication. They are resistant to most conventional chemical and disinfecting agents (Pawlowski and Murrel, 2001). A recent study demonstrating experimental inactivation of *T. hydatigena* eggs after exposure to 60 °C for 5 min supports heating as the most reliable treatment (Buttar et al., 2013a).

14.7.2 Trichinella *spp.*

Heat treatment, using different time/temperature/meat thickness combinations applied to *T. spiralis*-infected pork, has been validated to reliably destroy the parasite. The thermal death point for *T. spiralis* is 54–57 °C and heating meat products to 71 °C will ensure food safety. Although data for other host species and *Trichinella* genotypes are limited, it is likely that thorough cooking will effectively inactivate all *Trichinella*, and is therefore currently the most widely recommended method to ensure food safety. No curing or smoking processes are currently recommended to reliably inactivate *Trichinella* larvae in meat (Gajadhar et al., 2009). Freezing at −15 °C for at least 3 weeks for meat up to 15 cm thickness and for at least 4 weeks for meat up to 50 cm thickness, can kill *T. spiralis* in pork. In lieu of testing, this is the most frequent treatment applied to pork destined for international markets requiring *Trichinella* mitigation for imported meat. However, other *Trichinella* genotypes, such as *T. nativa*, *T. murrelli*, and *T. britovi* occurring in other hosts such as horses and wild game are freeze tolerant (OIE, 2014b). Therefore meat from game or other susceptible hosts of these genotypes should be thoroughly cooked. Irradiation, where permitted and acceptable to the consumer, can also render meat safe for human consumption, since levels of at least 0.3 kGy have been proven to inactivate *Trichinella* (Gamble et al., 2000; FAO, 2013b). Further information on inactivation of *Trichinella* is provided in Chapter 11.

14.7.3 Opisthorchiidae

Treatments to destroy FBTs in harvested fish can be implemented at the processing and/or consumer level and are the only practical control intervention for wild-caught fish. Heat inactivation is the most reliable method and is time/temperature dependent, with the thickest part of the product reaching an internal minimum temperature of 63 °C for at least 15 s. Freezing at −35 °C for 15 h or at −20 °C for 7 days is also effective. Irradiation has been proposed but has issues relating to the palatability of the final product after administration of levels required to kill the parasite and to consumer acceptance. Other methods such as smoking and pickling are not reliable (Adams et al., 1997). Further details on the inactivation of these parasites are provided in Chapter 12.

Praziquantel is currently the most common drug used for individual or mass treatment of humans or nonhuman definitive hosts with FBT infection. In localities where the prevalence of infection is more than 20%, the WHO recommends that mass treatment of all residents be done annually; for infection rates less than 20%, treatment can be administered biannually (WHO, 2014). Although these interventions can be effective in reducing the transmission of FBTs, they are also one of the most costly interventions and may not be sustainable in poorer regions (Clausen et al., 2012). To help address this, in its recent efforts to include foodborne trematodiases in its mainstream preventative chemotherapy strategy, the WHO has negotiated agreements with pharmaceutical companies to donate and ship free of charge anthelmintics such as triclabendazole to ministries of health in endemic countries that request them (WHO, 2014).

14.7.4 Coccidian protozoa

Oocysts are highly resistant to environmental conditions and to disinfectants commonly used in food and water processing. Use of two conventional disinfectants, chlorine and ozone, at much higher concentrations than typically used for water treatment, failed to inactivate *T. gondii* occysts (Wainwright et al., 2007). Gaseous chlorine dioxide at 4.1 mg/L will inactivate *Cryptosporidium*, but will not affect sporulation of *Cyclospora* (Ortega et al., 2008). Relatively low doses of UV have been shown to inactivate *C. parvum* oocysts (Craik et al., 2001). Removal of oocysts, with or without disinfection, can be more effective and includes such processes as coagulation, flocculation, sedimentation, filtration, and membrane technology (Betancourt and Rose, 2004). A 1-μ filter is required to exclude *Cryptosporidium* oocysts (Orlandi et al., 2002). Although washing of produce is recommended, it will not reliably remove all oocysts. *Cryptosporidium* oocysts can survive within, and be protected by, the stoma of fresh fruits and leafy vegetables. There are also apparent higher binding affinities for particular produce such as raspberries, which have fine hairlike projections that entrap oocysts. The degree of adhesion of *Cyclospora* appears to be stronger than that for other occysts (Ortega and Sanchez, 2010). Freezing will not reliably inactivate oocysts, although *Cryptosporidium* is reported to be inactivated at −20 °C for greater than 24 h or at −15 °C for at least a week (Fayer and Nerad, 1996). However, blast freezing representative of that used on a commercial scale by industry (−20 °C for 4 min) inactivated less than 20% of *Cryptosporidium* oocysts inoculated onto green peppers (Duhain et al., 2012). *Cyclospora* oocysts appear even more resistant to freezing, surviving −20 °C for 2 days (Ortega and Sanchez, 2010). Freezing at −12 °C or lower should reliably kill *Toxoplasma* tachyzoites and bradyzoites within tissue cysts, although it has been suggested that some strains may be resistant to freezing (Kotula et al., 1991; Tenter, 2009). Both oocysts and *Toxoplasma* tissue stages can be reliably destroyed by thorough cooking to temperatures of at least 67 °C. Other treatments such as gamma and UV irradiation, as well as high hydrostatic pressure, have been applied to oocysts and *Toxoplasma* tissue cysts, with varying degrees of success and consumer acceptance. For example, for *Toxoplasma*, irradiation at greater or equal to 0.4 kGy can inactivate tissue cysts in meat and render oocysts noninfective (Kijlstra and Jongert, 2008; Dubey et al., 1998). High hydrostatic pressure of 340 MPa for 60 s applied to raspberries inoculated with *Toxoplasma* oocysts was reported to render the oocysts noninfectious (Lindsay et al., 2008). Salting, curing, smoking, and other processing of meat can reduce the viability of *Toxoplasma* tissue cysts, but there is too much variability for reliable recommendations (Kijlstra and Jongert, 2008; Jones and Dubey, 2012). Further information on treatments to inactivate *Toxoplasma* in pork is provided in Chapter 11.

Mass chemotherapy of humans for *Cyclospora* or *Cryptosporidium*, or of animals for *Cryptosporidium* or *Toxoplasma*, has not been implemented as a control measure to reduce transmission of these parasites. This is presumably due to the usually transient and self-limiting nature of infections with *Cyclospora* and *Cryptosporidium*, and the overall lack of effective or practical treatment regimes.

14.8 Prevention of infection and contamination

Prevention of infection in food animals and of the contamination of foods is the ultimate goal of any foodborne parasite control program. This includes the establishment of physical barriers and biosecurity measures to reduce or prevent exposure of food animals and produce to parasites, biological control measures, and vaccination. The prophylactic use of chemicals and drugs has public health and environmental implications and should be regarded as a last measure only (Hastein, 2000). Parasitic infections of food animals at the farm level are transmitted via a variety of feeding behaviors, such as garbage feeding, scavenging, and cannibalism (Gajadhar et al., 2006). In developed countries, modern production practices for livestock such as swine, which are typically housed indoors, fed highly processed feed, and raised under a high level of biosecurity have precluded the transmission of parasites such as *Trichinella*. However, the increasing popularity of more extensive husbandry and organic practices for food production increases the risk of exposure. In these cases, particular attention must be paid to the risks of parasite transmission posed by other domestic and wild animals, feed, and the environment. Preventative measures include installing barriers, such as fencing, to wildlife or domestic pets involved in parasite transmission, and sourcing uncontaminated water and feed. The transmission stages of most parasites are disseminated via the host's feces, including humans; thus, proper hygiene and sanitation are important, and regular removal and proper disposal of animal manure is recommended, particularly in intensive production systems (Bolin et al., 2004; Gajadhar et al., 2006). The environmental stages of many parasites are able to survive relatively long term, particularly under cool and moist conditions. Fallowing pastures to expose parasites to the effects of UV irradiation and dessication prior to grazing livestock, particularly after human sewage or manure has been applied as fertilizer, and ensilage of feeds will help reduce transmission. Biological control approaches include the introduction of nonsusceptible species to displace, or prey upon, susceptible intermediate hosts such as snails. Another potential approach is the introduction of a relatively benign parasite species to competitively exclude or offer cross-protective immunity against the foodborne parasite being targeted. Vaccination has the potential to be one of the most effective preventative measures for controlling foodborne parasites. However, only a few effective vaccines have been developed in this realm, and most are not available commercially (Innes et al., 2011; Jones and Dubey, 2012; Lightowlers, 2013).

14.8.1 Taenia *spp.*

Housing of pigs and cattle will reduce their exposure to *Taenia* eggs. Use of latrines will reduce the numbers of eggs contaminating the environment, and the hygienic preparation of foods will reduce the risk of their being contaminated with *T. solium* eggs. For reasons indicated earlier, screening of food handlers or farm employees as a prophylactic measure against cysticercosis is likely not feasible. For suspected sources of contamination, measures can be taken to inactivate any eggs present. If sewage must be used as fertilizer, lagooning of sludge prior to application, and delayed grazing of cattle on treated pastures can be used to decrease survivability and the number of viable *T. saginata* eggs (Bruce et al., 1990; Moussavou-boussougou et al., 2005). Ensilation of contaminated potato waste or hay for specified time periods has been demonstrated to inactivate *Taenia* eggs (Buttar et al., 2013b). Sentinel pigs have been used to reduce or monitor environmental contamination with *T. solium* eggs and to assess the efficacy of control measures (Devleesschauwer et al., 2013).

Effective vaccines exist for both bovine and porcine cysticercosis, but are not yet commercially available. Current limitations include the requirement for multiple vaccine injections to confer immunity, and the lack of any effect on preexisting infections. However, a recent control scheme consisting of single-dose chemotherapy with oxfendazole combined with two injections of TSOL 18 vaccine shows promise as an effective and sustainable strategy to reduce the burden of porcine cysticercosis (Lightowlers, 2013). A recent study of pigs in Laos indicates that cross-protective immunity to *T. solium* may be conferred by natural infection with the relatively non-pathogenic and nonzoonotic *T. hydatigena* (Conlan et al., 2012). This invites speculation on the future possibility of biological control of pathogenic *Taenia* via the introduction and competitive effect of less pathogenic species.

14.8.2 Trichinella *spp.*

Because there is no environmental stage in the life cycle of *Trichinella*, and infected humans are essentially dead-end hosts, transmission occurs solely via the consumption of infected animal tissues. Prevention of garbage feeding and access to domestic animal and wildlife carcasses, rodent control, and enhanced management practices including indoor housing will therefore interrupt transmission of *Trichinella* at the producer level. Although rats have long been implicated in perpetuating the pastoral cycle of *T. spiralis* in domestic swine, it is debatable whether the infection in rats can persist long term in the absence of pigs (Takumi et al., 2010). Therefore the importance of promptly removing pig carcasses to prevent pig-to-pig, and pig-to-rat, transmission should not be overlooked. Current OIE guidelines stipulate the controlled management conditions required to establish compartments with negligible risk of *Trichinella* infection, including introducing only pigs with similar status into the compartment. Because controlled housing is so integral to establishing negligible risk for *Trichinella*, more extensive, organic management practices for domestic swine make prevention of infection much more difficult. This is also true for horses ultimately slaughtered for human consumption as horses are not typically raised as food animals under controlled management conditions. Practices such as those reported from Eastern Europe, whereby raw pork is fed to horses to condition them prior to sale, should be discouraged (Murrell et al., 2004). For obvious reasons, there is little that can be done to prevent infection with sylvatic *Trichinella* genotypes among wildlife.

14.8.3 Opisthorchiidae

The following practices will help prevent the transmission of FBTs: the provision and implementation of latrines, the placement of barriers around ponds to prevent access by dogs, cats, and other potential definitive hosts, the erection of walls to prevent surface water runoff from entering ponds, no use of human and livestock feces for fertilizing ponds, no consumption of raw or inadequately cooked fish, and no feeding of these materials to dogs, cats, or pigs. Interventions have also included practices to control the snail populations. Physical approaches, such as the periodic draining of ponds and removal of surface mud from the pond floor, and removal of vegetation in and around the ponds to reduce snail habitat have been recommended. However, effects of such efforts to control snail populations in fish ponds are usually minimal; in a recent intervention study where these measures were applied to fish nurseries in northern Vietnam, no subsequent reduction in snails occurred when compared to nonintervention ponds (Clausen et al., 2012). Biological and chemical control may be more effective. However, most molluscicides are toxic to fish as well as to snails and have other environmental implications. The introduction of competitor snails not susceptible to infection has been demonstrated to displace those transmitting schistosomes in the field (Hung et al., 2013b). Species of mollusk-eating fishes also have potential for snail control (Hung et al., 2013a).

14.8.4 Coccidian protozoa

Preventative measures to reduce the likelihood of oocyst contamination of produce at the preharvest stage include the use of good quality water for irrigation and mixing of pesticides, restricting access of cats, livestock, and other animals to croplands and surface waters, monitoring the health of farm workers and encouraging good hygiene, and using only composted (or otherwise treated) manure as fertilizer. Removal of feces before sporulation of *C. cayetanensis* or *T. gondii* and inactivation in sewage lagoons or by solar UV will help reduce environmental contamination (King et al., 2008; Jenkins et al., 2013b). Postharvest measures include the use of good quality water for washing and processing produce, monitoring and enforcing good personal hygiene in food handlers, prevention of cross-contamination, and the incorporation of a HACCP system.

Housing of livestock to prevent exposure to cats, wildlife, domestic animal carcasses, and environmental oocysts, and the prompt removal of manure will similarly reduce the overall transmission of *Cryptosporidium* and *Toxoplasma* to food animals. Initiatives such as the establishment of serological herd profiles and risk categorization for *Toxoplasma* will facilitate the application of these preventative measures where they are needed most (Meemken et al., 2014). Preventative control programs for humans have focused primarily on maternal screening to reduce the incidence of congenital toxoplasmosis, but the overall benefits of such programs are still unclear (Jones et al., 2014).

Efforts to develop safe and effective vaccines continue. Although a live vaccine for cats to reduce oocyst shedding was available commercially at one time, it has since been discontinued (Jones and Dubey, 2012). A live vaccine for toxoplasmosis to reduce abortions in sheep is currently the only commercial vaccine for this parasite worldwide (Innes et al., 2011; Jones and Dubey, 2012). Live vaccines have proven most effective so far, but have limited application, particularly to developing regions, due to safety risks, short shelf life, and the need for refrigerated storage prior to delivery in the field (Innes et al., 2011).

14.9 Education and training

Educating people at risk of infection with foodborne parasites and those involved in food production is fundamental to sustained foodborne parasite control. This should include education on the life cycle and epidemiology of the parasite(s) of concern, on basic health, hygiene, and sanitation, and on specific risk factors and preventative measures. Education can also play an important role in establishing political engagement in control programs at all levels of society. However, changing human behavior through education, even to simply encourage the proper cooking of food, continues to be a major challenge, undermined by the long prepatent periods and insidious subclinical nature of most of these parasitoses (Macpherson, 2005). The role of human behavior in the transmission of foodborne parasites is discussed in Chapter 4. Thus, in many cases where education has been used as the basis for an intervention strategy, the impact on perceptions, knowledge, and practices has been limited or is difficult to assess (Lightowlers, 2013). Another of the ongoing challenges to this approach is cost and subsequent difficulty in sustainability, particularly in those endemic developing regions where it is needed most (Pawlowski et al., 2005; Lightowlers, 2013). Standardized and measurable training is also required for capacity building when developing and implementing control programs for foodborne parasites. This includes training of public health and veterinary professionals and other qualified personnel in food safety, surveillance, quality assurance, and proficiency in diagnostic testing. As relevant, these activities should be conducted under the oversight of the responsible competent authority (OIE, 2014a).

14.9.1 Taenia *spp.*

The effect of health education as an effective intervention for control of *Taenia* spp. has been difficult to assess due to limited data, but where evaluated has not proven to have led to a major sustained impact of reducing *T. solium* transmission (Lightowlers, 2013). A computer-based interactive education tool called "The Vicious Worm" has recently been developed to provide evidence-based knowledge about the control and prevention of *T. solium* cysticercosis. It can be downloaded from a website for free and has simplified and made more accessible the health messages that are needed for the various stakeholders across disciplines and sectors. It is hoped that its implementation as a specific intervention measure will prove more productive than have past attempts in this realm (Johansen et al., 2014).

14.9.2 Trichinella *spp.*

In general, producers of commercial swine in developed countries are well aware of the biosecurity risks posed by *Trichinella* and other pathogens. Therefore, education and increased awareness should focus on backyard and organic pig producers and consumers of their products. After trichinellosis outbreaks in France, attempts to educate consumers on the risk of eating raw or undercooked horsemeat have not been effective (Boireau et al., 2000). A program initiated in Nunavik in the Canadian Arctic in 1992 to prevent trichinellosis due to the consumption of raw walrus meat infected with *T. nativa* appears to have been more successful at engaging consumers. Accepting that the long-established practice of eating uncooked walrus meat in northern communities is unlikely to be changed, the program has focused on providing residents with information about the parasite and the disease, providing training to hunters in sample-collection procedures, testing of all harvested carcasses, and communication of results back to the community prior to distribution and consumption of the meat (Proulx et al., 2002). Since 1997, no locally acquired outbreaks of trichinellosis linked to walrus have occurred (Larrat et al., 2012).

14.9.3 Opisthorchiidae

A successful control program for FBTs must include knowledge of the social and anthropological determinants of people's raw-fish consumption and hygiene practices. A recent follow-up study of *O. viverrini* infection in a rural community in Thailand found no change in the incidence of infection after several years of implementing a control program, which included health education. The limited success of such educational campaigns to achieve a sustained reduction in FBT prevalence may be because they have not been based on the people's awareness, attitudes, and eating practices, and their perceptions of raw fish and the associated health risks. For example, in northern Vietnam, even though there was awareness in local communities of the risks of eating raw fish, people continued to do so because they believed they could be easily treated and cured if infected (Phan et al., 2011). Although inspectors in Vietnam have been trained in the recognition and detection of FBT infections in cultivated fish under the international FIBOZOPA project initiative described in Section 14.2.1.3 of this chapter, there are, unfortunately, no indications that these methods are being routinely used (Lima dos Santos and Howgate, 2011).

14.9.4 Coccidian protozoa

Education on these parasites' biology and transmission is most critical, but also most challenging, in impoverished endemic regions where veterinary and public health infrastructure and resources are limited. Surveys in the United States and in other developed countries indicate a decreasing seroprevalence of *Toxoplasma*, likely due to better biosecurity practices for livestock production, improved cat-care hygiene, and education of the population at risk (Jones et al., 2014). However, even for developed countries, a recent systematic review found very little rigorous scientific evidence for the effectiveness of prenatal education in reducing congenital toxoplasmosis (Di Mario et al., 2013). It is interesting to note, however, that a survey of pregnant women in Italy indicated they perceived an apparent overestimation of the risk of foodborne toxoplasmosis that could lead them to exclude low-risk foods from their diet (Pezzoli et al., 2009).

14.10 Conclusions and future trends

Although many countries have adopted regulations to minimize contamination of food with some specific parasites, other foodborne parasites continue to be overlooked. When implemented, systems for routine surveillance or reporting are often inadequate and underestimate the occurrence of foodborne parasites as well as the incidence of human disease (Slifko et al., 2000). Conventional methodologies to control foodborne parasites will continue to be valid, with ongoing advances in more sensitive, specific, and rapid tests, chemotherapeutic agents, and alternative vaccination strategies lending further improvements. Although in the past most efforts to control foodborne pathogens were focused on preventing contamination of human food with sewage or animal manure, future success will likely increasingly depend on controlling contamination of feed and water consumed by the animals themselves (Tauxe, 1997). Because establishing and maintaining countrywide freedom from particular foodborne parasites in food animals may be impractical, international disease control standards are trending toward zoning and compartmentalization of subpopulations with a distinct and verifiable health status, as per the general recommendations provided in Chapter 4.3 of the OIE terrestrial code (OIE, 2014c).

Globalization of our food systems has occurred, and in much of the developed world an increasing proportion of the food supply is outsourced. In many cases this is from countries endemic for foodborne parasites. Increasing global demand for meat and fresh produce is driving increased production and trade, but inspection of these commodities, and the availability of international standardized testing for parasites, has not kept pace (Robertson et al., 2014). However, globalization might also prove to be the greatest resource for combating these pathogens by enabling researchers from a range of disciplines to collaborate and disseminate their knowledge, in a "One Health" approach (Robertson et al., 2014).

International food and health organizations need to provide consolidated safety guidelines for the most important foodborne parasites, linking parasites, people, animals, and food, to galvanize international efforts to reduce the risks from globalization (Robertson et al., 2014). In this regard, OIE, FAO/WHO/Codex, and ISO are working more closely than ever toward harmonized standards for pre- and postharvest control and quality assurance, respectively. Such new international codes increasingly recognize risk-assessment methodologies as the scientific process to address public health globally. Environmental monitoring of food and water using new technologies, along with molecular epidemiology, and facilitated by the development of an online global database of foodborne parasite occurrences, will be one of the best approaches to identifying and mitigating risks in the future (Slifko et al., 2000; Robertson et al., 2014).

References

Abuseir, S., Kuhne, M., Schnieder, T., Klein, G., Epe, C., 2007. Evaluation of a serological method for the detection of *Taenia saginata* cysticercosis using serum and meat juice samples. Parasitol. Res. 101, 131–137.

Acar, J.F., Moulin, G., 2013. Integrating animal health surveillance and food safety: the issue of antimicrobial resistance. Rev. Sci. Tech Off. Int. Epiz. 32, 383–394.

Adams, A.M., Murrell, K.D., Cross, J.H., 1997. Parasites of fish and risks to public health. Rev. Sci. Tech Off. Int. Epiz. 16, 652–660.

Al-Adhami, B.H., Gajadhar, A.A., 2014. A new multi-host species indirect ELISA using protein A/G conjugate for detection of anti-*Toxoplasma gondii* IgG antibodies with comparison to ELISA-IgG, agglutination assay and Western blot. Vet. Parasitol. 200, 66–73.

Alban, L., Pozio, E., Boes, J., Boireau, P., Boue, F., Claes, M., Cook, A.J.C., Dorny, P., Enemark, H.L., van der Giessen, J., Hunt, K.R., Howell, M., Kirjusina, M., Nockler, K., Rossi, P., Smith, G.C., Snow, L., Taylor, M.A., Theodoropoulos, G., Vallee, I., Viera-Pinto, M.M., Zimmer, I.A., 2011. Towards a standardised surveillance for *Trichinella* in the European Union. Prev. Vet. Med. 99, 148–160.

Alexander, A., John, K.R., Jayaraman, T., Oommen, A., Raghava, M.V., Dorny, P., Rajshekhar, V., 2011. Economic implications of three strategies for the control of taeniasis. Trop. Med. Int. Health 16, 1410–1416.

Alvarado-Esquivel, C., Pacheco-Vega, S.J., Hernandez-Tinoco, J., Centeno-Tinoco, M.M., Beristain-Garcia, I., Sanchez-Anguiano, L.F., Liesenfeld, O., Rabago-Sanchez, E., Berumen-Segovia, L.O., 2014. Miscarriage history and *Toxoplasma gondii* infection: a cross-sectional study in women in Durango City, Mexico. Eur. J. Microbiol. Immunol. 4, 117–122.

Armignacco, O., Ferri, F., Gomez-Morales, M.A., Caterini, L., Pozio, E., 2013. Short report: cryptic and asymptomatic *Opisthorchis felineus* infections. Am. J. Trop. Med. Hyg. 88, 364–366.

Bellamy, J.E.C., 2004. Quality assurance considerations for detection of waterborne zoonotic parasites using *Cryptosporidium* oocyst detection as the main example. Vet. Parasitol. 126, 235–248.

Berman, E.M., Shimshony, A., 2013. Integrating animal health and foodborne disease surveillance. Rev. Sci. Tech Off. Int. Epiz. 32, 337–346.

Betancourt, W.Q., Rose, J.B., 2004. Drinking water treatment processes for removal of *Cryptosporidium* and *Giardia*. Vet. Parasitol. 126, 219–234.

Boireau, P., Vallee, I., Roman, T., Perret, C., Mingyuan, L., Gamble, H.R., Gajadhar, A., 2000. *Trichinella* in horses: a low frequency infection with high human risk. Vet. Parasitol. 93, 309–320.

Bolin, C., Brown, C., Rose, J., 2004. Emerging zoonotic diseases and water. In: Cotruvo, J.A., Dufour, A., Rees, G., Bartram, J., Carr, R., Cliver, D.O., Craun, G.F., Fayer, R., Gannon, V.P.J. (Eds.), Waterborne Zoonoses: Identification, Causes and Control. WHO, IWA Publishing, London, UK, ISBN: 1 84339 058 2.

Boyaci, I.H., Temiz, H.T., Uysal, R.S., Velioglu, H.M., Yadegari, R.J., Rishkan, M.M., 2014. A novel method for discrimination of beef and horsemeat using Raman spectroscopy. Food Chem. 148, 37–41. http://dx.doi.org/10.1016/j.foodchem.2013.10.006.

Britt, A.G., Bell, C.M., Evers, K., Paskin, R., 2013. Linking live animals and products: traceability. Rev. Sci. Tech Off. Int. Epiz. 32, 571–582.

Bruce, A.M., Pike, E.B., Fisher, W.J., 1990. A review of treatment process options to meet the EC sludge directive. J. Inst. Water Environ. Manage. 4, 1–13.

Bruschi, F., 2012. Trichinellosis in developing countries: is it neglected? J. Infect. Dev. Ctries. 6, 216–222.

Buttar, B.S., Nelson, M.L., Busboom, J.R., Hancock, D.D., Walsh, D.B., Jasmer, D.P., 2013a. Effect of heat treatment on viability of *Taenia hydatigena* eggs. Exp. Parasitol. 133, 421–426.

Buttar, B.S., Nelson, M.L., Busboom, J.R., Hancock, D.D., Walsh, D.B., Jasmer, D.P., 2013b. Effect of ensilation of potato on viability of *Taenia hydatigena* eggs. Exp. Parasitol. 133, 483–486.

CAC (Codex Alimentarius Commission), 2013. Codex Committee on Food Hygiene-Proposed draft guidelines for the control of specific zoonotic parasites in meat: *Trichinella* spp. and *Cysticercus bovis*. Available at: ftp://ftp.fao.org/codex/reports/reports2014/REP14/FHe.pdf.

Calcagno, M.A., Bourlot, I., Taus, R., Saracino, M.P., Venturiello, S.M., 2014. Description of an outbreak of human trichinellosis in an area of Argentina historically regarded as *Trichinella*-free: the importance of surveillance studies. Vet. Parasitol. 200, 251–256.

Calvo-Artavia, F.F., Nielsen, L.R., Alban, L., 2013. Epidemiologic and economic evaluation of risk-based meat inspection for bovine cysticercosis in Danish cattle. Prev. Vet. Med. 108, 253–261.

Cann, K.J., Chalmers, R.M., Nichols, G., O'Brien, S.J., 2000. *Cyclospora* infections in England and Wales: 1993 to 1998. Commun. Dis. Public Health 3, 46–49.

Cantey, P.T., Coyle, C.M., Sorvillo, F.J., Wilkins, P.P., Starr, M.C., Nash, T.E., 2014. Neglected parasitic infections in the United States: cysticercosis. Am. J. Trop. Med. Hyg. 90, 805–809.

Carneiro, A.C., Andrade, G.M., Costa, J.G., Pinheiro, B.V., Vasconcelos-Santos, D.V., Ferreira, A.M., Su, C., Januario, J.N., Vitor, R.W., 2013. Genetic characterization of *Toxoplasma gondii* revealed highly diverse genotypes for isolates from newborns with congenital toxoplasmosis in southeastern Brazil. J. Clin. Microbiol. 51, 901–907.

Carr, R., Bartram, J., 2004. The control envelope and risk management. In: Cotruvo, J.A., Dufour, A., Rees, G., Bartram, J., Carr, R., Cliver, D.O., Craun, G.F., Fayer, R., Gannon, V.P.J. (Eds.), Waterborne Zoonoses: Identification, Causes and Control. WHO, IWA Publishing, London, UK, ISBN: 1 84339 058 2.

Clausen, J.H., Madsen, H., Murrell, K.D., Phan, V.T., Ha, T.T.N., Trung Dung, D., Lan, T.N.A., Hung, M.N., Dalsgaard, A., 2012. Prevention and control of fish-borne zoonotic trematodes in fish nurseries, Vietnam. Emerg. Infect. Dis. 18, 1438–1445.

Clementino Andrade, M.M., Pinheiro, B.V., Cunha, M.M., Carneiro, A.C.A.V., Andrade Neto, V.F., Vitor, R.W.A., 2013. New genotypes of *Toxoplasma gondii* obtained from farm animals in Northeast Brazil. Res. Vet. Sci. 94, 587–589.

Collett, S.R., 2013. Principles of disease prevention, diagnosis, and control. In: Swayne, D.E. (Ed.), Diseases of Poultry, thirteenth ed. John Wiley and Sons. Etobicoke, Ontario, Canada. ISBN: 978-1-118-71973-2 (Chapter 1).

Conlan, J.V., Vongxay, K., Khamlome, B., Dorny, P., Sripa, B., Elliot, A., Blacksell, S.D., Fenwick, S., Thompson, R.C.A., 2012. A cross-sectional study of *Taenia solium* in a multiple taeniid-endemic region reveals competition may be protective. Am. J. Trop. Med. Hyg. 87, 281–291.

Coral-Almeida, M., Rodriguez-Hidalgo, R., Celi-Erazo, M., Garcia, H.H., Rodriguez, S., Devleesschauwer, B., Benitez-Ortiz, W., Dorny, P., Praet, N., 2014. Incidence of human *Taenia solium* larval infections in an Ecuadorian endemic area: implications for disease burden assessment and control. PLoS Negl. Trop. Dis. 8, 1–9.

Craig, P., Ito, A., 2007. Intestinal cestodes. Curr. Opin. Infect. Dis. 20, 524–532.

Craik, S.A., Weldon, D., Finch, G.R., Bolton, J.R., Belosevic, M., 2001. Inactivation of *Cryptosporidium parvum* oocysts using medium and low pressure ultraviolet radiation. Water Res. 35, 1387–1398.

De Cassia Paulan, S., Gonzales, R.M.H., Peralta, L.A., Vicentini-Oliveira, J.C., Biondi, G.F., Conde, E.S., Parkhouse, R.M.E., Nunes, C.M., 2013. Usefulness of serological ELISA assay for *Taenia saginata* to detect naturally infected bovines. Rev. Bras. Parasitol. Vet. 22, 270–275.

De Liberato, C., Scaramozzino, P., Brozzi, A., Lorenzetti, R., Di Cave, D., Martini, E., Lucangeli, C., Pozio, E., Berrilli, F., Bossu, T., 2011. Investigation on *Opisthorchis felineus* occurrence and life cycle in Italy. Vet. Parasitol. 177, 67–71.

DeGiorgio, C., Pietsch-Escueta, S., Tsang, V., Corral-Leyva, G., Ng, L., Medina, M.T., Astudillo, S., Padilla, N., Leyva, P., Martinez, L., Noh, J., Levine, M., del Villasenor, R., Sorvillo, F., 2005. Sero-prevalence of *Taenia solium* cysticercosis and *Taenia solium* taeniasis in California, USA. Acta Neurol. Scand. 111, 84–88.

Devleesschauwer, B., Aryal, A., Tharmalingam, J., Joshi, D.D., Rijal, S., Speybroeck, N., Gabriel, S., Victor, B., Dorny, P., 2013. Complexities in using sentinel pigs to study *Taenia solium* transmission dynamics under field conditions. Vet. Parasitol. 193, 172–178.

Devleesschauwer, B., Praet, N., Speybroeck, N., Torgerson, P.R., Haagsma, J.A., De Smet, K., Murrell, K.D., Pozio, E., Dorny, P., 2014. The low global burden of trichinellosis: evidence and implications. Int. J. Parasitol. 45, 95–99. http://dx.doi.org/10.1016/j.ipara.2014.05.006 [Epub ahead of print].

Dewhirst, L.W., Cramer, J.D., Sheldon, J.J., 1967. An analysis of current inspection procedures for detecting bovine cysticercosis. J. Am. Vet. Med. Assoc. 150, 412–417.

Di Mario, S., Basevi, V., Gagliotti, C., Spettoli, D., Gori, G., D'Amico, R., Magrini, N., 2013. Prenatal education for congenital toxoplasmosis. Cochrane Database Syst. Rev, CD006171.

Diaz, J.H., 2013. Paragonimiasis acquired in the United States: native and non-native species. Clin. Microbiol. Rev. 26, 493–504.

Dixon, B., Parrington, L., Cook, A., Pollari, F., Farber, J., 2013. Detection of *Cyclospora*, *Cryptosporidium*, and *Giardia* in ready-to-eat packaged leafy greens in Ontario, Canada. J. Food Prot. 76, 307–313.

Dorny, P., Praet, N., 2007. *Taenia saginata* in Europe. Vet. Parasitol. 149, 22–24.

Dorny, P., Vercammen, F., Brandt, J., Vansteenkiste, W., Berkvens, D., Geerts, S., 2000. Sero-epidemiological study of *Taenia saginata* cysticercosis in Belgian cattle. Vet. Parasitol. 88, 43–49.

Dowdle, W.R., 1999. The principles of disease elimination and eradication. Centres for Disease Control and Prevention. Morb. Mortal. Wkly. Rep. 48 (SU01), 23–27, December 31.

Dubey, J.P., Thayer, D.W., Speer, C.A., Shen, S.K., 1998. Effect of gamma irradiation on unsporulated and sporulated *Toxoplasma gondii* oocysts. Int. J. Parasitol. 28, 369–375.

Duhain, G.L.M.C., Minnaar, A., Buys, E.M., 2012. Effect of chlorine, blanching, freezing, and microwave heating on *Cryptosporidium parvum* viability inoculated on green peppers. J. Food Prot. 75, 936–941.

Dupouy-Camet, J., 2000. Trichinellosis: a worldwide zoonosis. Vet. Parasitol. 93, 191–200.

Dupuy, C., Morlot, C., Gilot-Fromont, E., Mas, M., Grandmontagne, C., Gilli-Dunoyer, P., Gay, E., Callait-Cardinal, M.-P., 2014. Prevalence of *Taenia saginata* cysticercosis in French cattle in 2010. Vet. Parasitol. 203, 65–72.

Fabiani, S., Bruschi, F., 2013. Neurocysticercosis in Europe: still a public health concern not only for imported cases. Acta Trop. 128, 18–26.

FAO (Food and Agriculture Organisation), 2013a. Summary risk profile on *C. bovis* in meat from domestic cattle. http://www.fao.org/fileadmin/user_upload/agns/pdf/Foodborne_parasites/RiskProfTaeniasaginataOct2013.pdf.

FAO (Food and Agriculture Organisation), 2013b. Summary risk profile on *Trichinella* in meat. http://www.fao.org/fileadmin/user_upload/agns/pdf/Foodborne_parasites/RiskProfTrichinellaOct2013.pdf.

FAO/WHO (Food and Agriculture Organisation/World Health Organisation), 2014a. Multicriteria-Based Ranking for Risk Management of Food-Borne Parasites. In: Microbiological Risk Assessment, No. 23. FAO/WHO, Rome, 302 pp.

FAO/WHO (Food and Agriculture Organisation/World Health Organisation), 2014b. Risk-based examples for control of *Trichinella* spp. and *Taenia saginata* in meat. Preliminary report of a joint FAO/WHO expert meeting, 22–25 October 2013. Geneva, Switzerland: WHO Headquarters. http://www.fao.org/fileadmin/user_upload/agns/pdf/Foodborne_parasites/Risk-based_Control_Trich_and_Taenia_17June_Eng.pdf.

FAO/WHO/OIE (Food and Agriculture Organisation/World Health Organisation/World Organisation for Animal Health), 2007. In: Dupouy-Camet, J., Murrell, K.D. (Eds.), Guidelines for the Surveillance, Management, Prevention and Control of Trichinellosis. FAO/WHO/OIE, Paris, France, 119 p.

Farkas, J., 1998. Irradiation as a method for decontaminating food. A review. Int. J. Microbiol. 44, 189–204.

Fayer, R., Nerad, T., 1996. Effects of low temperatures on viability of *Cryptosporidium parvum* oocysts. Appl. Environ. Microbiol. 62, 1431–1433.

Fichi, G., Stefanelli, S., Pagani, A., Luchi, S., De Gennaro, M., Gomez-Morales, M.A., Selmi, M., Rovai, D., Mari, M., Fishetti, R., Pozio, E., 2014. Trichinellosis outbreak caused by meat from a wild boar hunted in an Italian region considered to be at negligible risk for *Trichinella*. Zoonoses Public Health. http://dx.doi.org/10.1111/zph.12148.

Forbes, L.B., Rajic, A., Gajadhar, A.A., 1998. Proficiency samples for quality assurance in *Trichinella* digestion tests. J. Food Prot. 61, 1396–1399.

Forbes, L.B., Gajadhar, A.A., 1999. A validated *Trichinella* digestion assay and an associated sampling and quality assurance system for use in testing pork and horsemeat. J. Food Prot. 62, 1308–1313.

Forbes, L.B., Parker, S.E., Scandrett, W.B., 2003. Comparison of a modified digestion assay with trichinoscopy for the detection of *Trichinella* larvae in pork. J. Food Prot. 66, 1043–1046.

Fried, B., Abruzzi, A., 2010. Food-borne trematode infections of humans in the United States of America. Parasitol. Res. 106, 1263–1280.

Gajadhar, A.A., Forbes, L.B., 2010. A 10-year wildlife survey of 15 species of Canadian carnivores identifies new hosts or geographic locations for *Trichinella* genotypes T2, T4, T5, and T6. Vet. Parasitol. 168, 78–83. http://dx.doi.org/10.1016/j.vetpar.2009.10.012.

Gajadhar, A.A., Scandrett, W.B., Forbes, L.B., 2006. Overview of food- and water-borne zoonotic parasites at the farm level. Rev. Sci. Tech Off. Int. Epiz. 25, 595–606.

Gajadhar, A.A., Pozio, E., Gamble, H.R., Nockler, K., Maddox-Hyttel, C., Forbes, L.B., Vallee, I., Rossi, P., Marinculic, A., Boireau, P., 2009. *Trichinella* diagnostics and control: mandatory and best practices for ensuring food safety. Vet. Parasitol. 159, 197–205.

Gallie, G.J., Sewell, M.M.H., 1983. Duration of immunity and absorption of cysticerci in calves after treatment of *Taenia saginata* cysticercosis with praziquantel. Res. Vet. Sci. 34, 127–130.

Gamble, H.R., Bessonov, A.S., Cuperlovic, K., Gajadhar, A.A., van Knapen, R., Nockler, K., Schenone, H., Zhu, X., 2000. International Commission on Trichinellosis: recommendations on methods for the control of *Trichinella* in domestic and wild animals intended for human consumption. Vet. Parasitol. 93, 393–408.

Garcia, H.H., Gonzalez, A.E., Del Brutto, O.H., Tsang, V.C., Llanos-Zavalaga, F., Gonzalvez, G., Romero, J., Gilman, R.H., 2007. Strategies for the elimination of taeniasis/cysticercosis. J. Neurol. Sci. 262, 153–157.

Garcia, H.H., Gonzalez, A.E., Rodriguez, S., Gonzalvez, G., Llanos-Zavalaga, F., Tsang, V.C., Gilman, R.H., 2010. Epidemiology and control of cysticercosis in Peru. Rev. Peru. Med. Exp. Salud Publica 27, 592–597.

Goodgame, R.W., 1996. Understanding intestinal spore-forming protozoa: Cryptosporidia, Microsporida, Isospora and Cyclospora. Ann. Intern. Med. 124, 429–441.

Gottstein, B., Pozio, E., Nockler, K., 2009. Epidemiology, diagnosis, treatment, and control of trichinellosis. Clin. Microbiol. Rev., 127–145. http://dx.doi.org/10.1128/CMR. 00026-08.
Hastein, T., 2000. Principles of prevention and control of aquatic animal diseases. Conf. OIE, 27–49. Available at: http://www.oie.int/doc/ged/D2973.PDF.
Hill, D.E., Dubey, J.P., 2013. *Toxoplasma gondii* prevalence in farm animals in the United States. Int. J. Parasitol. 43, 107–113.
Hill, D.E., Forbes, L.B., Kramer, M., Gajadhar, A.A., Gamble, H.R., 2007. Larval viability and serological response in horses with long-term infection of *Trichinella spiralis* infection. Vet. Parasitol. 146, 107–116.
Hilwig, R.W., Cramer, J.D., Forsyth, K.S., 1978. Freezing times and temperatures required to kill *Taenia saginata* in beef. Vet. Parasitol. 4, 215–219.
Holec-Gasior, L., 2013. *Toxoplasma gondii* recombinant antigens as tools for serodiagnosis of human toxoplasmosis: current status of studies. Clin. Vacc. Immunol. 20, 1343–1351.
Hung, M.N., Duc, V.N., Stauffer Jr., J.R., Madsen, H., 2013a. Use of black carp (*Mylopharyngodon piceus*) in biological control of intermediate host snails of fish-borne zoonotic trematodes in nursery ponds in the Red River Delta, Vietnam. Parasit. Vectors 6 (142), 1–9. http://www.parasitesandvectors.com/contents/6/1/142.
Hung, M.N., Madsen, H., Fried, B., 2013b. Global status of fish-borne zoonotic trematodiasis in humans. Acta Parasit. 58, 231–258.
ICT (International Commission on Trichinellosis), 2014. ICT recommendations for quality assurance in digestion testing programs for *Trichinella*. Available at: www.trichinellosis.org.
Innes, E.A., Bartley, P.M., Rocchi, M., Benavidas-Silvan, J., Burrells, A., Hotchkiss, E., Chianini, F., Canton, G., Katzer, F., 2011. Developing vaccines to control protozoan parasites in ruminants: dead or alive? Vet. Parasitol. 180, 155–163.
Jenkins, D.J., Brown, G.K., Traub, R.J., 2013a. 'Cysticercosis storm' in feedlot cattle in northwest New South Wales. Aust. Vet. J. 91, 89–93.
Jenkins, M.B., Liotta, J.L., Bowman, D.D., 2013b. Inactivation kinetics of *Cryptosporidium parvum* oocysts in a swine waste lagoon and spray field. J. Parasitol. 99, 337–342.
Johansen, M.V., Sithithaworn, P., Bergquist, R., Utzinger, J., 2010. Towards improved diagnosis of zoonotic trematode infections in southeast Asia. Adv. Parasitol. 73, 171–195 (Chapter 7).
Johansen, M.V., Trevisan, C., Braae, U.C., Magnussen, P., Ertel, R.L., Mejer, H., Saarnak, F.L., 2014. The Vicious Worm: a computer-based *Taenia solium* education tool. Trends Parasitol. 30, 372–374. http://dx.doi.org/10.1016/j.pt.2014.06.003.
Jones, J.L., Dubey, J.P., 2012. Foodborne toxoplasmosis. Clin. Infect. Dis. 55, 845–851.
Jones, J.L., Parise, M.E., Fiore, A.E., 2014. Neglected parasitic infections in the United States: toxoplasmosis. Am. J. Trop. Med. Hyg. 90, 794–799.
Kapel, C.M.O., 2000. Host diversity and biological characteristics of the *Trichinella* genotypes and their effect on transmission. Vet. Parasitol. 93, 263–278.
Kijlstra, A., Jongert, E., 2008. Control of the risk of human toxoplasmosis transmitted by meat. Int. J. Parasitol. 38, 1359–1370.
King, B.J., Hoefel, D., Daminato, D.P., Fanok, S., Monis, P.T., 2008. Solar UV reduces *Cryptosporidium parvum* oocyst infectivity in environmental waters. J. Appl. Microbiol. 104, 1311–1323.
Kotula, A.W., Dubey, J.P., Sharar, A.K., Andrews, C.D., Shen, S.K., Lindsay, D.S., 1991. Effect of freezing on infectivity of *Toxoplasma gondii* tissue cysts in pork. J. Food Prot. 54, 687–690.
Larrat, S., Simard, M., Lair, S., Belanger, D., Proulx, J.-F., 2012. From science to action and from action to science: the Nunavik Trichinellosis Prevention Program. Int. J. Circumpolar Health 71, 18595.

Lass, A., Pietkiewicz, H., Szostakowska, B., Myjack, P., 2012. The first detection of *Toxoplasma gondii* DNA in environmental fruits and vegetables samples. Eur. J. Clin. Microbiol. Infect. Dis. 31, 1101–1108. http://dx.doi.org/10.1007/s10096-011-1414-8.

Lightowlers, M.W., 2010. Eradication of *Taenia solium* cysticercosis: a role for vaccination of pigs. Int. J. Parasitol. 40, 1183–1192. http://dx.doi.org/10.1016/j.ijpara.2010.05.001.

Lightowlers, M.W., 2013. Control of *Taenia solium* taeniasis/cysticercosis: past practices and new possibilities. Parasitology 140, 1566–1577.

Lima dos Santos, C.A.M., Howgate, P., 2011. Fishborne zoonotic parasites and aquaculture. Aquaculture 318, 253–261.

Lin, R.-Q., Tang, J.-D., Zhou, D.-H., Song, H.-Q., Huang, S.-Y., Chen, J.-X., Chen, M.-X., Zhang, H., Zhu, X.-Q., Zhou, X.-N., 2011. Prevalence of *Clonorchis sinensis* infection in dogs and cats in subtropical southern China. Parasit. Vectors 4, 180. http://www.parasitesandvectors.com/content/4/1/180.

Lindsay, D.S., Holliman, D., Flick, G.J., Goodwin, D.G., Mitchell, S.M., Dubey, J.P., 2008. Effects of high pressure processing on *Toxoplasma gondii* oocysts on raspberries. J. Parasitol. 94, 757–758.

Macpherson, C.N.L., 2005. Human behaviour and the epidemiology of parasitic zoonoses. Int. J. Parasitol. 35, 1319–1331. http://dx.doi.org/10.1016/j.ijpara.2005.06.004.

Meemken, D., Tangermann, A.H., Meermeier, D., Gundlach, S., Mischok, D., Greiner, M., Klein, G., Blaha, T., 2014. Establishment of serological herd profiles for zoonoses and production diseases in pigs by "meat juice multi-serology." Prev. Vet. Med. 113, 589–598.

Moussavou-boussougou, M.-N., Geerts, S., Madeline, M., Ballandonne, C., Barbier, D., Cabaret, J., 2005. Sewage sludge or cattle slurry as pasture fertilisers: comparative cysticercosis and trichostrongylosis risk for grazing cattle. Parasitol. Res. 97, 27–32.

Murrell, K.D., 2013. Zoonotic foodborne parasites and their surveillance. Rev. Sci. Tech Off. Int. Epiz. 32, 559–569.

Murrell, K.D., Djordjevic, M., Cuperlovic, K., Sofronic, Lj, Savic, M., Djordjevic, M., Damjanovic, S., 2004. Epidemiology of *Trichinella* infection in the horse: the risk from animal product feeding practices. Vet. Parasitol. 123, 223–233.

Nga, V.T., Dung, D.T., Litzroth, A., Praet, N., Huong, N.T., Hien, N.T., Hung, N.M., Dorny, P., 2013. The hidden burden of trichinellosis in Vietnam: a postoutbreak epidemiological study. BioMed Res. Int. 2013, 4. Article ID 149890. http://dx.doi.org/10.1155/2013/149890.

Nkouawa, A., Sako, Y., Nakao, M., Nakaya, K., Ito, A., 2009. Loop-mediated isothermal amplification method for differentiation and rapid detection of *Taenia* species. J. Clin. Microbiol. 47, 168–174.

OIE (World Organisation for Animal Health), 2014a. Guidelines for animal disease control. Available at: www.oie.int/fileadmin/Home/eng/Our_scientific_expertise/docs/pdf/A_Guidelines_for_Animal_Disease_Control_final.pdf.

OIE (World Organisation for Animal Health), 2014b. Manual of diagnostic tests and vaccines for terrestrial animals. Available at: www.oie.int/international-standard-setting/terrestrial-manual/access-online/.

OIE (World Organisation for Animal Health), 2014c. Terrestrial animal health code. Available at: www.oie.int/international-standard-setting/terrestrial-code/access-online/.

Orlandi, P.A., Chu, D.-M.T., Bier, J.W., Jackson, G.J., 2002. Parasites and the food supply. Food Technol. 56, 72–81.

Ortega, Y.R., Mann, A., Torres, M.P., Cama, V., 2008. Efficacy of gaseous chlorine dioxide as a sanitizer against *Cryptosporidium parvum*, *Cyclospora cayetanensis*, and *Encephalitozoon intestinalis* on produce. J. Food Prot. 71, 2410–2414.

Ortega, Y.R., Sanchez, R., 2010. Update on *Cyclospora cayetanensis*, a food-borne and water-borne parasite. Clin. Microbiol. Rev. 23, 218–234.

Pawlowski, Z.S., Murrel, K.D., 2001. Taeniasis and cysticercosis. In: Hui, Y.H., Sattar, S.A., Murrell, K.D., Nip, W.-K., Stanfield, P.S. (Eds.), Foodborne Disease Handbook. second ed., 2. Marcel Dekker, New York, USA, pp. 217–227.

Pawlowski, Z., Allan, J., Sarti, E., 2005. Control of *Taenia solium* taeniasis/cysticercosis: from research towards implementation. Int. J. Parasitol. 35, 1221–1232.

Petroff, D., Hasenclever, D., Makrutzki, G., Riehn, K., Lucker, E., 2014. Assessing laboratory performance in Trichinella ring trials. Parasitol. Res. 113, 2837–2843.

Pezzoli, L., Marotta, V., Sattanino, G., Griglio, B., 2009. Toxoplasmosis in Italian pregnant women: results of a survey on perception of foodborne risks. J. Food Prot. 72, 680–684.

Phan, V.T., Ersboll, A.K., Do, D.T., Dalsgaard, A., 2011. Raw-fish-eating behavior and fish-borne zoonotic trematode infection in people of Northern Vietnam. Foodborne Pathog. Dis. 8, 255–260. http://dx.doi.org/10.1089/fpd.2010.0670.

Pomares, C., Ajzenberg, D., Bornard, L., Bernardin, G., Hasseine, L., Darde, M.-L., Marty, P., 2011. Toxoplasmosis and horse meat, France. Emerg. Infect. Dis. 17, 1327–1328.

Pozio, E., Armignacco, O., Ferri, F., Gomez Morales, M.A., 2013. *Opisthorchis felineus*, an emerging infection in Italy and its implication for the European Union. Acta Trop. 126, 54–62.

Praet, N., Verweij, J.J., Mwape, K.E., Phiri, I.K., Muma, J.B., Zulu, G., van Lieshout, L., Rodriguez-Hidalgo, R., Benitez-Ortiz, W., Dorny, P., Gabriel, S., 2013. Bayesian modelling to estimate the test characteristics of coprology, coproantigen ELISA and a novel real-time PCR for the diagnosis of taeniasis. Trop. Med. Int. Health 18, 608–614.

Proulx, J.-F., Maclean, D., Gyorkes, T.W., Leclair, D., Richter, A.-K., Serhir, B., Forbes, L., Gajadhar, A.A., 2002. Novel prevention program for trichinellosis in Inuit communities. Clin. Infect. Dis. 34, 1508–1514.

Pyburn, D.G., Gamble, H.R., Wagstrom, E.A., Anderson, L.A., Miller, L.E., 2005. Trichinae certification in the United States pork industry. Vet. Parasitol. 132, 179–183.

Robertson, L.J., Chalmers, R.M., 2013. Foodborne cryptosporidiosis: is there really more in Nordic countries? Trends Parasitol. 29, 3–9.

Robertson, L.J., Sprong, H., Ortega, Y.R., van der Giessen, J., Fayer, R., 2014. Impacts of globalisation on foodborne parasites. Trends Parasitol. 30, 37–52.

Ryan, U., Fayer, R., Xiao, L., 2014. Cryptosporidium species in humans and animals: current understanding and research needs. Parasitology 141, 1667–1685. http://dx.doi.org/10.1017/S0031182014001085.

Saini, P.K., Webert, D.W., McCaskey, P.C., 1997. Food safety and regulatory aspects of cattle and swine cysticercosis. J. Food Prot. 60, 447–453.

Scandrett, W.B., Gajadhar, A.A., 2004. Recovery of putative taeniid eggs from silt in water associated with an outbreak of bovine cysticercosis. Can. Vet. J. 45, 758–760.

Scandrett, W.B., Haines, D.M., Parker, S.E., Robinson, Y., Forbes, L.B., Brandt, J., Geerts, S., Dorny, P., Gajadhar, A.A., 2012. Validation of an immunohistochemical assay for bovine cysticercosis, with comparison to a standard histological method. Vet. Parasitol. 186, 301–311.

Schantz, P.M., Moore, A.C., Munoz, J.L., Hartman, B.J., Schaefer, J.A., Aron, A.M., Persaud, D., Sarti, E., Wilson, M., Flisser, A., 1992. Neurocysticercosis in an Orthodox Jewish community in New York City. N. Engl. J. Med. 327, 692–695.

Slifko, T.R., Smith, H.W., Rose, J.B., 2000. Emerging parasite zoonoses associated with water and food. Int. J. Parasitol. 30, 1379–1393.

Steinparzer, R., Reisp, K., Grunberger, B., Kofer, J., Schmoll, F., Sattler, T., 2014. Comparison of different commercial serological tests for the detection of *Toxoplasma gondii* antibodies in serum of naturally exposed pigs. Zoonoses Public Health 15, 1–6.

Sturbaum, G.D., Ortega, Y.R., Gilman, R.H., Sterling, C.R., Cabrera, L., Klein, D.A., 1998. Detection of *Cyclospora cayetanensis* in wastewater. Appl. Environ. Microbiol. 64, 2284–2286.

Suwannahitatorn, P., Klomjit, S., Naaglor, T., Taamasri, P., Rangsin, R., Leelayoova, S., Mungthin, M., 2013. A follow-up study of *Opisthorchis viverrini* infection after the implementation of control program in a rural community, central Thailand. Parasit. Vectors 6, 188. http://www.parasitesandvectors.com/content/6/1/188.

Takumi, K., Franssen, F., Fonville, M., Grasset, A., Vallee, I., Boireau, P., Teunis, P., van der Giessen, J., 2010. Within-host dynamics of *Trichinella spiralis* predict persistent parasite transmission in rat populations. Int. J. Parasitol. 40, 1317–1324.

Tauxe, R.V., 1997. Emerging foodborne diseases: an evolving public health challenge. Emerg. Infect. Dis. 3, 425–434.

Tenter, A.M., 2009. *Toxoplasma gondii* in animals used for human consumption. Mem. Inst. Oswaldo Cruz 104, 364–369.

Thompson, R.C.A., 2014. Parasites and food: ripe for exploitation. Trends Parasitol. 30, 1–3.

Toledo, R., Esterban, J.G., Fried, B., 2012. Current status of food-borne trematode infections. Eur. J. Clin. Microbiol. Infect. Dis. 31, 1705–1718.

Traub, R.J., Macaranas, J., Mungthin, M., Leelayoova, S., Cribb, T., Murrell, K.D., Thompson, R.C.A., 2009. A new PCR-based approach indicates the range of *Clonorchis sinensis* now extends to Central Thailand. PLoS Negl. Trop. Dis. 3 (1), e367. http://dx.doi.org/10.1371/journal.pntd.0000367.

Turk, M., Kaptan, F., Turker, N., Korkmaz, M., El, S., Ozkaya, D., Ural, S., Vardari, I., Alkan, M.Z., Coskun, N.A., Turker, M., Pozio, E., 2006. Clinical and laboratory aspects of a trichinellosis outbreak in Izmir, Turkey. Parasite 13, 65–70.

Uga, S., Hoa, N.T., Noda, S., Moji, K., Cong, L., Aoki, Y., Rai, S.K., Fujimaki, Y., 2009. Parasite egg contamination of vegetables from a suburban market in Hanoi, Vietnam. Nepal Med. Coll. J. 11, 75–78.

Vallee, I., Mace, P., Forbes, L., Scandrett, B., Durand, B., Gajadhar, A., Boireau, P., 2007. Use of proficiency samples to assess diagnostic laboratories in France performing a *Trichinella* digestion assay. J. Food Prot. 70, 1685–1690.

Van Der Logt, P.B., Hathaway, S.C., Vose, D.J., 1997. Risk assessment model for human infection with the cestode *Taenia saginata*. J. Food Prot. 60, 1110–1119.

Vanderstichel, R., Christensen, J., Stryhn, H., Hurnik, D., 2013. Standards for reporting surveillance information in freedom from infection models by example of *Trichinella* in Canadian market hogs. Prev. Vet. Med. 111, 176–180.

Wainwright, K.E., Miller, M.A., Barr, B.C., Gardner, I.A., Melli, A.C., Essert, T., Packham, A.E., Truong, T., Lagunas-Solar, M., Conrad, P.A., 2007. Chemical inactivation of *Toxoplasma gondii* oocysts in water. J. Parasitol. 93, 925–931.

Whittaker, M., Berquist, R., Buttsworth, M., 2013. Strengthening control of neglected tropical diseases in the Asia-Pacific region: implications for health information system priorities and strategies. Working Paper Series Number 32, Health Information Systems, School of Population Health, University of Queensland, Australia. www.uq.edu.au/hishub.

WHO (World Health Organisation), 1995. Food technologies and public health. Available at: www.who.int/entity/foodsafety/publications/fs_management/en/foodtech.pdf.

WHO (World Health Organisation), 2008a. Section 3. Surveillance to detect foodborne disease outbreaks. In: Foodborne Disease Outbreaks: Guidelines for Investigation and Control. WHO Press, Geneva, Switzerland, 146 p.

WHO (World Health Organisation), 2008b. Section 4. Investigation of foodborne disease outbreaks. In: Foodborne Disease Outbreaks: Guidelines for Investigation and Control. WHO Press, Geneva, Switzerland, 146 p.

WHO (World Health Organisation), 2014. Foodborne trematodiases. Fact sheet No. 368. Available at: http://www.who.int/mediacentre/factsheets/fs368/en/.

WHO/FAO (World Health Organisation/Food and Agriculture Organisation), 2002. Food-borne trematode infections in Asia. Report of a joint FAO/WHO workshop, 26–28 November 2002, Ha Noi, Viet Nam, 54 pp.

WHO/FAO/OIE (World Health Organisation/Food and Agriculture Organisation/World Organisation for Animal Health), 2005. In: Murrell, K.D. (Ed.), Guidelines for the Surveillance, Prevention and Control of Taeniosis/Cysticercosis. WHO/FAO/OIE, Paris, France, 139 p.

Wiriya, B., Clausen, J.H., Inpankaew, T., Thaenkham, U., Jittapalapong, S., Satapornvanit, K., Dalsgaard, A., 2013. Fish-borne trematodes in cultured Nile tilapia (*Oreochromis niloticus*) and wild-caught fish from Thailand. Vet. Parasitol. 198, 230–234.

Yossepowitch, O., Gotesman, T., Assous, M., Marva, E., Zimlichman, R., Dan, M., 2004. Opisthorchiasis from imported raw fish. Emerg. Infect. Dis. 10, 2122–2126.

Zarlenga, D.S., Chute, M.B., Martin, A., Kapel, C.M., 1999. A multiplex PCR for unequivocal differentiation of all encapsulated and non-encapsulated genotypes of *Trichinella*. Int. J. Parasitol. 29, 1859–1867.

Zhang, R., Gao, S., Geng, Y., Huang, D., Yu, L., Zhang, S., Cheng, J., Fu, Y., 2007. Epidemiological study on *Chlonorchis sinensis* infection in Shenzhen area of Zhujiang delta in China. Parasitol. Res. 101, 179–183.

Modeling as an approach to identify and manage food safety risks related to parasites in the food chain

15

P. Delaquis, S. Bach
Pacific Agri-Food Research Centre, Summerland, BC, Canada

15.1 Introduction

Historical deficiencies in disease data quality and quantity hinder the measurement of the public health and economic impact of foodborne parasitic infections. It has been suggested, however, that rates of infection for some species or taxa may approach those attributed to common bacterial or viral pathogens in the developed world (Macpherson et al., 2000; Newell et al., 2010). Statistics from underdeveloped or developing nations are often incomplete, but meta-analysis of available data suggests that foodborne parasitic disease is endemic in some regions (Dawson, 2005; Torgerson et al., 2014; Fürst et al., 2012). A recent expert solicitation and call for data requested by the Codex Committee on Food Hygiene led to a review of the current status of knowledge on parasites in food, their public health impact, and their trade impact (FAO/WHO, 2014). This exercise included a global ranking for foodborne parasites based on the several criteria, including the number of global illnesses, distribution, acute morbidity, chronic morbidity, and economic impact. Results of the analysis illustrate the range of taxa associated with foodborne parasitic diseases and the variety of foods involved in their transmission (see Chapter 1). Some of the pathogen–food associations are well-established, and implicated foods, commodities are subject to regulatory scrutiny in some jurisdictions. There is little doubt, however, that intensifying trade in increasingly varied foodstuffs across international borders, changing dietary habits, and shifts in geographic distribution due to climate change are promoting the spread of new taxa to previously unexposed populations (Rogers and Randolph, 2006; Broglia and Kapel, 2011; Robertson et al., 2013b; Garza et al., 2014). The emergence or potential reemergence of foodborne parasitic diseases has prompted recommendations to improve control measures on an international scale (Dorny et al., 2009). Clearly, improved means to identify and manage risks will be required to mitigate the implied threat to the safety of foods delivered to current and future consumers through increasingly complex food chains.

The capacity to forecast the spread and measure the public health outcomes of disease are important objectives in infectious disease epidemiology. Consequently, mathematical analysis and modeling are used extensively to predict and map disease

Foodborne Parasites in the Food Supply Web. http://dx.doi.org/10.1016/B978-1-78242-332-4.00015-1

progression on a population scale. Early models consisted of simple mathematical descriptions of disease incidence or mortality data that were used to gain insight into the dynamics and progression of epidemics. Considerable advances in the field over the past 50 years have led to the development of more functional modeling tools that may be used to characterize disease spread or to generate and test hypotheses about the transmission of infectious agents (Brauer et al., 2008; Grassly and Fraser, 2008; Keeling and Rohani, 2008; Temime et al., 2008; Hollingsworth, 2009). The advent of computer-assisted representations has vastly enhanced practical applications, and computerized modeling tools are now used routinely to monitor disease outbreaks, for surveillance purposes, in response planning, and to design control measures. Modeling techniques and tools have also been applied in the study of infectious parasitic diseases. Details of complex life cycles and transmission dynamics of the various foodborne parasites are described in several chapters of this book, and we refer the reader to examples in Michael and Spear (2010) and Basanez (2014), which demonstrate how these life cycles, changeable behavior along transmission routes, and multiple host exposure factors introduce unique challenges in the design of apposite models.

Epidemiological model development and usage have primarily been directed at the resolution of problems caused by infectious parasitic taxa or species associated with high case fatality rates and chronic public health problems, such as malaria. There have been comparatively fewer attempts to model factors that contribute to the spread and incidence of disease caused by foodborne parasites. Misdiagnosis owing to the range of disease outcomes and analytical limitations that hinder the detection of infectious forms in heterogeneous sample matrices have undoubtedly contributed to the historical scarcity of parasitic foodborne disease statistics and food prevalence data. However, advances in the design of pertinent analytical equipment and in molecular biology over the past 20 years have fueled the development of progressively more practical, sensitive, and reliable methods for the detection and characterization of parasites in clinical, environmental, and food samples. Improved analytical capability has led to a parallel rise in the reliability of data stemming from disease reports, clinical studies, and findings from outbreak investigations. Wider recognition of the associated food safety risks has also promoted increased surveillance of food supplies and research to examine parasite occurrence and behavior along complete food chains. More importantly, expanding knowledge about the origin, fate, and distribution of infectious foodborne parasites is contributing indispensable data and information for the development of models to characterize consequent risks at specific stages along the chain.

Risk analysis, comprising risk assessment, management, and communication, is widely applied to the control of known or potentially adverse effects of exposure to foodborne microbiological hazards (FAO/WHO, 2008). Microbiological risk assessment (MRA), or the comprehensive and systematic scientific evaluation of the risks implied by specific pathogens, has emerged as an important tool for the analysis of risks along food chains. General principles for conducting MRAs are defined in the Codex Alimentarius (CAC, 1999, 2004; Lammerding and Fazil, 2000). The four "cornerstones" of MRA include hazard identification, hazard characterization, exposure assessment, and risk characterization. Hazard identification is primarily a qualitative process wherein information about the disease agent is gathered from available sources.

Here data from epidemiological studies, outbreak investigations, or field reports may be used to define the range of associated illness, potential disease dynamics (endemic, epidemic), vulnerable populations, severity of consequences (morbidity, mortality), and food associations to clearly identify major sources of exposure. Hazard characterization requires a qualitative and/or quantitative description of the nature, severity, and duration of illness to establish a dose–response relationship. The latter describes the probability of illness resulting from exposure to the hazard in a given population as a function of ingested dose. In turn, qualitative and/or quantitative exposure assessments are derived from rates of food intake to estimate the likelihood and level of ingestion in the population. Information from each step is then integrated for risk characterization, which is defined by the Codex Alimentarius Commission as "[t]he qualitative and/or quantitative estimation, including attendant uncertainties, of the probability of occurrence and severity of known potential adverse effects in a given population based on hazard identification, hazard characterization and exposure assessment" (CAC, 1999).

Where the availability of data is limiting, qualitative MRAs may be developed to express risk in descriptive terms. Quantitative microbial risk assessments (QMRAs) that provide numerical expressions of risk, uncertainty, and variability that account for the potential multiplication or decay of microorganisms at different stages along the chain are preferable in food risk analysis. Key stages in the implementation of a QMRA are illustrated in Figure 15.1. QMRAs can be either deterministic, wherein parameters that influence risk are represented by single-point estimates, or stochastic and include probability distributions to describe the effect of individual or multiple variables. The latter yield the most accurate measures but tend to be more data-demanding and require mathematical modeling to accommodate random fluctuations in variables. The QMRA approach has been applied to the assessment of risks along farm-to-fork chains for several pathogen-food combinations, primarily enteric bacterial species in animal products (Boone et al., 2010; Chen et al., 2012; Vågsholm, 2012). Practical tools are now available to facilitate assessments for specific pathogen–food combinations. For example, the FAO/WHO has developed a risk-management simulation tool for *Campylobacter* and *Salmonella* in chicken meat that is accessible to public or industry interests through

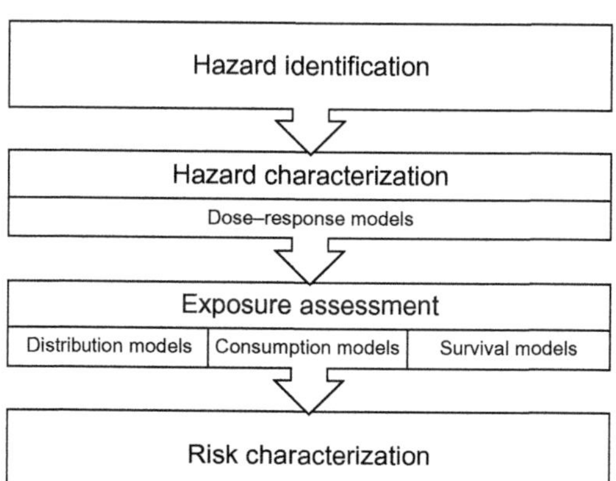

Figure 15.1 Key stages and relevant models for QMRAs of foods.

a user-friendly website (FAO/WHO, 2009). The tool consists of modules (farm and transport, processing, storage, and preparation) incorporating models that predict the fate of target pathogens and provide measures of risk at specific stages or in the complete chain. Uncertainty introduced by the aforementioned knowledge and data gaps, notably those that are essential for hazard characterization and exposure assessment, has undoubtedly hindered past attempts to adapt the approach for the analysis of risks associated with infectious foodborne parasites. However, contemporary growth in the prerequisite knowledge base and the expanding availability of adaptable modeling tools favor renewed attempts to adapt MRA principles for the identification and management of risks associated with these pathogens in modern food chains.

15.2 Framework for the development of models

A framework aligned with the principles of MRA for the development of models to identify risks from infectious parasites in food chains is outlined below. For the purpose of this exercise it will be assumed that the spectrum of disease, types of clinical outcomes, and routes of transmission for the species under consideration are known. Characterization of the associated risks should provide a quantitative measure of the relationship between ingested dose and the probability of health outcomes (infection, disease, or death) (FAO/WHO, 2003). Data needed to derive mathematical expressions of the dose–response relationship for some foodborne parasites is available from several sources. For example, analysis of records from outbreak investigations suggests that the infective dose for *Cyclospora cayetanensis* may be as low as 10 oocysts (Smith, 2007). More recently, Teunis et al. (2012) used data from well-characterized outbreaks to develop as dose–response model for *Trichinella* spp. which predicts a rapid rise in the probability of infection after exposure to a few pairs of larvae. Where outbreak data are scant the dose–response may be estimated from animal feeding trials, provided that a suitable animal model is available. Using this approach, Dubey et al. (1996) showed that one sporulated *Toxoplasma gondii* oocyst led to clinical manifestations of infection in pigs. However, dose–response estimates derived from animal feeding trials are subject to uncertainty induced by the assumption that infectivity is similar in humans and test animal species. Human feeding trials eliminate such uncertainty, although bioethical considerations restrict the use of this approach. A limited number of studies have been carried out with species such as *Cryptosporidium parvum* and *Entamoeba coli*, which yielded infectious doses as low as 10 oocysts and 1 cyst, respectively (Kothary and Babu, 2007). Human feeding trials with *Cryptosporidium* spp. have also provided information about variability in health outcomes due to species (Chappell et al., 2006), strain (Teunis et al., 2002a), and host-associated differences in response (Teunis et al., 2002b). More importantly, they have contributed critical data to support the development of dose–response models for *C. parvum* and *Cryptosporidium hominis* (Enger, 2013). The latter is available through a web-based portal sponsored by the Center for Advancing Microbial Risk Assessment (Michigan State University) that provides an evolving repository for current quantitative information and knowledge developed for MRA, including dose–response models for several human pathogens to support quantitative analysis (accessible at: http://qmrawiki.msu.edu/index.php?title=Quantitative_Microbial_Risk_Assessment_(QMRA)_Wiki). At the time of writing dose–response models for the food-transmissible species *C. parvum* and *C. hominis*, *E. coli* and *Giardia duodenalis* were available from this source. In the future, such community-based initiatives undoubtedly will improve the range and availability of data and dose–response models for the characterization of hazards caused by other species of foodborne parasites.

The objective of exposure assessment is to determine the probability and magnitude of exposure to a microbiological hazard in a given population resulting from the consumption of contaminated food. Various modeling approaches may be employed to achieve this objective depending on the nature of the hazard, potential pathways of exposure, behavior of the hazard in food, patterns of consumption, and overall intake (FAO/WHO, 2008). Comparatively simple models that assume linearity and constancy in the supply chain can be developed to anticipate exposure in settled populations where foods are sourced locally and consumption patterns are stable. For example, local growers may deliver fresh vegetables to community markets a short distance from a production site. Under such a scenario the level of exposure to pathogens at the point of consumption can be estimated using prevalence data. In contrast, the delivery of fresh vegetables to urban consumers may incorporate several supply lines, processing and packaging steps, transport under refrigeration to distribution centers, and delivery to multiple retail outlets where batches of similar products can be mixed. Modeling population exposure for commodities distributed under such a scenario requires the ability to predict intake against changeable factors that govern survival of the pathogen, consumer access to the contaminated food, and the amount and frequency at which it is consumed.

When consumer level data is unavailable, indirect estimates of intake can be deduced from food production statistics compiled by national governments or international agencies, such as the Statistics Division of the FAO. Far more detailed food intake data, including anticipated serving sizes and frequency of consumption on a daily basis, is obtainable from consumer surveys. Detailed statistics for some populations are available from public sources (see, for example, the United States Department of Agriculture (USDA) Food Commodity Intake Databases, accessible at: http://www.ars.usda.gov/Services/Services.htm?modecode=12-35-50-00&locpubs=yes).

Simple exposure models for linear supply chains can be developed from such food intake and pathogen prevalence data. Where foods are distributed through complex chains that encompass multiple supply channels subject to spatial and temporal variation, dynamic mathematical modeling is essential to accommodate supply variances and factors that influence consumption.

The means to describe the movement to foods through the chain and to anticipate the size of populations affected by contaminated food are essential for the development of exposure models. A systematic approach for the description of food chains and the development of distribution models that can be adapted to any commodity was proposed by Hashemi Beni et al. (2012). Description of the various stages in the chain requires the assembly of a relational database to include data on food origin; location of processing/packing facilities and quantities supplied on a seasonal basis; location and probability of shipment to distribution centers on a seasonal basis; locations of retail stores, and quantities and probability of shipment from individual distribution centers. Once assembled, the database can be used to develop space–time models to estimate consumer accessibility, or the ease with which a particular outlet where food is sold may be reached by an individual at that location (Kwan and Weber, 2003). Computerized geographic information systems (GIS) are well-suited to this purpose and enable detailed analysis of food dissemination to a point of sale along temporal and geographic planes against predictable (e.g., seasonal) or random (e.g., changes in a supply route) events. In the approach suggested by Hashemi Beni et al. (2012), spatial analytical tools within GIS are used to overlay mapped points of sale and fixed geographic "zones of influence" with corresponding census data to estimate the size of population that may purchase a specified food item. Distance traveled to purchase food is influenced by additional factors, however, such as the location of the point of sale in relation to other commercial activity and the socioeconomic status of resident populations. Shopping behavior models that consider the influence of these factors on estimates of distance traveled to shop may be applied to increase the accuracy of predictions about the size of populations likely to shop in a given location (Nakanishi and Cooper, 1974). Distribution models that incorporate predictions about the size of populations likely to purchase a specified food product deliver the most reliable estimates of consumption.

The assessment of exposure through extended supply chains mandates consideration of time and temperature factors and variances that may also affect pathogen survival at different stages along the production to consumption pathway. Time spent in storage or transit between stages and temperature profiles may be included in the relational databases proposed by Hashemi Beni et al. (2012) to accommodate the integration of mathematical equations to calculate time and/or temperature effects on pathogen survival. The fate of bacterial foodborne pathogens such as *Salmonella* spp. during the production, processing, and distribution of major food commodities (e.g., milk, meat) has been studied extensively and predictive mathematical equations have been developed to support exposure assessments. With few exceptions, considerably less effort has been devoted to the examination of infectious foodborne parasite behavior in foods or to the mathematical analysis of survival data. Consequently, models that accommodate time or temperature effects on parasite survival are presently scarce, although assumptions about the stability of some species can be deduced from survival data obtained through experimentation in foods. For example, *Cryptosporidium* oocysts or the cyst stage of *G. duodenalis* have been shown to resist dehydration, refrigeration, or freezing and are presumed to remain stable in number and to remain infectious for extended periods of time in diverse foods of animal or plant origin (Smith et al., 2007). In contrast, the effects of food processing and storage on the fate of many species of foodborne parasite, *Echinococcus* spp., for example, are poorly characterized. When such data are unavailable, persistence in foods may be implied on the basis of survival characteristics in other media or environments, such as water or soil.

Distribution, consumption, and survival models are typically integrated to assess risks of exposure in an epidemiological context, principally to determine the public health impact of food contamination events on a population scale. Their value and utility extend well beyond the quantification of disease impact, however, increasingly for the simulation and analysis of complex phenomena that influence risks at discrete stages along food chains. Risk factors such as rates of pathogen survival or the probability of exposure in human populations are often difficult or impossible to measure *in situ* or to duplicate in the laboratory. *In silico* simulation provides a means to project changes in these factors due to independent or simultaneous variation in supply, level of processing, time, temperature, or alterations in consumption patterns. Information derived from the analysis of scenarios that replicate the effect of variation on risk factors can therefore be used to guide investigations aimed at the measurement of actual risks in food chains. More importantly, *in silico* simulations provide insight on the evolution of risk in response to events that occur at specific stages along a food supply chain. At a functional level, the latter is central to the recognition of critical control points where mitigation efforts can deliver the greatest reduction in overall risk.

15.3 Future prospects

Deficiencies in key biological knowledge required to fully satisfy a risk-based approach to the identification of hazards associated with foodborne parasites have long hampered the development of tools to support control and prevention programs. Although the transmission of classical parasitic diseases such as trichinellosis and taeniosis tends to follow direct routes (e.g., consumption of tissues from infected food animals), many infections such as cysticercosis are spread through the indirect fecal–oral route of transmission. Routes of transmission may be evident where there is a strong correlation between disease and poor hygienic practices. In contrast, routes of transmission are difficult to define for species with multiple infectious forms of variable infectivity and resistance to stresses in the natural environment or in foods. Analytical difficulties alluded to previously in this work have contributed much to deficiencies in data required to identify reservoirs and to track parasites along potential routes of transmission. Data gaps are gradually receding, however, because of the increasing availability of cost-effective and reliable molecular methods to facilitate the detection of infectious forms in clinical and other materials. Furthermore, genomic, transcriptomic, and proteomic approaches are increasingly applied to the resolution of fundamental problems in parasitology. Exploration of datasets derived from the various omic research is vastly improving our fundamental understanding of parasite development, host interactions, virulence, infectivity, and pathogenicity (Cantacessi et al., 2012). The increasing availability of omic data has promoted the development of analytical techniques to discriminate between species or variants within species with a high degree of precision. It is now possible to track the movement of distinct pathotypes through hosts and environmental reservoirs to facilitate the characterization of transmission routes. From a risk-assessment perspective, the capacity to identify relevant phenotypes in complex samples, to discriminate between virulent and avirulent forms, and to link this information to disease outcome is of immense value. Most methods currently used to detect parasites provide little or no information about phenotype, and none about virulence. Consequently, risk measurements are usually based on the assumption that the presence of the pathogen signals a high probability of infection and disease. Improvements in the ability to forecast disease outcomes stemming from the availability of data that incorporate information about virulence will undoubtedly stimulate the development of increasingly accurate modeling tools for the identification of risks associated with infectious parasites in food chains.

References

Basanez, M.G., 2014. Mathematical models for parasites and vectors. In: Basanez, M.G. (Ed.), Parasites & Vectors. Springer, New York. Accessed at: http://www.parasitesandvectors.com/series/modelling.

Boone, I., Van der Stede, Y., Aerts, M., Mintiens, K., Dube, G., 2010. Quantitative microbial risk assessment: methods and quality assurance. Vlaams Diergen Tijds 79, 367–380.

Brauer, F., van den Driessche, P., Wu, J., 2008. Mathematical Epidemiology. Lecture Notes in Mathematics, Mathematical Biosciences Subseries, vol. 1945. Springer, Berlin/Heidelberg.

Broglia, A., Kapel, C., 2011. Changing dietary habits in a changing world: emerging drivers for the transmission of foodborne parasitic zoonoses. Vet. Parasitol. 182, 2–13.

CAC (Codex Alimentarius Commission, FAO/WHO), 1999. Principles and guidelines for the conduct of microbiological risk assessment. CAC/GL-30. World Health Organization/Food and Agriculture Organization of the United Nations, Rome. Available at: http://www.who.int/foodsafety/publications/micro/cac1999/en/.

CAC (Codex Alimentarius Commission, FAO/WHO), 2004. Procedural Manual, fourteenth ed. Available at: http://www.fao.org/docrep/007/y5817e/y5817e00.htm.

Cantacessi, C., Campbell, B.E., Jex, A.R., Young, N.D., Hall, R.S., Ranganathan, S., Gasser, R.B., 2012. Bioinformatics meets parasitology. Parasite Immunol. 34, 265–275.

Chappell, C.L., Okhuysen, P.C., Langer-Curry, R., Widmer, G., Akiyoshi, D.E., Tanriverdi, S., et al., 2006. *Cryptosporidium hominis*: experimental challenge of healthy adults. Am. J. Trop. Med. Hyg. 75, 851–857.

Chen, Y., Danyluk, M.D., Schaffner, D.W., 2012. Microbial quantitative risk assessment. In: Yan, X., Juneja, V.K., Fratamico, P.M., Smith, J.L. (Eds.), Omics, Microbial Modelling and Technologies for Foodborne Pathogens. DEStenc Publications, Inc., Lancaster, PA, 423–446.

Dawson, D., 2005. Foodborne protozoan parasites. Int. J. Food Microbiol. 103, 207–227.

Dorny, P., Praet, N., Deckers, N., Gabriel, S., 2009. Emerging food-borne parasites. Vet. Parasitol. 163, 196–206.

Dubey, J.P., Lunney, J.K., Shen, S.K., Kwok, O.C., Ashford, D.A., Thulliez, P., 1996. Infectivity of low numbers of *Toxoplasma gondii* oocysts to pigs. J. Parasitol. 82, 438–443.

Enger, K.S., 2013. *Cryptosporidium parvum* and *Cryptosporidium hominis*: dose response. QMRAWiki. Accessed at: http://qmrawiki.msu.edu/index.php?oldid=10896.

FAO/WHO, 2003. Hazard Characterization for Pathogens in Food and Water. Microbiological Risk Assessment Series No. 3. World Health Organization, Geneva.

FAO/WHO, 2008. Exposure Assessment of Microbiological Hazards in Foods—Guidelines. Microbiological Risk Assessment Series No. 7. World Health Organization, Geneva.

FAO/WHO, 2009. Risk Management Tool for the Control of *Campylobacter* and *Salmonella* in Chicken Meat. World Health Organization, Geneva. Accessed at: http://www.fstools.org/poultryRMTool/.

FAO/WHO, 2014. Multicriteria-Based Ranking for Risk Management of Foodborne Parasites. Microbiological Risk Assessment Series No. 23. World Health Organization, Geneva.

Fürst, T., et al., 2012. Global burden of human food-borne trematodiasis: a systematic review and meta-analysis. Lancet Infect. Dis. 12, 210–221.

Garza, M., Feria Arroyo, T.P., Casillas, E.A., Sanchez-Cordero, V., Rivaldi, C.-L., et al., 2014. Projected future distributions of vectors of *Trypanosoma cruzi* in North America under climate change scenarios. PLoS Negl. Trop. Dis. 8 (5), e2818.

Grassly, N.C., Fraser, C., 2008. Mathematical models of infectious disease transmission. Nat. Rev. Microbiol. 6, 477–487.

Hashemi Beni, L., Villeneuve, S., LeBlanc, D.I., Côté, K., Fazil, A.M., Otten, A., McKellar, R., Delaquis, P.J., 2012. Spatio-temporal assessment of food safety risks in Canadian food distribution systems using GIS. Spat. Spatiotemporal Epidemiol. 3, 215–223.

Hollingsworth, D.T., 2009. Controlling infectious disease outbreaks: lessons from mathematical modelling. J. Public Health Policy 30, 328–341.

Keeling, M.J., Rohani, P., 2008. Modeling Infectious Diseases in Humans and Animals. Princeton University Press, Princeton, NJ, USA.

Kothary, M.H., Babu, U.S., 2007. Infectious dose of foodborne pathogens in volunteers: a review. J. Food Saf. 21, 49–68.

Kwan, M., Weber, J., 2003. Individual accessibility revisited: implications for geographical analysis in the twenty-first century. Geogr. Anal. 35, 341–353.

Lammerding, A.M., Fazil, A., 2000. Hazard identification and exposure assessment for microbial food safety risk assessment. Int. J. Food Microbiol. 58, 147–158.

Macpherson, C.N.L., Gottstein, B., Geerts, S., 2000. Parasitic food-borne and water-borne zoonoses. Rev. Sci. Tech. Off. Int. Epiz. 19, 240–258.

Michael, E., Spear, R.C., 2010. Modeling parasite transmission and control. Adv. Exp. Med. Biol. 673, 212.

Nakanishi, M., Cooper, L.G., 1974. Parameter estimation for a multiplicative competitive interaction model: least squares approach. J. Mark. Res. 11, 303–311.

Newell, D.G., Koopmans, M., Verhoef, L., et al., 2010. Food-borne diseases—the challenges of 20 years ago still persist while new ones continue to emerge. Int. J. Food Microbiol. 139 (Suppl. 1), S3–S15.

Robertson, L.J., Sprong, H., Ortega, Y.R., van der Giessen, J.W.B., Fayer, R., 2013a. Impacts of globalisation on foodborne parasites. Trends Parasitol. 30, 37–52.

Robertson, L.J., van der Giessen, J.W.B., Batz, M.B., Kojima, M., Cahill, S., 2013b. Have foodborne parasites finally become a global concern? Trends Parasitol. 29, 101–103.

Rogers, D.J., Randolph, S.E., 2006. Climate change and vector-borne diseases. Adv. Parasitol. 62, 345–381.

Smith, H.V., 2007. Cyclospora. In: Simjee, S. (Ed.), Foodborne Diseases. Humana Press, Totowa, pp. 277–301 (Chapter 10).

Smith, H.V., Caccio, S.M., Cook, N., Nichols, R.A.B., Tait, A., 2007. *Cryptosporidium* and *Giardia* as foodborne zoonoses. Vet. Parasitol. 149, 29–40.

Temime, L., Hejblum, G., Setbon, M., Valleron, A.J., 2008. The rising impact of mathematical modelling in epidemiology: antibiotic resistance research as a case study. Epidemiol. Infect. 136, 289–298.

Teunis, P.F.M., Chappell, C.L., Ockhuysen, P.C., 2002a. *Cryptosporidium* dose–response studies: variation between isolates. Risk Anal. 22, 175–183.

Teunis, P.F.M., Chappell, C.L., Ockhuysen, P.C., 2002b. *Cryptosporidium* dose–response studies: variation between hosts. Risk Anal. 22, 475–485.

Teunis, P.F.M., Koningstein, M., Takumi, K., Van Der Giesen, J.W.B., 2012. Human beings are highly susceptible to low doses of *Trichinella* spp. Epidemiol. Infect. 140, 210–218.

Torgerson, P.R., de Silva, N.R., Fèvre, E.M., Kasuga, F., Rokni, M.B., Zhou, X.N., Sripa, B., Gargouri, N., Willingham, A.L., Stein, C., 2014. The global burden of foodborne parasitic diseases: an update. Trends Parasitol. 30, 20–26.

Vågsholm, I., 2012. Quantitative microbial risk assessments in the food chain context—examples, advantages and challenges. In: International Conference, Biological Food Safety and Quality BFSQ 2012, 4–5 October 2012, Belgrade, pp. 38–40.

Laboratory diagnostic methods

16

R.J. Traub[1], L. Cuttell[2]

[1]The University of Melbourne, Parkville, VIC, Australia; [2]Safe Food Production Queensland, Spring Hill, QLD, Australia

16.1 Introduction

The prevention and control of foodborne parasites, as they relate to the protection of public health, are highly dependent on laboratory diagnosis as well as the accuracy, sensitivity, and specificity of the methods used for detection and quantification throughout the food supply chain. The overarching aim of microbiological testing is to inform risk assessment and assure food safety by verifying that components and processes of the overall food safety management system, from farm-to-fork, comply with regulatory guidelines and protect consumers. Ideally, diagnostic tests allow (i) monitoring and surveillance of parasite stages in environmental/food samples (plant and animal) and identification of risk factors at a preharvest or primary production level; (ii) validation of food safety/microbiological criteria at each process step; (iii) disease outbreak and trace-back investigations; and (iv) estimation of disease incidence and burden in consumers and economic impacts to the community.

Foodborne parasites have not always received the attention they deserve based on their public health, trade, and socioeconomic importance, and many are classified under the umbrella of "neglected" diseases by the World Health Organization (WHO). Parasites are biologically diverse, often with complex life cycles involving multiple hosts and multiple routes of infection. Some are transmitted through the ingestion of infective stages within host tissue and/or the parasites themselves contaminate food via the production of environmentally stable oocysts, cysts, or ova shed in feces.

Prevention and control of foodborne parasites have also been hampered by unique diagnostic challenges. As a general rule, parasites are not capable of replicating outside the host, and, unlike bacteria, this fact makes their amplification into easily detectable populations by simple culture methods impractical or impossible. The ability of parasites to "encyst" or infect within host tissue or adhere to surfaces of fruit and fresh produce (Fayer et al., 2013), coupled with their relatively low infectious dose, provides further challenges to the detection limits or sensitivity of conventional parasitological tests. In addition, morphologically identical species and genotypes of infectious stages make differentiation of those that are infectious to humans (zoonotic) versus those that are animal-specific, challenging. Simple, high-throughput measurement of parasite viability is also a major limitation as is the inability to discriminate between viable and dead cells. Combined, these factors limit the ability to detect, characterize, and enumerate parasites at different levels of the production process in a practical and economical manner that can accurately estimate risk (Haas, 2000). At the consumer level, parasitic diseases can present with prolonged incubation periods (e.g.,

Foodborne Parasites in the Food Supply Web. http://dx.doi.org/10.1016/B978-1-78242-332-4.00016-3

hydatid disease, *Taenia solium* neurocysticercosis) and in many instances be subclinical (e.g., giardiasis, fishborne liver flukes, toxoplasmosis), making epidemiological or trace-back studies associating illness with a specific food type impossible.

To overcome some of these diagnostic challenges, an increased effort has led to the development of new, rapid, high-throughput methods for specific parasite detection in various food sources for purposes of surveillance, management, and control. A wide range of methods, both direct and indirect, are available including the use of molecular diagnostic tools such as quantitative real-time polymerase chain reaction (PCR) and microarray assays that allow for multiplex monitoring of a greater number of foodborne pathogens. In many instances, however, conventional parasitological methods of diagnosis still prevail due to the lack of funding toward validation and standardization of "newer" tests, as well as the cost and impracticability of monitoring and enumerating all known pathogens in a food. Furthermore, cost, especially those associated with the purchase and maintenance of equipment and appropriate training of laboratory personnel in some regions, limits their adoption.

16.2 Current laboratory methods for meatborne parasites

Zoonotic, meatborne parasites are primarily transmitted to humans through deliberate or accidental ingestion of raw or undercooked meat that may be infected with a variety of parasites including nematodes (e.g., *Trichinella* spp.), cestodes (e.g., *Taenia saginata*, *T. solium*, *Spirometra* sp.), and protozoa (e.g., *Toxoplasma gondii*, *Sarcocystis* spp.). In the human food supply chain, postslaughter meat inspection forms the cornerstone of consumer protection from parasitic stages present in meat. Meat inspection can refer to incision and visual examination of meat or meat products for any visible parasitic life stages at the slaughterhouse, or laboratory examination of meat samples for microscopic parasites using histopathology. Historically, meat inspection for parasites is primarily directed at the prevention and control of *Taenia* spp., namely *T. saginata* (beef) and *T. solium* (pork), as well as *Trichinella* spp. (pork), although inspection may also be conducted for other parasites such as hydatids, ascarids, and in fish, *Anisakis* (see Section 16.3). Important protozoan parasites, particularly *T. gondii*, but also *Sarcocystis* spp., may also be transmitted to humans through meat, but control or diagnosis of these microscopic pathogens in the food chain is rarely practiced, if at all. Macroscopic *Sarcocystis* spp. cysts or metacestode larvae of *Spirometra* sp. may be incidentally controlled through visual inspection (Gracey and Collins, 1999).

Ongoing needs to improve the economic performance of meat supply chains have seen a trend toward meat inspection reform around the world (Webber et al., 2012). Among other drivers, the low sensitivity of meat inspection that can negatively impact food safety, as well as low specificity that reduces economic profitability, are key attributes that processors and food safety managers seek to improve. The development and enhancement of laboratory diagnostic methods that improve sensitivity and specificity, but also increasingly meet the important producer and processor requirements of fast turnaround times and increased throughput, are leading to greater involvement of laboratories in the prevention and control of meatborne parasites. For end-stage testing, nucleic acid detection (synonymous with molecular) and immunological methods are at the forefront of this laboratory contribution. Indirect immunological methods are also increasingly being relied on for antemortem herd or on-farm surveillance.

16.2.1 *Direct methods of detection for* Trichinella *in meat*

Globally, one of the most costly parasites to control in the meat supply chain is *Trichinella*. Meat certification in susceptible animal species, mainly pork but also horse and game meats, is a food safety standard in many developed parts of the world and high costs are associated with testing individual carcasses to reduce the risk of trichinellosis in humans (Pozio, 1998). Although numerous diagnostic methods have been used over the past 150 years, the need to harmonize methods to meet increasing international trade requirements has seen the pooled sample, magnetic-stirrer artificial digestion (AD) assay becomes the most internationally recognized technique for routine meat inspection (Gajadhar et al., 2009). Documented standards of the recommended method have been published by the OIE and ICT, as well as elsewhere, although a universally accepted digestion test protocol for trade and food safety purposes is not yet available (World Organisation for Animal Health, 2014c; European Commission, 2005).

The recommended AD method involves the enzymatic digestion of pooled muscle samples followed by selective screening, sedimentation (or filtration) procedures, and microscopic examination for free *Trichinella* muscle larvae. The method offers advantages of being simple to perform with little training and the ability to pool samples for higher throughput. The performance of the method is strongly influenced by sample size, selection of muscle predilection sites, as well as adequate validation (Nöckler et al., 2000; p. 420). For routine meat inspection, examination of 1 g of muscle from a predilection site using current methods can achieve a test sensitivity of approximately three larvae per gram whereas testing of a 5 g sample increases sensitivity to one larva per gram (Nöckler and Kapel, 2007; World Organisation for Animal Health, 2014c). The AD method is also commonly applied in wildlife for monitoring the environmental prevalence of *Trichinella* parasites.

16.2.2 *Direct methods of detection for cysticeri of* Taenia *spp. in meat*

Larval metacestodes of *Taenia* spp. in cattle and swine are the agents of bovine or porcine cysticercosis and the infective stages to humans when they consume undercooked meat containing viable cysts. Humans acquire the disease taeniosis when the larva develops into an adult tapeworm. Postslaughter, the main diagnostic procedure for cysticercosis is also meat inspection, which requires examination of all animal carcasses by incision and visual inspection for grossly visible cysts. Common predilection sites of cysts in bovines include the heart, skeletal muscle and diaphragm and in porcines, muscle, the central nervous system, and liver (World Organisation for Animal Health, 2014a). In light infestations, detections are dealt with by freeze certification to render infectious cysts nonviable or condemnation of affected parts. In systemic or heavy infestations, whole condemnation of the carcass is required. The accuracy and efficiency of meat inspection has been documented to be low, particularly in light infections in which cysts are easily overlooked on palpation and incision. In cattle, several studies have reported efficacies as low as 50–54% for the detection of cysts at meat inspection, with the heart the most commonly reported site of cyst predilection (Scandrett et al., 2012; Wanzala et al., 2003). The accuracy of meat inspection is also limited, as misdiagnoses of suspect cysts are common with morphologically similar etiologies that may not even be zoonotic (Berends et al., 1993; Abuseir et al., 2006).

Meat inspection for cysticercosis has increasingly been recognized as time-consuming, costly, and of limited value in countries with low prevalence (Calvo-Artavia et al., 2013; Webber et al., 2012). With current, global reforms toward more risk-based approaches in meat inspection, efforts to enhance laboratory diagnostic methods for suspect *Taenia* spp. cysticerci have been a focus of research in recent years. Traditional laboratory diagnosis for cysticerci has relied on histological examination of haematoxylin and eosin-stained sections for evidence of parasite structures or infections of cestode origin. This method has not been used extensively in food safety management systems because of a slow turnaround time for results; also the method lacks accuracy in degenerated cysts, which are the most commonly encountered types at meat inspection. Immunohistochemical (IHC) techniques that build on histological methods have promise as powerful diagnostic tools because they combine morphologic detail of histological sections with concurrent visualization of target antigens (Ogunremi et al., 2004; Scandrett et al., 2012). In an applicability study, a mouse monoclonal IgG1 antibody directed against excretory–secretory *T. saginata* cysticerci identified significantly more positive bovine cysticerci than the histological method (91.7% and 38.5%, respectively), although there was some evidence of cross-reactivity with metacestode larvae of *Taenia ovis* and *Echinococcus granulosus*, which are not of significance in bovine muscle (Scandrett et al., 2012).

16.2.3 Direct methods of detection for Toxoplasma gondii *in meat*

T. gondii is an intracellular, parasitic protozoan that causes toxoplasmosis and is often overlooked as an important meatborne parasite. Humans become infected with *T. gondii* through the consumption of soil, food, or water contaminated with infective oocysts shed by felines, but also through the consumption of raw or undercooked meat from intermediate hosts containing cysts with bradyzoites. *T. gondii* can infect all domestic food-producing and game animals. Small ruminants and pigs in particular are attributed as important sources of meatborne infection (Cook et al., 2000; Jones and Dubey, 2012), especially when they are free range or extensively raised. Detection of infected animals destined for human consumption is a challenge for toxoplasmosis control and, at present, there is no internationally standardized approach for its diagnosis. Animal bioassays involving inoculation of fresh *T. gondii*-infected tissue into mice or cats (preferred) remains the preferred method for parasite isolation, despite prolonged turnaround times of up to 23 days in cats and 6–8 weeks in mice (Dubey,

1995). Direct methods such as PCR, histological, or IHC detection of bradyzoites in tissue sections using commercially available anti-*Toxoplasma* antibodies has been restricted to clinical use for the diagnosis of toxoplasmosis in aborted fetuses or at postmortem (Jokelainen and Nylund, 2012; Kim et al., 2009). Limitations of molecular-based diagnosis of *T. gondii* in meat are discussed in Section 16.5.1.

16.2.4 Indirect methods of detecting parasites in meat

Indirect detection methods for meatborne parasites using serum diagnostics have not yet reached the point of individual diagnosis or large-scale detection of infected carcasses in routine meat inspection. These methods are desirable, however, because of the potential for automation, ready standardization, reduced costs of damage to carcasses, and ability to provide acceptable test sensitivity and specificity if properly validated. Methods using antibodies directed against antigenic products of *viable* cysts or current infections offer further benefits to the meat supply chain by potentially eliminating detections of nonviable or past infections that no longer constitute a food safety issue (Ferrer et al., 2003; Harrison et al., 1989). Despite several decades of investigation, meatborne parasite immunodiagnostics have been variable in their success. For *Taenia* spp. serological tests, numerous methods have been described using antiparasite antibodies raised against excretory–secretory antigens, metacestode antigens as well as against secreted antigens of *viable* metacestodes for detection (Ogunremi and Benjamin, 2010; Onyango-Abuje et al., 1996; Sciutto et al., 1998). For the detection of *T. solium* cysticerci in pigs, an enzyme-linked immunosorbent assay (ELISA) using purified glycoproteins from *T. solium* cyst fluid purified by isoelectric electrophoresis or using recombinant chimeric proteins allows detection of *T. solium* antibody responses in pigs harboring 16 or more cysts within 30 days of infection (Sato et al., 2003). The major advantage of this assay is the lack of observed cross-reactions with pigs infected with *Taenia hydatigena*, however, the assay has yet to be validated for potential cross-reactivity with *Taenia asiatica*, present in pigs in some parts of Southeast Asia. For *T. saginata*, an antibody ELISA using excretory–secretory antigens of *T. saginata* metacestodes demonstrated a test sensitivity of 92.9% for cattle inoculated with 1000 or fewer eggs (Ogunremi and Benjamin, 2010) and shows promise for future field application. Further proteomic approaches aimed at discovery of highly species-specific antigens for measuring exposure to *Taenia* spp. metacestodes will help pave the way for the development of commercial assays for meat inspection purposes.

In *Trichinella* control, serological techniques have been most commonly used to monitor animals or systems for immunological evidence of transmission of parasites and are applied on serum or muscle fluids collected pre- or postslaughter (Nöckler and Kapel, 2007; Gamble et al., 2004). False negatives can occur in animals in the early stages of infection as most of the identified *Trichinella*-specific antigens originate from L1 muscle larvae, and there may be a lag between the time of infection and production of detectable antibodies. As such, serological methods are currently unsuitable for routine meat inspection although they have important applications for surveillance of transmission of *Trichinella* parasites on-farm as well as epidemiological investigations in wild porcine populations (Gajadhar et al., 2009). Research into alternative antigens, such as those from adult worms or newborn larvae has the potential to improve the detection of *Trichinella* parasite infection as early as 15 days postinfection (Liu et al., 2013). The ELISA is the most commonly used method for system or herd monitoring and can offer substantial increases in test sensitivity compared to AD methods. Larval burdens as low as 0.01 larva per gram in domestic pigs have been reported as detectable (Gamble et al., 1983) by ELISA. Commercially produced kits for monitoring purposes include PrioCHECK *Trichinella* Ab (Prionics).

In Europe, a risk-based approach for the control of *T. gondii* in naturally infected food animals is currently under proposal based on serological testing of blood and muscle fluids at the preharvest or abattoir level, respectively (European Food Safety Authority, 2013). Several serological tests are available for the detection of *T. gondii* antibodies in food animals, including the immunofluorescent antibody test, modified agglutination test (MAT), indirect haemaggluination test, and the ELISA (World Organisation for Animal Health, 2014d). The MAT is not host-specific and is considered superior in terms of sensitivity and specificity compared to the "gold standard" method of bioassays in mice and cats (Dubey and Desmonts, 1987; Dubey et al., 1995). A growing number of commercial kits for the detection of *T. gondii* antibodies are now available and show promise toward the standardization of *T. gondii* serodiagnostics in food-producing animals. In general, ELISA-based kits compare favorably with MAT and IFA for the detection of *T. gondii* antibodies in experimentally and naturally infected pig (Steinparzer et al., 2014; Glor et al., 2013) and sheep sera (Mainar-Jaime and Barberan, 2007). Moreover, incorporation of a protein A/G–peroxidase conjugate into the assay may allowed added advantage for *T. gondii*-specific IgG antibody detection from multiple-host species (Al-Adhami and Gajadhar, 2014). However, unlike the MAT, the ELISA's ability to detect *T. gondii* antibodies in meat juice, considered a logistically favorable matrix for abattoir-based surveillance systems, varies considerably depending on the muscle used (Villena et al., 2012), the burden of infection (Forbes et al., 2012), and the selected test kit (Glor et al., 2013; Basso et al., 2013). The length of time needed to perform the MAT, as well as the subjective nature of test result interpretations, however, may render the MAT impractical for widespread application at slaughter or for epidemiological surveys performed at different labs. The commercial serum ELISA thus appears to be a more useful test for the routine screening of animals on the farm or at slaughter facilities (Hill et al., 2006) but will require further validation for meat juice matrix in pigs and sheep infected with low burdens of *T. gondii*. Low antibody titers to *T. gondii* (<64) using any immunodiagnostic test must be interpreted with caution due to the potential for cross-reactivity with other tissue coccidia such as *Hammondia hammondi* (Munday and Dubey, 1986; Riahi et al., 1998).

16.3 Current laboratory methods for the detection of parasites in fish and crustaceans

Meat of reptiles, amphibians, and fish can also be infected with trematodes such as *Opisthorchis* spp., *Clonorchis sinensis*, intestinal flukes, *Paragonimus* spp., cestodes (*Diphyllobothrium* spp., *Spirometra*), and nematodes (nonencapsulated *Trichinella* spp., *Gnathostoma* spp., anisakine parasites). For detailed information on the foodborne trematodes see Chapter 10.

Several methods for the detection of anisakine larvae and *Diphyllobothrium* pleurocercoid stages in fresh fish have been described. According to Codex Standard 165-1989, certification requires that the entire fish filet be examined nondestructively by placing appropriate portions of the thawed skinless sample unit on a 5-mm-thick acrylic sheet with 45% translucency and candled with a light source giving 1500 lux 30 cm above the sheet. Any visible parasites found by spot testing during the industrial processing of fish intended for human consumption must be removed. The detection efficacy for candling, however, is regarded as highly variable and dependant on the thickness and size of the filet, the texture and color of the flesh, the species of fish, larval size, and site of predilection (Levsen et al., 2005). Detection efficacy of candling ranges from 7% to 10% in herring, mackerel, and blue whiting to 43–76% for white-fleshed fish such as rockfish, flounder, and Pacific cod (Adams et al., 1997). Glass plate compression techniques, in which filets are pressed by hand between two large glass plates (18 cm × 10 cm × 0.8 cm) and observed under a stereomicroscope have also been used for the detection of *Diphyllobothrium* pleurocercoids in fish, albeit at a lower sensitivity than candling (Torres and Puga, 2011). The attempt has been made to replace the expensive manual labor associated with candling with methods such as ultrasound, computer tomography, and spectroscopy (Stormo et al., 2007). Although these techniques have equivocal or better detection rates than the candling technique, they have been impractical and are difficult to implement in the industry, especially when manual inspection by candling is conducted on average at one filet per second. Due to the poor detection efficacy of fishborne helminth infections, adequate deep-freezing of any fresh fish product, especially if it is intended for consumption in a raw or semiraw state, is therefore recommended. For salted herring and sprat, Codex Standard 244-2004 stipulates that 200 g of the sample unit must be digested in an aqueous acidic solution of pepsin and any recovered larvae examined for viability. Pepsin digestion followed by microscopic identification of metacercarial morphology have been widely used to distinguish among species of Opisthorchid and Heterophyid trematodes in fish and *Paragonimus* spp. in crustaceans (Wiriya et al., 2013; Devi et al., 2010). However, the procedure is currently limited by its time-consuming nature and the need for highly skilled personnel. Moreover, the presence of multiple species of trematode metacercariae, including those of no zoonotic interest, makes this procedure notoriously difficult and unfeasible for routine postharvest inspection of fishborne trematodes.

16.4 Current laboratory detection methods for parasite in fresh produce, herbs, and berries

16.4.1 Indirect indicators of fecal parasites

Some of the hygienic principles to avoid bacterial contamination of food will also reduce the likelihood of parasite infestations that are transmitted by the fecal–oral route. Therefore, the common risk-management options somewhat justify the use of indirect detection and enumeration of fecal–oral transmitted indicator pathogens in foods, particularly fresh produce. The method of assessing the risk of parasite contamination by using an indirect measure of ubiquitous fecal contamination is widely applied but has significant limitations. For example, composted manure and water used to fertilize and wash fresh vegetables and berries may be enumerated for total coliforms, thermotolerant coliforms, *Escherichia coli*, and enterococci, *Clostridium perfringens*, *Bacteroides* spp., and coliphages as indirect gauges of the presence of parasites. The effectiveness of these bacterial indicators for parasitic contamination, however, has delivered poor results owing primarily to the superior environmental stability of helminth ova and protozoan cysts and oocysts and their relative resistance to temperature- and chemical-based disinfection (Paul et al., 1997).

Nevertheless, significantly positive correlations between the abundance of *Giardia* and *Cryptosporidium* and thermotolerant coliforms, *C. perfringens*, enterococci, and *E. coli* demonstrated by some studies (Cheng et al., 2012; Wu et al., 2011; Julio et al., 2012), support the need to carry out specific procedures for the detection of *Giardia* and *Cryptosporidium* whenever the values of fecal indicators approach the maximum allowed level. These factors, combined with the low infectious dose of parasites, translate to the presence of bacterial indicator organisms as significant for parasites, but the absence of bacterial indicator organisms as not necessarily so.

16.4.2 Direct detection of fecal parasites in fresh produce, herbs, and berries

For the detection and enumeration of *Giardia* and *Cryptosporidium* from water used to irrigate or wash fresh produce, the methods of choice include the US Environmental Protection Agency method 1623 and the Standard Operating Protocol 1999, SI No. 1524 (Genera Filta-Max, Dynal IMS, and Cellab FITC) in the United Kingdom. Both methods rely on immunofluorescence assays for the detection of cysts and oocysts and confirmation through vital dye staining [4V6-diamidino-phenylindole (DAPI)] and differential interference contrast microscopy.

Detection procedures for helminth ova and protozoan oocysts of *Toxoplasma*, *Cyclospora*, and *Cryptosporidium* and cysts of *Giardia* from fresh fruits and vegetables present yet another challenge. Detection of these parasites relies on effectively removing and then concentrating potentially minute quantities of parasite ova, oocysts, or cysts since as little as 10–30 *Giardia duodenalis*, *Cryptosporidium parvum*, and *Cryptosporidium hominis* organisms per average meal portion may result in illness (Rendtorff and Holt, 1954; DuPont et al., 1995; Chappell et al., 2006). Successful preliminary interlaboratory collaborative trials (Cook et al., 2006a,b) have strongly advocated for the development of a standard for the detection and enumeration of *Cryptosporidium* and *Giardia* in fresh leafy green vegetables and berry fruits (ISO/DIS 18744), which is currently in its final stages of development (http://www.iso.org).

The sensitivity of parasite ova, cysts, and oocysts detection is highly dependent on the first step of parasite detachment by washing, which, in turn, can be influenced by food matrix, the extraction solution and method, and duration of agitation (stomacher, rolling, pulsifying, and shaking) (Cook et al., 2006a). For example, using identical wash techniques, recovery rates of *Ascaris* ranged from 41% in bean sprouts to 76% in strawberries. Increasing the duration of a single wash step from 1 to 5 min, in turn, significantly decreased the recovery rate of *Ascaris* on strawberries to 6% (Robertson and Gjerde, 2000). Recovery rates are also highly dependent on extraction media used with 1 M glycine, pH 5.5, and 0.1% Alconox® (Shields et al., 2012), demonstrating superior recovery performances for oocysts of *Cryptosporidium* and *Cyclospora*. Concentration of the parasite stages by centrifugation and then a further "clarification" step then allows for a superior capture efficiency of organisms from other food debris, results in cleaner slide preparations for microscopic examination, and reduces the number of false positives. For *Giardia* and *Cryptosporidium*, commercial immunomagnetic separation kits (e.g., Crypto-Scan® IMS, Dynabeads® GC-Combo, Idexx) are available, but for other parasite ova, cysts, and oocysts, isolation may be achieved using flotation gradients for further clarity. One-color and two-color fluorescence-activated cell-sorting assays (employing competing surface monoclonal antibodies) have also been used to improve purification of *Cryptosporidium* oocysts prior to further processing (Ferrari et al., 2000). A proof of concept study using transparent double-sided adhesive tape has also shown potential as an alternative method for parasite detection on smooth-skinned fruits and vegetables, detecting as few as 10 *C. parvum* oocysts per 5 mm diameter area by both PCR and immunofluorescence microscopy (Fayer et al., 2013). Staining of cyst and oocysts with fluorescein isothiocyanate (FITC)-labeled monoclonal antibodies (e.g., MeriFluor®, Meridian Diagnostics, Cellab FITC, Aqua-Glo™ Waterborne Inc. EasyStain™BTF Pty. Limited) prior to microscopic confirmation also aids parasite detection. These techniques are not available for *Cyclospora*, however, microscopic detection may be enhanced by the use of an ultraviolet filter as oocysts are autofluorescent (Berlin et al., 1998) if parasitological expertise is capable of differentiating oocysts of *Cyclospora* from other autofluorescent coccidia. The major limitations of manual microscopic enumeration techniques include low sample throughput, operator subjectivity, and operator fatigue. Laser scanning cytometry (ChemScanRDI) for the enumeration of *Giardia* and *Cryptosporidium* has been used to partially overcome these drawbacks (de Roubin et al., 2002).

Inherent problems with both microscopy and DNA-based detection assays are their inability to differentiate between viable and nonviable parasites. Traditionally, animal infectivity assays, *in vitro* cell culture (Rochelle et al., 1997), *in vitro* sporulation (Sturbaum et al., 1998), and excystation assays (Campbell et al., 1992; Finch et al., 1993) were used to determine viability of parasite ova, cysts, and oocysts. Although these methods remain the best available to date, they are significantly limited by time and expense. Moreover, *in vitro* excystation assays, although more rapid than the cell culture often result in an overestimation of the total number of viable oocysts in water samples (Black et al., 1996; Bukhari et al., 2000). Fluorogenic vital dyes, 4′,6-diamidino-2-phenylindole (DAPI) as DAPI inclusion and propidium iodide (PI) exclusion, SYTO-9, and other nucleic acid stains may be used as reasonable indicators for determining the viability and infectivity of *Cryptosporidium* (Campbell et al., 1992; Jenkins et al., 1997) and *Giardia* (Thiriat et al., 1998), although they too appear to overestimate the number of viable cysts. As an alternative, fluorescent-labeled oligonucleotide probes targeted to specific sequences of cell ribosomal RNA (rRNA) in metabolically active cells (fluorescence *in situ* hybridization, FISH) are now routinely used. FISH was first applied to detect *Cryptosporidium* oocysts in water samples that used a probe specific to a sequence of rRNA present in all Eukarya (Vesey et al., 1998; Deere et al., 1998). More recently, a two-color microscopy-based FISH assay for the simultaneous detection of *C. parvum* and *C. hominis*, the two major species detected in humans, was developed and proved highly specific (Alagappan et al., 2009).

16.5 Molecular-based laboratory detection techniques: Future options

16.5.1 Molecular-based methods for the direct detection of parasites in meat

Although many molecular methods for parasite species identification of isolated stages have been developed in recent decades, efforts to obviate manual inspection have also focused on parasite DNA detection directly from meat samples. These *in situ* methods, including real-time PCR and loop-mediated isothermal amplification technology (LAMP), offer advantages of increased sensitivity as well as streamlined detection and species identification processes compared to more conventional techniques dependent on direct visualization of parasites.

Real-time PCR products can be monitored in real time through the use of fluorescent dyes. The superior specificity achieved through incorporation of sequence-specific fluorescent hybridization probes or post-PCR high-resolution melt curve analysis using nonspecific double-stranded DNA-intercalating dyes overcomes the requirement for post-PCR validation of products using DNA-sequencing or restriction-profiling techniques. High-throughput automated, robotic platforms may be used for both DNA extraction and for the PCR assay set-up steps and offers further advantages including lower labor costs, higher consistency, reduced probability for manual errors, and a quick turnaround of results. Real-time PCR assays also have the advantage of displaying significantly superior sensitivities to standard PCRs, which negates the requirement for further post-PCR amplification steps. Another alternative to conventional PCR is LAMP, which amplifies DNA with high sensitivity relying on an enzyme with strand displacement activity under isothermal conditions. The technology uses four to six specially designed primers recognizing six to eight regions of the target DNA sequence, hence a high specificity. The auto-cycling reactions lead to the accumulation of a large amount of the target DNA and other reaction by-products, such as magnesium pyrophosphate, that allow rapid detection using varied formats (reviewed by Njiru, 2012). LAMP has additional advantages to real-time PCR, as the isothermal reaction can be conducted in the field without specialized laboratory equipment, hence a potentially greatly reduced turnaround time for results.

For parasite species where labor-intensive detection methods are currently the best methods used, molecular methods have been investigated as a possible solution. Such has been the case with real-time PCR to replace AD in meat inspection for *Trichinella* parasites. Several real-time PCR methods have been developed experimentally for *Trichinella* muscle larvae detection and to allow qualitative detection and/or quantitative measurements of infection intensity in porcine or wildlife muscle samples (Guenther et al., 2008; Tantrawatpan et al., 2012; Cuttell et al., 2012). These assays have focused on genus-specific amplification or differentiation of regional *Trichinella* species (e.g., European or Southeast Asian species) for purposes of both meat inspection and wildlife surveillance. Assays have shown high specificity and, although establishing the actual diagnostic sensitivity attained, are difficult due to variations in experimental design and the common analysis of serial dilutions of extracted *Trichinella* DNA (which is not an accurate depiction of diagnostic sensitivity), test sensitivities appear in the range of 0.5–1.0 larva per gram (Atterby et al., 2009; Guenther et al., 2008). Validation data in these assays are still limited and in their current format, they do not offer the high-throughput capability or cost efficiency of AD methods. Development of pooled-sample testing, as well as more rapid and cost-effective methods for sample homogenization and digestion, still needs to be developed.

Molecular methods could also be usefully applied to unambiguously classify suspect *Taenia* spp. metacestodes isolated at meat inspection. Although many PCR assays have previously been described for the differentiation of adult taeniids in humans, methods using conventional nested PCR, PCR–RFLP, multiplex PCR, and real-time PCR have also recently been developed experimentally for meat inspection purposes (Chiesa et al., 2010; Geysen et al., 2007; Abuseir et al., 2006; Cuttell et al., 2013; Gonzalez et al., 2006). Generally, PCR methods have demonstrated better or equal sensitivity and specificity compared to abattoir and histological diagnosis, although PCR sensitivity has decreased with increasing degrees of cyst degeneration. Selection of target loci has been variable, but methods targeting HDP1/HDP2, although sensitive, have shown some difficulty in interpretation (Abuseir et al., 2006; Gonzalez et al., 2006). The mitochondrial cytochrome *c* oxidase subunit 1 (mtCOI) loci have performed well in *T. saginata*-specific assays, offering ease of interpretation and sensitivity (Cuttell et al., 2013; Chiesa et al., 2010). Multiplex assays that allow species-specific identification of *Taeniid* spp. cysticerci, as well as differentiation from other commonly misdiagnosed etiologies (e.g., *Sarcocystis* spp.), provide the greatest information, but by requiring multiple PCR rounds or reactions, they have not yet reached rapid, streamlined laboratory workflows (Gonzalez et al., 2006). Assays that use internal control targets for examining bovine or porcine DNA targets, and closed systems such as real-time PCR, offer additional quality assurance for experimental procedures and results (Cuttell et al., 2013). Major incentives to pursue molecular methodologies include improved public health outcomes and significant economic benefits to be gained by rapid differentiation of zoonotic *Taenia* spp. from nonzoonotic parasites, allowing retained carcasses/parts back into the food supply chain.

Several conventional and real-time PCR-based assays based on the high copy number genes, such as the B1 and 529 bp repetitive regions (Burg et al., 1989; Homan et al., 2000) and 18S rRNA gene (Jauregui et al., 2001), have been valuable as a screening tool for tissue and fluid from clinical cases of toxoplasmosis (Gutierrez et al., 2012; Scheepers et al., 2013). In contrast, the use of PCR assays has been limited for meat-inspection purposes owing to poor sensitivity compared to serological methods and animal bioassays (Garcia et al., 2006; Hill et al., 2006; da Silva and Langoni, 2001). Low sensitivity is generally attributed to the low burdens of randomly distributed tissue cysts in naturally infected animals (less than one cyst per 50 g in pigs), coupled with the small size of tissue sampled. These factors limit the parasite's detection both histologically (Dubey, 1988) and by PCR. Increasing the quantity of sample subjected to DNA extraction via the use of magnetic capture methods (Opsteegh et al., 2010) or use of pelleted filtrates of whole organ digests (Boughattas et al., 2014) obviates these limitations, to the detriment of time and costs of assay performance.

Although molecular methods have the potential for enhancing sensitivity and aiding multiple-pathogen detection and trace-back investigations in routine meat inspection, disadvantages of high costs and low sample throughput need to be circumvented before they can be considered suitable for this purpose.

16.5.2 Molecular- and immunological-based methods for the direct detection of parasites in fish and crustaceans

Several PCR-based molecular techniques have been developed to detect and differentiate between species of isolated *Anisakis* nematodes to assess zoonotic risk. Genetic analysis of *Anisakis simplex* complex, the principal causative agent of anisakiasis, comprising *Anisakis pegreffii*, *A. simplex* sensu stricto, and *A. simplex* C can be accomplished by analyses of the ribosomal ITS data, the mitochondrial cytochrome *c* oxidase 2 gene as well as allozyme electrophoretic data (Mattiucci et al., 2011; Arizono et al., 2012). The detection of the zoonotic species of anisakids in fresh and processed fish products has been successful at detecting as little as 1–40 pmol anisakid DNA in 25–30 g fish using real-time PCR (Fang et al., 2011; Lopez and Pardo, 2010) and shows promise in replacing AD techniques. ELISAs for the detection of crude proteins (Werner et al., 2011), or more specifically the primary heat-stable allergen Ani s 4 of *A. simplex* (Rodríguez-Mahillo et al., 2010) in fish muscle have also been developed as alternatives to conventional testing. These immunodiagnostic assays have reported detection rates of as little as one larva in 100 g of fish meat (Werner et al., 2011) and a recovery rate of 82.5% for *A. simplex* allergens (Rodríguez-Mahillo et al., 2010).

A number of molecular-based detection methods targeting ribosomal, mitochondrial, microsatellite, repetitive elements, and mobile elements within the genome of liver, lung, and intestinal flukes have been developed for their specific detection from clinical samples and host tissue (Petney et al., 2013; Tantrawatpan et al., 2013). Real-time PCRs have been developed for the detection of *O. viverrine* metacercarial DNA in fish and are capable of detecting as little as one metacercaria inoculated in a pool of 30 noninfected caudal fins of 100 mg each (Intapan et al., 2008). Similarly, a LAMP approach for the detection of *C. sinensis* metacercariae in fish based on the cathepsins B3 gene boasts of having a 100-fold increase in sensitivity compared to conventional PCR; however, validation was performed only on samples with intensities of three metacercariae per gram of fish (Cai et al., 2010). Further validation and standardization of these molecular-based techniques show promise for the routine detection of metacercaria of fish and crustacean foodborne trematode infections.

16.5.3 Molecular-based methods for the direct detection of parasites in fresh produce, herbs, and berries

DNA-based real-time quantitative PCRs capable of enumerating foodborne parasites with a high degree of sensitivity and specificity have been developed for most parasites capable of contaminating various fresh produce and herbs. These include the protozoa *Cyclospora* (Lalonde and Gajadhar, 2011; Shields et al., 2013) and *T. gondii* (Yu et al., 2013), but also other potentially neglected parasites that may be sourced from fresh produce, such as *Echinococcus multilocularis* (Knapp et al., 2014).

Premixed automated LAMP-based assays also show promise for the highly sensitive detection of *Toxoplasma* oocysts in water samples boasting a higher sensitivity for the detection of oocysts compared with nested PCR and immunofluorescence microscopy (Gallas-Lindemann et al., 2013). Similar LAMP assays have been developed for the detection of *Cryptosporidium* and *Giardia* (Plutzer and Karanis, 2009; Bakheit et al., 2008).

DNA oligonucleotide microarray assays have also emerged as a promising alternative for high-throughput monitoring of multiple pathogens in parallel. Broad-range PCR is initially used that targets conserved regions within the rRNA genes prior to microarray analysis, which quantifies hybridization events between target DNA with specific fluorescently labeled probes that are bound on the array (Sibley et al., 2012). Microarray assays targeting multiple species of bacterial pathogens (Lee et al., 2008) and six protozoal pathogens including *Acanthamoeba castellanii*, *C. parvum*, and *G. duodenalis* (Lee et al., 2010) have been developed for monitoring pathogens in wastewater. Several commercial microarray platforms are available that can be analyzed using bioinformatics software on an automated system. These commercial suppliers now offer researchers and industry support in designing and validating a broad range of custom-genotyping array options.

These assays, which have yet to be trialed and validated from a food matrix, allow for multiplex high-throughput detection and in the case of qPCR, enumeration of parasite ova, cysts, and oocysts from concentrated washings. Moreover, they potentially allow differentiation of anthroponotic and zoonotic pathogens, which aid risk assessment and trace-back investigations.

16.5.4 Molecular-based detection of parasite viability in food matrices

Reverse transcriptase real-time quantitative PCR (qRT-PCR) has aimed to replace vital dye staining as a measure of cyst and oocyst viability by detecting and quantifying changes in gene expression by measuring the level of heat-induced hsp70 mRNA, as well as other molecular viability indicators such as beta tubulin mRNA and 18S rRNA, in *Cryptosporidium* (Liang and Keeley, 2012) and *Giardia* (Baque et al., 2011). The labile nature of quantifying rRNA and especially mRNA, however, makes working with it more challenging. Degradation can occur by inadequate sample processing and storage or as a result of sample contamination with RNA-degrading enzymes (Fittipaldi et al., 2012). Ethidium monoazide and propidium monoazide treatments coupled with traditional or real-time PCR or LAMP have been extensively used in bacteriology for the differentiation of viable and nonviable cells and, more recently, protozoa (Brescia et al., 2009). These photoactive vital dyes can only penetrate into membrane-compromised or dead cells, intercalate into DNA, and form a stable covalently bounded dye–DNA complex due to exposure to bright white light, thus rendering the DNA inaccessible for PCR amplification (Nocker et al., 2007). A good correlation between what is now called *viability PCR* and RT-qPCR for viability detection of fresh *Cryptosporidium* oocysts was reported following disinfection of oocysts in water samples (Liang and Keeley, 2012). Viability PCR is a promising technique because it makes use of the speed and sensitivity of the molecular detection while at the same time providing information on potential infectivity. Nevertheless, a number of factors and variables, such as choice of the dye, its concentration, the incubation conditions, the light source, the presence of a high number of dead cells, suspended solids, the length of the target gene, and the sequence of the target gene, can influence the outcome of the results (Fittipaldi et al., 2012). Moreover, based on the low rates of recovery of most parasite concentration methods coupled with their low infectious dose, it seems unlikely that regulatory agencies would declare a sample as safe or low risk, even if these methods classify the ova, cyst, or oocyst as nonviable.

16.6 Ensuring quality assurance in laboratory diagnostic testing

Valid laboratory results, in terms of accuracy and reproducibility, are essential for the diagnosis and control of foodborne pathogens in the food supply chain and to support the efficacy and competency of a food safety management system. Attaining valid laboratory results is critically dependent on a number of factors, starting with the appropriate collection, storage, and transport of samples, appropriateness and validity of the diagnostic method used, as well as the use of a laboratory-quality management system including documentation, standard operating procedures, and quality assurance (Farrell-Evans and Warren, 2014). The International Organization for Standardization (ISO) has developed international laboratory standards (ISO/IEC 17025-2005) that also incorporates standards for quality assurance (QA) management systems. Several veterinary diagnostic authorities have produced guidelines for ensuring suitable and standardized laboratory diagnostic testing and these concepts are also well summarized well in the World Organisation for Animal Health (OIE)'s *Manual of Diagnostic Tests and Vaccines for Terrestrial Animals 2014* (http://www.oie.int/international-standard-setting/terrestrial-manual/access-online/). The US Centers for Disease Control and Prevention offer an excellent online resource for laboratory diagnosis of parasitic diseases of public health concern (http://www.cdc.gov/dpdx/diagnosticProcedures/index.html).

16.6.1 Sample collection and processing

The starting point for any laboratory investigation is the collection of relevant samples for the purpose of the investigation, and the suitable selection of the diagnostic test to be performed. In a food inspection system, different samples may be required for different purposes including monitoring system compliance for a food safety management program, health certification at end-stage inspection, or diagnosis of human and animal infections. For example, management systems for the prevention and control of *Trichinella* spp. in pig production systems can include collection of herd-level blood/sera samples for monitoring purposes, whereas meat inspection of individual carcasses for public health certification requires samples of skeletal muscle for the direct isolation of infectious *Trichinella* larvae. When samples are collected for a particular testing purpose, they should be provided in sufficient quantity, both in amount and number, for the method to be carried out, as well as to produce statistically valid results (World Organisation for Animal Health, 2014b). Sample quality is critical in many diagnostic assays, and precautions should be taken in correct collection and storage conditions during transport to the laboratory. All samples should be carefully packed, labeled, and transported to the laboratory according to specific requirements for packing and shipping of infectious substances and/or biological samples.

For human or animal diagnosis of enteric parasite infections, fresh or fixed stool specimens are the most common sample type examined for the presence of oocysts or other life stages (Ash and Orihel, 1991). Fresh samples should be transported directly to the laboratory as soon as possible and examined, processed, or fixed immediately. If samples are to be fixed, consideration to the choice of preservative should be given with respect to the diagnostic method, or the specimens split and fixed in multiple preservatives. In most cases, specimens preserved in 10% buffered formalin can be successfully examined by direct wet mount (helminths and protozoa), immunoassays (*Giardia* and *Cryptosporidium*) (Flanagan, 1992; Rosoff et al., 1989), and chromatrope stain, or undergo concentration or fecal flotation procedures prior to examination. Poly vinyl alcohol (PVA) is useful for permanent staining with trichrome but is not conducive to many other applications (Agrawal et al., 2006). Neither formalin nor PVA are optimal for preserving samples to be used in molecular assays. Samples for downstream molecular applications should be processed by freezing or fixing in 2.5% potassium dichromate (Centers for Disease Control and Prevention, 2013).

Serum/plasma from clotted blood samples or tissue fluids are collected for immunodiagnostic methods for foodborne parasites including enzyme immunoassays and immunoblots. Cerebral spinal fluid for use in immunoblot can also be collected for suspect human neurocysticercosis cases (Del Brutto, 2012). For transport to the laboratory, serum should be removed from the blood clot following centrifugation and shipped within 1–2 days at room temperature. For longer transport periods, serum samples can be protected from bacterial overgrowth by the addition of 0.1% sodium azide or another antimicrobial. Samples with long-term storage requirements can be stored by deep freezing (less than −60 °C) or freeze-drying (World Organisation for Animal Health, 2014b).

Tissue samples are examined for life stages such as larvae or cysts of meatborne parasites and are usually collected postmortem. To allow for an appropriate level of sensitivity for the purpose of the testing, samples should be taken from predilection sites and in sufficient quantity. For examination of tissues or excised cysts/lesions (e.g., *Taenia* metacestodes) by histopathology, specimens fixed in 10% buffered formalin for sectioning and staining are most commonly used in investigations and follow-up testing (McFadden et al., 2011). For *Trichinella* larvae digestion assays, fresh muscle samples from the diaphragm are preferred, although frozen tissue can also be tested with some loss of sensitivity (International Commission for Trichinellosis, 2012). Molecular assays for parasitic stages in tissue perform best with fresh or frozen samples.

The sample types described thus far relate to clinical samples for diagnosis of parasitic infections or health certification; however, an important tool in the prevention of parasite occurrence in the food supply chain relates to hygiene monitoring of the food safety inspection system or end-stage testing of finished product. Hygiene monitoring is conducted by testing environmental samples taken throughout the food supply chain. Both environmental sampling and end-stage product testing are particularly important for helminth ova or protozoan oocysts that are common contaminants of fresh produce via fecally contaminated water, food handlers, or manure used as fertilizer (Quintero-Betancourt et al., 2002). Samples for the detection of parasites include washes or rinses from fresh produce or samples of produce (Shields et al., 2013). For monitoring hygiene and processing steps, samples are taken at critical control points, for example, at water sources, filtration, or finished product. Because of the typically low concentration of helminth ova or protozoan oocysts in water or the environment, laboratory processing of samples usually includes filtration, concentration, and sedimentation steps to improve assay sensitivity. Submission of bulk water samples, food washes, or produce should be transported to the laboratory on ice rapidly (as soon as possible) to ensure best results. For fresh produce such as leafy greens or berries, chilled transportation is preferred as freezing or overheating can deteriorate the sample and affect test sensitivity.

16.6.2 Test method selection and validation

The abundance of diagnostic methods available in laboratories today, both traditional and those developed with advancing technology, means managers have a broad range of tests to choose from when implementing food safety inspection systems. When selecting a diagnostic method, the test should be ensured it is "fit for purpose," meaning that the test has performance capabilities consistent with the application's requirements (World Organisation for Animal Health, 2014b). Additionally, the type and number of samples required for the selected method should be realistically and economically obtainable. For example, the application of PCR to routine water testing for enteric protozoa offers several major advantages, but disadvantages have slowed the uptake of this method for bulk or routine analysis (Quintero-Betancourt et al., 2002). On the one hand, PCR techniques have offered benefits of genotyping to delineate the complex relationships and assemblages of isolates that can aid in trace-back investigations. However, PCR can amplify nonviable as well as viable oocysts so that results may overestimate the level of risk to food safety. Common PCR inhibitors such as humic acid and inefficient lysis of oocysts or cysts can also lead to nondetectable levels of DNA (Gillbride, 2014; Quintero-Betancourt et al., 2002).

Once a "fit for purpose" test has been selected, regulators or food safety managers must ensure the test has been adequately validated. Test validation refers to establishing and evaluating test performance characteristics that provide information about the appropriateness of the method under various testing and sample conditions. These characteristics can include determining the optimal sample for testing, size for sampling, sensitivity, specificity, range, accuracy, capacity, as well as other test limitations. Important considerations also include the availability of reference tests with which to compare the method being validated. Using a properly validated test is essential for producing accurate and reliable test results on which food safety inspection systems rely. In recent decades, international efforts to improve the methodological quality and standard of reporting of diagnostic test evaluations have led to the development of protocols and guidelines that can be followed or "checked" off when assessing the validity of a diagnostic method. Although primarily developed for clinical research, the Standards for the Reporting of Diagnostic Accuracy (STARD) statement was an important precursor to other guidelines and allows users of a diagnostic method to assess the internal validity and applicability of the test (Bossuyt et al., 2003). Recently, the OIE has produced guidelines for the principles and methods of validation of diagnostic assays for infectious diseases in its Terrestrial Manual. An extensive list of standard, guidelines, and validation methods specific to food safety has also been prepared and published by the Codex Alimentarius.

16.6.3 Laboratory QA management systems

Laboratory QA management systems are important for maintaining food safety as their integration in food safety management systems confirm the laboratory's capability for producing valid test results, minimization of errors, and evidence of technical competence and associated data (Gajadhar and Forbes, 2002; Bellamy, 2004; Farrell-Evans and Warren, 2014). In recent decades, concern regarding the lack of validity and accuracy of methods and results in laboratory testing precipitated the development of guidelines to standardize the competence of diagnostic laboratories. A number of internationally recognized guidelines have been developed by the ISO for quality assurance and testing purposes including ISO/IEC 17025:2005 General requirements for the competence of testing and calibration laboratories, "a standard that covers testing and calibration performed using standard methods, nonstandard methods, and laboratory-developed methods." Adherence to this standard will also assure that the laboratory is operating within the ISO standard for QA systems (ISO 9001-2008). The OIE *Manual of Diagnostic Tests and Vaccines*, Part 1, Chapter 1 also describes accepted methods and minimum requirements for the implementation and use of QA systems. Adherence to these guidelines can enable an effective and reliable food inspection system and possible international accreditation with authorized accrediting bodies such as the Australian National Association of Testing Authorities (NATA), the Standards Council of Canada (SCC), or the American Association for Laboratory Accreditation (A2LA). The essential components of a reliable QA system include appropriate test methods, method validation, confirmation of laboratory capability, documentation, reporting, and monitoring of the test system (Gajadhar and Forbes, 2002; Bellamy, 2004). Continual monitoring of the test system is an important requirement to measure the ongoing accuracy of test results and sustainability of the QA system as it provides indicators of the laboratory's performance as well as quality of the results. Examples of monitoring include internal and external audits, proficiency testing using known positive and negative samples, and monitoring of the critical control points and critical equipment (i.e., calibration data).

16.7 Conclusion

As global food trade expands, harmonization of international food safety standards to assure consumer protection is becoming increasingly imperative. Breaches in regulations can lead to negative impacts on consumer and economic health. To date, testing for parasites in food has been largely restricted to conventional postslaughter inspection methods for meat and fish, which remain limited by cost, are labor intensive, and lack sensitivity. Freeze certification to render the parasite noninfectious remains the ultimate protector in cases where risk is perceived to be high, albeit at cost to industry and the consumer. A risk-based approach to testing is being suggested as a method of making end-stage meat inspection testing more efficient. This approach has been recently implemented as an international trade requirement for some foodborne parasites. The growing recognition of fresh produce as an important source of protozoan pathogens has, for the first time, led to the development of an international standard for their detection, due for release in early 2015. A plethora of immunodiagnostic- and molecular-based parasite detection methods are being trialed or employed for the purpose of providing alternative or more efficient testing of parasites in foods. These methods show potential for automated high-throughput testing of multiple pathogens in food, and a move toward their standardization should now be priority.

References

Abuseir, S., Epe, C., Schnieder, T., Klein, G., Kuhne, M., 2006. Visual diagnosis of *Taenia saginata* cysticercosis during meat inspection: is it unequivocal? Parasitol. Res. 99, 405–409.

Adams, A.M., Murrell, K.D., Cross, J.H., 1997. Parasites of fish and risks to public health. Rev. Sci. Tech. 16, 652–660.

Agrawal, N., Sharma, U., Sharma, A.K., 2006. Trichrome staining for detection of intestinal protozoa a better screening method. J. Commun. Dis. 38, 351–354.

Al-Adhami, B.H., Gajadhar, A.A., 2014. A new multi-host species indirect ELISA using protein A/G conjugate for detection of anti-*Toxoplasma gondii* IgG antibodies with comparison to ELISA-IgG, agglutination assay and Western blot. Vet. Parasitol. 200, 66–73.

Alagappan, A., Bergquist, P.L., Ferrari, B.C., 2009. Development of a two-color fluorescence in situ hybridization technique for species-level identification of human-infectious *Cryptosporidium* spp. Appl. Environ. Microbiol. 75, 5996–5998.

Arizono, N., Yamada, M., Tegoshi, T., Yoshikawa, M., 2012. *Anisakis simplex* sensu stricto and *Anisakis pegreffii:* biological characteristics and pathogenetic potential in human anisakiasis. Foodborne Pathog. Dis. 9, 517–521.

Ash, L.R., Orihel, T.C., 1991. Formalin-ethyl acetate or formalin-ether sedimentation technique for fresh material. In: Ash, L.R. (Ed.), Parasites: A Guide to Laboratory Procedure and Identification. American Society of Clinical Pathologists, Chicago, pp. 23–25.

Atterby, H., Learmount, J., Conyers, C., Zimmer, I., Boonham, N., Taylor, M., 2009. Development of a real-time PCR assay for the detection of *Trichinella spiralis* in situ. Vet. Parasitol. 161, 92–98.

Bakheit, M.A., Torra, D., Palomino, L.A., Thekisoe, O.M., Mbati, P.A., Ongerth, J., Karanis, P., 2008. Sensitive and specific detection of *Cryptosporidium* species in PCR-negative samples by loop-mediated isothermal DNA amplification and confirmation of generated LAMP products by sequencing. Vet. Parasitol. 158, 11–22.

Baque, R.H., Gilliam, A.O., Robles, L.D., Jakubowski, W., Slifko, T.R., 2011. A real-time RT-PCR method to detect viable *Giardia lamblia* cysts in environmental waters. Water Res. 45, 3175–3184.

Basso, W., Hartnack, S., Pardini, L., Maksimov, P., Koudela, B., Venturini, M.C., Schares, G., Sidler, X., Lewis, F.I., Deplazes, P., 2013. Assessment of diagnostic accuracy of a commercial ELISA for the detection of *Toxoplasma gondii* infection in pigs compared with IFAT, TgSAG1-ELISA and Western blot, using a Bayesian latent class approach. Int. J. Parasitol. 43, 565–570.

Bellamy, J.E., 2004. Quality assurance considerations for detection of waterborne zoonotic parasites using *Cryptosporidium* oocyst detection as the main example. Vet. Parasitol. 126, 235–248.

Berends, B.R., Snijders, J.M., Van Logtestijn, J.G., 1993. Efficacy of current EC meat inspection procedures and some proposed revisions with respect to microbiological safety: a critical review. Vet. Rec. 133, 411–415.

Berlin, O.G., Peter, J.B., Gagne, C., Conteas, C.N., Ash, L.R., 1998. Autofluorescence and the detection of *Cyclospora* oocysts. Emerg. Infect. Dis. 4, 127–128.

Black, E.K., Finch, G.R., Taghi-Kilani, R., Belosevic, M., 1996. Comparison of assays for *Cryptosporidium parvum* oocysts viability after chemical disinfection. FEMS Microbiol. Lett. 135, 187–189.

Bossuyt, P.M., Reitsma, J.B., Bruns, D.E., Gatsonis, C.A., Glasziou, P.P., Irwig, L.M., Lijmer, J.G., Moher, D., Rennie, D., De Vet, H.C., 2003. Towards complete and accurate reporting of studies of diagnostic accuracy: the STARD initiative. BMJ 326, 41–44.

Boughattas, S., Ayari, K., Sa, T., Aoun, K., Bouratbine, A., 2014. Survey of the parasite *Toxoplasma gondii* in human consumed ovine meat in Tunis City. PLoS One 9, e85044.

Brescia, C.C., Griffin, S.M., Ware, M.W., Varughese, E.A., Egorov, A.I., Villegas, E.N., 2009. *Cryptosporidium* propidium monoazide-PCR, a molecular biology-based technique for genotyping of viable *Cryptosporidium* oocysts. Appl. Environ. Microbiol. 75, 6856–6863.

Bukhari, Z., Marshall, M.M., Korich, D.G., Fricker, C.R., Smith, H.V., Rosen, J., Clancy, J.L., 2000. Comparison of *Cryptosporidium parvum* viability and infectivity assays following ozone treatment of oocysts. Appl. Environ. Microbiol. 66, 2972–2980.

Burg, J.L., Grover, C.M., Pouletty, P., Boothroyd, J.C., 1989. Direct and sensitive detection of a pathogenic protozoan, *Toxoplasma gondii*, by polymerase chain reaction. J. Clin. Microbiol. 27, 1787–1792.

Cai, X.Q., Xu, M.J., Wang, Y.H., Qiu, D.Y., Liu, G.X., Lin, A., Tang, J.D., Zhang, R.L., Zhu, X.Q., 2010. Sensitive and rapid detection of *Clonorchis sinensis* infection in fish by loop-mediated isothermal amplification (LAMP). Parasitol. Res. 106, 1379–1383.

Calvo-Artavia, F.F., Nielsen, L.R., Alban, L., 2013. Epidemiologic and economic evaluation of risk-based meat inspection for bovine cysticercosis in Danish cattle. Prev. Vet. Med. 108, 253–261.

Campbell, A.T., Robertson, L.J., Smith, H.V., 1992. Viability of *Cryptosporidium parvum* oocysts: correlation of in vitro excystation with inclusion or exclusion of fluorogenic vital dyes. Appl. Environ. Microbiol. 58, 3488–3493.

Centers for Disease Control and Prevention, 2013. DPDx Laboratory identification of parasitic diseases of public health concern. Available from: http://www.cdc.gov/dpdx/diagnosticProcedures/index.html (accessed 23.11.13.).

Chappell, C.L., Okhuysen, P.C., Langer-Curry, R., Widmer, G., Akiyoshi, D.E., Tanriverdi, S., Tzipori, S., 2006. *Cryptosporidium hominis:* experimental challenge of healthy adults. Am. J. Trop. Med. Hyg. 75, 851–857.

Cheng, H.W., Broaders, M.A., Lucy, F.E., Mastitsky, S.E., Graczyk, T.K., 2012. Determining potential indicators of *Cryptosporidium* oocysts throughout the wastewater treatment process. Water Sci. Technol. 65, 875–882.

Chiesa, F., Dalmasso, A., Bellio, A., Martinetti, M., Gili, S., Civera, T., 2010. Development of a biomolecular assay for postmortem diagnosis of *Taenia saginata* Cysticercosis. Foodborne Pathog. Dis. 7, 1171–1175.

Cook, A.J., Gilbert, R.E., Buffolano, W., Zufferey, J., Petersen, E., Jenum, P.A., Foulon, W., Semprini, A.E., Dunn, D.T., 2000. Sources of *Toxoplasma* infection in pregnant women: European multicentre case-control study. European Research Network on Congenital Toxoplasmosis. BMJ 321, 142–147.

Cook, N., Paton, C.A., Wilkinson, N., Nichols, R.A., Barker, K., Smith, H.V., 2006a. Towards standard methods for the detection of *Cryptosporidium parvum* on lettuce and raspberries. Part 1: development and optimization of methods. Int. J. Food Microbiol. 109, 215–221.

Cook, N., Paton, C.A., Wilkinson, N., Nichols, R.A., Barker, K., Smith, H.V., 2006b. Towards standard methods for the detection of *Cryptosporidium parvum* on lettuce and raspberries. Part 2: validation. Int. J. Food Microbiol. 109, 222–228.

Cuttell, L., Corley, S.W., Gray, C.P., Vanderlinde, P.B., Jackson, L.A., Traub, R.J., 2012. Real-time PCR as a surveillance tool for the detection of *Trichinella* infection in muscle samples from wildlife. Vet. Parasitol. 188, 285–293.

Cuttell, L., Owen, H., Lew-Tabor, A.E., Traub, R.J., 2013. Bovine cysticercosis—development of a real-time PCR to enhance classification of suspect cysts identified at meat inspection. Vet. Parasitol. 194, 65–69.

Da Silva, A.V., Langoni, H., 2001. The detection of *Toxoplasma gondii* by comparing cytology, histopathology, bioassay in mice, and the polymerase chain reaction (PCR). Vet. Parasitol. 97, 191–198.

De Roubin, M.R., Pharamond, J.S., Zanelli, F., Poty, F., Houdart, S., Laurent, F., Drocourt, J.L., Van Poucke, S., 2002. Application of laser scanning cytometry followed by epifluorescent and differential interference contrast microscopy for the detection and enumeration of *Cryptosporidium* and *Giardia* in raw and potable waters. J. Appl. Microbiol. 93, 599–607.

Deere, D., Vesey, G., Milner, M., Williams, K., Ashbolt, N., Veal, D., 1998. Rapid method for fluorescent in situ ribosomal RNA labelling of *Cryptosporidium parvum.* J. Appl. Microbiol. 85, 807–818.

Del Brutto, O.H., 2012. Diagnostic criteria for neurocysticercosis, revisited. Pathog. Glob. Health 106, 299–304.

Devi, K.R., Narain, K., Agatsuma, T., Blair, D., Nagataki, M., Wickramasinghe, S., Yatawara, L., Mahanta, J., 2010. Morphological and molecular characterization of animal *Paragonimus westermani* in northeastern India. Acta Trop. 116, 31–38.

Dubey, J.P., 1988. Long-term persistence of *Toxoplasma gondii* in tissues of pigs inoculated with *T. gondii* oocysts and effect of freezing on viability of tissue cysts in pork. Am. J. Vet. Res. 49, 910–913.

Dubey, J.P., 1995. Duration of immunity to shedding of *Toxoplasma gondii* oocysts by cats. J. Parasitol. 81, 410–415.

Dubey, J.P., Desmonts, G., 1987. Serological responses of equids fed *Toxoplasma gondii* oocysts. Equine Vet. J. 19, 337–339.

Dubey, J.P., Thulliez, P., Weigel, R.M., Andrews, C.D., Lind, P., Powell, E.C., 1995. Sensitivity and specificity of various serologic tests for detection of *Toxoplasma gondii* infection in naturally infected sows. Am. J. Vet. Res. 56, 1030–1036.

Dupont, H.L., Chappell, C.L., Sterling, C.R., Okhuysen, P.C., Rose, J.B., Jakubowski, W., 1995. The infectivity of *Cryptosporidium parvum* in healthy volunteers. N. Engl. J. Med. 332, 855–859.

European Commission, 2005. Regulation (EC) 2075/2005 of the European Parliament and of the Council of 5 December 2005 laying down the specific rules on official controls for *Trichinella* in meat. Off. J. EC L338, 60–82.

European Food Safety Authority, 2013. Scientific opinion on the public health hazards to be covered by inspection of meat from sheep and goats. EFSA J. 11 (6), 3265. Available from: http://www.efsa.europa.eu/en/efsajournal/doc/3265.pdf (accessed 05.09.14.).

Fang, W., Liu, F., Zhang, S., Lin, J., Xu, S., Luo, D., 2011. *Anisakis pegreffii:* a quantitative fluorescence PCR assay for detection in situ. Exp. Parasitol. 127, 587–592.

Farrell-Evans, M., Warren, W., 2014. Food safety assurance systems: quality assurance and good laboratory practice. In: Mortarjemi, Y. (Ed.), Encyclopedia of Food Safety. Academic Press, Waltham, pp. 293–300.

Fayer, R., Santin, M., Macarisin, D., Bauchan, G., 2013. Adhesive-tape recovery combined with molecular and microscopic testing for the detection of *Cryptosporidium* oocysts on experimentally contaminated fresh produce and a food preparation surface. Parasitol. Res. 112, 1567–1574.

Ferrari, B.C., Vesey, G., Davis, K.A., Gauci, M., Veal, D., 2000. A novel two-color flow cytometric assay for the detection of *Cryptosporidium* in environmental water samples. Cytometry 41, 216–222.

Ferrer, E., Cabrera, Z., Rojas, G., Lares, M., Vera, A., De Noya, B.A., Fernandez, I., Romero, H.U., Harrison, L.J., Parkhouse, R.M., Cortez, M.M., 2003. Evidence for high seroprevalence of *Taenia solium* cysticercosis in individuals from three rural communities in Venezuela. Trans. R. Soc. Trop. Med. Hyg. 97, 522–526.

Finch, G.R., Black, E.K., Gyurek, L., Belosevic, M., 1993. Ozone inactivation of *Cryptosporidium parvum* in demand-free phosphate buffer determined by in vitro excystation and animal infectivity. Appl. Environ. Microbiol. 59, 4203–4210.

Fittipaldi, M., Nocker, A., Codony, F., 2012. Progress in understanding preferential detection of live cells using viability dyes in combination with DNA amplification. J. Microbiol. Methods 91, 276–289.

Flanagan, P.A., 1992. *Giardia*—diagnosis, clinical course and epidemiology. A review. Epidemiol. Infect. 109, 1–22.

Forbes, L.B., Parker, S.E., Gajadhar, A.A., 2012. Performance of commercial ELISA and agglutination test kits for the detection of anti-*Toxoplasma gondii* antibodies in serum and muscle fluid of swine infected with 100, 300, 500 or 1000 oocysts. Vet. Parasitol. 190, 362–367.

Gajadhar, A.A., Forbes, L.B., 2002. An internationally recognized quality assurance system for diagnostic parasitology in animal health and food safety, with example data on trichinellosis. Vet. Parasitol. 103, 133–140.

Gajadhar, A.A., Pozio, E., Gamble, H.R., Nöckler, K., Maddox-Hyttel, C., Forbes, L.B., Vallee, I., Rossi, P., Marinculic, A., Boireau, P., 2009. *Trichinella* diagnostics and control: mandatory and best practices for ensuring food safety. Vet. Parasitol. 159, 197–205.

Gallas-Lindemann, C., Sotiriadou, I., Mahmoodi, M.R., Karanis, P., 2013. Detection of *Toxoplasma gondii* oocysts in different water resources by loop mediated isothermal amplification (LAMP). Acta Trop. 125, 231–236.

Gamble, H.R., Anderson, W.R., Graham, C.E., Murrell, K.D., 1983. Diagnosis of swine trichinosis by enzyme-linked immunosorbent assay (ELISA) using an excretory–secretory antigen. Vet. Parasitol. 13, 349–361.

Gamble, H.R., Pozio, E., Bruschi, F., Nöckler, K., Kapel, C.M., Gajadhar, A.A., 2004. International Commission on Trichinellosis: recommendations on the use of serological tests for the detection of *Trichinella* infection in animals and man. Parasite 11, 3–13.

Garcia, J.L., Gennari, S.M., Machado, R.Z., Navarro, I.T., 2006. *Toxoplasma gondii*: detection by mouse bioassay, histopathology, and polymerase chain reaction in tissues from experimentally infected pigs. Exp. Parasitol. 113, 267–271.

Geysen, D., Kanobana, K., Victor, B., Rodriguez-Hidalgo, R., De Borchgrave, J., Brandt, J., Dorny, P., 2007. Validation of meat inspection results for *Taenia saginata* cysticercosis by PCR-restriction fragment length polymorphism. J. Food Prot. 70, 236–240.

Gillbride, K., 2014. Molecular methods for the detection of waterborne pathogens. In: Bridle, H. (Ed.), Waterborne Pathogens. Academic Press, Amsterdam, pp. 231–290 (Chapter 8).

Glor, S.B., Edelhofer, R., Grimm, F., Deplazes, P., Basso, W., 2013. Evaluation of a commercial ELISA kit for detection of antibodies against *Toxoplasma gondii* in serum, plasma and meat juice from experimentally and naturally infected sheep. Parasit. Vectors 6, 1–11.

Gonzalez, L.M., Villalobos, N., Montero, E., Morales, J., Sanz, R.A., Muro, A., Harrison, L.J., Parkhouse, R.M., Garate, T., 2006. Differential molecular identification of Taeniid spp. and *Sarcocystis* spp. cysts isolated from infected pigs and cattle. Vet. Parasitol. 142, 95–101.

Gracey, J.F., Collins, D.S., 1999. Meat Hygiene. Bailliere Tindall, London, UK.

Guenther, S., Nöckler, K., Von Nickisch-Rosenegk, M., Landgraf, M., Ewers, C., Wieler, L.H., Schierack, P., 2008. Detection of *Trichinella spiralis*, *T. britovi* and *T. pseudospiralis* in muscle tissue with real-time PCR. J. Microbiol. Methods 75, 287–292.

Gutierrez, J., O'donovan, J., Proctor, A., Brady, C., Marques, P.X., Worrall, S., Nally, J.E., Mcelroy, M., Bassett, H., Fagan, J., Maley, S., Buxton, D., Sammin, D., Markey, B.K., 2012. Application of quantitative real-time polymerase chain reaction for the diagnosis of toxoplasmosis and enzootic abortion of ewes. J. Vet. Diagn. Invest. 24, 846–854.

Haas, C.N., 2000. Epidemiology, microbiology, and risk assessment of waterborne pathogens including *Cryptosporidium*. J. Food Prot. 63, 827–831.

Harrison, L.J., Joshua, G.W., Wright, S.H., Parkhouse, R.M., 1989. Specific detection of circulating surface/secreted glycoproteins of viable cysticerci in *Taenia saginata* cysticercosis. Parasite Immunol. 11, 351–370.

Hill, D.E., Chirukandoth, S., Dubey, J.P., Lunney, J.K., Gamble, H.R., 2006. Comparison of detection methods for *Toxoplasma gondii* in naturally and experimentally infected swine. Vet. Parasitol. 141, 9–17.

Homan, W.L., Vercammen, M., De Braekeleer, J., Verschueren, H., 2000. Identification of a 200- to 300-fold repetitive 529 bp DNA fragment in *Toxoplasma gondii*, and its use for diagnostic and quantitative PCR. Int. J. Parasitol. 30, 69–75.

Intapan, P.M., Thanchomnang, T., Lulitanond, V., Phongsaskulchoti, P., Maleewong, W., 2008. Real-time fluorescence resonance energy transfer PCR with melting curve analysis for the detection of *Opisthorchis viverrini* in fish intermediate hosts. Vet. Parasitol. 157, 65–71.

International Commission for Trichinellosis, 2012. Recommendations for quality assurance in digestion testing programs for *Trichinella*. In: ICT Quality Assurance Committee Appendix 1 (Part 3). International Commission for Trichinellosis.

Jauregui, L.H., Higgins, J., Zarlenga, D., Dubey, J.P., Lunney, J.K., 2001. Development of a real-time PCR assay for detection of *Toxoplasma gondii* in pig and mouse tissues. J. Clin. Microbiol. 39, 2065–2071.

Jenkins, M.B., Anguish, L.J., Bowman, D.D., Walker, M.J., Ghiorse, W.C., 1997. Assessment of a dye permeability assay for determination of inactivation rates of *Cryptosporidium parvum* oocysts. Appl. Environ. Microbiol. 63, 3844–3850.

Jokelainen, P., Nylund, M., 2012. Acute fatal toxoplasmosis in three Eurasian red squirrels (*Sciurus vulgaris*) caused by genotype II of *Toxoplasma gondii*. J. Wildl. Dis. 48, 454–457.

Jones, J.L., Dubey, J.P., 2012. Foodborne toxoplasmosis. Food Safety 55, 845–851.

Julio, C., Sa, C., Ferreira, I., Martins, S., Oleastro, M., Angelo, H., Guerreiro, J., Tenreiro, R., 2012. Waterborne transmission of *Giardia* and *Cryptosporidium* at river beaches in Southern Europe (Portugal). J. Water Health 10, 484–496.

Kim, J.H., Kang, K.I., Kang, W.C., Sohn, H.J., Jean, Y.H., Park, B.K., Kim, Y., Kim, D.Y., 2009. Porcine abortion outbreak associated with *Toxoplasma gondii* in Jeju Island, Korea. J. Vet. Sci. 10, 147–151.

Knapp, J., Millon, L., Mouzon, L., Umhang, G., Raoul, F., Ali, Z.S., Combes, B., Comte, S., Gbaguidi-Haore, H., Grenouillet, F., Giraudoux, P., 2014. Real time PCR to detect the environmental faecal contamination by *Echinococcus multilocularis* from red fox stools. Vet. Parasitol. 201, 40–47.

Lalonde, L.F., Gajadhar, A.A., 2011. Detection and differentiation of coccidian oocysts by real-time PCR and melting curve analysis. J. Parasitol. 97, 725–730.

Lee, D.Y., Lauder, H., Cruwys, H., Falletta, P., Beaudette, L.A., 2008. Development and application of an oligonucleotide microarray and real-time quantitative PCR for detection of wastewater bacterial pathogens. Sci. Total Environ. 398, 203–211.

Lee, D.Y., Seto, P., Korczak, R., 2010. DNA microarray-based detection and identification of waterborne protozoan pathogens. J. Microbiol. Methods 80, 129–133.

Levsen, A., Lunestad, B.T., Berland, B., 2005. Low detection efficiency of candling as a commonly recommended inspection method for nematode larvae in the flesh of pelagic fish. J. Food Prot. 68, 828–832.

Liang, Z., Keeley, A., 2012. Comparison of propidium monoazide-quantitative PCR and reverse transcription quantitative PCR for viability detection of fresh *Cryptosporidium* oocysts following disinfection and after long-term storage in water samples. Water Res. 46, 5941–5953.

Liu, P., Wu, X.P., Bai, X., Wang, X.L., Yu, L., Rosenthal, B., Blaga, R., Lacour, S., Vallee, I., Boireau, P., Gherman, C., Oltean, M., Zhou, X.N., Wang, F., Zhao, Y., Liu, M.Y., 2013. Screening of early antigen genes of adult-stage Trichinella spiralis using pig serum from different stages of early infection. Vet. Parasitol. 194, 222–225.

Lopez, I., Pardo, M.A., 2010. Evaluation of a real-time polymerase chain reaction (PCR) assay for detection of *Anisakis simplex* parasite as a food-borne allergen source in seafood products. J. Agric. Food Chem. 58, 1469–1477.

Mainar-Jaime, R.C., Barberan, M., 2007. Evaluation of the diagnostic accuracy of the modified agglutination test (MAT) and an indirect ELISA for the detection of serum antibodies against *Toxoplasma gondii* in sheep through Bayesian approaches. Vet. Parasitol. 148, 122–129.

Mattiucci, S., Paoletti, M., Borrini, F., Palumbo, M., Palmieri, R.M., Gomes, V., Casati, A., Nascetti, G., 2011. First molecular identification of the zoonotic parasite *Anisakis pegreffii* (Nematoda: Anisakidae) in a paraffin-embedded granuloma taken from a case of human intestinal anisakiasis in Italy. BMC Infect. Dis. 11, 82.

Mcfadden, A.M., Heath, D.D., Morley, C.M., Dorny, P., 2011. Investigation of an outbreak of *Taenia saginata* cysts (cysticercus bovis) in dairy cattle from two farms. Vet. Parasitol. 176, 177–184.

Munday, B.L., Dubey, J.P., 1986. Serological cross-reactivity between *Hammondia hammondi* and *Toxoplasma gondii* in experimentally inoculated sheep. Aust. Vet. J. 63, 344–345.

Njiru, Z.K., 2012. Loop-mediated isothermal amplification technology: towards point of care diagnostics. PLoS Negl. Trop. Dis. 6, e1572.

Nocker, A., Sossa, K.E., Camper, A.K., 2007. Molecular monitoring of disinfection efficacy using propidium monoazide in combination with quantitative PCR. J. Microbiol. Methods 70, 252–260.

Nöckler, K., Pozio, E., Voigt, W.P., Heidrich, J., 2000. Detection of *Trichinella* infection in food animals. Vet. Parasitol. 93, 335–350.

Nöckler, K., Kapel, C.M., 2007. Detection and Surveillance for *Trichinella:* meat inspection and hygiene, and legislation. In: Camet, J., Murrell, D. (Eds.), FAO/WHO/OIE Guidelines for the Surveillance, Management, Prevention and Control of Trichinellosis. World Organisation for Animal Health Press, Paris, France, pp. 69–98.

Ogunremi, O., Benjamin, J., 2010. Development and field evaluation of a new serological test for *Taenia saginata* cysticercosis. Vet. Parasitol. 169, 93–101.

Ogunremi, O., Macdonald, G., Geerts, S., Brandt, J., 2004. Diagnosis of *Taenia saginata* cysticercosis by immunohistochemical test on formalin-fixed and paraffin-embedded bovine lesions. J. Vet. Diagn. Invest. 16, 438–441.

Onyango-Abuje, J.A., Hughes, G., Opicha, M., Nginyi, K.M., Rugutt, M.K., Wright, S.H., Harrison, L.J., 1996. Diagnosis of *Taenia saginata* cysticercosis in Kenyan cattle by antibody and antigen ELISA. Vet. Parasitol. 61, 221–230.

Opsteegh, M., Langelaar, M., Sprong, H., Den Hartog, L., De Craeye, S., Bokken, G., Ajzenberg, D., Kijlstra, A., van der Giessen, J., 2010. Direct detection and genotyping of *Toxoplasma gondii* in meat samples using magnetic capture and PCR. Int. J. Food Microbiol. 139, 193–201.

Paul, J.H., Rose, J.B., Jiang, S.C., London, P., Xhou, X., Kellogg, C., 1997. Coliphage and indigenous phage in Mamala Bay, Oahu, Hawaii. Appl. Environ. Microbiol. 63, 133–138.

Petney, T.N., Andrews, R.H., Saijuntha, W., Wenz-Mucke, A., Sithithaworn, P., 2013. The zoonotic, fish-borne liver flukes *Clonorchis sinensis*, *Opisthorchis felineus* and *Opisthorchis viverrini*. Int. J. Parasitol. 43, 1031–1046.

Plutzer, J., Karanis, P., 2009. Rapid identification of *Giardia duodenalis* by loop-mediated isothermal amplification (LAMP) from faecal and environmental samples and comparative findings by PCR and real-time PCR methods. Parasitol. Res. 104, 1527–1533.

Pozio, E., 1998. Trichinellosis in the European Union: epidemiology, ecology and economic impact. Parasitol. Today 14, 35–38.

Quintero-Betancourt, W., Peele, E.R., Rose, J.B., 2002. *Cryptosporidium parvum* and *Cyclospora cayetanensis*: a review of laboratory methods for detection of these waterborne parasites. J. Microbiol. Methods 49, 209–224.

Rendtorff, R.C., Holt, C.J., 1954. The experimental transmission of human intestinal protozoan parasites. IV. Attempts to transmit *Endamoeba coli* and *Giardia lamblia* cysts by water. Am. J. Hyg. 60, 327–338.

Riahi, H., Bouteille, B., Darde, M.L., 1998. Antigenic similarity between *Hammondia hammondi* and *Toxoplasma gondii* tachyzoites. J. Parasitol. 84, 651–653.

Robertson, L.J., Gjerde, B., 2000. Isolation and enumeration of *Giardia* cysts, *Cryptosporidium* oocysts, and *Ascaris* eggs from fruits and vegetables. J. Food Prot. 63, 775–778.

Rochelle, P.A., Ferguson, D.M., Handojo, T.J., De Leon, R., Stewart, M.H., Wolfe, R.L., 1997. An assay combining cell culture with reverse transcriptase PCR to detect and determine the infectivity of waterborne *Cryptosporidium parvum*. Appl. Environ. Microbiol. 63, 2029–2037.

Rodríguez-Mahillo, A., González-Muñoz, M., de las Heras, C., Tejada, M., Moneo, I., 2010. Quantification of *Anisakis simplex* allergens in fresh, long-term frozen and cooked fish muscle. Foodborne Pathog. Dis. 7, 967–973.

Rosoff, J.D., Sanders, C.A., Sonnad, S.S., De Lay, P.R., Hadley, W.K., Vincenzi, F.F., Yajko, D.M., O'hanley, P.D., 1989. Stool diagnosis of giardiasis using a commercially available enzyme immunoassay to detect *Giardia*-specific antigen 65 (GSA 65). J. Clin. Microbiol. 27, 1997–2002.

Sato, M.O., Yamasaki, H., Sako, Y., Nakao, M., Nakaya, K., Plancarte, A., Kassuku, A.A., Dorny, P., Geerts, S., Benitez-Ortiz, W., Hashiguchi, Y., Ito, A., 2003. Evaluation of tongue inspection and serology for diagnosis of *Taenia solium* cysticercosis in swine: usefulness of ELISA using purified glycoproteins and recombinant antigen. Vet. Parasitol. 111, 309–322.

Scandrett, W.B., Haines, D.M., Parker, S.E., Robinson, Y., Forbes, L.B., Brandt, J., Geerts, S., Dorny, P., Gajadhar, A.A., 2012. Validation of an immunohistochemical assay for bovine cysticercosis, with comparison to a standard histological method. Vet. Parasitol. 186, 301–311.

Scheepers, M.A., Lecuona, K.A., Rogers, G., Bunce, C., Corcoran, C., Michaelides, M., 2013. The value of routine polymerase chain reaction analysis of intraocular fluid specimens in the diagnosis of infectious posterior uveitis. ScientificWorldJournal 2013, 545149.

Sciutto, E., Martinez, J.J., Villalobos, N.M., Hernandez, M., Jose, M.V., Beltran, C., Rodarte, F., Flores, I., Bobadilla, J.R., Fragoso, G., Parkhouse, M.E., Harrison, L.J., De Aluja, A.S., 1998. Limitations of current diagnostic procedures for the diagnosis of *Taenia solium* cysticercosis in rural pigs. Vet. Parasitol. 79, 299–313.

Shields, J.M., Joo, J., Kim, R., Murphy, H.R., 2013. Assessment of three commercial DNA extraction kits and a laboratory-developed method for detecting *Cryptosporidium* and *Cyclospora* in raspberry wash, basil wash and pesto. J. Microbiol. Methods 92, 51–58.

Shields, J.M., Lee, M.M., Murphy, H.R., 2012. Use of a common laboratory glassware detergent improves recovery of *Cryptosporidium parvum* and *Cyclospora cayetanensis* from lettuce, herbs and raspberries. Int. J. Food Microbiol. 153, 123–128.

Sibley, C.D., Peirano, G., Church, D.L., 2012. Molecular methods for pathogen and microbial community detection and characterization: current and potential application in diagnostic microbiology. Infect. Genet. Evol. 12, 505–521.

Steinparzer, R., Reisp, K., Grunberger, B., Kofer, J., Schmoll, F., Sattler, T., 2014. Comparison of different commercial serological tests for the detection of *Toxoplasma gondii* antibodies in serum of naturally exposed pigs. Zoonoses Public Health 62, 119–124.

Stormo, S.K., Sivertsen, A.H., Heia, K., Nilsen, H., Elvevoll, E., 2007. Effects of single wavelength selection for Anisakid roundworm larvae detection through multispectral imaging. J. Food Prot. 70, 1890–1895.

Sturbaum, G.D., Ortega, Y.R., Gilman, R.H., Sterling, C.R., Cabrera, L., Klein, D.A., 1998. Detection of *Cyclospora cayetanensis* in wastewater. Appl. Environ. Microbiol. 64, 2284–2286.

Tantrawatpan, C., Intapan, P.M., Thanchomnang, T., Lulitanond, V., Boonmars, T., Wu, Z., Morakote, N., Maleewong, W., 2012. Differential detection of *Trichinella papuae*, *T. spiralis* and *T. pseudospiralis* by real-time fluorescence resonance energy transfer PCR and melting curve analysis. Vet. Parasitol. 185, 210–215.

Tantrawatpan, C., Intapan, P.M., Thanchomnang, T., Sanpool, O., Janwan, P., Lulitanond, V., Anamnart, W., Maleewong, W., 2013. Application of a real-time fluorescence resonance energy transfer polymerase chain reaction assay with melting curve analysis for the detection of *Paragonimus heterotremus* eggs in the feces of experimentally infected cats. J. Vet. Diagn. Invest. 25, 620–626.

Thiriat, L., Sidaner, F., Schwartzbrod, J., 1998. Determination of *Giardia* cyst viability in environmental and faecal samples by immunofluorescence, fluorogenic dye staining and differential interference contrast microscopy. Lett. Appl. Microbiol. 26, 237–242.

Torres, P., Puga, S., 2011. Comparative efficacy of candling and glass plate compression for detection of diphyllobothriosis in rainbow trout (*Oncorhynchus mykiss*) musculature. Rev. Sci. Tech. 30, 831–837.

Vesey, G., Ashbolt, N., Fricker, E.J., Deere, D., Williams, K.L., Veal, D.A., Dorsch, M., 1998. The use of a ribosomal RNA targeted oligonucleotide probe for fluorescent labelling of viable *Cryptosporidium parvum* oocysts. J. Appl. Microbiol. 85, 429–440.

Villena, I., Durand, B., Aubert, D., Blaga, R., Geers, R., Thomas, M., Perret, C., Alliot, A., Escotte-Binet, S., Thebault, A., Boireau, P., Halos, L., 2012. New strategy for the survey of *Toxoplasma gondii* in meat for human consumption. Vet. Parasitol. 183, 203–208.

Wanzala, W., Onyango-Abuje, J.A., Kang'ethe, E.K., Zessin, K.H., Kyule, N.M., Baumann, M.P., Ochanda, A.H., Harrison, L.J., 2003. Control of *Taenia saginata* by post-mortem examination of carcasses. Afr. Health Sci. 3, 68–76.

Webber, J., Dobrenov, B., Lloyd, J., Jordan, D., 2012. Meat inspection in the Australian red-meat industries: past, present and future. Aust. Vet. J. 90, 363–369.

Werner, M., Fæste, C., Levsen, A., Egaas, E., 2011. A quantitative sandwich ELISA for the detection of *Anisakis simplex* protein in seafood. Eur. Food Res. Technol. 232, 157–166.

Wiriya, B., Clausen, J.H., Inpankaew, T., Thaenkham, U., Jittapalapong, S., Satapornvanit, K., Dalsgaard, A., 2013. Fish-borne trematodes in cultured Nile tilapia (*Oreochromis niloticus*) and wild-caught fish from Thailand. Vet. Parasitol. 198, 230–234.

World Organisation for Animal Health, 2014a. Cysticercosis. In: Manual of Diagnostic Tests and Vaccines for Terrestrial Animals. World Organisation for Animal Health, Paris, France. Available from: http://www.oie.int/international-standard-setting/terrestrial-manual/access-online/ (accessed 12.09.14) (Chapter 2.9.5).

World Organisation for Animal Health, 2014b. Part 1: general standards. In: Manual of Diagnostic Tests and Vaccines for Terrestrial Animals. World Organisation for Animal Health, Paris, France. Available from: http://www.oie.int/international-standard-setting/terrestrial-manual/access-online/ (accessed 12.09.14.).

World Organisation for Animal Health, 2014c. Trichinellosis [Online]. In: Manual of Diagnostic Tests and Vaccines for Terrestrial Animals 2014. World Organisation for Animal Health, Paris, France. Available from: http://www.oie.int/international-standard-setting/terrestrial-manual/access-online/ (accessed 12.09.14) (Chapter 2.1.16).

World Organisation for Animal Health, 2014d. Toxoplasmosis. In: Manual of Diagnostic Tests and Vaccines for Terrestrial Animals 2014. Available from: http://www.oie.int/international-standard-setting/terrestrial-manual/access-online/ (accessed 12.09.14) (Chapter 2.9.10).

Wu, J., Long, S.C., Das, D., Dorner, S.M., 2011. Are microbial indicators and pathogens correlated? A statistical analysis of 40 years of research. J. Water Health 9, 265–278.

Yu, H., Huang, B., Zhuo, X., Chen, X., Du, A., 2013. Evaluation of a real-time PCR assay based on the single-copy SAG1 gene for the detection of *Toxoplasma gondii*. Vet. Parasitol. 197, 670–673.

The role of regulatory and standard-setting organizations in the control of neglected foodborne parasites

17

P. Boireau[1], *I. Vallée*[1], *A.A. Gajadhar*[2], *X. Wang*[3], *L. Mingyuan*[3]
[1]ANSES, Animal Health Laboratory, OIE Collaborating Centre Foodborne Zoonotic Parasites, Maisons-Alfort, France; [2]Canadian Food Inspection Agency, Saskatoon, SK, Canada; [3]Jilin University, Institute of Zoonosis, OIE Collaborating Centre Foodborne Zoonotic Parasites, Changchun, PR China

17.1 Introduction

In the next two decades meat consumption is expected to double in the world with a rise in pork and poultry production in developing countries. In addition to environmental considerations, harmful effects on public health can occur. Particularly, meatborne parasites can emerge or reemerge in countries whose residents are consuming more meat without an effective control system (Dorny et al., 2009a). In 2012, the Food and Agriculture Organization (FAO) of the United Nations with Codex *Alimentarius*, under the auspices of World Organization for Animal Health (OIE) and World Health Organization (WHO), performed an expert ranking exercise on neglected foodborne zoonotic parasites of global importance (FAO/WHO, 2014) (Figures 17.1 and 17.2). Food and food products that are at greatest risk of harboring the most important parasites are described. An overview of the risk management options and approaches available for the control of the most highly ranked foodborne parasites are reported. Subsequently, in 2014 WHO developed training for stakeholders and officers in charge of foodborne parasites throughout the world. Agencies such as the European Centre for Disease Prevention and Control (ECDC) sustained this effort (2014) and participated in disseminating the training globally. Among these parasites *Trichinella* has a unique position. It is obviously one of the two main meatborne parasites with *Cysticercus* at the world level with a strong economic impact (Murrell, 2013). Even if *Trichinella* is no longer an important public health problem in developed countries, this nematode parasite has an economic burden particularly in the cost for meat production to be exported. Conversely, several endemic countries (such as some countries in Asia, Eastern Europe, and South America) cannot avoid human infection due to inadequate quality control in meat production.

In this chapter, we will describe the role of national and international organizations to control foodborne parasites with emphasis on the nematode parasite *Trichinella*. The

Foodborne Parasites in the Food Supply Web. http://dx.doi.org/10.1016/B978-1-78242-332-4.00017-5

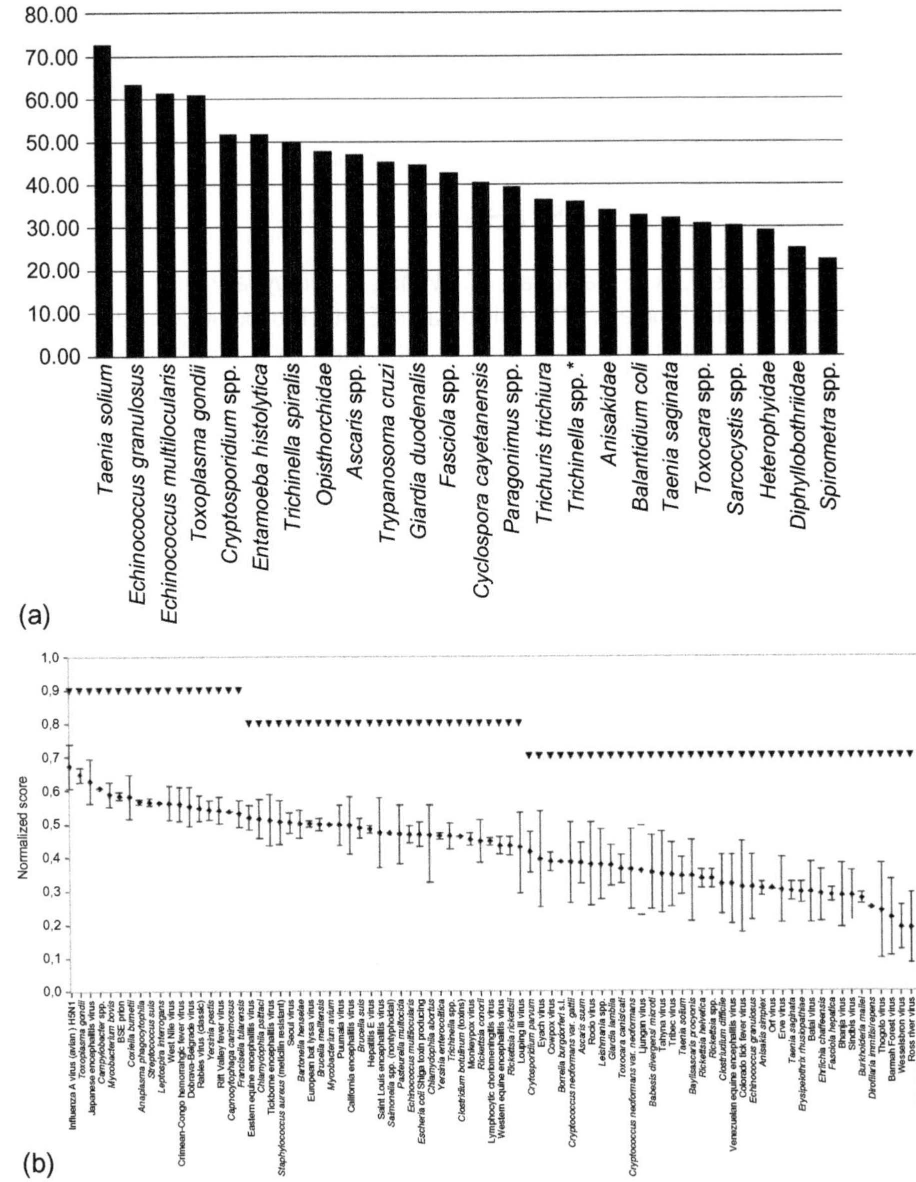

Figure 17.1 Global ranking of foodborne parasites by FAO/WHO, 2014 (a) and regional ranking of all zoonotic pathogens by Havelaar et al. (2010) (b). (a) Ranking of parasites performed by an international panel of experts using a normalized score. Several of these parasites were already identified as a causative agent of neglected tropical diseases (NTD) by WHO. *Cysticercus suis/Taenia solium* is the major public health threat at the world level. (b) Ranking of zoonotic pathogens relevant for the Netherlands area (Havelaar et al., 2010). The score for each pathogen was determined by using seven risk criteria that are similar to those used by FAO-ranking parasites. Interestingly, in this country *Cysticercus suis/Taenia solium* is "eradicated" and considered as "no risk," whereas *Toxoplasma* is considered to be the major zoonotic parasite.

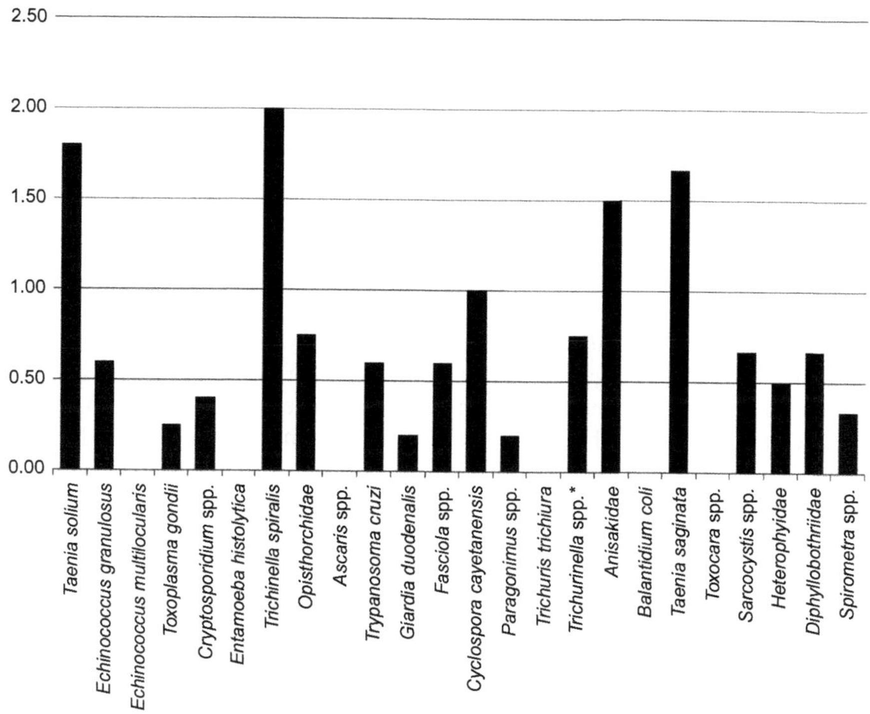

Figure 17.2 Trade scores for foodborne parasites (FAO/WHO, 2014). Only the weighted trade criterion data are displayed to suggest that there may be additional or separate trade issues that may be considered by risk regulators and managers, such as Codex and national competent authorities. The parasites *T. spiralis* and *T. saginata/C. bovis* were considered important for trade, based on the criterion scores (in this analysis the weight of "trade" parameter is deeply emphasized by comparison to other parameters). *Trichinella spiralis*, *Taenia saginata*, *Taenia solium*, and/or *Echinococcus granulosus* were mentioned in the regional reports as current or potential trade concerns for Africa, Australia, Europe, the Near/ Middle East, and South America.

chapter will be divided into four parts to describe successively the risk management organization, the risk assessment, the standardization, and the reference laboratory activities.

17.2 Regulations and veterinary services (competent authority): Risk management and organization

The regulatory management of animal diseases or foodborne zoonotic pathogens, including parasites, is often the role of government and more precisely official veterinary services that are designated as a "competent authority." Most nations have regulation and official acts that regulate the inspection and control of food to detect and manage specific pathogens. In this chapter, we use *Trichinella* to illustrate the role of regulation and competent authority starting at the end of the nineteenth century with the establishment of veterinary services in several countries and the implementation of regulatory organizations. In the United States, the "pork war" (1879–1889) was responsible in part for establishing a federal meat inspection service. Meanwhile in Europe the official control of meat was organized during this period by veterinary services. Trichinelloscopy (syn. trichinoscopy) was used for the first time in Germany in 1863 for the direct detection of *Trichinella* larvae in meat. The number of inspected carcasses in this country reached 27,000 in 1895. Even though there were criticisms on the cost of such systematic controls, in most European and other countries, including the United States, a similar monitoring system was implemented by the respective veterinary services.

The US Food and Drug Administration (FDA), which was created in 1848 (www.fda.gov), is an example of an organization that has as its major mission to protect consumers at the level of risk management and with a strong influence on food protection. The FDA became a part of the public health service, and recently the Food Safety Modernization Act of 2010 yielded new authority to regulate the manner in which foods are grown, harvested, and processed. The act's main objective was to prevent food safety problems rather than to react to related public health crises. The US Department of Agriculture (USDA) is the authority that develops safety standards and preventive controls plans for food production; it also organizes and performs inspections. These USDA services are performed by the Animal and Plant Health Inspection Services (APHIS) and the Food Safety and Inspection Service (FSIS). The FDA works in synergy with these agencies, particularly the FSIS, which regulates meats, poultry, and fish.

This underlines a key integration and communication problem for the regulatory and inspection roles of competent authorities in many countries. The efficacy of the system depends on the efficient cooperation and collaboration between authorities. To overcome these organizational and jurisdictional challenges, the Canadian Food Inspection Agency (CFIA) is an integrated federal organization with combined regulatory and inspection responsibilities similar to those typically held in multiple ministries or departments such as Agriculture, Food and Drugs, and Fisheries. In other countries the department of agriculture and veterinary services may have similar roles with multiple variation of organization and responsibilities.

The primary goal of all the present regulations in the world is to facilitate release of parasite-free meat into the market. For example, it is under the responsibility of each state to certify that exported meat (primarily pork, but also meat from other susceptible animals) is free of *Trichinella*. To reach this goal, compulsory controls on individual carcasses are still organized by veterinary and inspection services with the help of routine meat testing laboratories (often linked with slaughterhouses). EU regulation (Commission, 2005, 2014), for example, requires that all meat that comes from susceptible hosts be individually tested by the digestion test, which is considered to be the highest standard of testing. An exception is if the animal is raised in a negligible risk category as stipulated by the OIE. For other foodborne parasites such as *Echinococcus/Hydatidosis* and *Cysticercus*, a surveillance test in endemic countries is necessary, and a visual inspection is compulsory on all carcasses.

Modern systems of pig raising have dramatically reduced the occurrence of *Trichinella* in pork. In the early 2000s, experts from various countries, including

Australia and Denmark, suggested that the cost of testing individual carcasses is no longer justified because of the reduced risk for human trichinosis. Following considerable risk assessments and other considerations, regulations were amended to reduce or eliminate laboratory testing of individual carcasses to certify the meat as free of *Trichinella*: (i) Based on a hazard analysis and critical control points (HACCPs)-based process, the United States Department of Agriculture (USDA) or EU regulations allowed an on-farm approach. Under this process it was possible to certify as *Trichinella*-safe some meat based on the absence of the risk of infection (periodic audit) and negative serological tests for newly introduced animal. By extension, piglets under 5 weeks are not controlled, as they cannot be "at risk" (EFSA, 2005). (ii) It was also possible to certify a geographic area as having a low-risk status and, under these conditions, all of animal production that maintains the necessary standards to avoid any environmental contamination can be certified as *Trichinella*-safe. This concept emerged from the "zoning concept" described in an earlier version of the OIE Animal Health Code.

To facilitate the control of many serious outbreaks in China arising from the foodborne transmission of parasites such as *Clonorchis sinensis*, *Trichinella*, and *Echinococcus*, new food safety legislation was implemented in 2009 to replace the older food hygiene laws. Food safety in China is comanaged by several government agencies, including the Ministry of Health, the Ministry of Agriculture, the State General Administration of Quality Supervision and Inspection and Quarantine (AQSIQ), the Certification and Accreditation Administration (CNCA), and the State Food and Drug Administration (SFDA). However, the responsibility for auditing and certifying food products belongs to the Ministry of Health. Ensuring the implementation of good agriculture practice (GAP) for the processing of agricultural products is a main task of the Ministry of Agriculture. AQSIQ is responsible for the quality and safety of imported and exported food. The management of inspection, certification, and accreditation is the main function of CNCA. SFDA organizes each department in food safety management. The organization of the foodborne parasites in China belongs to four levels of organization: county, city, province, and national levels. The compulsory inspection of *Trichinella* in pigs is usually performed by microscopy at slaughterhouses and is under the responsibility of the Chinese Ministry of Agriculture. Sero-epidemiological surveys of *Trichinella spiralis* have been carried out for humans and pigs in 10 out of 34 provinces/autonomous regions/municipals (P/A/Ms) of China (Cui et al., 2011). Similar surveys were organized for *C. sinensis* in various provinces (personal communication, Dr. Zhou Xiaonong, Chinese Center for Disease Control and Prevention, Shanghai).

17.3 Agencies, nonregulatory bodies, and experts on foodborne zoonotic parasites: From risk assessment toward risk communication

Agencies play a pivotal role in several countries to give some specific up-to-date data on foodborne zoonotic parasites for ministries. They are performing independent expertise for stakeholders and citizens (transparency for the public is a common duty for all these agencies) in some countries. The European Food Safety Authority (EFSA) is an example of a multicountry organization in charge of the scientific expertise and communication on risk associated within the food chain. The EFSA gives scientific support for a risk management decision but is not involved in inspection or regulation as is the FDA and FSIS in the United States. The EFSA was established for the European Union in 2002 (Commission, 2002) to give confidence to consumers and stakeholders "in the decision-making processes underpinning food law" based on scientific support. This independent organization is intended to provide coherence between risk assessment and risk management. Comparable organizations exist in other countries, such as Japan (Food Safety Commission of Japan) and EU member states: Germany (*Bundesinstitute für Risikobewertung* (BfR)), United Kingdom (Food Standards Agency (FSA)), Netherlands (National Institute for Public Health and the Environment (RIVM)), Spain (*La Agencia Espanola de Consumo, Seguridad Alimentaria y Nutricion* (AECOSAN)), and France (*Agence Française de sécurité sanitaire alimentaire, environnement, travail* (ANSES)). In China, the Chinese Food and Drug Administration (CFDA) is in charge of risk management and the Chinese Food Safety Agency (CFSA) evaluates the risk for foodborne pathogens and contaminants in food. The EFSA supports several scientific opinions on the management of foodborne zoonotic parasites, including *Trichinella* (Alban et al., 2011), *Cysticercus* (Dorny et al., 2009b), *Echinococcus* (Boue et al., 2009), *Sarcocystis* (Taylor et al., 2009), and *Toxoplasma* (EFSA, 2007). An EFSA report on the definition of the geographic area with negligible risk for *Trichinella* allowed the European Directorate-General for Health and Consumers Affairs (DG SANCO) to write the new regulations on foodborne parasites in 2005 (2075) (EFSA, 2005). In summary, various government agencies are involved in risk analysis and, in some countries, in risk management. They provide scientific support for the regulation of food and food inspection. They can act as independent bodies for consumers and professionals and can be in charge of the risk communication related to food safety in coordination with risk management bodies. In such situations these agencies also conduct public meetings to exchange information with stakeholders including food producers and consumers.

Noninspection regulatory bodies have an important role in the surveillance of food safety. According to the EU Directive (Commission, 2003), member states are required to establish a system of monitoring zoonoses and zoonotic agents. Toxoplasmosis and trichinellosis are on the list of diseases and agents for epidemiological monitoring when warranted. The data collected by the competent authority are forwarded to the appropriate organization for risk analysis. Following a review of available information, the EFSA has recommended increased monitoring for *Toxoplasma* infection in animals, especially sheep, pigs, and cattle. In particular, in the framework of the *Scientific Opinion* on the inspection of pork, the EFSA invited member states to support national studies to help clarify the risk factors for infection in pigs, as well as the role of meat as a source of human infections (EFSA, 2011).

Many government agencies are also involved in the management of human diseases due to foodborne parasites. Centers or agencies for disease control and prevention exist in various countries (European ECDC, Chinese CDC, US CDC, Public Health Agency of Canada (PHAC), etc.). Centers for Disease Control investigate and work to prevent human diseases. In China, an animal CDC defines standards to control animal diseases including zoonoses. Chinese CDC can collect samples of foodborne parasites (particularly *Cysticercus*, *C. sinensis*, *Toxoplasma*, and *Cryptosporidium*) from all provinces of China. The Chinese CDC has the capabilities and skills to provide training, expertise, scientific, technical, and diagnostic support to provincial laboratories.

In many jurisdictions there is interest and some effort to organize a clear chain of command to sustain local to national levels of foodborne parasites surveillance at key points in the food chain. To have an effective monitoring and control food safety system, it is important for cooperation among all stakeholders, including government regulatory and inspection bodies, public health organizations, veterinary organizations, producers, and consumer groups.

17.4 International standards

International standard-setting organizations such as OIE, Codex, WHO, and FAO play an important role in the assessment of risk and in the control of foodborne parasites on a global basis. This is done through various efforts, including development and dissemination of guidelines, diagnostic methods, technician training, and reference activities.

17.4.1 World Organization for Animal Health

The OIE was originally created in Paris in 1924 as the *Organisation Internationale des Epizooties* by an international agreement initially signed by 28 countries; there are now 178 member countries. This world organization has three main tasks. The OIE collects and disseminates to governments and their veterinary services all data concerning the advance of emerging animal diseases. It develops and publishes animal health and welfare standards for international trade in animal and animal products. Its guidelines and directives are included in the *Codes for Terrestrial and Aquatic Animal Health* (OIE, 2013a,c) and the *Manuals of Diagnostic Tests and Vaccines for Terrestrial and Aquatic Animals* (OIE, 2009, 2013b). These normative works are recognized by the World Trade Organization and facilitate animal (or products from animal origin) exchanges between countries. The OIE stimulates and coordinates research and surveillance on animal pathogens for prophylaxis purposes and induces international cooperation (twinning). The OIE promotes food safety and veterinary services throughout the world. This role of world reference for animal diseases and their control is a major responsibility of OIE that is accomplished by the use of international scientific and technical experts to develop and update guidelines and standards, with input from national experts through chief veterinary officers of member countries. The international Animal Health Code Commission ensures the suitability of each Code Chapter prior to publication in the OIE Animal Health Code (AHC). In 2013, two new code chapters included Infection with *Echinococcus granulosus* and Infection with *Echinococcus multilocularis*, and a replacement chapter for Trichinellosis.

The AHC defines the compartmentalization approach to managing a number of animal and zoonotic diseases. Using the guiding principles of the OIE, the procedures for zoning and compartmentalization fall under the responsibility of the member states, according to local situations. An infected zone is a defined geographic area where the pathogen (parasite) is present in an otherwise free country. This concept allows countries to define containment zones, which is particularly useful for large countries. For example, compulsory individual control can be suppressed in an area with a negligible risk for *Trichinella*, and with adequate containment and survey. More technical details to detect and control parasites are found in the OIE *Manual of Standards for Diagnostic Tests and Vaccines*. Several parasites including *Trichinella* (2.1.16), *Cysticercus* (2.4.4 and 2.8.6, 2.9.5), *Cryptopsoridium* (2.9.4), and *Toxoplama* (2.9.10) have monographs in the manual, which describes recommended diagnostic reagents and techniques (direct and indirect methods), as well as requirements for vaccines. One of the most important tasks of the OIE is to facilitate the international trade of animals and products of animal origin without incurring health risks dissemination. Therefore, official science-based tests that are accepted by the 178 member states for the monitoring and surveillance of foodborne parasites and/or their control are precisely described.

To promote elicitation of standards and research within its domain, the OIE designates reference laboratories and collaborating centers for various parasites or areas of parasitology (Figure 17.3).

17.4.2 Food and Agriculture Organization, World Health Organization, and Codex Alimentarius

The FAO and WHO were established by the United Nations (UN) to address issues related to food production and public health, respectively, in all areas of the world. The FAO faces major challenges in the security and safety of food in most areas of the world, and WHO's mandate includes support for the prevention and control of both established and emerging human diseases including foodborne parasitoses. To help address common areas of their mandates, FAO and WHO created Codex *Alimentarius* in 1963 to develop and harmonize science-based international food standards and other related guidelines for the production of safe food and the protection of consumers' health. At the 42nd session (December, 2010) of the Codex Committee on Food Hygiene (CCFH), the FAO and WHO were tasked to "review the current status of knowledge on parasites in food and their public health and trade impact." The anticipated increase of meat consumption in emerging countries was one of the triggering parameters for this review. An international panel of experts was organized by FAO and WHO in 2012 to address this task. It listed and ranked 24 foodborne parasites with *Cysticercus*, *Echinococcus*, and *Trichinella* as among the most important in the world. Various aspects of technical information on epidemiology, diagnosis, and management were developed for each of these 24 foodborne parasites (FAO/WHO, 2014). At the 44th session of the Codex Committee on Food Hygiene, (2012) the committee agreed that Australia would lead an electronic working group (EWG) to prepare a discussion paper on the occurrence and control of parasites in food, taking into account the previous work organized by FAO and WHO. Specific parasite control information is now suitable as an annex of the existing Codex Codes for *Trichinella* and *Cysticercus*. WHO subsequently organized the development of various forms of

Organizations	Roles	Level
International organizations: **OIE, FAO, WHO, ICT, CODEX ALIMENTARIUS, ISO**	Public health and Food security. Expertise Guidelines, standards setting and scientific	***World***
EU organizations: **EFSA, DG-SANCO**	Scientific expertise Risk assessment and management Risk communication	***European Union Multistates level***
Ministry of agriculture, **Ministry of health....**	Risk management Risk communication Organization of inspection and control	***National***
Agencies	Risk assessment Scientific expertise Opinions and advices on regulatory texts	
Reference laboratories	Expertise Research and development	
Stakeholders and professional organizations	Communication Information	
Food control visual detection — **Certified laboratories**	Routine diagnosis and inspection	***Province or state city***

Figure 17.3 Organisms involved on foodborne parasites. At the world level, international organizations such as OIE, FAO, and WHO bring together all available information on foodborne parasites, perform expert analyses, and coordinate surveillance with national and international health bodies. Risk management and risk communication are major responsibilities of the competent authorities; independent advice and expertise are provided as is communication by agencies in the field. At the local levels, such as provincial/state or city levels, routine inspections and/or laboratory analysis is organized to monitor and/or detect foodborne parasites and mitigate positive findings.

training on foodborne parasites, including e-learning modules and face-to-face teaching as a consequence of FAO expertise and EWG recommendations. The education module is presently under evaluation by agencies before being disseminated through the WHO website.

17.4.3 The International Commission on Trichinellosis

The International Commission on Trichinellosis (ICT, http://www.trichinellosis.org/) is an example of a scientific organization dedicated to various aspects of a foodborne parasite. The ICT is an organization of scientists from across the world working on aspects of *Trichinella* and Trichinellosis. Its purpose is to exchange knowledge on the biology, physiopathology, epidemiology, immunology, and clinical aspects of *Trichinella* infection in animals and humans and to provide guidance and recommendations on the prevention of exposure of humans to this foodborne parasite.

The ICT uses the best available scientific authorities in the development of guidelines and has issued its recommendations for the control of *Trichinella* and trichinellosis, including "Recommendations on Methods for the Control of *Trichinella* in Domestic and Wild Animals Intended for Human Consumption," "Recommendations for Quality Assurance in Digestion Testing Programs for *Trichinella*," "Recommendations on Essential Components and Minimum Requirements for a *Trichinella* Testing Laboratory Certification Program," and "Recommendations for Training and Qualifying Analysts to Perform the *Trichinella* Digestion Assay" (http://www.trichinellosis.org/). ICT efforts in developing control guidelines and recommendations have also resulted in several noteworthy publications, including *Opinion on the Diagnosis and Treatment of Human Trichinellosis*, and *Taxonimic Scheme of the Genus* Trichinella (see http://www.trichinellosis.org/Further_Reading.html).

17.5 International Standards Organization

As the international body for standardization, the International Standards Organization (ISO) develops and publishes international standards for methods. Among them are two standard methods for the detection of foodborne parasites. A digestion assay for *Trichinella* and a detection and enumeration of *Cryptosporidium* and *Giardia* in fresh products are expected to be finalized for publication by the time this book goes to print. Such standards will complement other guidelines such as those by the OIE and ICT, by providing a prescriptive set of technical details to ensure satisfactory quality assurance and performance of the assay.

17.6 The Organisation for Economic Co-operation and Development

The Organisation for Economic Co-operation and Development (OECD) is an international organization that promotes policies and practices to facilitate trade and economic development around the world. OECD sponsored a workshop by the ICT to establish a framework for recommendation on surveillance of *Trichinella* in 2013 for use in evaluating public health risk of pork in various situations.

17.7 Reference laboratories

Reference laboratories are fundamental elements in the infrastructure for the control of foodborne parasites on an international, national, or local level. Their roles are often multiple and may include any of the following: (i) Support and proposed reference diagnostic testing performed in routine laboratories to detect parasites in food; identify at species level, store and supply parasite strains and reagent standards; establish and maintain serum banks, parasites collection, and database of strains isolated across the country or the geographic area within its pursue; prepare and supply proficiency samples and administer proficiency testing to subordinate testing laboratories; characterize parasite strains by the most modern and reliable methods available to allow better understanding of the biology and epidemiology of foodborne parasites; provide scientific advice to competent authorities and others on surveillance program, epidemiology, and prevention. (ii) Reference laboratories facilitate harmonization of techniques throughout routine laboratories in particular defining standard test methodologies. (iii) Reference laboratories organize workshops for the benefit of routine laboratories and specific training of technicians, especially for the implementation of new analytical methods. (iv) Reference activities are directly linked with method developments and their validation. Reference laboratories coordinate research activities aimed at improving tests for the control of foodborne parasites and may be involved in the development of tools for the eradication of parasites in food (e.g., vaccine for porcine cysticercosis).

International organizations, such as the OIE, FAO, WHO, and ICT, as well as national, regional, or local authorities authenticate and support reference laboratories in performing their roles (Table 17.1). These laboratories may be specialized for one parasite or a group of pathogens (zoonoses, etc.). This is exemplified by OIE Reference Laboratories for *Trichinella* and OIE Collaborating Centers (OIE CC) for Foodborne Zoonotic Parasites. There are presently three OIE CC (Canada, France, and China) that have competence at the world level (see Table 17.1). Competent authorities usually designate national reference laboratories for support of the country's regulations. DG SANCO mandated Institute Superiore di Sanita (Italy) as the European Reference Laboratory (EU-RL) for parasites. As for all other EU-RL, its functions and duties consist of providing adequate analytical methods to identify parasite in hosts or food and to organize ring trials with the national reference laboratories within the European Union. It coordinates validation of future commercial kits for parasite detection; it can also coordinate research on new diagnostic methods and give expertise to the EU Commission. The EU-RL parasites is also the *Trichinella* Reference Laboratory for ICT where identification and traceability of all new isolates are performed.

Table 17.1 Examples of reference laboratories and collaborating centres for foodborne parasites

Organization or competent authority	Name	Geographic covering	Parasites name	Name of institute	Website
OIE	Reference laboratory	World	*Trichinella*	• ISS, Italy • Centre for Food-borne and Animal Parasitology, Canada	www.oie.org
OIE	Reference laboratory	World	Echinococcosis/ Hydatidosis	Rakuno-Gakuen University, Japan	www.oie.org
OIE	Reference laboratory	World	Echinococcosis/ Hydatidosis	Rabat Institute, Morocco	www.oie.org
OIE	Reference laboratory	World	Echinococcosis/ Hydatidosis	University of Salford Manchester, United Kingdom	www.oie.org
OIE	Collaborating center	Geographic area	Foodborne zoonotic parasites	• Center for Food-borne and Animal Parasitology, Canada • Anses, France • Jilin University, China	www.oie.org
WHO/FAO	Collaborating reference center	World	Foodborne parasites	University of Copenhagen, Denmark	http://www.ivs.ku.dk
DG SANCO	EU reference laboratory	Europe (28 countries)	Parasites	ISS, Rome	http://www.iss.it/crlp/
National	National reference laboratories	Country	Various	Various	
ICT		World	Trichinella	ISS, Rome	www.ict.org

17.8 Future trends

With the three main meatborne parasites (*Trichinella*, *Toxoplasma*, and *Cysticercus*) there can be various approaches to control management (Table 17.2) and assessment due to the coordinated action of involved competent authorities, laboratories, and agencies. For *Toxoplasma* there is no compulsory meat control risk despite a huge human contamination and high risk for pregnant women and especially to the health of their fetus. In many countries only cooking and freezing are recommended for at-risk persons. The competent authority for human health can organize a survey by serology of human populations at risk. The ministries of agriculture are usually not involved in *Toxoplasma* surveys in livestock except in countries where national surveys were performed to quantify the risk for human contamination, such as in France (Halos et al., 2010), in the United States (Hill et al., 2010), and in the Netherlands (van der Giessen et al., 2007).

Trichinella, however, is controlled by veterinary services. It is primarily the responsibility of the ministry of agriculture of each country to organize, if it sees fit, the compulsory control of individual carcasses. Routine laboratories and reference laboratories are involved in the diagnosis and the quality management with the help of international guidelines (ICT, OIE, etc.). Because there is no effective vaccine or treatment to prevent or eliminate *Trichinella* infection, current control strategies include adequate cooking of meat or producing food animals without access to potential sources of infection. The latter practice is used to certify meat as safe for trade. *Cysticercus suis*, identified as the most important neglected foodborne

Table 17.2 Objectives of the risk manager for three serious meatborne parasites

	Toxoplasma	*Trichinella*	*Cysticercus*/Teniasis
Human contamination	+++++	Endemic to low endemic area	Endemic, eradication
Human survey	+++	0	0
Animal survey	0	+++	+++
Diagnosis tests	+++	+++	+++
Vaccine to eradicate parasite from host	0	0	+++
Objectives of risk manager	Quantitative risk assessment and information/ education to avoid human contamination	Compulsory control on target species in endemic area to avoid human contamination	To eradicate

Concerning *Toxoplasma*, compulsory control is not possible on the meat, and only quantitative risk assessment is important to give practitioners up-to-date information. For *Trichinella*, veterinary services need to organize compulsory control on pig carcasses and other meat if necessary to avoid human contamination in endemic area. Concerning *Cysticercus*, all the tools exist to allow eradication.

parasites (see Figure 17.1), is endemic in several countries where the various competent authorities and their services can organize different strategies of prophylaxis. This may involve education to limit the spreading of the parasite between humans (*C. suis*) and the emergence of neurocysticercosis. Therapeutic treatment for cysticercosis in humans can be effective and should be sustained in poor highly endemic countries. A vaccine for pigs—the intermediate host—has been developed and shown to be useful, but it is not commercially available (OIE, 2013a). Support and implementation of a sustained widescale eradication plan are necessary to eliminate the infection from the single reservoir host species, humans. An example of an eradication plan for *C. suis* in Peru has been described (Gilman et al., 2012) where a global strategy for human and pig prevention was organized involving human chemoprophylaxis, detection of infected pigs, and survey by serology of newly introduced animals.

In brief, the joint efforts of multiple organizations (see Figure 17.3) are needed to be effective to control and eradicate foodborne zoonotic parasites. However, coordination at all levels can be difficult but not impossible and is necessary to ensure parasite-free food.

Acknowledgments

We are grateful to the FAO and WHO for authorization to duplicate Figures 17.1a and 17.2. We acknowledge Arie H. Havelaar from the Centre for Infectious Disease Control, National Institute for Public Health and the Environment (RIVM), Bilthoven, The Netherlands, for permission to reproduce Figure 17.1b (Havelaar et al., 2010).

References

Alban, L., Pozio, E., Boes, J., Boireau, P., Boue, F., Claes, M., Cook, A.J., Dorny, P., Enemark, H.L., van der Giessen, J., Hunt, K.R., Howell, M., Kirjusina, M., Nockler, K., Rossi, P., Smith, G.C., Snow, L., Taylor, M.A., Theodoropoulos, G., Vallee, I., Viera-Pinto, M.M., Zimmer, I.A., 2011. Towards a standardised surveillance for Trichinella in the European Union. Prev. Vet. Med. 99, 148–160.

Boue, F., Boes, J., Boireau, P., Claes, M., Cook, A.J., Dorny, P., Enemark, H.L., van der Giessen, J., Hunt, K.R., Howell, M., Kirjusina, M., Nockler, K., Pozio, E., Rossi, P., Smith, G.C., Snow, L., Taylor, M.A., Theodoropoulos, G., Vallee, I., Viera-Pinto, M.M., Zimmer, I.A., 2009. Development of harmonised schemes for the monitoring and reporting of *Echinococcus* in animals and foodstuffs in the European Union. Scientific report submitted to EFSA, 41 pp.

Commission E, 2002. Regulation (EC) No 178/2002 of the European Parliament and of the Council of t28 January 2002 laying down the general principles and requirements of food law, establishing the European Food Safety Authority and laying down procedures in matters of food safety. Off. J. Eur. Union L31, 22.

Commission E, 2003. Directive 2003/99/EC on the monitoring of zoonoses and zoonotic agents, amending Council decision 90/424/EEC and repealing Council Directive 92/117/EEC, pp. 31–40.

Commission E, 2005. Regulation no 2075/2005 of 5 December 2005 laying down specific rules on official controls for Trichinella in meat (text with EEA relevance). Off. J. Eur. Union 338, 21.

Commission E, 2014. Amending Regulation (EC) No 2075/2005 laying down specific rules on official controls for Trichinella in meat. Off. J. Eur. Union L69, 85–92.

Cui, J., Wang, Z.Q., Xu, B.L., 2011. The epidemiology of human trichinellosis in China during 2004–2009. Acta Trop. 118, 1–5.

Dorny, P., Praet, N., Deckers, N., Gabriel, S., 2009a. Emerging food-borne parasites. Vet. Parasitol. 163, 196–206.

Dorny, P., Vallee, I., Boes, J., Boireau, P., Boue, F., Claes, M., Cook, A.J., Enemark, H.L., van der Giessen, J., Hunt, K.R., Howell, M., Kirjusina, M., Nockler, K., Pozio, E., Rossi, P., Smith, G.C., Snow, L., Taylor, M.A., Theodoropoulos, G., Viera-Pinto, M.M., Zimmer, I.A., 2009b. Development of harmonised schemes for the monitoring and reporting of *Cysticercus* in animals and foodstuffs in the European Union. Scientific report submitted to EFSA, 30 pp.

EFSA, 2005. Feasibility of establishing Trichinella-free areas, and if feasible on the risk increase to public health of not examining pigs from those areas for Trichinella spp. EFSA J. 277, 4–37.

EFSA, 2007. Surveillance and monitoring of Toxoplasma in humans, food and animals: scientific opinion of the panel on biological hazards. EFSA J. 583, 1–64.

EFSA, 2011. Scientific opinion on the public health hazards to be covered by inspection of meat (swine). EFSA J. 9, 198.

FAO/WHO, 2014. Multicriteria-based ranking for risk management of food-borne parasites. In: Report of a Joint FAO/WHO Expert Meeting, 3–7 September 2012. Microbiological Risk Assessment Series. FAO and WHO (Food and Agriculture Organization of the United Nations/World Health Organization) Headquarters, Rome, Italy, p. 302.

Gilman, R.H., Gonzalez, A.E., Llanos-Zavalaga, F., Tsang, V.C., Garcia, H.H., Cysticercosis Working Group in Peru, 2012. Prevention and control of *Taenia solium* taeniasis/cysticercosis in Peru. Pathog. Glob. Health 106, 312–318.

Halos, L., Thebault, A., Aubert, D., Thomas, M., Perret, C., Geers, R., Alliot, A., Escotte-Binet, S., Ajzenberg, D., Darde, M.L., Durand, B., Boireau, P., Villena, I., 2010. An innovative survey underlining the significant level of contamination by *Toxoplasma gondii* of ovine meat consumed in France. Int. J. Parasitol. 40, 193–200.

Havelaar, A.H., van Rosse, F., Bucura, C., Toetenel, M.A., Haagsma, J.A., Kurowicka, D., Heesterbeek, J.H., Speybroeck, N., Langelaar, M.F., van der Giessen, J.W., Cooke, R.M., Braks, M.A., 2010. Prioritizing emerging zoonoses in the Netherlands. PLoS One 5, e13965.

Hill, D.E., Haley, C., Wagner, B., Gamble, H.R., Dubey, J.P., 2010. Seroprevalence of and risk factors for *Toxoplasma gondii* in the US swine herd using sera collected during the National Animal Health Monitoring Survey (Swine 2006). Zoonoses Public Health 57, 53–59.

Murrell, K.D., 2013. Zoonotic foodborne parasites and their surveillance. Rev. Sci. Tech. 32, 559–569.

OIE, 2009. Aquatic Manual. Office International des Epizooties, Paris, France.

OIE, 2013a. Aquatic Code. Office International des Epizooties, Paris, France.

OIE, 2013b. Manual of Diagnostic Tests and Vaccines for Terrestrial Animals (Mammals, Birds and Bees), seventh ed. Office International des Epizooties, Paris, France, 1467 pp.

OIE, 2013c. Terrestrial Animal Health Code. Office International des Epizooties, Paris, France, 800 pp.

Taylor, M.A., Boes, J., Boireau, P., Boue, F., Claes, M., Cook, A.J., Dorny, P., Enemark, H.L., van der Giessen, J., Hunt, K.R., Howell, M., Kirjusina, M., Nockler, K., Pozio, E., Rossi, P., Smith, G.C., Snow, L., Theodoropoulos, G., Vallee, I., Viera-Pinto, M.M., Zimmer, I.A., 2009. Development of harmonised schemes for the monitoring and reporting of *Sarcocystis* in animals and foodstuffs in the European Union. Scientific report submitted to EFSA, 28 pp.

van der Giessen, J., Fonville, M., Bouwknegt, M., Langelaar, M., Vollema, A., 2007. Seroprevalence of *Trichinella spiralis* and *Toxoplasma gondii* in pigs from different housing systems in The Netherlands. Vet. Parasitol. 148, 371–374.

Index

Note: Page numbers followed by *f* indicate figures and *t* indicate tables.

D

G

H

I